Cardiac Fibrosis and Heart Failure

Cardiac Fibrosis and Heart Failure

Editor: Kasandra Carney

AMERICAN
MEDICAL PUBLISHERS
www.americanmedicalpublishers.com

AMERICAN
MEDICAL PUBLISHERS
www.americanmedicalpublishers.com

Cataloging-in-Publication Data

Cardiac fibrosis and heart failure / edited by Kasandra Carney.
p. cm.
Includes bibliographical references and index.
ISBN 978-1-63927-960-9
1. Heart--Fibrosis. 2. Heart failure. 3. Fibrosis. 4. Heart--Diseases.
5. Cardiology. I. Carney, Kasandra.
RC682 .C37 2023
616.12--dc23

American Medical Publishers,
41 Flatbush Avenue,
1st Floor, New York,
NY 11217, USA

ISBN 978-1-63927-960-9 (Hardback)

Contents

Preface

Cardiac fibrosis is the excess deposition of extracellular matrix in the cardiac muscle. It can also be used to imply an abnormal thickening of the heart valves due to the multiplication of cardiac fibroblasts. Fibrocyte cells play a crucial role in providing structural support to the heart, apart from releasing collagen. In a situation where this process is over-activated, it produces an increased amount of collagen which leads to the thickening and fibrosis of the valve. The right-sided heart failure and valvular dysfunction are the major consequences of the thickening and loss of flexibility in the cardiac muscle. There are three different types of myocardial fibrosis, namely interstitial fibrosis, subepicardial fibrosis, and replacement fibrosis. The objective of cardiac fibrosis treatment is to prevent the production of serotonin, which is responsible for producing archetype pattern of right-sided cardiac fibrosis. This book provides significant information of this discipline to help develop a good understanding of cardiac fibrosis and heart failure. A number of latest researches have been included to keep the readers up-to-date with the global concepts in this area of study. This book will serve as a valuable source of reference for graduate and post graduate students.

This book unites the global concepts and researches in an organized manner for a comprehensive understanding of the subject. It is a ripe text for all researchers, students, scientists or anyone else who is interested in acquiring a better knowledge of this dynamic field.

I extend my sincere thanks to the contributors for such eloquent research chapters. Finally, I thank my family for being a source of support and help.

Editor

1

A Porcine Model of Heart Failure with Preserved Ejection Fraction Induced by Chronic Pressure Overload Characterized by Cardiac Fibrosis and Remodeling

Weijiang Tan[1†], Xiang Li[1†], Shuang Zheng[1†], Xiaohui Li[2†], Xiaoshen Zhang[2], W. Glen Pyle[3], Honghua Chen[1], Jian Wu[4], Huan Sun[5], Yunzeng Zou[4], Peter H. Backx[6,7] and Feng Hua Yang[1,2]*

[1] Guangdong Provincial Key Laboratory of Laboratory Animals, Guangdong Laboratory Animals Monitoring Institute, Guangzhou, China, [2] Department of Cardiovascular Surgery, The First Affiliated Hospital, Jinan University, Guangzhou, China, [3] Department of Biomedical Sciences, University of Guelph, Guelph, ON, Canada, [4] Shanghai Institute of Cardiovascular Diseases, Zhongshan Hospital and Institutes of Biomedical Sciences, Fudan University, Shanghai, China, [5] Cardiology Department, China-Japan Union Hospital of Jilin University, Changchun, China, [6] Department of Biology, York University, Toronto, ON, Canada, [7] Department of Physiology, University of Toronto, Toronto, ON, Canada

***Correspondence:**
Feng Hua Yang
fenghua.yang@gdlami.com

[†] These authors have contributed equally to this work

Heart failure is induced by multiple pathological mechanisms, and current therapies are ineffective against heart failure with preserved ejection fraction (HFpEF). As there are limited animal models of HFpEF, its underlying mechanisms have not yet been elucidated. Here, we employed the descending aortic constriction (DAC) technique to induce chronic pressure overload in the left ventricles of Tibetan minipigs for 12 weeks. Cardiac function, pathological and cellular changes, fibrotic signaling activation, and gene expression profiles were explored. The left ventricles developed concentric hypertrophy from weeks 4 to 6 and transition to dilation starting in week 10. Notably, the left ventricular ejection fraction was maintained at >50% in the DAC group during the 12-week period. Pathological examination, biochemical analyses, and gene profile analysis revealed evidence of inflammation, fibrosis, cell death, and myofilament dephosphorylation in the myocardium of HFpEF model animals, together with gene expression shifts promoting cardiac remodeling and downregulating metabolic pathways. Furthermore, we noted the activation of several signaling proteins that impact cardiac fibrosis and remodeling, including transforming growth factor-β/SMAD family members 2/3, type I/III/V collagens, phosphatidylinositol 3-kinase, extracellular signal-regulated kinase, matrix metalloproteinases 2 and 9, tissue inhibitor of metalloproteinases 1 and 2, interleukins 6 and 1β, and inhibitor of κBα/nuclear factor-κB. Our findings demonstrate that this chronic pressure overload-induced porcine HFpEF model is a powerful tool to elucidate the mechanisms of this disease and translate preclinical findings.

Keywords: porcine model, pressure overload, heart failure with preserved ejection fraction, fibrosis, signal transduction, cardiac remodeling

INTRODUCTION

Although survival and hospitalization rates for patients with heart failure (HF) have greatly improved over the past three decades, HF remains one of the leading causes of death worldwide. European data reported that the 12-month all-cause mortality rate for hospitalized patients with HF is approximately 24% (1). In the USA, an estimated 6.2 million adults 20 years of age or older had HF between 2013 and 2016 (2). In China, among the 290 million patients with cardiovascular disease, approximately 2.5 million suffer from HF (3). The European Society of Cardiology (ESC) guidelines on the diagnosis and treatment of acute and chronic HF classify the disease as either heart failure with reduced ejection fraction [HFrEF, with a left ventricular ejection fraction (LVEF) ≤40%], mid-range EF (HFmrEF, LVEF 40–49%), or preserved EF (HFpEF, LVEF ≥50%) (4). The USA and Japan have adopted similar guidelines (5, 6). Based on studies of multiple diverse community-based cohorts in the USA, HFpEF accounts for 51–63% of HF cases (7); however, the prevalence is lower in Asian countries, at ~30% (8). Clinically, the criteria for HFpEF diagnosis in the 2016 ESC guidelines include symptoms and signs, LVEF ≥50%, elevated natriuretic peptides [brain natriuretic peptide (BNP) and N terminal proBNP], and relevant structural heart disease and/or diastolic dysfunction (4). Additionally, patients with HFpEF display cardiac vasculature abnormalities, inflammation, fibrosis, ischemia, metabolic disorder, myocyte hypertrophy, and detrimental cellular signal transduction (7, 9, 10). However, because of limitations in available animal models, these mechanisms remain hypothetical.

To explore safe and more effective strategies to treat and manage HF, numerous approaches have been used to generate animal models that mimic its phenotypes (11, 12). Aortic constriction-induced HF in rodents has been one of the most widely used models since its development in the early 1990s (13–15). Aortic constriction mimics high blood pressure, inducing chronic pressure overload in the left ventricles and ventricular hypertrophy or dilation (13, 16). Experimental pressure overload can induce all three types of HF. Recently, researchers successfully developed a HFpEF model by controlling the degree of vessel narrowing or blood flow. By using a constriction ring of a specific size (inner diameter: 0.71 mm), they could induce cardiac hypertrophy with preserved EF (>50%) in mice for 8–20 weeks (17). In pigs, an HF model with cardiac hypertrophy and preserved EF can be generated by placing an inflatable cuff at the aortic root to increase left ventricle pressure (18). However, compared with mice, the phenotypes and mechanisms of pig HFpEF models remain relatively unreported.

In this study, we employed the aortic constriction technique to induce chronic pressure overload in porcine ventricles. The pigs developed left ventricular concentric hypertrophy, followed by left ventricle dilation with a preserved ejection fraction. Cardiac remodeling, histology, gene expression profiles, and fibrotic signaling were explored. This is the first study to use descending aortic constriction (DAC) to model HFpEF, providing a powerful tool to study this condition.

METHODS

Ethical Statement and Animals

All animal experiments were performed in accordance with the Guide for the Care and Use of Laboratory Animals (8th Ed., 2011, The National Academies, USA). The protocol was approved by the Institutional Animal Care and Use Committee of the Guangdong Laboratory Animals Monitoring Institute (approval no. IACUC2017009). Ten Tibetan minipigs (male, 25–30 kg) were purchased from a licensed laboratory animal facility [license no. SCXK (YUE) 2015-0036, China]. Minipigs were randomly assigned to two groups ($n = 5$ each). One group underwent sham surgery; the second underwent DAC surgery. During the experimental period, the animals were housed in an AAALAC-accredited facility at the Guangdong Laboratory Animals Monitoring Institute [license no. SYXK (YUE) 2016-0122, China]. At this facility, the ambient temperature and humidity were 20–26°C and 40–70%, respectively, and the light cycle was 12 h day/12 h night.

Before (week 0) and after surgery (weeks 2, 4, 6, 8, 10, and 12), echocardiography was performed to evaluate cardiac morphology and function. Twelve weeks after surgery, animals were euthanized, and cardiac tissues were collected for histopathological and expression analyses.

DAC Model

Surgical Procedure

The descending aorta segment was selected as the constriction site. All surgical instruments were autoclaved, and aseptic techniques were applied during the surgical procedure. The operating room was located in the AAALAC-accredited facility of the Guangdong Laboratory Animals Monitoring Institute. The minipigs were fasted overnight before surgery. Ketamine hydrochloride (6 mg/kg) and midazolam (0.5 mg/kg) were used for basal anesthesia, propofol (5 mg/kg) was used for induction anesthesia, and volatile anesthetic with isoflurane (1.5–2.5%) was used to maintain general anesthesia. The animals were placed in the right lateral position and connected to a veterinary monitor (iPM12Vet; Mindray, China). After pre-operative skin preparation, a ~15 cm-long incision was made on the thoracic skin. Electrosurgical and blunt dissection techniques were used in combination to separate the muscle layers, and the constriction site (the descending segment of the aorta, located under the fourth to fifth intercostal space) was exposed.

Pressure Determination at the Constriction Site

After determining the constriction site, two pressure sensors were placed on the segment proximal to the heart (S1) and after the constriction site (on the segment distal to the heart, S2; **Figure 1**). The pressures at S1 and S2 were equal and designated P0. At the constriction site, three layers of sterile gauze were wrapped around the aorta, and surgical sutures (size 7–0) were placed. Pressure was monitored as the sutures were gradually tightened. When the pressure at S1 (PS1) reached 120% of that at S2 (PS2), this condition was stabilized for 30 s, and the sutures were secured with surgical knots. After inserting an indwelling chest tube, the muscles and skin were closed layer by layer.

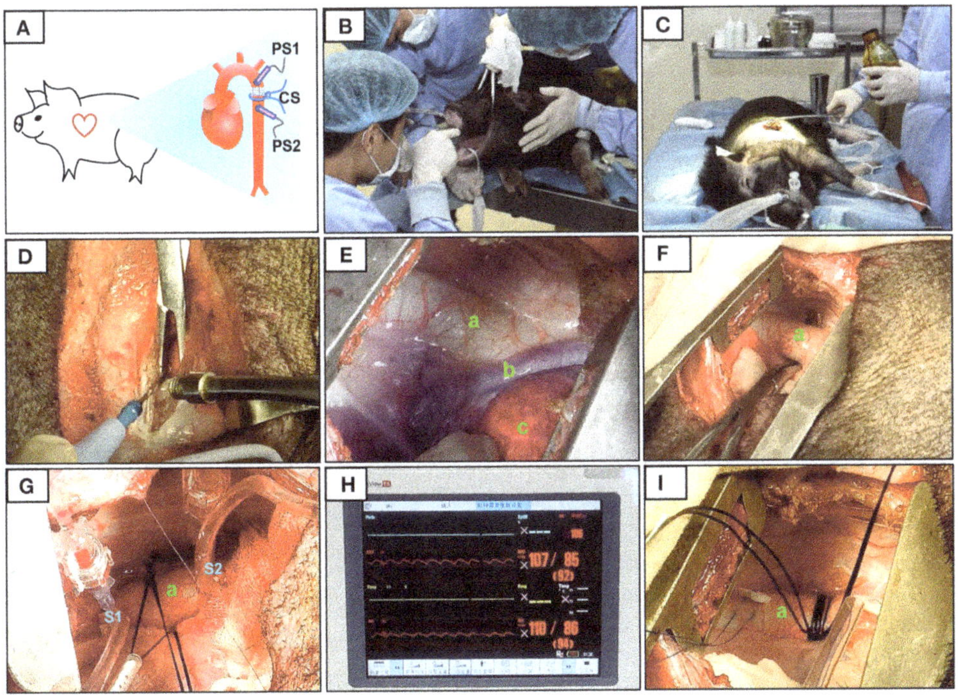

FIGURE 1 | Surgical procedure and pressure determination at the constriction site. The constriction site (CS) was at the descending aorta segment **(A)**. During the surgery, volatile anesthetic with isoflurane was used for the maintenance of general anesthesia **(B)**. After pre-operative skin preparation **(C)**, an incision was made and a combination of electrosurgical and blunt dissection techniques was used to separate muscle layers **(D)**. The descending segment of the aorta located under the fourth to fifth intercostal space was exposed **(E,F)**. After determining the constriction site, two pressure sensors were placed on the segment proximal to the heart (S1) and after (on the segment distal to the heart, S2) the constriction site **(G)**. The pressures at S1 and S2 were displayed over the ECG monitor **(H)**. When the pressure at S1 (PS1) reached 120% of that at S2 (PS2), the sutures were then secured with surgical knots **(I)**. The aorta (a), accessory hemiazygos vein (b), and lung (c) were shown in **(E–G,I)**.

Penicillin was applied to the operation site post-surgery and daily for 1 week afterwards (20,000 U/kg). Animals in the sham group also underwent thoracotomy, but no aortic constriction was performed.

Echocardiography

An ultrasound diagnostic imaging system equipped with a Cardiac PA122 phased array transducer (3–8 MHz, MyLab30; Esatoe, Italy) was used to evaluate cardiac morphology and function at weeks 0, 2, 4, 6, 8, 10, and 12. Following anesthesia with ketamine hydrochloride (50 mg/kg), a transducer was placed in the left or right intercostal area to obtain both B-mode and M-mode images of the left ventricular long axis, and internal aortic dimensions. The measured indices of the M-mode images included the left ventricular dimensions at the end of systole and diastole (LVIDs and LVIDd, respectively), the ventricular septum thickness at the end of systole and diastole (VSTs and VSTd, respectively), the posterior wall thickness at the end of systole and diastole (PWTs and PWTd, respectively), and the aortic root diameter at the end of systole and diastole (ARDs and ARDd, respectively). The left ventricular EF and fraction shortening (FS) were analyzed using software provided by Esaote Inc.

Serum Biochemistry

After overnight fasting, blood samples (5 mL) were collected from the minipigs and allowed to clot for 60 min at room temperature. Serum was separated by centrifugation at 2,150 $\times$ g at 4°C for 30 min. For serum biochemistry tests, an automatic biochemistry analyzer (LX20; Beckman, USA) and corresponding reagents were used. Laboratory parameters measured included creatine kinase (CK), lactate dehydrogenase (LDH), and creatinine.

Hematoxylin and Eosin (HE) and Sirius Red Staining

HE staining was used to examine tissue damage to the main organs, and Sirius red staining was used to determine cardiac fibrosis. Animals were euthanized with ketamine hydrochloride at the end of the experimental period. Heart tissues (left ventricle, right ventricle, left atrium, right atrium, and interventricular septum), aortic vessels, and the lungs, liver, and kidneys were collected. Tissue blocks were fixed overnight in 4% paraformaldehyde. The tissues were embedded in paraffin and sectioned to 3 μm, then sequentially treated with xylene, absolute ethanol, 95% absolute ethanol, 80% absolute ethanol, 70% absolute ethanol, and pure water for dewaxing. For HE staining, the sections were incubated in hematoxylin solution (cat. no. H3136; Sigma-Aldrich, USA) for 10 min and then with alcohol-soluble eosin (cat. no. E4009; Sigma-Aldrich, USA) for 25 s. For Sirius red staining to detect the myocardial collagen content, left ventricle sections were incubated in Sirius red solution for 1 h and then washed with acidified water. Following dehydration and mounting, the tissue sections were observed under a microscope (DM2500; Leica, Germany).

Enzyme-Linked Immunosorbent Assay (ELISA)

A commercial ELISA kit (Cusabio Biotech Co., China) was used to determine serum concentrations of cardiac troponin I (cTnI) at week 12. Blood samples from the minipigs were centrifuged at 2,500 × *g* at 4°C for 30 min, and the supernatants were collected. The ELISA was performed according to the manufacturer's instructions. Optical density was measured at 450 nm using a microplate reader (Multiskan FC; Thermo Fisher Scientific, USA).

RNA Sequencing, Raw Data Processing, and Gene Set Enrichment Analysis (GSEA)

RNA sequencing was used to profile gene expression following DAC treatment as previously described (19). Briefly, total RNA was extracted using TRIzol reagent (cat. no.15596026; Invitrogen, USA). RNA concentrations were determined using an Invitrogen Qubit RNA Assay Kit on a Qubit 2.0 Fluorometer (cat. no. Q10210; Thermo Fisher Scientific, USA), and RNA integrity was tested using an RNA Nano 6000 Assay Kit (cat. no. 5067-1511; Agilent, USA) with the Bioanalyzer 2100 system (Agilent Technologies, USA). For RNA library generation, 3 μg of RNA per sample was used as input material After the addition of index codes and sample cluster generation, the libraries were sequenced on an Illumina HiSeq platform, and 125-bp/150-bp paired-end reads were generated. Gene reads from the sham and DAC groups were compared, and fold changes in expressed genes were log2-transformed. Differentially expressed genes (DEGs) were identified by *P*-values <0.05. Furthermore, DEGs with log2 (fold change) values >0 and <0 were considered upregulated and downregulated, respectively. Gene expression profiles are presented using volcano plots. Up- and downregulated DEGs were inputted into the web-accessible gene annotation and analysis tool Metascape (https://metascape.org) to analyze enrichment in biological processes, and Database for Annotation, Visualization and Integrated Discovery (DAVID) v6.8 (https://david.ncifcrf.gov) to analyze Kyoto Encyclopedia of Genes and Genomes (KEGG) pathways in chronic pressure-overloaded hearts. Raw RNA-seq data were deposited in the National Center for Biotechnology Information Gene Expression Omnibus (https://www.ncbi.nlm.nih.gov/geo/) with accession number GSE167643.

Terminal Deoxynucleotidyl Transferase (TdT) dUTP Nick-End Labeling (TUNEL) Staining

To examine myocardial apoptosis, left ventricle tissues were embedded in paraffin wax. After dewaxing and sectioning, the slices were incubated with proteinase K (20 μg/mL) at 37°C for 30 min. Sections were then washed with phosphate-buffered saline (pH 7.4) and treated with 0.5% Triton X-100 at room temperature for 5 min. A TUNEL cell apoptosis detection kit containing TdT (cat. no. Bio-C1088; Biyuntian, China) was used to fully cover the tissue, and samples were incubated in the dark for 60 min. The sections were then mounted with a 4′, 6-diamidino-2-phenylindole reagent containing an antifluorescence quencher (cat. no. P36966; Thermo Fisher Scientific, USA) and observed under a microscope (DM2500; Leica, Germany).

TABLE 1 | RT-qPCR Primers used in this study.

Gene	Forward	Reverse
MMP9	AGCCGCTCAGCAAGAAGATT	GCCCAGGCCCAACTTATCC
TIMP2	TTTTGCAATGCAGACGTAGTGA	GGGTTGCCGTAGATGTCGTT
α-SMA	CTGCCCTGGTGTGTGACAAT	TCCCACAATGGACGGGAAAA
ANP	GACCACTTGGAGGACAAGATG	TCCTCATTCTGCTCGCTTAGT
BNP	CTCAGAACTGCCAGGGATAC	GAGGACTTGGAAGATGCTACTG
β-actin	GACGATATTGCTGCGCTCGTG	TCAGGATGCCTCTCTTGCTCT

Reverse Transcription Quantitative Polymerase Chain Reaction (RT-qPCR)

RT-qPCR was used to determine the expression of atrial natriuretic peptide (ANP), BNP, α-smooth muscle actin (SMA), tissue inhibitor of metalloproteinase 2 (TIMP2), and matrix metalloproteinase 9 (MMP9), which are associated with HF or fibrosis. Briefly, total RNA extracted from left ventricle tissue was subjected to RT-qPCR using the primers listed in **Table 1**. TB Green Premix Ex Taq II (cat. no. RR820; Takara Bio Inc., Japan) was used for qPCR as follows: 95°C for 30 s, then 40 cycles of 95°C for 5 s and 60°C for 34 s, then a final extension at 72°C for 10 min. Transcript levels were normalized to the expression of β-actin, and the results are expressed as ratios of the DAC group to the sham group.

Western Blotting

The cytosolic fraction was extracted from cardiac tissues of the sham and DAC groups to detect the expression levels of proteins involved in fibrosis, cellular proliferation, and inflammatory responses. Briefly, cytosolic proteins (40 μg) were resolved by 10% sodium dodecyl sulfate-polyacrylamide gel electrophoresis (SDS-PAGE) and transferred to polyvinylidene difluoride membranes (Millipore, USA). After blocking with 5% skim milk, the membranes were incubated with primary antibodies overnight at 4°C, followed by incubation with a species-appropriate secondary antibody. All primary and secondary antibodies were purchased from Cell Signaling Technology (Danvers, USA). The bands were detected with Immobilon Western Chemiluminescent HRP Substrate (Millipore, USA). Band density was analyzed using ImageJ (National Institutes of Health, Bethesda, MD, USA). Primary antibodies used were as follows: anti-collagen α1 (COL1α1; cat. no. 91144), anti-phospho-SMAD family member (SMAD)2 (p-SMAD2; cat. no. 18338T), anti-phospho-SMAD2/SMAD3 (p-SMAD2/3; cat. no. 8828S), anti-transforming growth factor β (TGF-β; cat. no. 3709S), anti-phospho-nuclear factor-κB p65 (p-NFκB; cat. no. 3033), anti-phospho-inhibitor of κBα (p-IκBα; cat. no. 2859), anti-phospho-extracellular signal-regulated kinase (p-ERK; cat. no. 4370T), anti-interleukin (IL)6 (cat. no. 12912), anti-IL-1β (cat. no. 12703S), anti-phospho-phosphatidylinositol 3-kinase (p-PI3K; cat. no. 4228S), and anti-glyceraldehyde 3-phosphate dehydrogenase (GAPDH; cat. no. 2118).

Myofilament Phosphorylation

Myofilament phosphorylation levels were analyzed to examine their responses to chronic pressure overload. Myofilaments were extracted as previously described, with modifications (19–21). The hearts were homogenized in an ice-cold cell lysis buffer comprising 60 mM KCl, 30 mM imidazole (pH 7.0), 2 mM $MgCl_2$, and proteinase inhibitors, and then centrifuged at 12,000 × *g* at 4°C for 15 min. Pellets were extracted with the same ice-cold lysis buffer containing 1% Triton X-100 and centrifuged at 1,100 × *g* to obtain myofilaments. Phosphorylation levels of myofilaments [myosin binding protein C (MyBP-C), desmin, cardiac troponin T (cTnT), tropomyosin, cardiac troponin I (cTnI), and myosin light chain 2 (MLC2)] were measured using Pro-Q Diamond Phosphoprotein Gel Stain according to the manufacturer's instructions (Molecular Probes, USA). Briefly, myofilaments (60 μg) were resolved by SDS-PAGE on 12% gels. After fixation with 50% methanol/10% acetic acid for 30 min twice, the gels were incubated with Pro-Q Diamond solution for 90 min. Phosphorylated bands were visualized using a Gel Doc XR+ gel documentation system (Bio-Rad Laboratories Ltd., USA). Total protein was stained with Coomassie brilliant blue (cat. no. 112553; Sigma-Aldrich, USA), and actin bands were used as loading controls.

Statistical Analysis

All experimental data are presented as means ± standard errors of the means (SEMs). Raw data of the sham and TAC groups were input into GraphPad Prism 8.0 (GraphPad Software, USA) for statistics analysis. Unpaired *t*-tests and a two-sided *P*-value with a confidence level of 95% were used to determine the differences between the groups. $P < 0.05$ was considered significant. The graphs showing each individual data point were presented.

RESULTS

Left Ventricles Display Concentric Hypertrophy and Then Dilation After DAC Surgery, With Preserved EF

In this study, we developed a surgical procedure to induce an HF model in Tibetan minipigs (**Figure 1**). Several key steps were performed, including localization of the descending aorta, analysis of the degree of aortic narrowing, and pressure measurements. One animal in each group did not have stable heart rates during the recording of echocardiography, so these two animals were excluded from experiments. Transmitral Doppler showed that the E: A ratio and the left atrial diameter were significantly higher in the DAC group than in the sham group. In addition, compared with the sham group, serum cTnI, CK, and LDH levels were significantly increased in the DAC group at week 12 (**Table 2**). These changes indicate diastolic dysfunction of the left ventricles.

TABLE 2 | Indices of heart failure of the sham and DAC groups.

Groups		Sham	DAC
Transmitral Doppler			
	E (m/s)	0.58 ± 0.02	0.67 ± 0.07
	A (m/s)	0.48 ± 0.01	0.27 ± 0.03***
	E/A	1.22 ± 0.05	2.49 ± 0.14***
Left atrial size			
	LA (mm)	34.05 ± 0.57	42.43 ± 0.81***
Laboratory parameters			
	cTnI (pg/mL)	149.10 ± 28.92	340.06 ± 56.32*
	CK (U/L)	366.80 ± 34.40	546.25 ± 48.58*
	LDH (U/L)	255.40 ± 10.00	373.25 ± 15.53***
	Creatinine (μmol/L)	90.00 ± 12.52	85.00 ± 5.31

*All data are presented as the means ± SEMs. Sham, the sham group; DAC, the descending aortic constriction group; E, the peak early filling velocity; A, the velocity at atrial contraction; E/A, ratio of early diastolic blood flow peak E and late diastolic peak A; BNP, brain natriuretic peptide; cTnI, cardiac troponin I; CK, creatine kinase; LDH, lactate dehydrogenase. *P < 0.05; ***P < 0.001 vs. the sham group.*

Echocardiography showed that the aortic roots of minipigs gradually expanded over time after surgery (**Figure 2A**). The ARDd was also significantly larger in the DAC group than in the sham group at weeks 2, 4, 6, 8, 10, and 12 following DAC surgery (**Figures 2B,C, Table 3**). Left ventricles were remodeled after the DAC surgery (**Figure 2D**). Specifically, VST values were significantly altered at each of the post-surgical time points. Increases in VSTs (**Figure 2E**) and VSTd (**Figure 2F**) started at week 2, while changes in the PWTs and PWTd started at week 4. VSTs and VSTd hypertrophy remained at week 4, 6, and 8, but posterior wall hypertrophy was not observed at these time points. After 10 and 12 weeks, the PWTd was significantly decreased in the DAC group compared with the sham group (**Figures 2G,H**). The results were summarized in **Table 3**.

Changes in the LVID displayed a V-shaped pattern over time after surgery (**Figures 2I,J, Table 3**). At week 2, the LVID at systole or diastole was decreased in DAC animals, with the smallest diameter at week 6. At week 10, the LVID started to enlarge, resulting in a significant difference compared with the LVID in sham animals at week 12. At the stage of ventricular hypertrophy in the DAC animals, EF and FS were increased, and at weeks 4 and 6, the increases were significantly different compared with the two indices in the pre-surgery group and the sham group at the corresponding time points. However, in dilated ventricles, the EF and FS were preserved in the DAC group compared with those observed in the sham group at the corresponding time points (**Figures 2K,L, Table 3**).

DAC Induces Pulmonary and Cardiovascular Damage, Including Fibrosis, Inflammatory Cell Infiltration, and Cardiomyocyte Hypertrophy

Pathological examination was performed on the aortas, atria, ventricles, lungs, livers, spleens, and kidneys of sham and DAC minipigs 12 weeks after surgery (**Figures 3A,B**). In DAC animals,

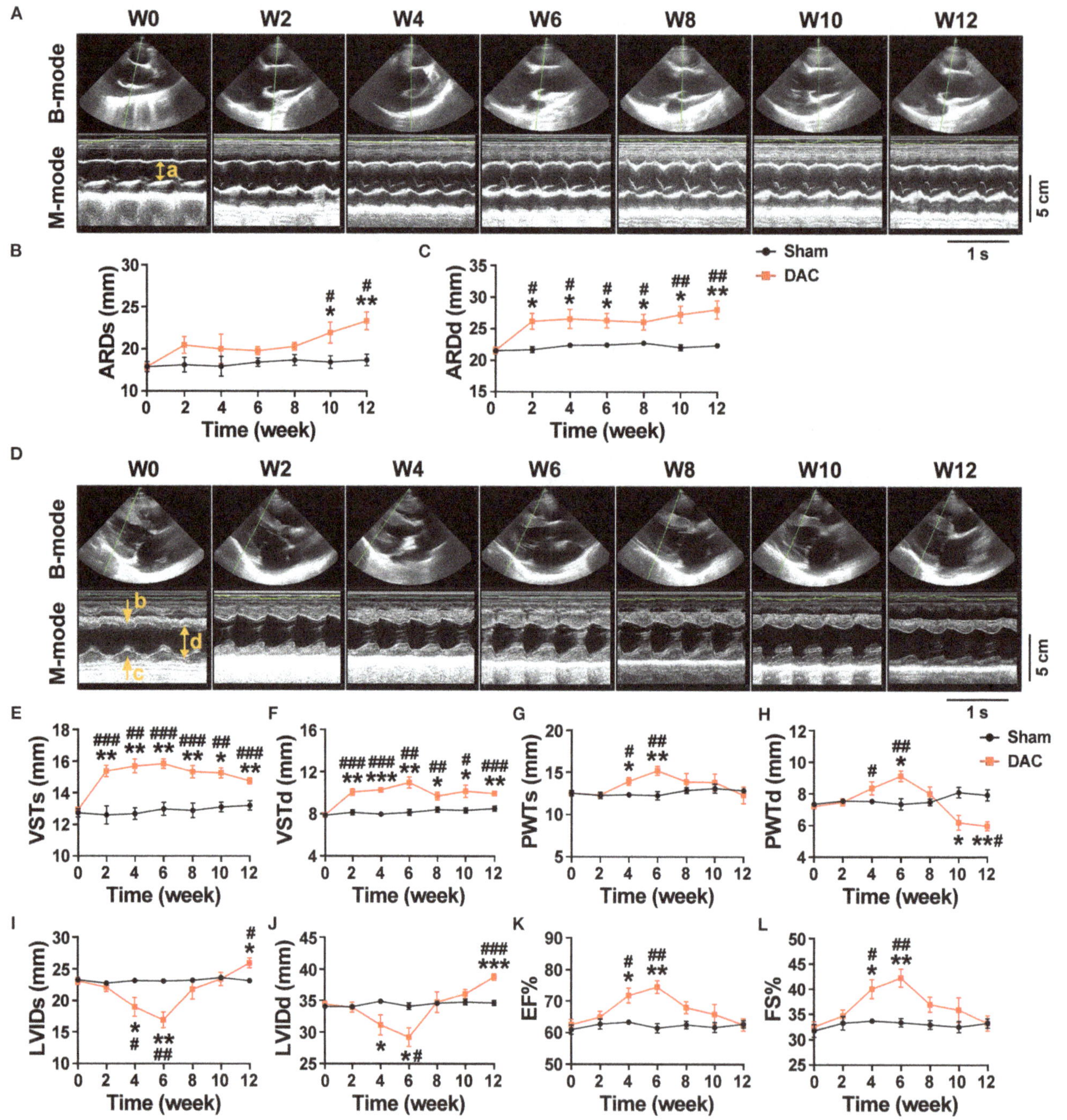

FIGURE 2 | Echocardiography of the sham and DAC animals. B-mode and M-mode of the aortic root **(A)** and left ventricle **(D)** at weeks 0, 2, 4, 6, 8, 10, and 12. Following DAC surgery, the diameters of aortic roots at systole (ARDs) and diastole (ARDd) were increased following DAC **(B,C)**. The thicknesses of the intraventricular septum at systole (VSTs) and diastole (VSTd) and were significantly increased over time **(E,F)**. The thickness of posterior wall at systole (PWTs) and diastole (PWTd) in the DAC group were gradually increased after week 2, but decreased after week 8 **(G,H)**. Changes in the left ventricular internal dimension at systole (LVIDs) and diastole (LVIDd) displayed a pattern with a "V" shape over time after surgery **(I,J)**. The left ventricular ejection fraction (EF) and fractional shortening (FS) in the DAC groups were preserved, compared with those of the sham groups at the corresponding time points **(K,L)**. ARD (a), VST (b), PWT (c), and LVID (d) were indicated in M mode images of **(A)** and **(D)**. $n = 4$ minipigs per group. All data are presented as the means ± SEMs. $^{*}P < 0.05$, $^{**}P < 0.01$, $^{***}P < 0.001$ vs. the sham group; $^{\#}P < 0.05$, $^{\#\#}P < 0.01$, $^{\#\#\#}P < 0.001$ vs. the week 0.

the intima of the proximal aorta displayed hyperplasia, mainly manifested as an increase in collagen fibers in the subendothelial layer. The alveolar wall was thickened. In addition, hepatic tissues displayed hepatocellular edema, congestion in the central vein, and hepatic sinusoids. There were no obvious lesions caused by DAC in the kidneys or spleen.

TABLE 3 | Echocardiographic analysis of the sham and DAC groups.

Time		Week 0	Week 2	Week 4	Week 6	Week 8	Week 10	Week 12
ARDd (mm)	Sham	21.5 ± 0.3	21.7 ± 0.5	22.4 ± 0.3	22.5 ± 0.4	22.8 ± 0.1	22.1 ± 0.5	22.4 ± 0.3
	DAC	21.6 ± 0.5	$26.2 \pm 1.3^{*\#}$	$26.6 \pm 1.5^{*\#}$	$26.3 \pm 1.2^{*\#}$	$26.1 \pm 1.2^{*\#}$	$27.3 \pm 1.3^{*\#\#}$	$28.1 \pm 1.4^{**\#\#}$
ARDs (mm)	Sham	17.9 ± 0.6	18.1 ± 0.9	18.0 ± 1.2	18.5 ± 0.5	18.7 ± 0.6	18.5 ± 0.8	18.7 ± 0.7
	DAC	17.9 ± 0.4	20.5 ± 1.0	20.0 ± 1.7	19.8 ± 0.5	20.3 ± 0.5	$22.0 \pm 1.3^{*\#}$	$23.4 \pm 1.1^{**\#}$
VSTs (mm)	Sham	12.7 ± 0.3	12.6 ± 0.6	12.7 ± 0.4	13.0 ± 0.4	12.9 ± 0.5	13.1 ± 0.3	13.2 ± 0.3
	DAC	12.9 ± 0.2	$15.4 \pm 0.4^{**\#\#\#}$	$15.7 \pm 0.4^{**\#\#}$	$15.9 \pm 0.3^{**\#\#\#}$	$15.3 \pm 0.4^{**\#\#\#}$	$15.3 \pm 0.3^{*\#\#}$	$14.8 \pm 0.2^{**\#\#\#}$
VSTd (mm)	Sham	7.9 ± 0.2	8.2 ± 0.2	8.0 ± 0.1	8.2 ± 0.3	8.4 ± 0.2	8.4 ± 0.3	8.5 ± 0.2
	DAC	7.9 ± 0.1	$10.1 \pm 0.3^{**\#\#\#}$	$10.3 \pm 0.2^{***\#\#\#}$	$11.0 \pm 0.5^{**\#\#}$	$9.7 \pm 0.4^{*\#\#}$	$10.2 \pm 0.6^{*\#}$	$10.0 \pm 0.2^{**\#\#\#}$
PWTs (mm)	Sham	12.5 ± 0.3	12.3 ± 0.4	12.4 ± 0.2	12.3 ± 0.5	12.9 ± 0.3	13.1 ± 0.5	12.9 ± 0.3
	DAC	12.5 ± 0.2	12.3 ± 0.2	$13.9 \pm 0.5^{*\#}$	$15.2 \pm 0.5^{**\#\#}$	13.9 ± 1.0	13.8 ± 1.0	12.3 ± 1.0
PWTd (mm)	Sham	7.4 ± 0.1	7.6 ± 0.1	7.5 ± 0.1	7.4 ± 0.4	7.5 ± 0.2	8.1 ± 0.3	7.9 ± 0.4
	DAC	7.2 ± 0.2	7.5 ± 0.2	$8.4 \pm 0.4^{\#}$	$9.1 \pm 0.3^{*\#\#}$	8.0 ± 0.5	$6.2 \pm 0.5^{*}$	$6.0 \pm 0.3^{**\#}$
LVIDs (mm)	Sham	23.3 ± 0.2	22.8 ± 0.4	23.2 ± 0.4	23.1 ± 0.4	23.2 ± 0.2	23.6 ± 0.4	23.2 ± 0.3
	DAC	23.1 ± 0.6	22.1 ± 0.7	$19.0 \pm 1.5^{*\#}$	$16.9 \pm 1.2^{**\#\#}$	21.8 ± 1.6	23.4 ± 1.0	$25.9 \pm 0.8^{*\#}$
LVIDd (mm)	Sham	34.1 ± 0.3	34.0 ± 0.4	34.9 ± 0.4	34.1 ± 0.5	34.6 ± 0.4	34.8 ± 0.5	34.7 ± 0.4
	DAC	34.4 ± 0.5	33.9 ± 0.8	$31.1 \pm 1.6^{*}$	$29.2 \pm 1.5^{*\#}$	34.8 ± 1.7	36.1 ± 0.7	$38.8 \pm 0.5^{***\#\#\#}$
EF (%)	Sham	61.0 ± 1.5	62.8 ± 1.6	63.4 ± 0.7	61.5 ± 1.4	62.5 ± 1.2	61.8 ± 1.6	62.8 ± 1.2
	DAC	62.5 ± 1.7	64.9 ± 1.9	$71.8 \pm 2.4^{*\#}$	$74.5 \pm 2.0^{**\#\#}$	68.0 ± 1.9	65.8 ± 3.2	62.5 ± 1.9
FS (%)	Sham	31.8 ± 1.3	33.3 ± 1.3	33.7 ± 0.5	33.4 ± 0.8	33.0 ± 0.9	32.5 ± 1.1	33.3 ± 0.9
	DAC	32.5 ± 1.0	34.7 ± 1.2	$40.0 \pm 1.9^{*\#}$	$42.3 \pm 1.8^{**\#\#}$	37.0 ± 1.5	35.9 ± 2.5	33.3 ± 1.5

All data are presented as the means ± SEMs. DAC, descending aortic constriction group; ARDs and ARDd, aortic root diameter at the end of systole and diastole, respectively; VSTs and VSTd, thickness of the ventricular septum at the end of systole and diastole, respectively; PWTs and PWTd, thickness of the posterior wall at the end of systole and diastole, respectively; LVIDs and LVIDd, left ventricular internal dimension at the end of systole and diastole, respectively; EF, left ventricular ejection fraction; FS, left ventricular fraction shortening. $^{*}P < 0.05$; $^{**}P < 0.01$; $^{***}P < 0.001$ *vs. the sham group;* $^{\#}P < 0.05$; $^{\#\#}P < 0.01$; $^{\#\#\#}P < 0.001$ *vs. the week 0.*

Next, the ventricles, atria, and ventricular septa were examined (**Figure 4**). There was widespread fibrosis in the myocardium of the left and right atria. Eosinophil infiltration was observed in the right atrium. Cardiomyocyte hypertrophy and nuclear pyknosis were observed in the internal ventricular septum. Moreover, fibrosis was widely present in the left ventricular myocardium, accompanied by dissolved cardiomyocyte nuclei and scarring. The right ventricle revealed cardiomyocyte hypertrophy and interstitial fibrosis. Overall, cardiac damage induced by DAC was characterized by fibrosis, eosinophil infiltration, and cardiomyocyte hypertrophy.

The Myocardium of the HFpEF Model Exhibits Evidence of Fibrosis

Overall gene expression profiles demonstrated that 543 genes were downregulated and 405 genes were upregulated in the DAC myocardium compared with in the sham myocardium (**Figure 5A**). Biological process enrichment analysis identified eight upregulated biological processes, including regulation of vasculature development (26 genes), regulation of cytokine production (25 genes), maintenance of location (15 genes), mitogen-activated protein kinase cascade (27 genes), negative regulation of translation (10 genes), positive regulation of cell migration (25 genes), RNA splicing (20 genes), and extracellular structure organization (19 genes; **Figure 5B**). In addition, we identified 10 downregulated biological processes, including response to oxidative stress (21 genes), regulation of G-protein-coupled receptor signaling (11 genes), regulation of lipid metabolic process (21 genes), carbohydrate metabolic process (28 genes), positive regulation of programmed cell death (31 genes), protein exit from the endoplasmic reticulum (7 genes), mitochondrion organization (26 genes), tricarboxylic acid metabolic process (7 genes), oxidation-reduction process (31 genes), and generation of precursor metabolites and energy (30 genes; **Figure 5C**). KEGG pathway analysis showed that two pathways were upregulated, including the PI3K/Akt signaling pathway and extracellular matrix/receptor interactions, and 9 pathways were down regulated (**Figure 5D**). Among these downregulated pathways, 7 pathways were involved in cellular metabolisms, including the carbon metabolism, metabolic pathways, citrate cycle, glycolysis/gluconeogenesis, biosynthesis of amino acids, pyruvate metabolism, and tryptophan metabolism. Thus, enrichment analyses suggested that heart cells in HFpEF suffer from inflammatory and oxidative stress and have altered remodeling, proliferation, apoptosis, and metabolic signaling. Furthermore, cluster analysis identified 10 genes associated with fibrosis, including *COL1A1*, *COL1A2*, *COL3A1*, *COL5A2*, *MMP16*, *MMP2*, *Fibronectin 1*, *Integrin Subunit Alpha V*, *Transforming Growth Factor Beta Receptor 3*, and *TIMP1* (**Figure 5E**). These findings suggest that fibrosis occurs in the myocardium of minipigs with HFpEF.

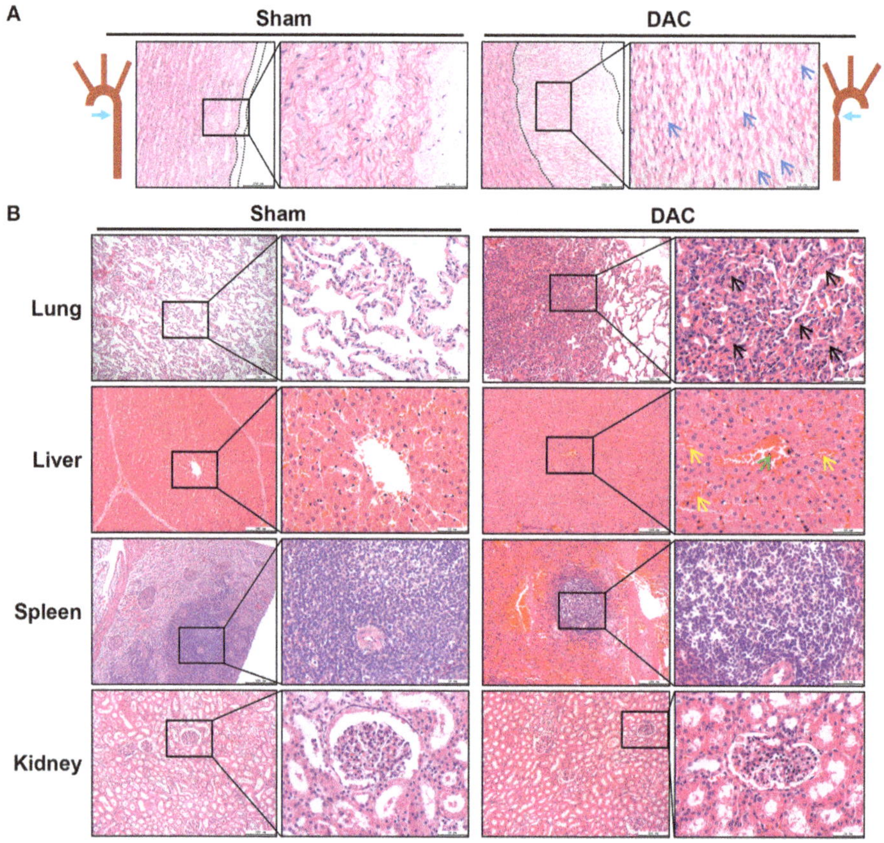

FIGURE 3 | Pathological changes of the aorta **(A)** and main organs **(B)** of lungs, livers, spleens, and kidneys of the sham and DAC minipigs. In DAC animals at 12 weeks after surgery, the intima of the proximal aorta displayed hyperplasia, indicated at **(A)**. The collagen fibers in the subendothelial layer were indicated (blue arrows). The alveolar wall thickened (black arrows). In addition, hepatic tissues displayed hepatocellular oedema, congestion in the central vein (green arrows), and hepatic sinusoids (yellow arrows).

Decreased Phosphorylation of Cardiac Myofilaments Is Associated With Cardiac Remodeling and Diastolic Dysfunction in HFpEF

Cardiac injuries in the left ventricles of the minipigs with HFpEF were observed at the cellular and molecular levels. RT-qPCR showed that expression levels of the heart failure markers (ANP and BNP) and the fibrotic markers (α-SMA, TIMP2, and MMP9) were significantly higher in the DAC group than in the sham group (**Figures 6A,B**). Sirius Red staining revealed that the fibrotic area was significantly greater in the DAC group than in the sham group (**Figure 6C**). Additionally, the cardiomyocytes displayed hypertrophy, and apoptosis was observed in the myocardium and epicardium of the DAC group (**Figures 6C,D**).

Upon examining alterations in myofilament phosphoproteins that regulate cardiac diastolic function, we found that the phosphorylation levels of myofilament proteins (MyBP-C, desmin, cTnT, tropomyosin, cTnI, and MLC2) were significantly suppressed in minipigs with HFpEF induced by chronic pressure overload compared to sham pigs (**Figure 7**). Study has shown that myofilament phosphorylation is essential for normal diastolic function in HFpEF hearts (22), and in the end stages of HF, aged dogs with HFpEF display lower levels of myofilament phosphorylation than healthy dogs (23). This suggested impaired diastolic function in the heart, and indicated that cardiomyocyte hypertrophy, apoptosis, and fibrosis contribute to cardiac remodeling in HFpEF.

Activation of Fibrotic and Inflammatory Pathways in Chronic Pressure Overload-Induced HFpEF

Both pathological examination and GSEA suggested that inflammatory responses were critical events in the impairment of heart cells. Secretion of cytokines upon mechanical overload is known to trigger the activation of fibroblasts. Therefore, we investigated inflammatory signaling pathways and found that DAC elevated the levels of p-IκBα, p-NFκB, IL6, and IL-1β in the minipig myocardium (**Figures 8A,B**). These results suggested that activation of fibrotic signaling pathways promotes the differentiation of myofibroblasts in hearts with chronic pressure overload.

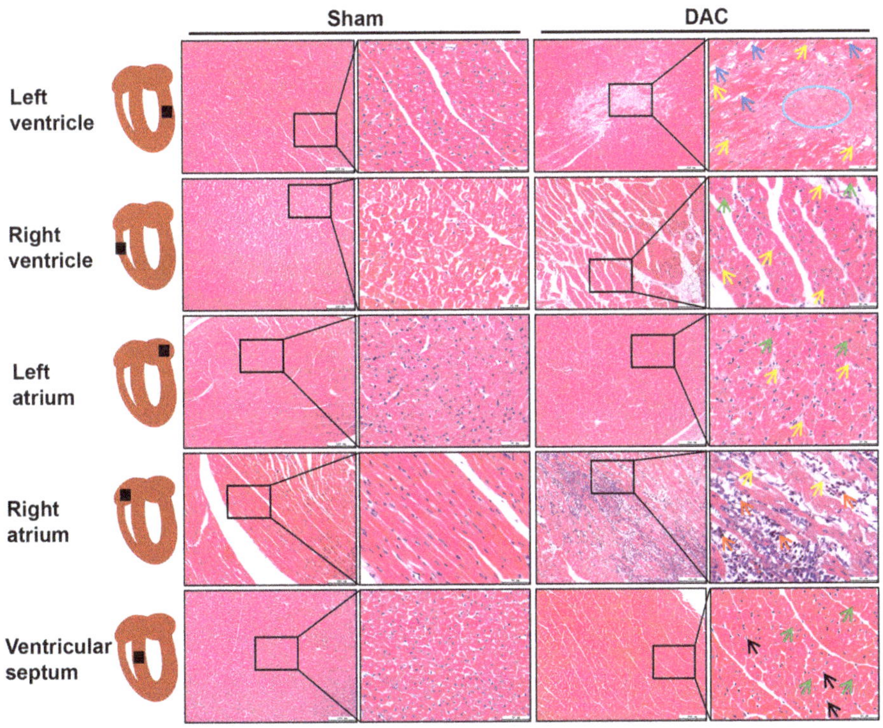

FIGURE 4 | Tissue damage of atria, ventricles, and interventricular septum induced by DAC. There was widespread fibrosis (yellow arrows) in the myocardium of the left and right atria. Cardiomyocyte hypertrophy (green arrows) and eosinophil infiltration (red arrows) were observed in the right atrium. Cardiomyocyte hypertrophy (green arrows) and nuclear pyknosis (black arrows) were observed in the internal ventricular septum. Fibrosis (yellow arrows) was present in the left ventricular myocardium, accompanied by dissolved cardiomyocyte nuclei (blue arrows) and scar (blue circle) appearance. The right ventricle showed cardiomyocyte hypertrophy (green arrows) and interstitial fibrosis (yellow arrows).

Next, we investigated whether fibrosis-associated molecular signals were activated in HFpEF. Importantly, we observed significant increases in the levels of fibroblast-secreted TGF-β, its downstream effectors p-SMAD2 and p-SMAD2/3, and proteins associated with cellular proliferation, including p-PI3K and p-ERK, following DAC (**Figures 8C,D**). Additionally, transcriptional sequencing analysis showed increases in MMP2 and TIMP1 levels in HFpEF hearts compared with sham hearts, accompanied by increases in collagen I protein expression (**Figures 8C,D**). These findings explain the fibrosis observed in the myocardium of HFpEF.

DISCUSSION

In this study, we successfully developed a novel HFpEF model using DAC-induced chronic pressure overload in minipigs. This model was characterized by cardiac remodeling, fibrosis, tissue damage, and impaired cellular signal transduction. Echocardiography was performed to trace the aortic and ventricular morphology and cardiac contractile function over 12 weeks, demonstrating the pattern of HFpEF disease progression. In our further investigation of the mechanisms underlying the pathological and cellular responses, the fibrotic signaling pathways in the myocardium of HFpEF were explored. Based on this, we can propose a potential regulatory mechanism underlying cardiac remodeling and functional impairment in HFpEF (**Figure 9**). Briefly, chronic pressure overload induces inflammatory responses, which in turn activate cytokines and intracellular NFκB signaling, resulting in tissue damage. In addition, inflammatory stimuli are also involved in fibrotic signaling. On the other hand, chronic pressure overload activates TGF-β/SMAD signaling, which together with inflammatory stimuli and PI3K/ERK activation, promotes proliferation and fibroblast differentiation. Furthermore, MMPs, TIMPs, and several other signals increase collagen production. The resultant tissue damage, fibrosis, cardiomyocyte hypertrophy, and myofilament dephosphorylation all contribute to cardiac remodeling and dysfunction. This is the first study to use DAC to model HFpEF, establishing a powerful tool for modeling this condition.

Assessment of Pathological and Cellular Responses of HFpEF Model

HFpEF is a heterogeneous cardiac phenotype with many patterns of cardiac remodeling. These structural phenotypes include normal cardiac tissue, concentric remodeling, concentric hypertrophy, and eccentric hypertrophy (24). We found that constriction at the descending aorta trunk was suitable for linear studies of structural and functional changes following chronic pressure overload. During the 12-week observation period,

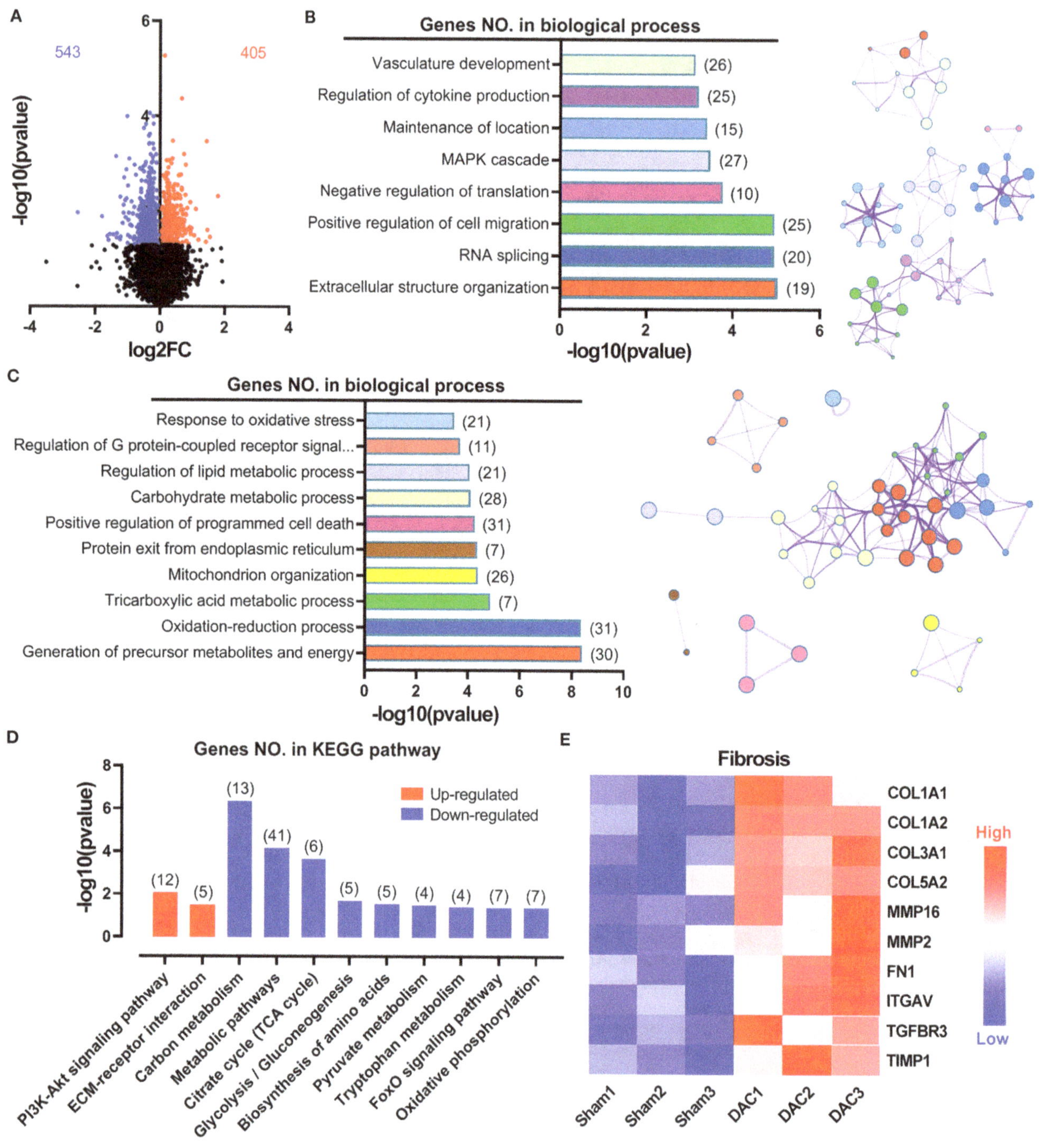

FIGURE 5 | Overall gene expression profiles in sham and DAC animals. Gene enrichment analyses suggested that heart cells in HFpEF suffer inflammatory stress, oxidative stress, remodeling, proliferation, apoptosis, and metabolic disorders. Specifically, 543 genes were downregulated, whereas 405 genes were upregulated in the DAC myocardium compared with that in the sham myocardium **(A)**. Biological process enrichment analysis identified eight upregulated biological processes **(B)** and 10 downregulated biological processes **(C)**. KEGG pathway analysis showed that two pathways were upregulated and night pathways were downregulated **(D)**. In addition, 10 genes associated with fibrosis were seen in **(E)**. $n = 3$ minipigs per group.

we detected concentric hypertrophy, hypertrophy with normal LVID, and left ventricle dilation with normal interventricular septum thickness, suggesting that our model mimics the conditions in human HFpEF. In addition, the results of our pathological examination were consistent with other studies describing cardiomyocyte hypertrophy (25). Here, we conclude

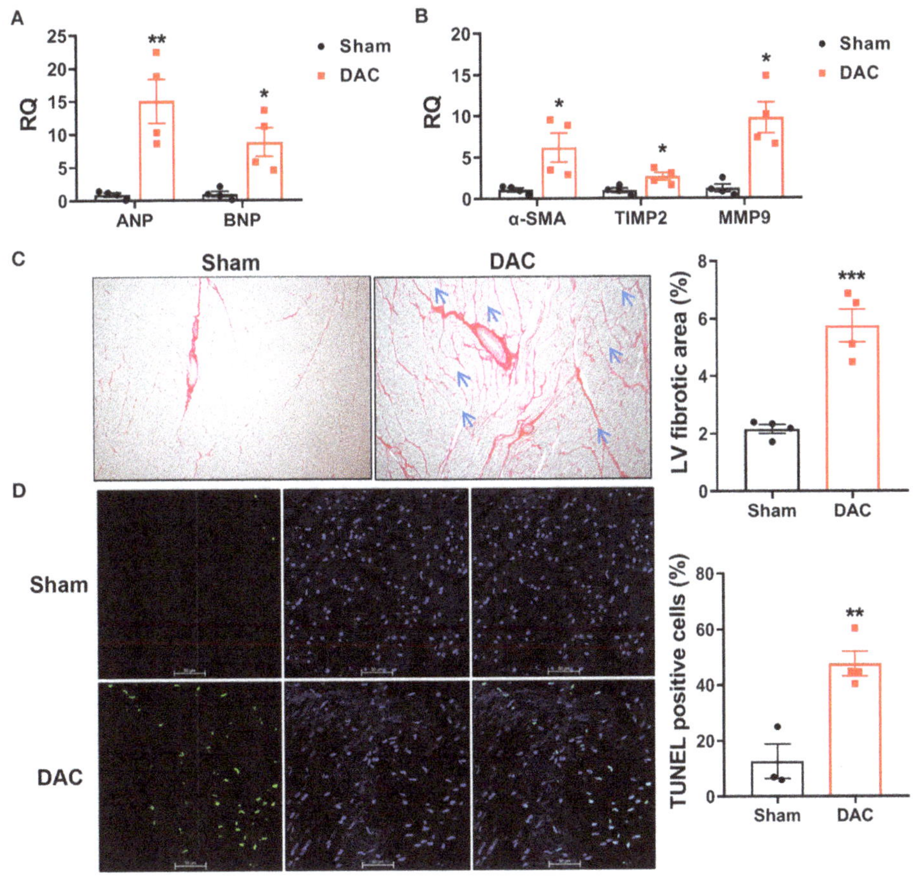

FIGURE 6 | Biomarkers of heart failure, fibrotic area, and apoptosis in the left ventricles. The cardiac injuries at the cellular and molecular levels were seen of the left ventricles of the minipigs with HFpEF. The expression levels of ANP and BNP **(A)** and α-SMA, TIMP2, MMP9 **(B)** were significantly higher in the DAC group than those in the sham group. $n = 4$ minipigs per group. Sirius Red staining showed the fibrotic area in the DAC group was significantly greater than that in the sham group **(C)**, and the cardiomyocytes in the DAC group displayed hypertrophy (blue arrows), and apoptosis **(D)** was observed in the myocardium and epicardium of HFpEF. $n =$ 3–4 minipigs per group. All data are presented as the means ± SEMs. $^*P < 0.05$, $^{**}P < 0.01$, $^{***}P < 0.001$ vs. the sham group.

that echocardiography is the appropriate imaging tool to evaluate cardiac structure and function in the laboratory study of large animal HFpEF models. Furthermore, consistent with the structural findings from echocardiography, gene ontology enrichment analysis demonstrated the upregulation of several biological processes associated with cardiac remodeling, including vasculature development, positive regulation of cell migration, and extracellular structure.

Regarding the selection of constriction sites for inducing pressure overload, the aortic root, and ascending, transverse, and descending trunks have been used in small and large animal models (13, 16, 18, 26). The ascending or transverse trunks are more favorable in small animal HF models. These sites are approachable by either using a medical needle to determine the constriction degree or placing a ring of fixed size (13, 16). In large animals, the internal aortic diameters are comparable with those of humans. With the aid of a catheter and angiogram technology, researchers can deliver medical stents (26) or inflatable cuffs (18) to any fragments of the aorta to execute vessel constriction. Thus, compared with small animals, aortic constriction sites are less restricted by thoracic anatomy in large animals. However, the high cost of angiography machines has hindered the use of catheters. In this study, we adopted the thoracotomy used in small animals, but applied the incision on the left chest. This strategy avoids sternum damage while clearly exposing the aortic descending trunk. More importantly, this large animal HFpEF model can be generated without the need for expensive instrument. Besides the descending aorta, banding at the ascending aorta was performed by two independent groups (27–29). In these cases, the third intercostal space was widened to locate the ascending aortic trunk (27).

Several methods have been used to develop HFpEF pig models. Deoxycorticosterone acetate (DOCA) combined with a Western diet was used to induce hypertension and hyperlipidemia in Landrace pigs for 12 weeks (22), and it was later shown that DOCA alone can induce the development of early stage HFpEF in pigs (30). A combination of a Western diet and pressure overload has been used to study HFpEF in rodent models, and this approach was recently introduced in a pig model (31). Compared with these methods, our model

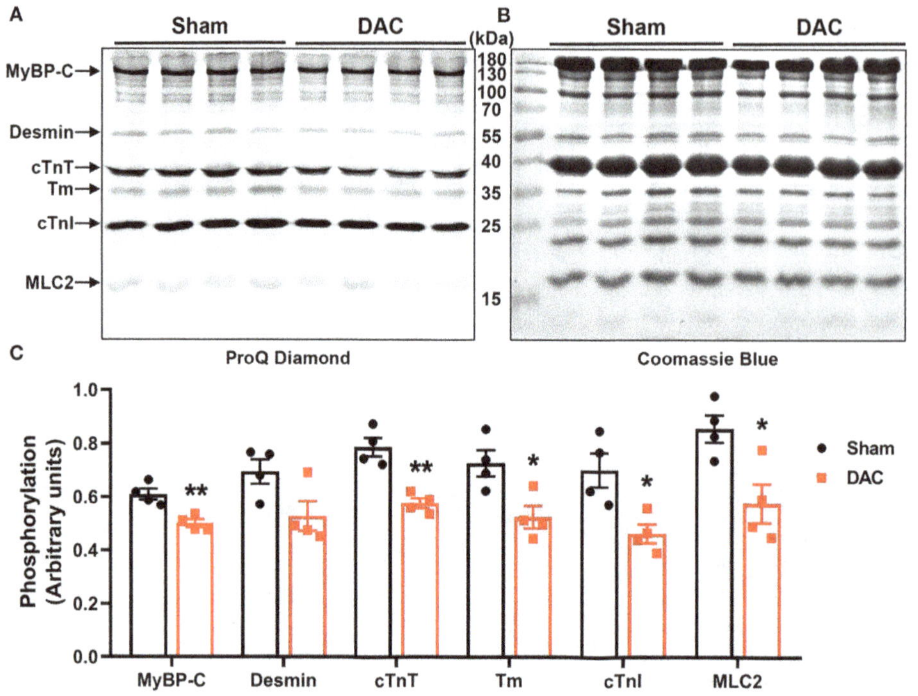

FIGURE 7 | Phosphorylation of contractile proteins. Phosphorylation levels of MyBP-C, desmin, cTnT, tropomyosin (Tm), cTnI, and MLC2 were significantly suppressed **(A,C)** in minipigs with HFpEF induced by chronic pressure overload. **(A)** Pro-Q phosphorylation staining image, each band represents an individual animal. $n = 4$ minipigs per group. $^{*}P < 0.05$, $^{**}P < 0.01$ vs. the sham group.

has the advantage of introducing chronic pressure overload as a condition of hypertension, one of the most common chronic diseases related to HFpEF.

Metabolic KEGG pathway analysis showed that the DEGs between healthy and HFpEF myocardia were involved in citrate cycle suppression, glycolysis, amino acid biosynthesis, and pyruvate metabolism, suggesting that metabolic changes are crucial in HFpEF. Our findings are consistent with a study in a murine HFpEF model of metabolic disorder, in which researchers found that β-hydroxybutyrate was an effective treatment, as it targets the acetyl-CoA pool and mitochondrial acetylation (32). Furthermore, a clinical study including 46 patients with new-onset HFpEF and 75 patients with new-onset HFrEF revealed 11 plasma metabolites that differed between the two groups, and proposed that the hearts of patients with HFpEF tended to show increased rates of fibrosis, oxidative stress, and inflammation compared with those of patients with HFrEF (33). Together, these results suggested that metabolic pathways could be effective targets for HFpEF therapy.

Cardiac Fibrosis Is a Key Response to Chronic Pressure Overload-Induced HFpEF

Fibrosis is a cellular response to harmful stimuli such as mechanical stress, and is mainly caused by the excessive deposition of extracellular matrix proteins. The key signal transduction pathways regulating the development of fibrous connective tissues include TGF-β signaling and growth-promoting PI3K signaling pathways. In the current study, we found that the TGF-β expression level was upregulated by chronic pressure overload, as were the phosphorylation levels of SMAD2 and SMAD3. However, we did not identify the distinct roles of each cellular signaling protein in the development of HF in this study. In pressure overload, deletion of the genes encoding TGF-β receptor and SMAD3 reduces the fibrotic response; additionally, deletion of the TGF-β receptor reduces the hypertrophic response, whereas deletion of *SMAD2/3* reduces cellular expansion (34). In future studies, identifying the different roles of these proteins will help to explain how hearts respond to biomechanical stress. In response to stimulation with TGF-β, cardiac fibroblasts switch to a myofibroblast phenotype expressing α-SMA, which is increased in pressure overload hearts displaying fibrosis (35). Consistent with their findings, we observed elevated gene expression of myofibroblast-derived α-SMA and protein expression of collagen I in the myocardium of HFpEF animals. Moreover, we found downregulated PI3K and upregulated ERK in the fibrotic myocardium. It has been known that PI3K and ERK signaling pathways are involved in the regulation of fibrosis. For example, suppression of α-SMA expression in cardiac fibroblasts is dependent upon PI3K signaling (36), and the suppression of cardiac fibrosis by chemical compounds (such as gentisic acid) occurs through the ERK signaling pathway (37). However, the regulatory mechanisms

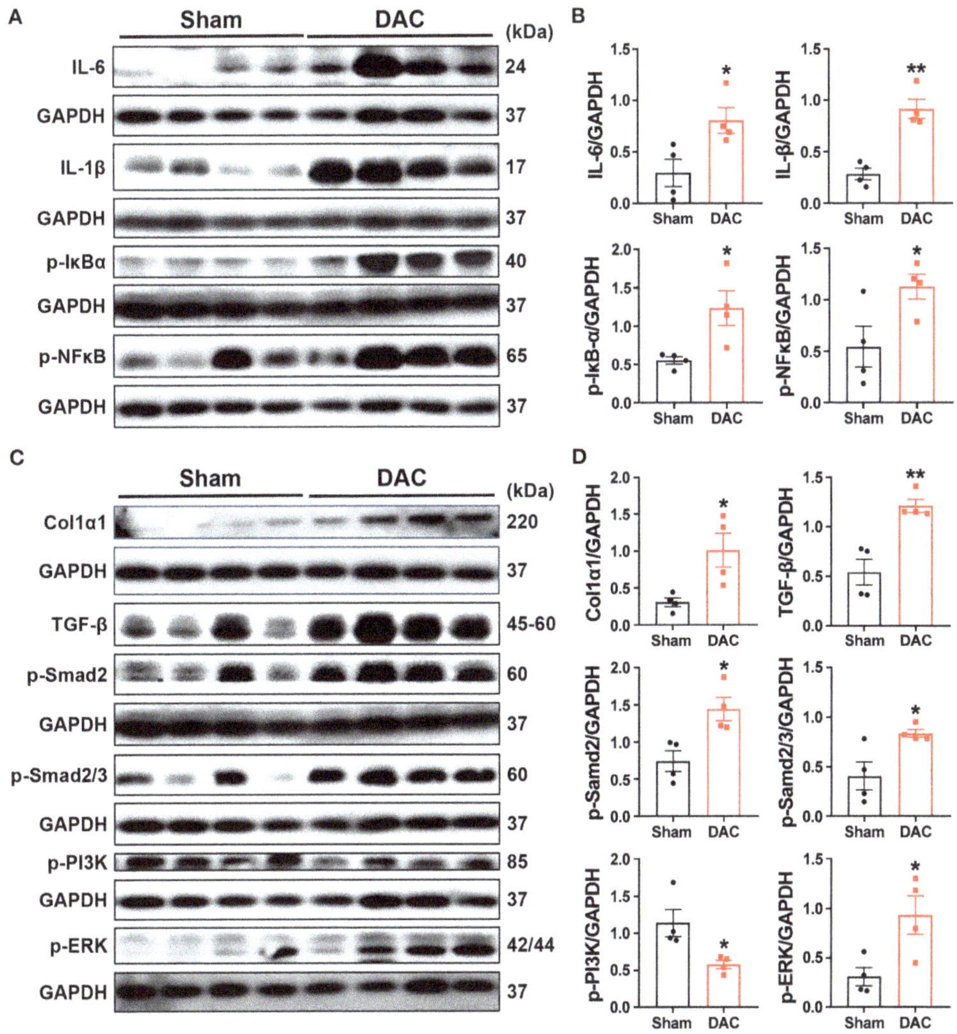

FIGURE 8 | Activation of the inflammatory and fibrotic pathways. This study demonstrates that myocardial fibrosis is associated with activation of inflammatory pathways as the evident elevation of p-IκBα, p-NFκB, IL-6, and IL-1β in the DAC myocardium **(A,B)** and significant increases in the levels of fibroblast-secreted TGF-β1, the downstream effectors p-Smad2 and p-Smad2/3, and p-PI3K and p-ERK linking to cellular proliferation following DAC **(C,D)**. $n = 4$ minipigs per group. Each band represent an individual animal. All data are presented as the means ± SEMs. $^{*}P < 0.05$, $^{**}P < 0.01$ vs. the sham group.

by which pathways affect the progression of HFpEF needs further investigation.

Enzymes such as MMP2, MMP9, and their inhibitors are known to regulate extracellular matrix turnover and induce cardiac fibrosis. Bergman et al. reported that MMP2 transgenics exhibit significant increases in interstitial and perivascular collagen in the heart, accompanied by marked ventricular remodeling (38). Moreover, deletion of *MMP2* or *TIMP1* minimizes fibrosis in pressure-overloaded mouse hearts (39). Notably, elevation of serum TIMP1 levels in the hypertensive heart is associated with left ventricular diastolic dysfunction and correlated with the elevation of other fibrotic markers, including plasma procollagen type I carboxy-terminal pro-peptide and the carboxy-terminal telopeptide of collagen type I (40). Similarly, in this study, we found that the expression levels of MMP2 and its inhibitor TIMP2, and MMP9 and its inhibitor TIMP1 were upregulated in the myocardium of HFpEF. These findings suggested that the porcine HFpEF model is an effective tool for studying the extracellular matrix turnover-dependent fibrotic mechanisms underlying this disease. However, we did not measure the protein expression levels of these enzymes and their inhibitors. Further studies are needed to elucidate the mechanisms underlying HFpEF.

Regarding the expression of MMP inhibitors, clinical studies have demonstrated that elevated TIMP1 is associated with fibrosis and cardiac remodeling in patients with hypertension; in contrast, in mechanistic studies in animal models, the inhibition of TIMP1 or TIMP2 effectively suppresses cardiac fibrosis and remodeling (39, 41). These differences may be due to analysis of samples from different stages (i.e., the compensatory and

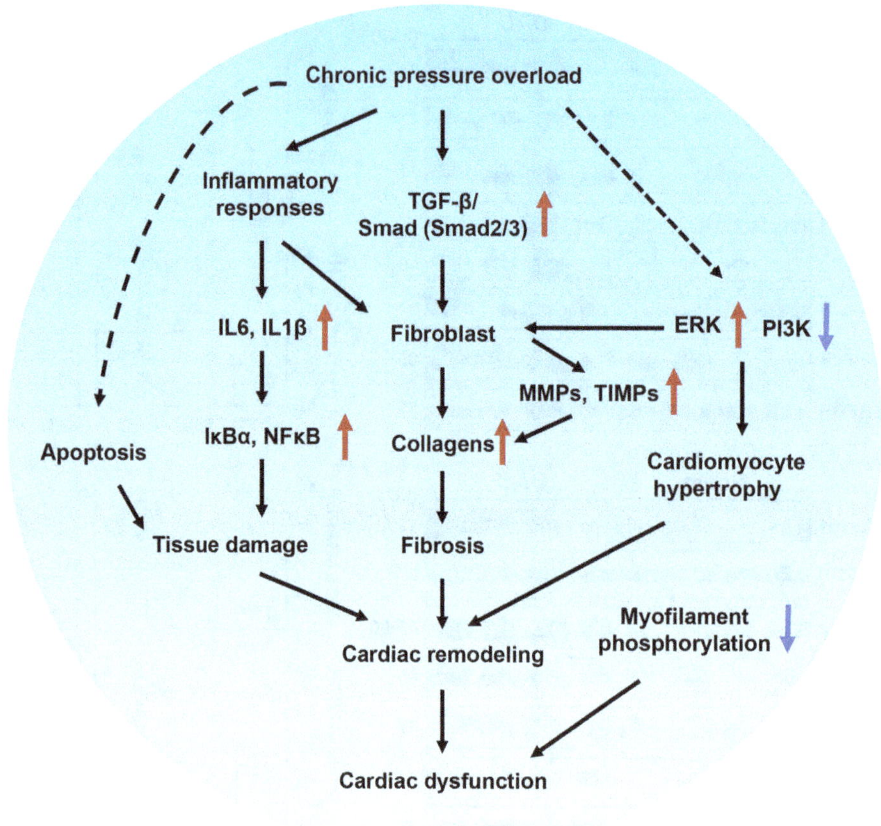

FIGURE 9 | Proposed molecular mechanisms underlying cardiac remodeling and functional impairment in HFpEF. Chronic pressure overload induces inflammatory responses, which in turn activates cytokines and intracellular NFκB signaling and associated with tissue damage. In addition, inflammatory stimuli also involved in the fibrotic signaling. On the other hand, chronic pressure overload activates TGF-β/Smad signaling pathways, which together with inflammatory stimuli, PI3K/ERK signaling promote proliferation and differentiation of fibroblast. Furthermore, MMPs, TIMPs and several other signals regulates the production of collagens. The tissue damage, fibrosis, cardiomyocyte hypertrophy, and myofilament dephosphorylation contribute to cardiac remodeling and diastolic dysfunction.

decompensatory stages) of cardiac remodeling. Importantly, in end-stage cardiomyopathy, higher levels of TIMP1 and TIMP2 are associated with cardiac fibrosis (42). However, further studies are needed to investigate the regulation of MMPs and their inhibitors.

The Impairment of Diastolic Function in HFpEF

Although HFpEF has discrete pathophysiologic phenotypes, diastolic dysfunction is among its key features. Consistent with observations in clinical and experimental studies (43, 44), several key changes indicating diastolic dysfunction exist in our HFpEF model. These include changes in the E: A ratio, left atrial size, and serum cTnI, CK, and LDH levels. However, the mechanisms underlying diastolic dysfunction in the development of HFpEF are still unclear. Fibrosis and inflammation can have marked effects on diastolic function. In addition to profibrotic signaling triggered by TGF-β, inflammatory cytokines also promote myofibroblast differentiation (45). Clinical research has shown that the inflammatory biomarkers IL6 and tumor necrosis factor α are strongly associated with HFpEF in older adults (46) and in HFpEF animals (25). Furthermore, treatment with anti-chemoattractant protein inhibits macrophage accumulation and fibroblast proliferation, and is associated with improved remodeling and diastolic dysfunction (47). Here, we have shown that IL6, IL-1β, NFκB, and IκBα are significantly upregulated in the fibrotic myocardium of minipigs with diastolic dysfunction. Gene ontology enrichment analysis also demonstrated effects on the regulation of cytokine production. Together with our other findings, we conclude that cardiomyocyte hypertrophy, inflammatory responses, and apoptosis synergistically determine cardiac diastolic dysfunction in this porcine HFpEF model.

Furthermore, the phosphorylation of myofilament proteins is essential for normal diastolic function. In a previous study, Rosas et al. reported that MyBP-C phosphorylation benefits relaxation, whereas decreased phosphorylation of this myofilament protein disrupts diastolic function, a characteristic of HFpEF (48). In this study, we found that the phosphorylation levels of myofilament proteins were significantly lower in the hearts of

HFpEF animals than in sham hearts, consistent with a study in a canine HFpEF model showing reduced phosphorylation of MyBP-C, TnT, TnI, and MLC2 (23). Hamdani et al. (23) further found that the phosphorylation levels of several titin sites were decreased, accompanied by corresponding changes in the expression levels of protein kinases and phosphatases. Our previous study revealed that myofilament phosphorylation is sensitive to all cardiac stresses (19, 21). However, myofilament phosphorylation is quite dynamic during cardiac stress. Further examination of the relationship between myofilament phosphorylation and cardiac diastolic dysfunction is required.

In conclusion, we have successfully developed a minipig HFpEF model characterized by cardiac fibrosis and remodeling. Our findings support the use of this porcine model of hypertension-induced HFpEF as a powerful tool to elucidate the mechanisms of this disease and translate preclinical findings.

LIMITATIONS

Although this HFpEF model has multiple advantages, there are still some unsolved questions that require further investigation. For example, the molecular changes associated with this model were not fully investigated. Notably, stimulation with angiotensin II promotes cardiac fibroblast and collagen production (49). Exploring this signaling mechanism may help elucidate the pathogenesis of HFpEF in our pig model. Furthermore, consistency in the surgical procedure across laboratories may make generalization challenging. Additionally, our model only used one type of minipig. Because many laboratory pig strains have been used in different studies, it may be necessary to optimize the degree of constriction when using other strains to generate the model. Finally, Melleby et al. (17) have shown that a constriction ring induces HFpEF phenotypes, whereas a smaller ring leads to HFrEF. Despite these limitations, our study has established an effective model for basic or translational medical research and has uncovered crucial changes that provide mechanistic insights into HFpEF.

AUTHOR CONTRIBUTIONS

FY, WT, and XianL designed and initiated the project. SZ, WT, XianL, XiaoL, FY, HS, XZ, JW, and HC were responsible for the laboratory experiments, data analysis, and/or animal care. WP, YZ, and PB provided critical comments during experiment design and manuscript preparation. All authors read and approved the final manuscript.

FUNDING

This work was supported by the Guangdong Science and Technology Program (2016A020216019), the National Natural Science Foundation of China (31672376 and 81941002), the Guangdong Science and Technology Program (2019A030317014, 2017A020215076, 2018A0303130208, 2018B030317001, 2017B020231001, 2008A08003, and 2020B1111490002), the Guangzhou Science and Technology Program (201804010206), and the Guangdong Provincial Key Laboratory of Laboratory Animals (2017B030314171). WP was supported with a Senior Investigator Award for Women's Heart Health from the Heart and Stroke Foundation of Canada. Laboratory Animal Science Foundation of Shanghai Committee of Science and Technology grant (201409005000).

ACKNOWLEDGMENTS

The authors thank the Large Animal Facility of the Guangdong Laboratory Animal Monitoring Institute for maintaining the animals used in this work.

REFERENCES

1. Maggioni AP, Dahlström U, Filippatos G, Chioncel O, Crespo Leiro M, Drozdz J, et al. EURObservational Research Programme: regional differences and 1-year follow-up results of the heart failure pilot survey (ESC-HF Pilot). *Eur J Heart Fail.* (2013) 15:808–17. doi: 10.1093/eurjhf/hft050
2. Virani SS, Alonso A, Benjamin EJ, Bittencourt MS, Callaway CW, Carson AP, et al. Heart disease and stroke statistics-2020 update: a report from the American Heart Association. *Circulation.* (2020) 141:e139–e596. doi: 10.1161/CIR.0000000000000757
3. Ma LY, Chen WW, Gao RL, Liu LS, Zhu ML, Wang YJ, et al. China cardiovascular diseases report 2018: an updated summary. *J Geriatr Cardiol.* (2020) 17:1–8. doi: 10.11909/j.issn.1671-5411.2020.01.001
4. Ponikowski P, Voors AA, Anker SD, Bueno H, Cleland JGF, Coats AJS, et al. 2016 ESC Guidelines for the diagnosis treatment of acute chronic heart failure: the task force for the diagnosis treatment of acute chronic heart failure of the European Society of Cardiology (ESC) developed with the special contribution of the Heart Failure Association (HFA) of the ESC. *Eur Heart J.* (2016) 37:2129–200. doi: 10.1093/eurheartj/ehw128
5. Yancy CW, Jessup M, Bozkurt B, Butler J, Casey DE Jr, Drazner MH, et al. 2013 ACCF/AHA guideline for the management of heart failure: a report of the American College of Cardiology Foundation/American Heart Association Task Force on practice guidelines. *Circulation.* (2013) 128:e240–327. doi: 10.1161/CIR.0b013e31829e8776
6. Tsutsui H, Isobe M, Ito H, Ito H, Okumura K, Ono M, et al. JCS 2017/JHFS 2017 guideline on diagnosis and treatment of acute and chronic heart failure- digest version. *Circ J.* (2019) 83:2084–184. doi: 10.1253/circj.CJ-19-0342
7. Pfeffer MA, Shah AM, Borlaug BA. Heart failure with preserved ejection fraction in perspective. *Circ Res.* (2019) 124:1598–617. doi: 10.1161/CIRCRESAHA.119.313572
8. Tromp J, Teng TH, Tay WT, Hung CL, Narasimhan C, Shimizu W, et al. Heart failure with preserved ejection fraction in Asia. *Eur J Heart Fail.* (2019) 21:23–36. doi: 10.1002/ejhf.1227
9. Cuijpers I, Simmonds SJ, Van Bilsen M, Czarnowska E, González Miqueo A, Heymans S, et al. Microvascular and lymphatic dysfunction in HFpEF and its associated comorbidities. *Basic Res Cardiol.* (2020) 115:39. doi: 10.1007/s00395-020-0798-y
10. Mishra S, Kass DA. Cellular and molecular pathobiology of heart failure with preserved ejection fraction. *Nat Rev Cardiol.* (2021). doi: 10.1038/s41569-021-00516-5. [Epub ahead of print].

11. Dixon JA, Spinale FG. Large animal models of heart failure: a critical link in the translation of basic science to clinical practice. *Circ Heart Fail.* (2009) 2:262–71. doi: 10.1161/CIRCHEARTFAILURE.108.814459
12. Riehle C, Bauersachs J. Small animal models of heart failure. *Cardiovasc Res.* (2019) 115:1838–49. doi: 10.1093/cvr/cvz161
13. Schunkert H, Dzau VJ, Tang SS, Hirsch AT, Apstein CS, Lorell BH. Increased rat cardiac angiotensin converting enzyme activity and mRNA expression in pressure overload left ventricular hypertrophy. Effects on coronary resistance, contractility, and relaxation. *J Clin Invest.* (1990) 86:1913–20. doi: 10.1172/JCI114924
14. Rockman HA, Ross RS, Harris AN, Knowlton KU, Steinhelper ME, Field LJ, et al. Segregation of atrial-specific and inducible expression of an atrial natriuretic factor transgene in an *in vivo* murine model of cardiac hypertrophy. *Proc Natl Acad Sci U.S.A.* (1991) 88:8277–81. doi: 10.1073/pnas.88.18.8277
15. Weinberg EO, Schoen FJ, George D, Kagaya Y, Douglas PS, Litwin SE, et al. Angiotensin-converting enzyme inhibition prolongs survival and modifies the transition to heart failure in rats with pressure overload hypertrophy due to ascending aortic stenosis. *Circulation.* (1994) 90:1410–22. doi: 10.1161/01.CIR.90.3.1410
16. Litwin SE, Katz SE, Weinberg EO, Lorell BH, Aurigemma GP, Douglas PS. Serial echocardiographic-Doppler assessment of left ventricular geometry and function in rats with pressure-overload hypertrophy. Chronic angiotensin-converting enzyme inhibition attenuates the transition to heart failure. *Circulation.* (1995) 91:2642–54. doi: 10.1161/01.CIR.91.10.2642
17. Melleby AO, Romaine A, Aronsen JM, Veras I, Zhang L, Sjaastad I, et al. A novel method for high precision aortic constriction that allows for generation of specific cardiac phenotypes in mice. *Cardiovasc Res.* (2018) 114:1680–90. doi: 10.1093/cvr/cvy141
18. Charles CJ, Lee P, Li RR, Yeung T, Ibraham Mazlan SM, Tay ZW, et al. A porcine model of heart failure with preserved ejection fraction: magnetic resonance imaging and metabolic energetics. *ESC Heart Fail.* (2020) 7:92–102. doi: 10.1002/ehf2.12536
19. Li X, Zheng S, Tan W, Chen H, Li X, Wu J, et al. Slit2 protects hearts against ischemia-reperfusion injury by inhibiting inflammatory responses and maintaining myofilament contractile properties. *Front Physiol.* (2020) 11:228. doi: 10.3389/fphys.2020.00228
20. Yang FH, Pyle WG. Reduced cardiac CapZ protein protects hearts against acute ischemia-reperfusion injury and enhances preconditioning. *J Mol Cell Cardiol.* (2012) 52:761–72. doi: 10.1016/j.yjmcc.2011.11.013
21. Zheng S, Tan W, Li X, Li B, Gong B, Pyle WG, et al. Aged monkeys fed a high-fat/high-sugar diet recapitulate metabolic disorders and cardiac contractile dysfunction. *J Cardiovasc Transl Res.* (2021). doi: 10.1007/s12265-021-10105-z. [Epub ahead of print].
22. Schwarzl M, Hamdani N, Seiler S, Alogna A, Manninger M, Reilly S, et al. A porcine model of hypertensive cardiomyopathy: implications for heart failure with preserved ejection fraction. *Am J Physiol Heart Circ Physiol.* (2015) 309:H1407–18. doi: 10.1152/ajpheart.00542.2015
23. Hamdani N, Bishu KG, Von Frieling-Salewsky M, Redfield MM, Linke WA. Deranged myofilament phosphorylation and function in experimental heart failure with preserved ejection fraction. *Cardiovasc Res.* (2013) 97:464–71. doi: 10.1093/cvr/cvs353
24. Shah AM, Pfeffer MA. The many faces of heart failure with preserved ejection fraction. *Nat Rev Cardiol.* (2012) 9:555–6. doi: 10.1038/nrcardio.2012.123
25. Glezeva N, Baugh JA. Role of inflammation in the pathogenesis of heart failure with preserved ejection fraction and its potential as a therapeutic target. *Heart Fail Rev.* (2014) 19:681–94. doi: 10.1007/s10741-013-9405-8
26. Gyöngyösi M, Pavo N, Lukovic D, Zlabinger K, Spannbauer A, Traxler D, et al. Porcine model of progressive cardiac hypertrophy and fibrosis with secondary postcapillary pulmonary hypertension. *J Transl Med.* (2017) 15:202. doi: 10.1186/s12967-017-1299-0
27. Bikou O, Miyashita S, Ishikawa K. Pig model of increased cardiac afterload induced by ascending aortic banding. *Methods Mol Biol.* (2018) 1816:337–42. doi: 10.1007/978-1-4939-8597-5_26
28. Hiemstra JA, Veteto AB, Lambert MD, Olver TD, Ferguson BS, Mcdonald KS, et al. Chronic low-intensity exercise attenuates cardiomyocyte contractile dysfunction and impaired adrenergic responsiveness in aortic-banded mini-swine. *J Appl Physiol.* (1985) 124:1034–44. doi: 10.1152/japplphysiol.00840.2017
29. Olver TD, Edwards JC, Ferguson BS, Hiemstra JA, Thorne PK, Hill MA, et al. Chronic interval exercise training prevents BK(Ca) channel-mediated coronary vascular dysfunction in aortic-banded miniswine. *J Appl Physiol.* (2018) 125:86–96.
30. Reiter U, Reiter G, Manninger M, Adelsmayr G, Schipke J, Alogna A, et al. Early-stage heart failure with preserved ejection fraction in the pig: a cardiovascular magnetic resonance study. *J Cardiovasc Magn Reson.* (2016) 18:63. doi: 10.1186/s12968-016-0283-9
31. Silva KS, Leary EV, Olver TD, Domeier TL, Padilla J, Rector RS, et al. Tissue-specific small heat shock protein 20 activation is not associated with traditional autophagy markers in Ossabaw swine with cardiometabolic heart failure. *Am J Physiol Heart Circ Physiol.* (2020) 319:H1036–43. doi: 10.1152/ajpheart.00580.2020
32. Deng Y, Xie M, Li Q, Xu X, Ou W, Zhang Y, et al. Targeting mitochondria-inflammation circuit by β-hydroxybutyrate mitigates HFpEF. *Circ Res.* (2021) 128:232–45. doi: 10.1161/CIRCRESAHA.120.317933
33. Hage C, Löfgren L, Michopoulos F, Nilsson R, Davidsson P, Kumar C, et al. Metabolomic profile in HFpEF vs HFrEF patients. *J Card Fail.* (2020) 26:1050–9. doi: 10.1016/j.cardfail.2020.07.010
34. Khalil H, Kanisicak O, Prasad V, Correll RN, Fu X, Schips T, et al. Fibroblast-specific TGF-β-Smad2/3 signaling underlies cardiac fibrosis. *J Clin Invest.* (2017) 127:3770–83. doi: 10.1172/JCI94753
35. Leslie KO, Taatjes DJ, Schwarz J, Vonturkovich M, Low RB. Cardiac myofibroblasts express alpha smooth muscle actin during right ventricular pressure overload in the rabbit. *Am J Pathol.* (1991) 139:207–16.
36. Phosri S, Arieyawong A, Bunrukchai K, Parichatikanond W, Nishimura A, Nishida M, et al. Stimulation of adenosine A(2B) receptor inhibits endothelin-1-induced cardiac fibroblast proliferation and α-smooth muscle actin synthesis through the cAMP/Epac/PI3K/Akt-signaling pathway. *Front Pharmacol.* (2017) 8:428. doi: 10.3389/fphar.2017.00428
37. Sun S, Kee HJ, Jin L, Ryu Y, Choi SY, Kim GR, et al. Gentisic acid attenuates pressure overload-induced cardiac hypertrophy and fibrosis in mice through inhibition of the ERK1/2 pathway. *J Cell Mol Med.* (2018) 22:5964–77. doi: 10.1111/jcmm.13869
38. Bergman MR, Teerlink JR, Mahimkar R, Li L, Zhu BQ, Nguyen A, et al. Cardiac matrix metalloproteinase-2 expression independently induces marked ventricular remodeling and systolic dysfunction. *Am J Physiol Heart Circ Physiol.* (2007) 292:H1847–60. doi: 10.1152/ajpheart.00434.2006
39. Heymans S, Lupu F, Terclavers S, Vanwetswinkel B, Herbert JM, Baker A, et al. Loss or inhibition of uPA or MMP-9 attenuates LV remodeling and dysfunction after acute pressure overload in mice. *Am J Pathol.* (2005) 166:15–25. doi: 10.1016/S0002-9440(10)62228-6
40. Lindsay MM, Maxwell P, Dunn FG. TIMP-1: a marker of left ventricular diastolic dysfunction and fibrosis in hypertension. *Hypertension.* (2002) 40:136–41. doi: 10.1161/01.HYP.0000024573.17293.23
41. Kandalam V, Basu R, Moore L, Fan D, Wang X, Jaworski DM, et al. Lack of tissue inhibitor of metalloproteinases 2 leads to exacerbated left ventricular dysfunction and adverse extracellular matrix remodeling in response to biomechanical stress. *Circulation.* (2011) 124:2094–105. doi: 10.1161/CIRCULATIONAHA.111.030338
42. Polyakova V, Loeffler I, Hein S, Miyagawa S, Piotrowska I, Dammer S, et al. Fibrosis in endstage human heart failure: severe changes in collagen metabolism and MMP/TIMP profiles. *Int J Cardiol.* (2011) 151:18–433. doi: 10.1016/j.ijcard.2010.04.053
43. Borlaug BA. The pathophysiology of heart failure with preserved ejection fraction. *Nat Rev Cardiol.* (2014) 11:507–15. doi: 10.1038/nrcardio.2014.83
44. Obokata M, Reddy YNV, Borlaug BA. Diastolic dysfunction and heart failure with preserved ejection fraction: understanding mechanisms by using noninvasive methods. *JACC Cardiovasc Imaging.* (2020) 13:245–57. doi: 10.1016/j.jcmg.2018.12.034
45. Bacmeister L, Schwarzl M, Warnke S, Stoffers B, Blankenberg S, Westermann D, et al. Inflammation and fibrosis in murine models of heart failure. *Basic Res Cardiol.* (2019) 114:19. doi: 10.1007/s00395-019-0722-5

46. Kalogeropoulos A, Georgiopoulou V, Psaty BM, Rodondi N, Smith AL, Harrison DG, et al. Inflammatory markers and incident heart failure risk in older adults: the health ABC (health, aging, and body composition) study. *J Am Coll Cardiol.* (2010) 55:2129–37. doi: 10.1016/j.jacc.2009.12.045
47. Kuwahara F, Kai H, Tokuda K, Takeya M, Takeshita A, Egashira K, et al. Hypertensive myocardial fibrosis and diastolic dysfunction: another model of inflammation? *Hypertension.* (2004) 43:739–45. doi: 10.1161/01.HYP.0000118584.33350.7d
48. Rosas PC, Liu Y, Abdalla MI, Thomas CM, Kidwell DT, Dusio GF, et al. Phosphorylation of cardiac Myosin-binding protein-C is a critical mediator of diastolic function. *Circ Heart Fail.* (2015) 8:582–94. doi: 10.1161/CIRCHEARTFAILURE.114.001550
49. Sadoshima J, Izumo S. Molecular characterization of angiotensin II–induced hypertrophy of cardiac myocytes and hyperplasia of cardiac fibroblasts. Critical role of the AT1 receptor subtype. *Circ Res.* (1993) 73:413–23. doi: 10.1161/01.RES.73.3.413

2

FABP3 Deficiency Exacerbates Metabolic Derangement in Cardiac Hypertrophy and Heart Failure via PPARα Pathway

Lingfang Zhuang [1,2†], Ye Mao [3†], Zizhu Liu [1,2], Chenni Li [1,2], Qi Jin [1,2], Lin Lu [1,2], Rong Tao [1,2], Xiaoxiang Yan [1,2*] and Kang Chen [1,2*]*

[1] Department of Vascular and Cardiology, Ruijin Hospital, Shanghai Jiao Tong University School of Medicine, Shanghai, China, [2] Institute of Cardiovascular Diseases, Shanghai Jiao Tong University School of Medicine, Shanghai, China, [3] Department of Health Management Center, Ruijin Hospital Lu Wan Branch, Shanghai Jiao Tong University School of Medicine, Shanghai, China

***Correspondence:**
Rong Tao
rongtao@hotmail.com
Xiaoxiang Yan
cardexyanxx@hotmail.com
Kang Chen
chenkang1978@163.com

† These authors have contributed equally to this work

Background: Cardiac hypertrophy was accompanied by various cardiovascular diseases (CVDs), and due to the high global incidence and mortality of CVDs, it has become increasingly critical to characterize the pathogenesis of cardiac hypertrophy. We aimed to determine the metabolic roles of fatty acid binding protein 3 (FABP3) on transverse aortic constriction (TAC)-induced cardiac hypertrophy.

Methods and Results: Transverse aortic constriction or Ang II treatment markedly upregulated Fabp3 expression. Notably, Fabp3 ablation aggravated TAC-induced cardiac hypertrophy and cardiac dysfunction. Multi-omics analysis revealed that Fabp3-deficient hearts exhibited disrupted metabolic signatures characterized by increased glycolysis, toxic lipid accumulation, and compromised fatty acid oxidation and ATP production under hypertrophic stimuli. Mechanistically, FABP3 mediated metabolic reprogramming by directly interacting with PPARα, which prevented its degradation and synergistically modulated its transcriptional activity on Mlycd and Gck. Finally, treatment with the PPARα agonist, fenofibrate, rescued the pro-hypertrophic effects of Fabp3 deficiency.

Conclusions: Collectively, these findings reveal the indispensable roles of the FABP3–PPARα axis on metabolic homeostasis and the development of hypertrophy, which sheds new light on the treatment of hypertrophy.

Keywords: cardiac hypertrophy, PPARα, HFABP, metabolism, FAO, glycolysis

INTRODUCTION

Cardiovascular diseases (CVDs) have become the primary cause of adult death worldwide (1). Of note, cardiac hypertrophy is induced by various CVDs, such as hypertension, hypertrophic cardiomyopathy (HCM), and storage diseases (associated with abnormal accumulation of lipid, glycogen, and misfolded proteins), and eventually lead to heart failure and death (2). Therefore, it becomes urgent to further elucidate the mechanism underlying the development of cardiac hypertrophy. To date, studies have confirmed that numerous mechanisms contribute to the onset and progression of cardiac hypertrophy, such as increased cell death and fibrosis, impaired protein and mitochondrial quality control, and reprogrammed metabolism (2, 3). Of note, the role of metabolic rewiring in hypertrophic progression has recently become a topic of research interest.

Through the use of advanced genomic technology, single-cell RNA sequencing (scRNA-seq), significant transcriptional differences in cellular metabolism have been described as one of the most profound aspects contributing to cardiac dysfunction (4). Specifically, an energy preference that shifted from fatty acid β-oxidation (FAO) to glucose metabolism, with the downregulation of FAO genes and subsequently the upregulation of glucose oxidation genes, has been described in pathophysiological conditions, such as hypertrophy and heart failure (5–7). Moreover, an increase in glucose consumption reportedly induced cardiac hypertrophy, while the preservation of FAO improved myocardial energetics and cardiac function (8, 9).

Fatty acid β-oxidation accounts for nearly 70% of ATP production in the postnatal heart, which underscores the pivotal role of fatty acid metabolism in maintaining heart function (10, 11). Unlike glucose, lipid species are insoluble and generally bind to lipid chaperones for transportation and utilization. Among them, fatty acid binding protein 3 (FABP3) is a small protein that is abundantly expressed in heart tissues and participates in cell metabolism by binding free long-chain fatty acids (LCFAs) and transporting them for cell metabolism, thereby protecting against lipid toxicity (12, 13). Additionally, FABP3 has been described in the context of cardiac hypertrophy, with a positive relationship being described between cellular and circulating levels of FABP3 and cardiac hypertrophy in patients and mice (14). However, the mechanism through which FABP3 affects cellular metabolic homeostasis and advances of cardiac hypertrophy remains poorly understood.

Accordingly, the present study aimed to determine the metabolic effects of FABP3 on transverse aortic constriction (TAC)-induced cardiac hypertrophy and heart failure using genetic mutant *Fabp3*-null mice. Our findings indicate that *Fabp3*-defect exacerbates cardiac hypertrophy and heart dysfunction, resulting in defective FAO, and increased glycolysis by impairing the PPARα signaling pathway. Furthermore, the agonist of PPARα, fenofibrate, attenuated TAC-induced cardiac hypertrophy in both wild-type (WT) and *Fabp3*-null mice. Collectively, this study for the first time demonstrates the indispensable role of FABP3 on metabolic homeostasis and the advance of hypertrophy and heart failure.

METHODS AND MATERIALS

Animals and Generation of FABP3-KO Mice

C57BL/6 male mice were purchased from SLAC Laboratory Animal Co., Ltd. (Shanghai, China). Global *Fabp3* knockout (F3-KO) mice were generated using the CRISPR-Cas9 method as described previously (15) and housed in cages at room temperature and a 12-h light/dark cycle. All animal experimental procedures were approved by the Animal Care Committee of Shanghai Jiao Tong University School of Medicine. All animal procedures performed also conform to the guidelines from Directive 2010/63/EU of the European Parliament on the protection of animals used for scientific purposes or the current NIH guidelines. Expanded materials and methods are available in **Supplementary Materials**.

Experimental Animals

The TAC model was conducted to induce pathological cardiac hypertrophy *in vivo*. Briefly, 8-week-old mice were anesthetized with isoflurane, intubated, and mechanically ventilated with a low concentration of isoflurane gas (1.0%), and the aortic arch was visualized and ligated with 6-0 silk suture against a 27-gauge needle, then the needle was removed and the chest was closed with 5-0 silk suture. For echocardiographic analysis, the mice were firstly anesthetized by inhalation of isoflurane (3%) at the beginning and continued without anesthetic to obtain a better heart rate. At the end of the experiments, the mice were sacrificed by intraperitoneally injecting a lethal dose of pentobarbital sodium (100 mg/kg) or were killed by cervical dislocation to obtain organs for further analysis.

Statistical Analysis

Data are presented as the mean ± *SEM* or mean ± *SD*, which were performed using the GraphPad Prism software (version 7.0a, San Diego, CA, USA) or Rstudio. The statistical differences between two groups were analyzed with two-sided Student's *t*-test. For experiments with more than two groups, after confirming normality and homogeneity of variance, one-way analysis of variance followed by Tukey's *post-hoc* test was used for comparison in the situation of equal variance assumption; otherwise, the Games–Howell *post-hoc* test was used. Additionally, the Dunnett *post-hoc* test was applied to compare a single control group with the others. All statistical analyses were performed using the SPSS software (version 23; SPSS Inc., Chicago, USA). To confirm the survival rate between WT and F3-KO mice, Kaplan–Meier survival curve and log-rank statistics tests were performed in Rstudio using the Survminer package. For all statistical analysis, a p-value of < 0.05 was considered significant.

RESULTS

Hypertrophic Stimuli Upregulate FABP3 Expression

Firstly, to gain an overall profile of FABP3 expression, we examined its mRNA and protein level in mouse tissues using quantitative polymerase chain reaction (qPCR) and western blotting assays. Our results showed that the FABP3 protein and *Fabp3* mRNA level was exclusively expressed in the hearts, BAT, and muscles, while its expression was rare in other organs (**Figures 1A–C**). Intriguingly, the hearts and BAT have been recognized for their distinct preference on fatty acids as energy sources (16), which underscores the important role of FABP3 in cardiac fatty acid metabolism. Then, by using TAC operation to induce cardiac hypertrophy *in vivo* and neurohormonal stimuli (NE or Ang II) *in vitro*, we observed increased FABP3 expression

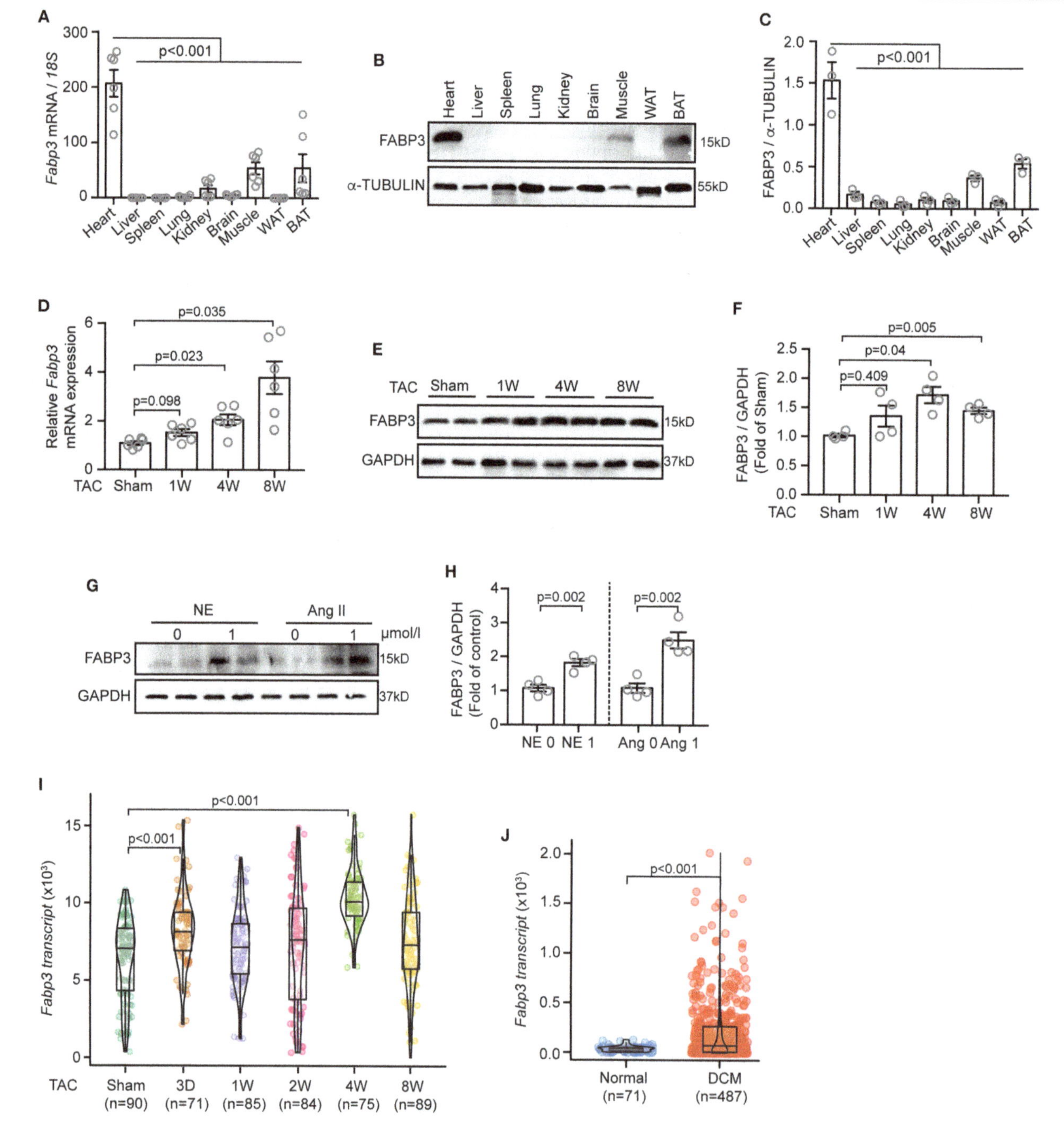

FIGURE 1 | TAC or Ang II upregulates the FABP3 expression *in vivo* and *in vitro*. **(A–C)** Mouse tissues were extracted for qPCR and western blot analyses to determine *Fabp3* levels. **(A)** qPCR analysis of *Fabp3* mRNA in the indicated organs; *18s* was used as the control. **(B)** The FABP3 protein level in the corresponding tissue was determined using western blotting. **(C)** Quantification of FABP3 expression in **(B)**. **(D)** The mRNA level of *Fabp3* after TAC operation, as determined using qPCR. **(E)** Representative western blot images showing the FABP3 expression. **(F)** Quantification results for **(E)**. **(G)** NRVMs treated with NE or Ang II were subjected to western blotting assay to determine the FABP3 protein expression. **(H)** Quantification results of **(G)**. **(I,J)** Single cell RNA sequencing of TAC-operated murine hearts or heart samples from DCM and normal patients were recalculated for the transcriptional expression of *Fabp3* (GEO accession code: *GSE95143*). [**A**, $n = 6$; **C**, $n = 3$; **(A,C)** Dunnett's *post-hoc* test; **D**, $n = 6$; **F**, $n = 4$; **(D,F)** Games–Howell *post-hoc* test; **H**, $n = 4$; **(H,J)** Student's *t*-test; **(I)** Dunnett's *post-hoc* test].

after TAC operations (**Figures 1D–F**) and after neurohormonal stimuli (**Figures 1G,H**).

Next, we assessed the transcriptional expression of *Fabp3* in the single-cell RNA-sequencing (scRNA-seq) datasets, which analyzed the transcriptional profile of murine cardiomyocytes after TAC surgery, and the scRNA-seq from dilated cardiomyopathy (DCM) or normal patients (17). Intriguingly, the scRNA-seq data in line with our *in vivo* and *in vitro* results showed significantly increased *Fabp3* expression at 4W after TAC surgery compared to the sham mice (**Figure 1I**) and more than five-fold higher *Fabp3* expression in DCM patients than their normal counterparts (**Figure 1J**). Taken together, these data suggest that FABP3 is expressed in heart tissues, which use fatty acids as a primary fuel substrate, and is upregulated *in vivo* and *in vitro* under hypertrophic stimuli.

Loss of FABP3 Aggravates Chronic Overload-Induced Cardiac Hypertrophy

To examine the effects of FABP3 on cardiac hypertrophy, we generated F3-KO mice using CRISPR/Cas9, and these *Fabp3*-null mice were viable and fertile. Homozygous, heterozygous allele, and WT mice were identified using PCR (**Supplementary Figures 1A–C**). Notably, cardiac FABP3 was completely abolished using this knockout strategy, which allowed for a direct examination for FABP3 on cardiac hypertrophy (**Supplementary Figures 1D,E**).

To explore whether FABP3 contributes to TAC-induced hypertrophy, F3-KO and WT mice were subjected to TAC or sham surgery and observed for 4 weeks (**Supplementary Figure 2A**). Firstly, to exclude the systemic differences among TAC-operated WT and F3-KO mice, which may exert extra effects on the development of cardiac hypertrophy, the organ mass to body weight ratio was measured, and similar spleen, kidney, BAT, and white adipose tissue (WAT) ratio was found between WT and F3-KO mice (**Supplementary Figure 2B**). Similarly, no difference was observed in liver mass among WT and F3-KO mice (**Supplementary Figure 2C**). Moreover, hematoxylin and eosin (H&E) staining of the above organs showed similar tissue morphology and structure between WT and F3-KO mice after TAC surgery, demonstrating that FABP3 deletion did not result in systemic abnormity after TAC operations (**Supplementary Figure 2D**).

Next, to determine the effects of *Fabp3*-null on cardiac function, echocardiography (echo) was performed on WT and F3-KO mice at 4W after surgery (**Figure 2A**). Compared with the WT mice, TAC surgery led to severer cardiac hypertrophy in the *Fabp3*-null mice, revealed as higher thickness of the interventricular septum (IVS; d: 1.56 ± 0.03 vs. 1.17 ± 0.04; IVS; s: 2.02 ± 0.05 vs. 1.63 ± 0.03; F3-KO vs. WT) and left ventricular posterior wall thickness (LVPW; d: 1.38 ± 0.08 vs. 1.11 ± 0.06; LVPW; s: 1.82 ± 0.07 vs. 1.60 ± 0.07; F3-KO vs. WT) in the F3-KO mice; meanwhile, these parameters were comparable in sham groups (**Figures 2B,C**). Although no statistical difference was observed in the lung weight to body weight ratio (LW/BW) between the WT and KO mice (**Supplementary Figure 2E**), we found an increased heart weight to body weight ratio (HW/BW) in the F3-KO mice after TAC surgery compared with the WT mice (**Figure 2D**).

Then, histological H&E and WGA staining was conducted to determine the degree of cardiac hypertrophy after echo analysis. A significant increase in left ventricular wall thickness was found in F3-KO hearts compared to WT littermates after TAC surgery (**Figure 2E**). In addition, *Fabp3*-null caused a significantly enlarged cell area compared to the WT counterparts after TAC surgery (**Figures 2F,G**). In line with the above hypertrophic phenotype, the mRNA levels of *Anp* and *Bnp* were upregulated in F3-KO hearts after surgery compared to WT hearts (**Figure 2H**). Similarly, ANP levels were increased in F3-KO hearts compared to WT hearts (**Figures 2I,J**). Altogether, we concluded that FABP3 deficiency promoted cardiac hypertrophy after TAC operations.

Loss of FABP3 Impairs Cardiac Remodeling After Hypertrophy

Cardiac hypertrophy contributes to heart failure under chronic overload, ultimately leading to adverse cardiovascular events and death. To determine whether *Fabp3* deficiency is associated with heart failure, the WT and F3-KO mice were observed over 8 weeks after TAC surgery. At the end of the observation period, a lower survival probability was observed in the F3-KO group compared to the WT group (**Supplementary Figure 3A**, $p = 0.3$), which was accompanied with increased heart size in the F3-KO mice after TAC surgery compared to the WT hearts (**Supplementary Figure 3B**). Consistent with the enlarged heart size in the *Fabp3*-defect mice, the decline in left ventricular ejection fraction (LVEF) and left ventricular fractional shortening (LVFS) was found in the F3-KO mice compared to their WT group at 8 weeks post-surgery, which was paralleled with higher left ventricular end diastolic volume (LVEDV) and left ventricular end systolic volume (LVESV) in the *Fabp3*-null mice (**Supplementary Figures 3C–E**).

Then, considering that fibrosis serves as a hallmark of cardiac dysfunction, by measuring the level of fibrosis-related genes via qPCR assay, we found that the mRNA expression of *Col3a1* was increased in the TAC-operated F3-KO hearts compared to the WT hearts. Moreover, *Fabp3* ablation reduced the mRNA expression of matrix metallopeptidase 2 (*Mmp2*) and matrix metallopeptidase (*Mmp9*) after TAC surgery, suggesting impaired collagen turnover and homeostasis in the *Fabp3*-KO mice (**Supplementary Figure 3F**). In agreement with the increased expression of fibrosis genes in the F3-KO hearts, Massons and Sirus red staining confirmed increased left ventricular collagen volume in the F3-KO hearts compared to the WT hearts (**Supplementary Figures 3G,H**). Cumulatively, these data suggest that the loss of FABP3 contributes to the progression of heart failure following TAC operation.

FABP3 Alleviates Ang II-Induced Cardiomyocyte Hypertrophy *in vitro*

To corroborate the above findings that FABP3 participates in TAC-induced hypertrophy, we knocked down the expression of *Fabp3 in vitro* using non-targeting small interfering RNA (siRNA) (**Supplementary Figure 4A**). The cell size was comparable in the PBS groups; however, knocking down *Fabp3* significantly enlarged the cell area after Ang II treatment compared with the Si-NC group (**Figures 3A,B**). Moreover, an increase in the *Anp* and *Bnp* mRNA expression in line with the upregulation of the ANP protein level was found in the Si-F3 group compared with the Si-NC group (**Figures 3C–E**).

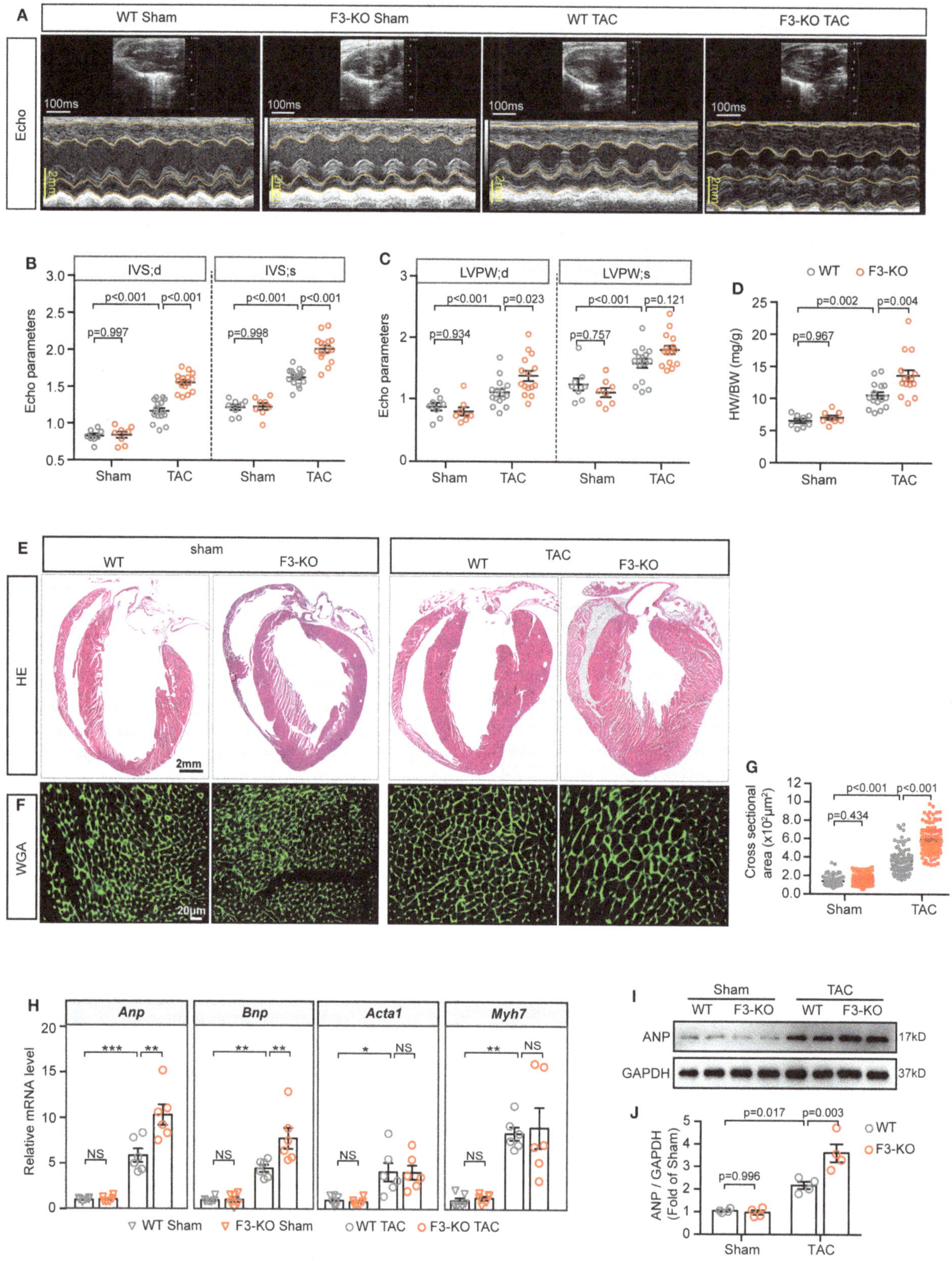

FIGURE 2 | Deficiency of FABP3 aggravates TAC-induced cardiac hypertrophy. **(A)** Representative echo images of the WT and F3-KO mice at 4 weeks after TAC or sham operation. **(B)** Quantification results for the interventricular septum (IVS) in **(A)**. **(C)** Quantification results for the left ventricular posterior wall thickness (LVPW)

(Continued)

FIGURE 2 | in **(A)**. **(D)** The ratio of heart weight to body weight from sham or TAC-operated WT or F3-KO mice. **(E)** Images of H&E stained longitudinal sections of the indicated hearts. **(F)** Heart sections stained with WGA to compare the size of the cardiomyocyte area. **(G)** Quantification results in **(F)**; a total of 100 cells/group were calculated. **(H)** qPCR assays compared the mRNA expression of *Anp*, *Bnp*, *Acta1*, and *Myh7* at 4 weeks after sham or TAC operation. NS, not significant, $^{*}p < 0.05$, $^{**}p < 0.01$, $^{***}p < 0.001$. **(I)** Representative western blot images of ANP in the indicated groups. (J) Quantification results of **(I)**. [**B–D**, $n = 8, 8, 15, 15$, respectively; **H**, $n = 6$; **J**, $n = 4$; **(B–D,G,H,J)** Tukey's *post-hoc* test].

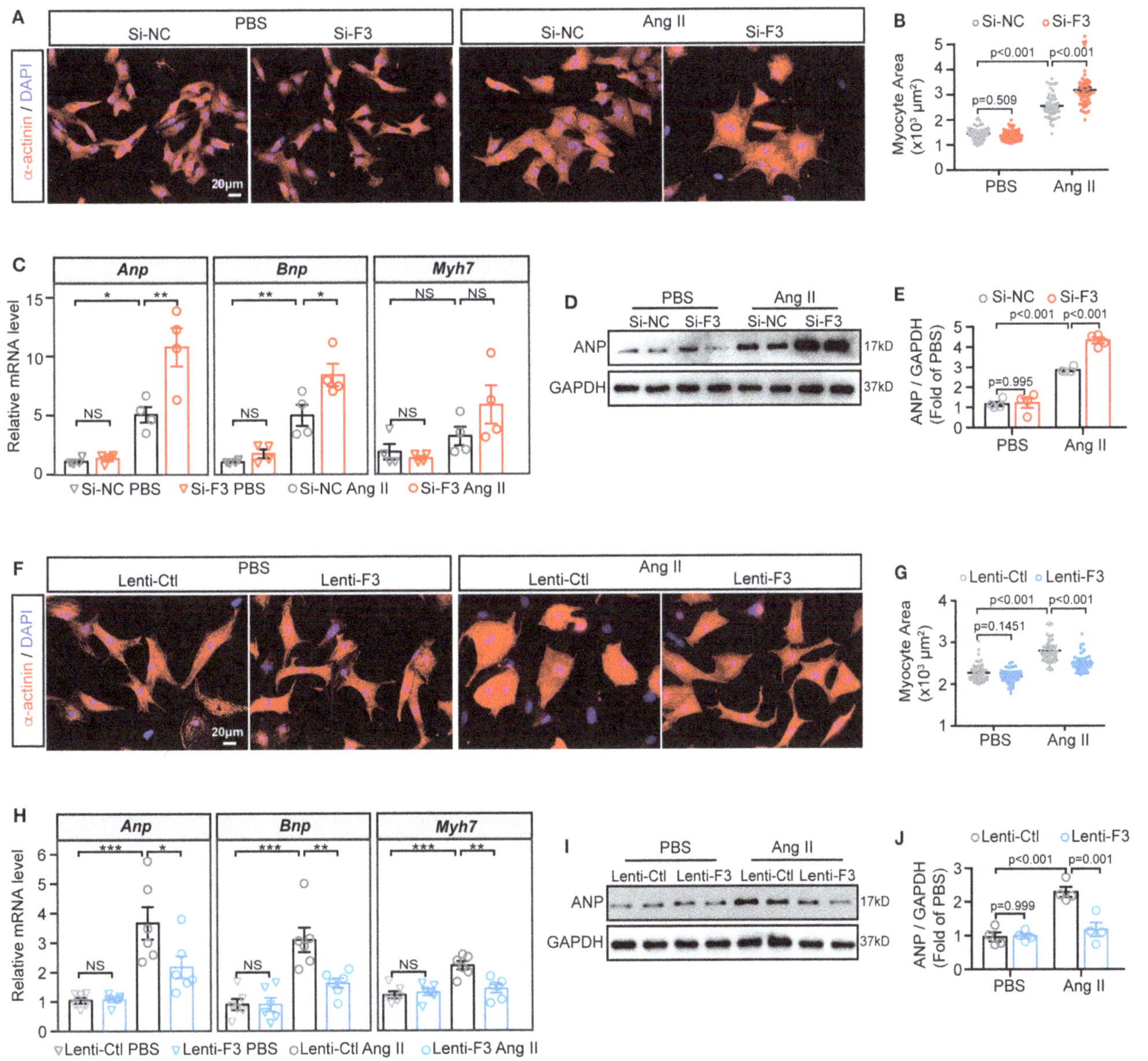

FIGURE 3 | FABP3 participates in Ang II induced cell hypertrophy. **(A–E)** NRVMs were treated with siRNA-targeting *Fabp3* (Si-F3) or its negative control (Si-NC) before PBS or Ang II treatment. **(A)** Immunofluorescence staining of α-actinin in NRVMs with or without Ang II treatment. **(B)** Quantification results of the cell area in (A); 50 cells/group were calculated. **(C)** mRNA expression of hypertrophic genes (*Anp, Bnp,* and *Myh7*) in indicated groups. NS, not significant, $^{*}p < 0.05$, $^{**}p < 0.01$. **(D)** Representative western blot images of ANP after *Fabp3* knocking-down. **(E)** Quantification of **(D)**. **(F–J)** NRVMs were transfected with lentivirus-encoding *Fabp3* (Lenti-F3) or its negative control (Lenti-Ctl) before PBS or Ang II treatment. **(F)** The cell area was determined by α-actinin staining in NRVMs. **(G)** Quantification results of the cell area in **(F)**; 50 cells/group were calculated. **(H)** The mRNA levels of *Anp, Bnp*, and *Myh7* were compared in the aforementioned groups. NS, not significant, $^{*}p < 0.05$, $^{**}p < 0.01$, $^{***}p < 0.001$. **(I)** Representative western blot images revealed reduced ANP protein levels in the Lenti-F3 group. **(J)** Quantification results of **(I)**. [**C,E,J**, $n = 4$; H, $n = 6$; **(B,G)**: Games–Howell *post-hoc* test; **(C,E,H,J)**: Tukey's *post-hoc* test].

Next, lentivirus vectors containing the full-length *Fabp3* transcript (NM_001320996) and green fluorescent protein (GFP) were constructed, transfected, and visualized with the fluorescence microscope to confirmed the transfection efficiency (**Supplementary Figure 4B**). After transfecting H9C2 cells with optimal multiplicity of infection (MOI) of 10 and 100, lentivirus carrying the *Fabp3* transcript (Lenti-F3) markedly increased FABP3 protein levels by more than four-fold compared to the empty control vector (Lenti-Ctl; **Supplementary Figures 4C,D**), which was supported by a higher FABP3 fluorescence value in the Lenti-F3 group (**Supplementary Figure 4E**). In contrast to the pro-hypertrophic effect of *Fabp3* ablation, the knocking-in expression of FABP3 prevented Ang II-induced cell hypertrophy *in vitro*. Specifically, Ang II stimulation resulted in enlarged cell sizes in the control group, which was markedly blunted with the overexpression of FABP3 (**Figures 3F,G**). Consistent with the reduction in the cell area, the overexpression of FABP3 curbed the increase in *Anp*, *Bnp*, and *Myh7* mRNA levels following Ang II treatment (**Figure 3H**), as well as the protein expression of ANP (**Figures 3I,J**). These *in vitro* data verified the protective effects of FABP3 on neurohormonal stimuli-induced hypertrophy. Altogether, these FABP3 loss- and gain-of-function results corroborate with *in vivo* phenotypes and reveal the important role of FABP3 in the development of cardiac hypertrophy.

Ablation of FABP3 Leads to Defective FA β-Oxidation and Lipid Homeostasis

To explore the mechanism through which FABP3 regulates cardiac hypertrophy, we collected F3-KO or WT hearts at 1-week post-sham or -TAC operation for RNA-seq analysis and liquid chromatography–mass spectrometry (LC-MS) analysis to determine differential genes and metabolites (**Figure 4A**). Principal component analysis (PCA) of RNA-seq revealed that the transcriptome of the F3-KO hearts was similar to those of the WT mice under sham conditions. However, TAC operation induced differentially expressed genes between WT and F3-KO hearts, which separated them on the PCA plot (**Supplementary Figure 5A**). Comparing the TAC-operated F3-KO hearts with the WT hearts, a total of 939 (upregulated: 772, downregulated: 167) differentially expressed genes were identified and analyzed in this study (**Figure 4A**). KEGG pathway analysis revealed that these differentially expressed genes were enriched for terms related to "lipid metabolism," "glycan metabolism," and "energy metabolism" (**Supplementary Figure 5B**). Next, gene set enrichment analysis (GSEA) revealed that pathways that involved "regulation of anatomical structure size," "wound healing," and "extracellular structure organization" were positively correlated with the TAC-operated F3-KO mice. These pathways, which were consistent with pro-hypertrophic phenotypes in the *Fabp3*-null hearts, suggested that ablation of *Fabp3* triggers maladaptive remodeling after TAC operation (**Supplementary Figure 5C**).

Intriguingly, GSEA indicated that *Fabp3* ablation resulted in impaired mitochondrial FAO and disrupted lipid homeostasis. Specifically, "fatty acid beta oxidation using acyl-CoA dehydrogenase" was negatively correlated with the F3-KO hearts (**Figure 4B**; **Supplementary Figure 5C**), while positively enriched "lipid biosynthetic process" and "lipid storage" were found in the F3-KO hearts compared with the WT hearts (**Figure 4C**; **Supplementary Figure 5D**). In line with the aforementioned pathways, suppressed FAO genes and upregulated lipid biogenesis genes were observed in the F3-KO TAC group than the WT TAC group in RNA-seq analysis and *in vivo* experiments (**Figures 4D,E**). However, these genes were comparable under sham conditions whether in RNA-seq analysis or their mRNA expression *in vivo* (**Figure 4D**; **Supplementary Figure 5E**), which manifested that *Fabp3* deficiency has no profound effect on cardiac lipid metabolism under physiological conditions; however, hypertrophic stimulation that occurred with higher energy demand magnified the effects of *Fabp3*-defect on energy homeostasis and resulted in imbalanced FAO and lipid biosynthesis processes.

Furthermore, to explore the effects of FABP3 on cardiomyocyte FAO activity under hypertrophic stimulation *in vitro*, mitochondrial stress assay was performed in NRVMs with or without the knocking-in expression of FABP3 to measure in real time the oxygen consumption rate (OCR). Compared with the negative control, overexpression of FABP3 resulted in significant increases in basal, maximal respiration, and spare respiratory capacity (**Figures 4F,G**). Relative to glucose, fatty acid required more oxygen for its β-oxidation; therefore, the OCR serves as a relative indicator of cell fuel preference. The higher OCR rate in the lenti-F3 group indicated that the overexpression of FABP3 resulted in the increase in FAO activity. Then, a supplement of etomoxir was used to evaluate the cell dependency on fatty acid as the energy substrate. We found that the application of etomoxir led to a marked drop of respiration in the FABP3 overexpressed group compared with its negative control groups, demonstrating that NRVMs with FABP3 overexpression have increased reliance on fatty acid as energy fuel (**Figures 4H,I**). Moreover, etomoxir treatment would reverse the protective effects of FABP3 on cardiac hypertrophy and upregulated the mRNA expression of *Bnp* and *Anp* (**Supplementary Figure 5F**). Taken together, these data point to the dependency of FABP3 on cardiomyocyte FA β-oxidation to meet an effective metabolic demand under hypertrophic stimulations.

FABP3-Null Hearts Exhibit Abnormal Lipid Accumulation

The RNA-seq analysis showed that FABP3 deletion led to increased lipid biogenesis (**Figures 4C,D**). Lipid-targeted metabolomics analysis was used to determine the differential metabolites in WT and F3-KO hearts. We found that rather than triglycerides (TAG, **Supplementary Figure 6B**) and Acyl-carnitine (ACar, **Supplementary Figure 6C**), the fatty acid (16:0) and diglyceride (DAG 18:2–22:5, 18:2–18:2) were significantly increased in the F3-KO hearts compared with the WT mice (**Figures 4J,K**), which was in line with an increase in neutral lipid in *Fabp3* knocking-down cells after Ang II treatment

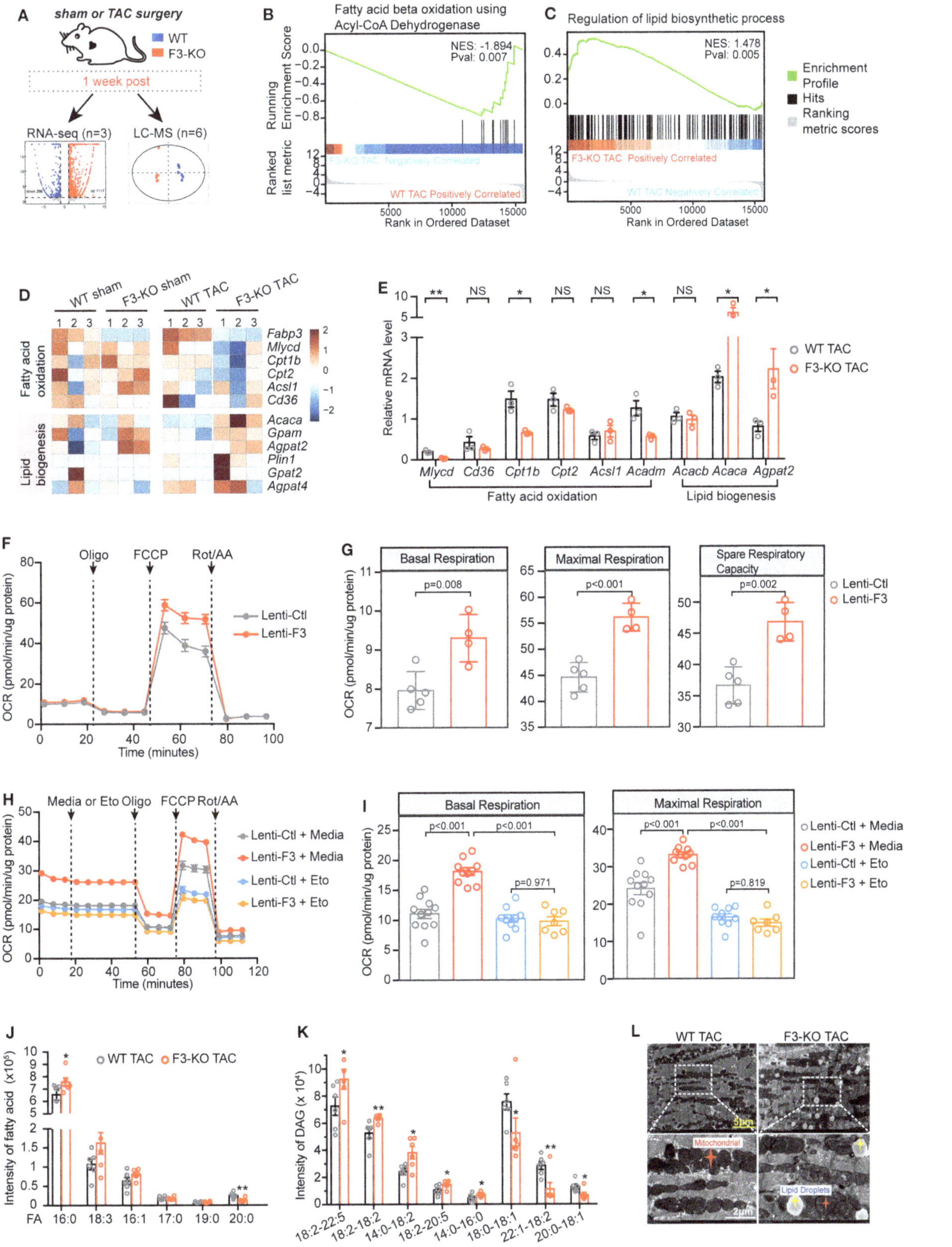

FIGURE 4 | FABP3-defect results to compromised fatty acid oxidation (FAO) and toxic lipid accumulation. **(A)** Experimental schematic of RNA-seq analysis and metabolomics analysis in WT and F3-KO hearts. **(B,C)** GSEA revealing that F3-KO negatively correlates with fatty acid beta oxidation using acyl-CoA dehydrogenase *(Continued)*

FIGURE 4 | (B), while positively correlating with the lipid biosynthetic process **(C)**. **(D)** Heatmap showed scaled expression of FAO and lipid biogenesis genes in indicated samples from RNA-seq analysis. **(E)** The mRNA expression of FAO and lipid biogenesis genes in TAC-operated WT and F3-KO hearts. NS, not significant, $^{*}p < 0.05$, $^{**}p < 0.01$. **(F)** Mitochondrial stress assay was performed in NRVMs transfected with *Fabp3* (Lenti-F3) or its negative control (Lenti-Ctl) after Ang II treatment to measure the oxygen consumption rates (OCR); data were presented as mean ± SD from individual experiments. **(G)** The parameters of basal respiration, maximal respiration, and spare respiration capacity were calculated from **(F)**; data were presented as mean ± SD from individual experiments. **(H)** LCFA oxidation stress assay was conducted in NRVMs with or without knocking-in expression of *Fabp3* after Ang II treatment; etomoxir (Eto) was applied to inhibit the mitochondrial FAO. Data were presented as mean ± SEM from individual experiments. **(I)** The parameters of basal respiration and maximal respiration were calculated from **(H)**; data were presented as mean ± SEM from individual experiments. (J and K) The level of fatty acid (FA) and diacylglycerol (DAG) in WT and F3-KO hearts determined by LC-MS analysis; six biological replicates per group. $^{*}p < 0.05$, $^{**}p < 0.01$. **(L)** Representative electron micrographs of WT and F3-KO hearts after TAC operation. (Bottom) Higher magnification images of the dashed rectangle from **(L)**. [**E**, $n = 3$, Student's *t*-test; **G**, $n = 5$, 4, respectively, Student's *t*-test; **I**, $n = 11$, 10, 9, 7, respectively, Tukey's *post-hoc* test; **(J,K)** Student's *t*-test].

(**Supplementary Figure 6A**). It is important to note that DGA and saturated fatty acid (especially palmitate) were closely associated with cellular toxicity for their direct actions as signaling lipids (18). Therefore, FABP3 deficiency not only blunted cardiac FA β-oxidation but also triggered the excessive accumulation of toxic lipids in hearts. Consistent with increased toxic lipid species and neutral lipid *in vivo* and *in vitro*, an excess of lipid droplet accumulation was observed in the *Fabp3*-null hearts after TAC surgery by using transmission electron microscopy (TEM), which was rare in the WT hearts (**Figure 4L; Supplementary Figure 6D**). To determine whether differences in lipid uptake accounted for the abnormal lipid accumulation in the F3-KO mice, plasma non-esterified fatty acid (NEFA) was measured at sham, 4W and 8W post-surgery; we found that the plasma concentration of NEFA was higher at 8W compared to the sham group; however, no significant difference was observed between WT and F3-KO mice (**Supplementary Figure 6E**). These data in line with comparable mRNA expression of fatty acid transporter *Cd36* between WT and F3-KO hearts (**Figures 4D,E**) revealed that abnormal lipid accumulation in the F3-KO hearts may arise from activated lipid biosynthesis rather than abnormal lipid uptake. Taken together, we showed that *Fabp3*-null contributes to defective FAO and increased lipid biogenesis and toxic lipid accumulation after cardiac hypertrophy (**Supplementary Figure 6F**).

FABP3 Defect Hearts Show Increased Reliance on Glycolysis

In the context of diminished capacity for FAO, we next sorted to determine whether the chief energy substrate shifted from fatty acids to glucose when FABP3 is defected. Intriguingly, GSEA revealed that the loss of FABP3 triggered abnormally activated glucose metabolic pathways, such as "glucan catabolic process" (**Supplementary Figure 7A**) and "regulation of gluconeogenesis" (**Supplementary Figure 7B**). In line with activated glucose oxidation and gluconeogenesis pathways, *Gck*, *Pfkfb2*, and *Pck1* were upregulated in the F3-KO TAC hearts (**Figure 5A**). A consistent mRNA expression profile *in vivo* confirmed the increased *Gck* and *Pck1* level in the *Fabp3* deficiency hearts after TAC surgery (**Figure 5B**). Intriguingly, "mitochondrial electron transport NADH to ubiquinone" was negatively correlated with the F3-KO hearts, which was consistent with markedly downregulated TCA cycle genes (*Ogdh*, *Idh2*, *Aco2*) in TAC-operated *Fabp3*-null hearts than in the WT mice (**Figure 5A; Supplementary Figure 7C**). These results indicated that rather than fuel-efficient aerobic respiration, the *Fabp3*-null hearts shifted toward inefficient anaerobic respiration (glycolysis) for ATP production. As increased glucose uptake would lead to higher glucose oxidation, we interrogated the expression glucose transporters (Slc2a1, Slc2a4), the concentration of blood glucose, and the glycogen content in liver and small intestine, and the results showed that the glucose uptake was comparable between the WT and F3-KO mice during cardiac hypertrophy (**Figures 5A,B; Supplementary Figures 7D,E**).

Furthermore, the gas chromatography–mass spectrometry (GC-MS) analysis was used to identify differential metabolites in WT and F3-KO hearts after TAC surgery. Principal component analysis showed that the F3-KO hearts were separated from the WT samples, which was consistent with the OPLS-DA analysis results (**Supplementary Figures 7F–H**). Notably, significantly increased glycolysis pathway related metabolites [glucose, glucose-6-phosphate (G6P), and fructose 2,6-biphosphate] and considerably downregulated TCA cycle metabolites (malic and fumaric acids) were observed in the *Fabp3*-deficient hearts as compared to the WT hearts (**Figure 5C**). Furthermore, by measuring the concentration of G6P, an indicator of cellular glycolytic flux, we showed a higher concentration of G6P in *Fabp3* knocking-down cells; however, overexpression of *Fabp3* resulted in dramatic decline in the G6P level (**Figure 5D**). These data confirmed that FABP3 defect contributed to the increased glycolysis under hypertrophic conditions.

Based on the results from the RNA-seq and metabolomics, we performed a glycolytic rate assay to analyze in real time the cellular glycolysis by calculating the proton efflux rate from glycolysis (glycoPER), a parameter that measures acidification from glycolysis without any contribution from mitochondrial respiration. NRVMs with *Fabp3* knocking-down exhibited a higher basal and compensatory glycolysis compared to its negative control after Ang II stimulation; however, the glycolytic rate showed no significant differences between these two groups under PBS treatment (**Figures 5E,F**). In striking contrast to increased glycolysis when knocking down the expression of *Fabp3*, *Fabp3* overexpression resulted in a marked drop of glycolysis than the control cells after Ang II treatment (**Figures 5G,H**). By combining with multi-omics analysis and glycolytic energetics analysis, we

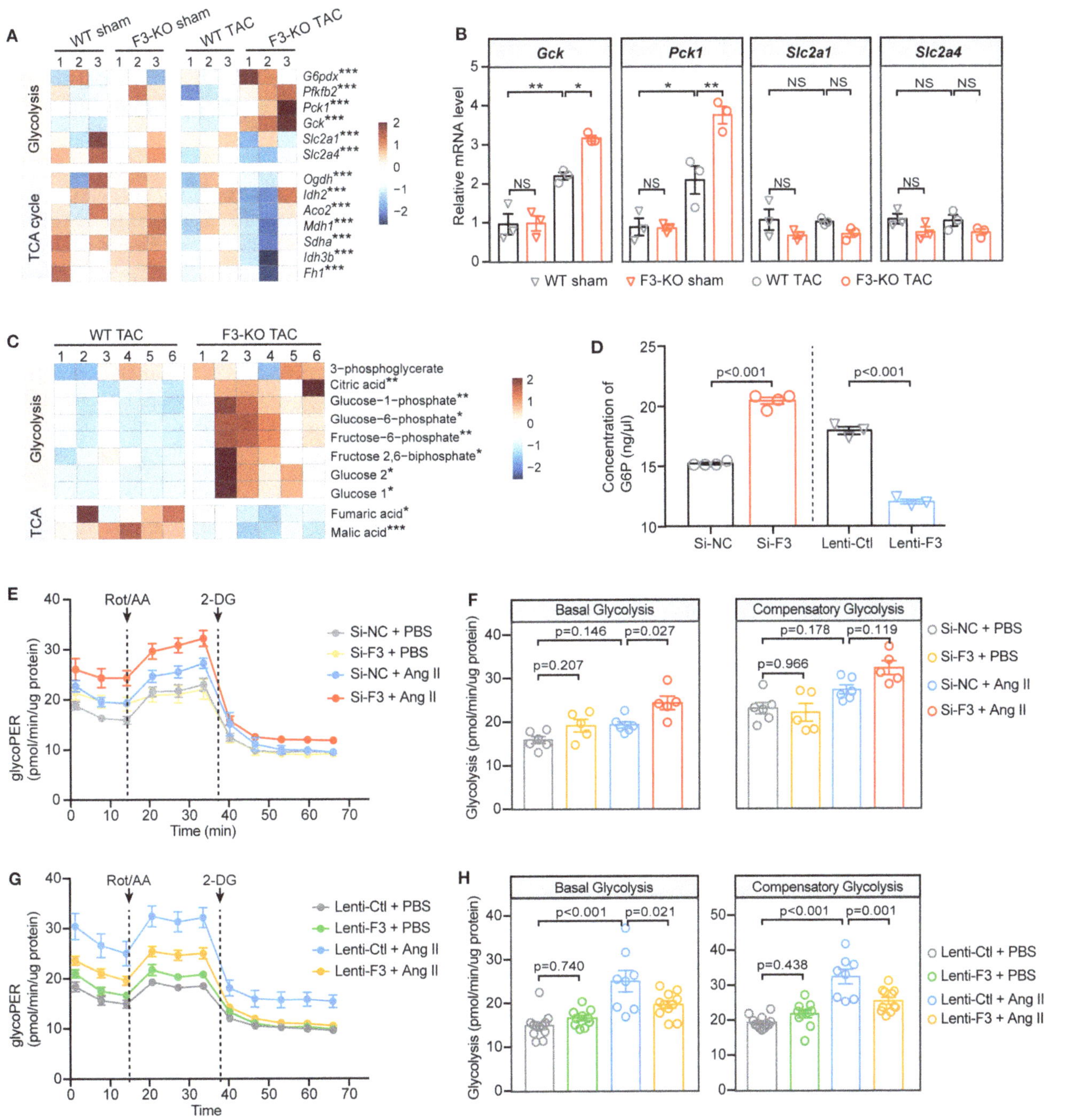

FIGURE 5 | FABP3-null contributes to increased glycolysis and reduced ATP production under hypertrophic stimulation. **(A)** Heatmap of glycolysis and TCA cycle genes from RNA-seq analysis. **(B)** The mRNA expression of *Gck*, *Pck1*, *Slc2a1*, and *Slc2a4* in indicated groups. NS, not significant, $^{*}p < 0.05$, $^{**}p < 0.01$. **(C)** Heatmap of differential metabolites from WT and F3-KO hearts. $^{*}p < 0.05$, $^{**}p < 0.01$, $^{***}p < 0.001$. **(D)** The intracellular concentration of glucose-6-phosphate (G6P) in NRVMs was measured after manipulating the expression of *Fabp3*. **(E)** Glycolytic rate assay was performed in NRVMs after knocking down the expression of *Fabp3* with siRNA to measure the OCR and extracellular acidification rates (ECAR) and converted to glycolytic proton efflux rate (glycoPER) in the Seahorse Report Generator. **(F)** The parameters of basal glycolysis and compensatory glycolysis were calculated from **(E)**. Data were presented as mean ± SEM from individual experiments. **(G)** Glycolytic rate assay was performed in NRVMs with or without *Fabp3* overexpression to measure glycoPER. **(H)** The parameters of basal glycolysis and compensatory glycolysis were calculated from **(G)**. Data were presented as mean ± *SD* from individual experiments. [**B**, $n = 3$, Tukey's *post-hoc* test; **D**, $n = 4$, 4, 3, 3, respectively, Student's *t*-test; **F**, $n = 6$, 5, 6, 5, respectively; **H**, $n = 12$, 10, 8, 11, respectively; **(F,H)** Tukey's *post-hoc* test].

demonstrated that *Fabp3* deficiency promoted the shift on glycolysis as the fuel source, which led to compromised TCA and ATP production (**Supplementary Figure 7I**). Taken together, these observations confirm that FABP3 defect contributes to compromised FAO and ATP production; on the other hand, it exacerbates glycolysis and toxic lipid accumulation, both of which ultimately aggravate metabolic derangement and heart failure.

FABP3 Mediates PPARα Level by Binding and Stabilizing PPARα, Further Enhances Its Transcriptional Activity Under Hypertrophic Stimuli

As mentioned before, *Fabp3* deficiency contributes to deranged metabolic milieu characterized by reduced FAO and increased glycolysis. Next, we sought to explore the mechanism through which *Fabp3* mediates metabolic derangement during cardiac hypertrophy. Firstly, our RNA-seq analysis verified that the "PPAR signaling pathway" was one of the top enriched pathways in the *Fabp3*-deficient hearts (**Supplementary Figure 8A**). Definitive evidence demonstrates the critical requirement of peroxisome proliferator activated receptor (PPAR), particularly PPARα, in myocyte metabolism and metabolic reprogramming under cardiac hypertrophy (19). Therefore, we postulated that FABP3 participates in cellular metabolism through the PPARα signaling pathway. Although the mRNA expression of *Ppara* showed no difference in WT and F3-KO hearts (**Supplementary Figure 8B**), its protein expression was marked downregulation in the *Fabp3* deficiency mice as compared to the WT hearts following TAC surgery (**Figures 6A,B**). Conversely, *in vitro* overexpression of *Fabp3* using a lentivirus vector rescued the protein level of PPARα following Ang II stimulation (**Figures 6A,B**). Immunofluorescence staining of PPARα at 4W post-surgery confirmed that TAC operation resulted in the decrease and perinuclear shuttling of PPARα, while *Fabp3* ablation accelerated its loss (**Figures 6C,D**). These findings indicate that FABP3 might participate in metabolic homeostasis during cardiac hypertrophy via PPARα signaling. However, the mechanism through which FABP3 targets PPARα for metabolic regulation remains elusive.

Next, by transfecting NRVMs with *Fabp3* or *Ppara* and co-immunoprecipitating with respective antibodies, we showed that FABP3 directly bond with PPARα, with or without Ang II stimulation (**Figures 6E,F**). As *Fabp3* deletion exerted no effect on the *Ppara* mRNA level, we postulated that FABP3 exerted a post-transcriptional modification on the protein level of PPARα. Expectedly, *Fabp3* overexpression markedly prolonged the half-life of PPARα compared with its negative control, suggesting that FABP3 increased the PPARα protein level by inhibiting its degradation (**Figures 6G,H**). Finally, to determine whether FABP3 affected PPARα transactivation, we performed luciferase gene transactivation assays in HEK 293T cells. The activation of PPARα was determined based on a reporter plasmid containing three PPAR-responsive elements ($PPRE_3$-TK-LUC). PPARα significantly increased the luciferase expression of $PPRE_3$-TK-LUC; moreover, cotransfection of FABP3 and PPARα induced higher PPRE-driven luciferase activity compared with PPARα alone (**Figure 6I**). Together, these findings indicate that FABP3 mediates hypertrophic response by interacting with PPARα, inhibiting its degradation, and modulating its transcriptional activity.

Required of PPARα on FABP3-Modulated FAO/Glycolysis Balance and Cardiac Hypertrophy

As regard the pleiotropic effects of PPARα on inhibiting glucose oxidation, while activating FAO, we aimed to determine whether FABP3 interacts with PPARα and modulates its transcriptional capacities on FAO/glycolysis genes, and further is involved in the advance of cardiac hypertrophy. Firstly, the PPARα target genes were curated based on our RNA-seq data and listed as **Supplementary Table 1**. In line with previous results in **Figures 4, 5**, *Fabp3* ablation led to a lower MLYCD and CPT1B protein level while upregulating ACC and GCK, suggesting a direct effect of FABP3 on MLYCD and CPT1B, and an inverse transcriptional effect of FABP3 on ACC and GCK via PPARα (**Figures 6J,K**). Therefore, to address the question of whether FABP3 participated in the transcriptional activation of FAO and glycolysis genes via PPARα, the plasmid containing firefly luciferase and *Mlycd* or *Gck* promoter (Mlycd-LUC, Gck-LUC, respectively) was constructed; after transfecting 293T cells with PPARα, FABP3, Mlycd-LUC, or Gck-LUC, we showed that PPARα increased the *Mlycd* transcriptional activity. However, higher luciferase activity was observed when it was cotransfected with FABP3 and PPARα (**Figure 6L**). In contrast to Mlycd-LUC, PPARα blunted the transactivation of Gck-LUC, which showed a severer inhibition in the presence of FABP3 (**Figure 6M**). These data suggest the metabolic regulatory role of FABP3 in transcriptionally activating FAO genes *Mlycd* and *Cpt1b* and curbing glycolysis and lipogenesis genes *Gck* and *Acaca* via PPARα (**Figure 6N**).

Finally, to demonstrate the requirement of PPARα in FABP3 mediated cardiac hypertrophy, PPARα was knocked down using siRNA methods as described previously (**Supplementary Figures 8C,D**) (20). We observed that PPARα downregulation abolished the protective effects of FABP3 on cardiomyocyte hypertrophy, resulting in an enlarged cell area (**Supplementary Figures 8E,F**) and the upregulation of *Bnp* and *Anp* (**Supplementary Figure 8G**). Notably, increased cellular neutral lipid was found after knocking down PPARα (**Supplementary Figure 8H**). Altogether, these data illustrate that FABP3 participates in cardiac hypertrophy by synergistically activating *Mlycd* and *Cpt1b* and repressing *Gck* and *Acaca* via PPARα.

Activation of PPARα With Fenofibrate Reverses FABP3-KO Induced Cardiac Hypertrophy

As observed previously, *Fabp3* deficiency contributes to hypertrophy and deranged metabolic milieu by impairing the PPARα pathway. We next sought to determine whether activating PPARα may rescue the pro-hypertrophic effects of *Fabp3* defect after TAC operation and search for clinical benefits on the treatment of cardiac hypertrophy. Firstly, NRVMs were

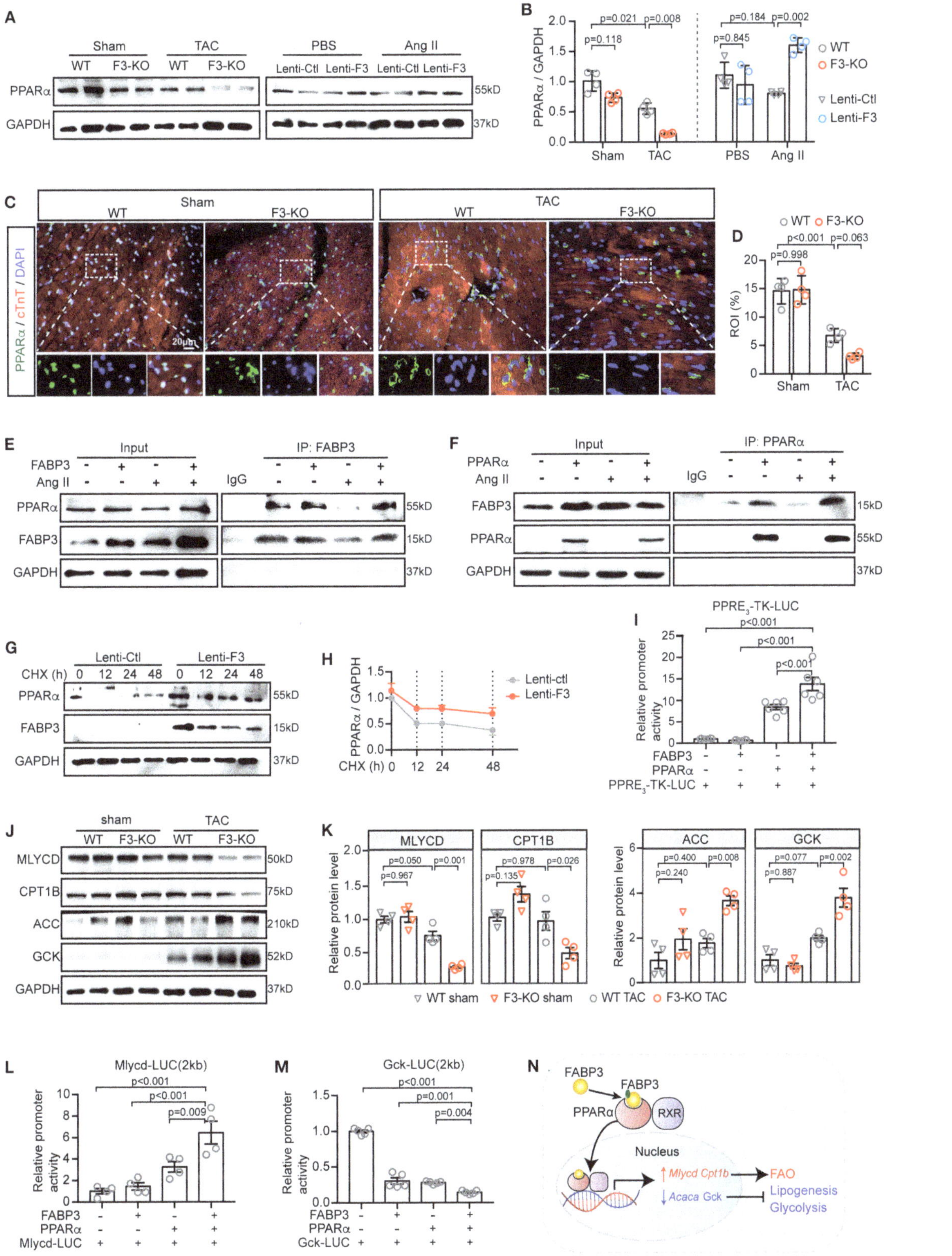

FIGURE 6 | FABP3 mediates metabolic reprogramming by directly interacting with PPARα, preventing its degradation and enhancing its transactivation. **(A)** Representative western blot images of PPARα from TAC-operated WT and F3-KO hearts, or from NRVMs transfected with *Fabp3* or its control virus with or without *(Continued)*

FIGURE 6 | Ang II treatment. **(B)** Quantification of **(A)**. **(C)** Immunofluorescence double-staining of PPARα (green) and cTnT (red) in WT and F3-KO hearts, with or without TAC surgery. (Bottom) Higher magnification of dashed rectangle in the upper panel. **(D)** Quantification results in **(C)**. **(E)** NRVMs with *Fabp3* overexpression were treated with or without Ang II for 24 h and then co-immunoprecipitated (co-IP) with FABP3. Western blotting assay was conducted with indicated antibodies. **(F)** NRVMs with *Pparα* overexpression were treated with or without Ang II for 24 h and then co-immunoprecipitated (co-IP) with PPARα. **(G)** NRVMs transfected with Lenti-F3 or Lenti-Ctl were treated with CHX for 0, 12, 24, or 48 h and the protein expression of PPARα was measured by western blotting. **(H)** Quantification of PPARα intensities by normalizing to those of GAPDH in **(G)**. **(I)** HEK 293T cells were transfected with a PPRE-driven luciferase reporter ($PPRE_3$-TK-LUC) and PPARα or FABP3 for 24 h. Relative activation of $PPRE_3$-TK-LUC was measured by normalizing its luminescence value to the renilla activity. **(J)** Representative western blot images of MLYCD, CPT1B, ACC, and GCK in WT and F3-KO mice after sham or TAC operation. **(K)** The quantification results of **(J)**. **(L,M)** HEK 293T cells were transfected with a *Mlycd*-promoter luciferase reporter (Mlycd-LUC, **L**) or a *Gck*-promoter luciferase reporter (Gck-Luc, **M**), PPARα, or FABP3 for 24 h. The relative expression of the *Mlycd*-promoter and *Gck*-promoter was measured by normalizing their luminescence value to the corresponding renilla luminescence value. **(N)** The schematic diagram shows FABP3 binds to PPARα and increases its transcriptional activity on *Mlycd* and *Cpt1b* while repressing *Acaca* and *Gck* to participate in cardiac FAO/glycolysis shift. [**B**, $n = 4$, Games–Howell *post-hoc* test; **D**, $n = 4$, Tukey's *post-hoc* test; **H**, $n = 2$; I, $n = 6$, Dunnett's *post-hoc* test; **K**, $n = 4$, Tukey's *post-hoc* test; **L**, $n = 4$; **M**, $n = 5$; (**L,M**) Dunnett's *post-hoc* test].

treated with fenofibrate, a PPARα-specific agonist, or vehicle (DMSO) for 24 h; knocking down of *Fabp3* with siRNA (Si-F3) resulted in an increased cell area compared to its control (Si-NC), while fenofibrate treatment markedly reduced the cell area in both the Si-NC and Si-F3 groups (**Figures 7A,B**).

Next, PPAR agonist studies were performed *in vivo* to investigate the effects of fenofibrate on hypertrophy. WT and *Fabp3*-KO mice were subjected to TAC surgery and randomly treated with fenofibrate (100 mg/kg/day) or vehicle by oral gavage daily for 4 weeks. Interestingly, compared with the vehicle group, fenofibrate treatment significantly rescued cardiac hypertrophy in WT and *Fabp3*-KO mice. More specifically, IVS and LVPW were markedly decreased following fenofibrate treatment (**Figures 7C–E**). Consistent with attenuated cardiac function, hypertrophic and fibrosis-related genes, such as *Anp*, *Bnp*, and *Col3a1*, were decreased after fenofibrate treatment, but not by the vehicle (**Figure 7F**). In addition, histochemical analysis showed that *Fabp3* deletion increased left ventricular wall thickness, cardiomyocyte size, and collagen volume, while fenofibrate supplement significantly rescued these effects whether in the WT or *Fabp3*-KO mice (**Figures 7G–K**).

Collectively, these results demonstrate an important role of the FABP3-PPARα pathway on fuel preference and cardiac hypertrophy, while treatment with fenofibrate may reverse hypertrophy, suggesting the potential clinical value for fenofibrate in hypertrophic treatment (**Figure 8**).

DISCUSSION

Herein, we observed an indispensable role of FABP3 in the incidence and advance of cardiac hypertrophy. *Fabp3* deficiency served to exacerbate TAC-induced hypertrophy and cardiac dysfunction, while its overexpression rescued cardiomyocyte hypertrophy. Mechanistically, *Fabp3* defect resulted in metabolic derangement characterized by defective FAO and increased glycolysis to elicit an imbalanced FAO/glycolysis rate and toxic lipid accumulation. Furthermore, *Fabp3* mediated the PPARα protein levels by directly binding to PPARα and preventing its degradation and underpinning its transactivation on *Mlycd* and *Gck*, which underscores the pivotal metabolic role of PPARα in FABP3-mediated cardiac hypertrophy. Additionally, treatment with the PPARα agonist, fenofibrate, effectively repressed *Fabp3*-KO induced cardiac hypertrophy, highlighting a potential clinical value of hypertrophic treatment by targeting cardiac energy metabolism.

FABP3, a small molecular weight protein, is abundantly expressed in the heart and muscle tissues (21). FABP3 can directly bind to cellular insoluble LCFAs and transport them to the mitochondrion, nucleus, or endoplasmic reticulum for utilization (12). Notably, single-cell RNA-sequencing research suggested that the increased expression of *Fabp3* from embryo to mature cardiomyocytes accounts for the developmental metabolic switch from embryonic glycolysis to postnatal mitochondrial fatty acid oxidation, underscoring its profound effects on fuel preference and cardiac metabolism (22). Besides that, the loss and gain function of FABP3 in brown adipocytes shows that FABP3 is a determinant of cellular fatty acid oxidation efficiency; brown adipocytes without FABP3 show defective capability to oxidize exogenously supplied fatty acids (16). These studies confirm the indispensable role of FABP3 on the maintenance of cardiac FAO and glucose homeostasis under physiological and pathological conditions.

In our previous studies, we reported that FABP3 plays an important role in myocardial infarction and in-stent restenosis (15, 23). Moreover, clinical studies have considered FABP3 to be a marker of cardiac ischemic injury, demonstrating that its expression is associated with major adverse cardiac outcomes and recurrent MI (24–28). As elevated FABP3 has been previously explored in the content of varied cardiac diseases, at least two mechanisms are involved in the regulation of FABP3 expression. Under stimulations, the myocardium shifts for higher energy demand, which occurs with the upregulation of IGF-1 and the decline of miR-1; (1) exposure to IGF-1 results in increased FABP3 expression, and (2) on the other hand, miR-1 downregulation is able to release its inhibitory role on FABP3 and eventually elicit the increase in FABP3 under cardiac hypertrophy (14). These literatures demonstrate a tight control of the FABP3 level by IGF-1 and miR-1. Consistently, we showed that FABP3 was increased in response to hypertrophic stimulations *in vivo* and *in vitro* to modulate cardiac metabolic homeostasis, especially the FAO and glucose oxidation processes under cardiac hypertrophy, a disease

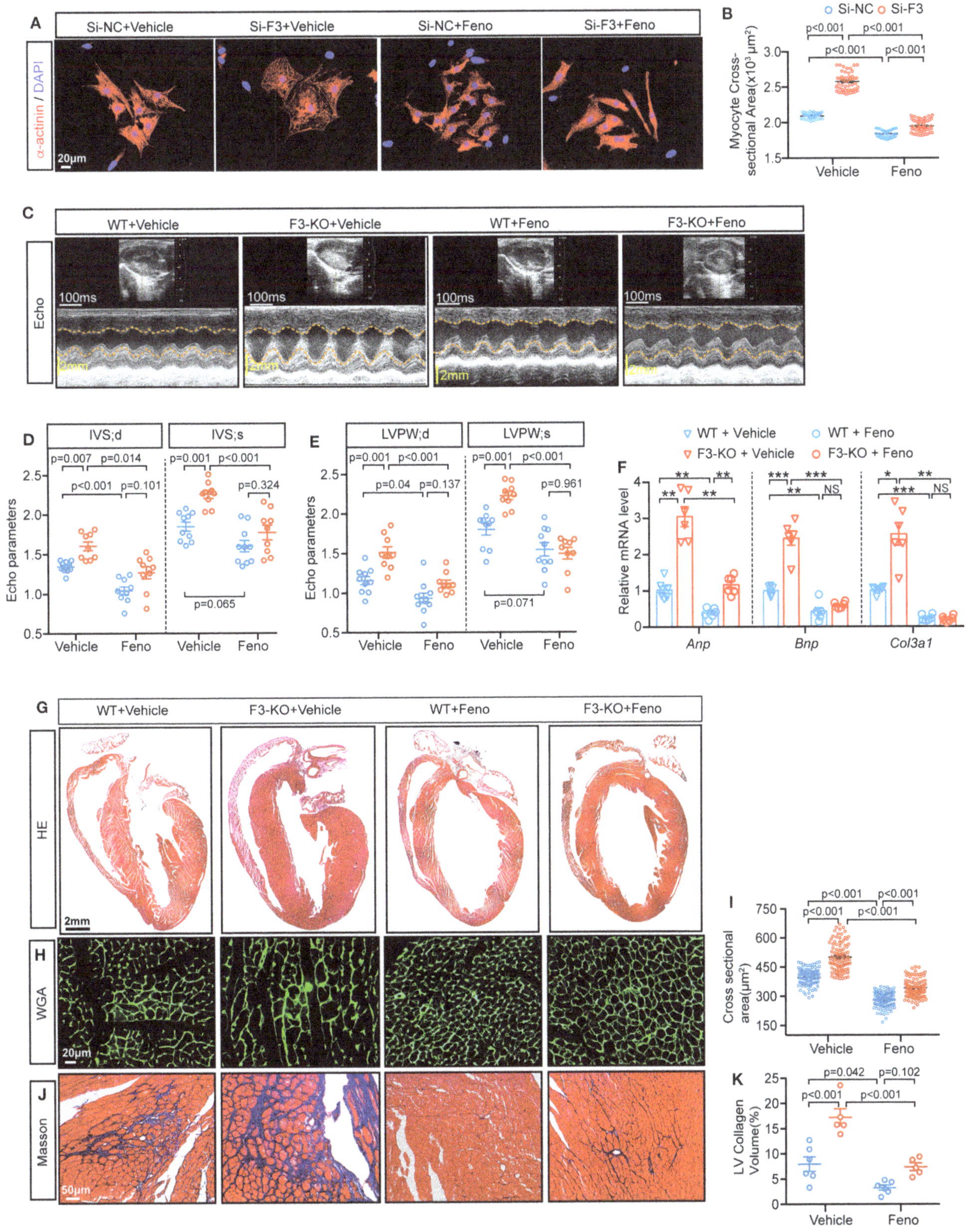

FIGURE 7 | Fenofibrate represses FABP3-null induced cardiac hypertrophy *in vivo* and *in vitro*. **(A)** NRVMs were treated with siRNA targeted *Fabp3* (Si-F3) or its negative control before fenofibrate or vehicle treatment. Immunofluorescence staining of α-actinin used to compare the myocyte area. **(B)** Quantification of **(A)**. **(C)** Representative echo images in WT or F3-KO mice with or without fenofibrate treatment (Feno or Vehicle, respectively) at 4 weeks after TAC surgery. **(D)** Quantification

(Continued)

FIGURE 7 | of IVS in **(C)**. **(E)** Quantification of LVPW in **(C)**. **(F)** Relative mRNA levels of *Anp, Bnp,* and *Col3a1*, as determined by qPCR in the indicated groups. NS, not significant, $^*p < 0.05$, $^{**}p < 0.01$, $^{***}p < 0.001$. **(G)** Images of H&E-stained longitudinal heart sections from WT or F3-KO mice with or without fenofibrate treatment. **(H)** Representative immunofluorescence images of WGA staining from WT or F3-KO mice with or without fenofibrate treatment. **(I)** Quantification of the cardiomyocyte cross-sectional area in **(I)** ($n = 100$). **(J)** Masson staining to determine cardiac fibrosis in the aforementioned groups. **(K)** Quantification of collagen volume in **(L)**. [**D, E**, $n = 10, 9, 10, 9$, respectively; (**B**, D-IVS; s): Games–Howell *post-hoc* test; (D-IVS; d, **E**): Tukey's *post-hoc* test; **F**, $n = 6$, (F-Anp, F-Col3a1, and **I**): Games–Howell *post-hoc* test; **K**, $n = 6, 5, 6, 5$; (F-Bnp, and **K**): Tukey's *post-hoc* test].

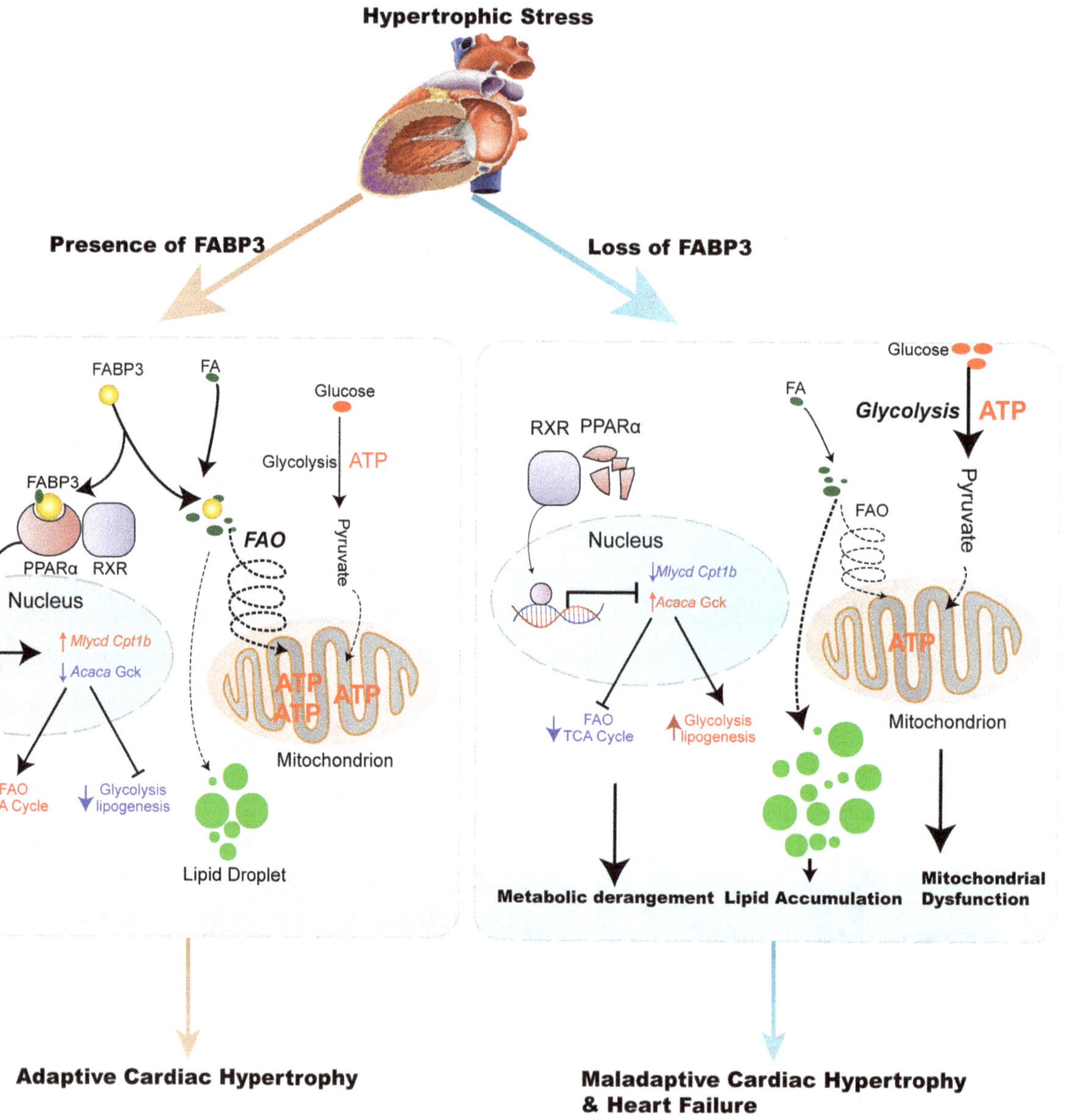

FIGURE 8 | Model of the FABP3-mediated PPARα pathway in cardiac metabolic reprogramming and progression of cardiac hypertrophy and heart failure. The schematic demonstrates that the FABP3-mediated PPARα pathway regulates cardiac metabolic reprogramming by directly interacting with PPARα, thereby stabilizing and inducing its transactivation, which triggers downstream Mlycd and Cpt1b gene expression, while suppressing Acaca and Gck gene expression. This results in increased FAO levels and mitochondrial ATP production, ultimately resulting in adaptive cardiac function. However, in mice lacking FABP3, the response of FABP3-mediated PPARα on FAO/Glycolysis balance is abolished, and leads to the degradation of PPARα, lower transcriptional activity on FAO genes accompanied by increased lipogenesis, and glycolysis gene expression, which contributes to the increase in the glycolysis rate, accumulation of toxic lipid species, and compromised mitochondrial ATP production, thereby aggravating the progression of cardiac hypertrophy and heart failure.

condition with higher energy demands. Here, we combined multi-omics analyses, such as RNA-seq and metabolomics, to reveal the indispensable role of FABP3 in governing the cardiac energy regulatory program by increasing FAO and inhibiting glycolysis under hypertrophic stimuli. Therefore, FABP3 has an important homeostatic role in the pathologically stressed mammalian heart. To the best of our knowledge, this is the first study to explore the role of FABP3 during cardiac hypertrophy.

As we have shown, *Fabp3* deletion contributes to dramatic abnormalities in myocardial metabolism by targeting PPARα pathways. Accumulating evidence has indicated that PPAR family members (PPARα, β/δ, and γ), a member of nuclear receptor superfamily of transcription factor (NR1C), play regulatory roles in cellular metabolism and cardiac hypertrophy, which was confirmed in loss- or gain-of-function mutated mice (29). Specifically, PPAR can directly bind to the promoter regions of metabolic-related genes and regulate their transcriptional levels (30). PPARγ is primarily expressed in adipose tissues, while PPARβ/δ is ubiquitously expressed. Of note, PPARα is exclusively expressed in tissues with higher capacity for fatty acid oxidation, such as the heart, liver, and BAT, which display a concordant expression profile with FABP3 (31). Cardiac-specific overexpression of PPARα resulted in the activation in FA transport genes and the suppression of glycolytic genes; however, these metabolic phenotypes were strikingly contrasted to the cardiac-specific overexpression of PPARβ/δ, which shows the increase in glycolysis and glucose uptake genes, indicating the reciprocal role of PPARα and PPARβ/δ on the regulation of cardiac metabolic homeostasis (32). Based on the expression profile and metabolic effects, the interactive effects of FABP3 and PPARα in cellular metabolism and cardiac hypertrophy were explored in this article. Previous studies show that the activation of PPARα exacerbates the uptake and utilization of FA and reduces glucose utilization (33, 34). Fasting or inhibiting mitochondrial FAO with etomoxir leads to markedly increased lipid accumulation in PPARα$^{-/-}$ heart and hepatocytes (19). These phenotypes were similar to the derangement of the FAO/glucose oxidation rate in our FABP3-deficient mice, corroborating a link between FABP3 and PPARα. Moreover, studies have demonstrated a direct interaction between PPARα and FABP family members, especially FABP1 and FABP4, reporting that FABP1 or FABP4 translocates from the plasma to the nucleus, where it binds to PPARα to stabilize and amplify its biological function by enhancing its transcriptional activities (35–37). Additionally, a luciferase assay containing FABP3 and PPARα plasmid suggests that FABP3 facilitates the transcriptional activity of PPARα in COS-7 cells (38). However, whether FABP3 could interact with PPARα and govern its transcriptional activity in cardiomyocytes during chronic hypertrophic stimulation has not been fully delineated. Here, our *in vivo* and *in vitro* results reveal the potential mechanism of the FABP3-mediated PPARα pathway in cardiac hypertrophy and in FAO/glycolysis balance by directly binding to PPARα, promoting its stability, and underpinning its transactivation in *Mlycd* and *Gck*.

In conclusion, we have provided a novel perspective into the relationship between FABP3 with cardiac hypertrophy and fuel preference. However, in relation to our observations, there are some problems that need further explorations. We have demonstrated a beneficial value of FABP3 on cardiac hypertrophy and heart failure by inhibiting PPARα degradation. However, whether FABP3 mediated PPARα stability by preventing its degradation from ubiquitylation proteasome or other pathways needed further in-depth investigation. In conclusion, in the present study, we provide novel insights into the regulatory role of FABP3 on cellular metabolism following TAC-induced cardiac hypertrophy. Meanwhile, targeting FABP3 with an agonist may represent an attractive approach to alleviate deranged metabolic milieu in cardiac hypertrophy and achieve the goal of improved heart function.

AUTHOR CONTRIBUTIONS

XY, KC, and RT designed the study. LZ, ZL, and CL participated in the experimental design, data interpretation, and manuscript preparation. LZ, ZL, CL, QJ, LL, and KC discussed, edited, and revised the manuscript. ZL and YM participated in the revising and polishing of the re-submitted manuscript. All authors contributed to the article and approved the submitted version.

FUNDING

This study was supported by the National Natural Science Foundation of China (81270004 to KC; 81970327 to RT; 81400362, 81670457, 81922007, and 91939103 to XY), Shanghai Municipal Education Commission–Gaofeng Clinical Medicine Grant Support (20191803 to XY), Shanghai Rising-Star Program grant (17QA1402300 to XY), Municipal Human Resources Development Program for Outstanding Young Talents in Medical and Health Sciences in Shanghai (2017YQ017 to XY), Shanghai Science and Technology Supporting Project (19411963400 to XY), and a Natural Science Research Funding from Shanghai Jiao Tong University School of Medicine (19XJ11002 to XY).

ACKNOWLEDGMENTS

We thank BGI Genomics procedures (BGI-SHENZHEN, China) for bulk RNA sequencing analysis and SHANGHAI BIOTREE Biomedical Technology Co., Ltd. for LS/GC-MS metabonomic analysis.

REFERENCES

1. Collaborators GM. Global, regional, and national under-5 mortality, adult mortality, age-specific mortality, and life expectancy, 1970-2016: a systematic analysis for the Global Burden of Disease Study 2016. *Lancet.* (2017) 390:1084–150. doi: 10.1016/S0140-6736(17)31833-0
2. Nakamura M, Sadoshima J. Mechanisms of physiological and pathological cardiac hypertrophy. *Nat Rev Cardiol.* (2018) 15:387–407. doi: 10.1038/s41569-018-0007-y
3. Shimizu I, Minamino T. Physiological and pathological cardiac hypertrophy. *J Mol Cell Cardiol.* (2016) 97:245–62. doi: 10.1016/j.yjmcc.2016.06.001
4. Wang L, Yu P, Zhou B, Song J, Li Z, Zhang M, et al. Single-cell reconstruction of the adult human heart during heart failure and recovery reveals the cellular landscape underlying cardiac function. *Nat Cell Biol.* (2020) 22:108–19. doi: 10.1038/s41556-019-0446-7
5. Pascual F, Coleman RA. Fuel availability and fate in cardiac metabolism: a tale of two substrates. *Biochem Biophys Acta.* (2016) 1861:1425–33. doi: 10.1016/j.bbalip.2016.03.014
6. Rijzewijk LJ, van der Meer RW, Lamb HJ, de Jong HW, Lubberink M, Romijn JA, et al. Altered myocardial substrate metabolism and decreased diastolic function in nonischemic human diabetic cardiomyopathy: studies with cardiac positron emission tomography and magnetic resonance imaging. *J Am Coll Cardiol.* (2009) 54:1524–32. doi: 10.1016/j.jacc.2009.04.074
7. Bertero E, Maack C. Metabolic remodelling in heart failure. *Nat Rev Cardiol.* (2018) 15:457–70. doi: 10.1038/s41569-018-0044-6
8. Ritterhoff J, Young S, Villet O, Shao D, Neto FC, Bettcher LF, et al. Metabolic remodeling promotes cardiac hypertrophy by directing glucose to aspartate biosynthesis. *Circ Res.* (2020) 126:182–96. doi: 10.1161/CIRCRESAHA.119.315483
9. Arumugam S, Sreedhar R, Thandavarayan RA, Karuppagounder V, Watanabe K. Targeting fatty acid metabolism in heart failure: is it a suitable therapeutic approach? *Drug Discov Today.* (2016) 21:1003–8. doi: 10.1016/j.drudis.2016.02.010
10. Lopaschuk GD, Ussher JR, Folmes CD, Jaswal JS, Stanley WC. Myocardial fatty acid metabolism in health and disease. *Physiol Rev.* (2010) 90:207–58. doi: 10.1152/physrev.00015.2009
11. Murashige D, Jang C, Neinast M, Edwards JJ, Cowan A, Hyman MC, et al. Comprehensive quantification of fuel use by the failing and nonfailing human heart. *Science.* (2020) 370:364–8. doi: 10.1126/science.abc8861
12. Furuhashi M, Hotamisligil GS. Fatty acid-binding proteins: role in metabolic diseases and potential as drug targets. *Nat Rev Drug Discov.* (2008) 7:489–503. doi: 10.1038/nrd2589
13. Lee SM, Lee SH, Jung Y, Lee Y, Yoon JH, Choi JY, et al. FABP3-mediated membrane lipid saturation alters fluidity and induces ER stress in skeletal muscle with aging. *Nat Commun.* (2020) 11:5661. doi: 10.1038/s41467-020-19501-6
14. Varrone F, Gargano B, Carullo P, Di Silvestre D, De Palma A, Grasso L, et al. The circulating level of FABP3 is an indirect biomarker of microRNA-1. *J Am Coll Cardiol.* (2013) 61:88–95. doi: 10.1016/j.jacc.2012.08.1003
15. Zhuang LF, Li CN, Chen QJ, Jin Q, Wu LQ, Lu L, et al. Fatty acid-binding protein 3 contributes to ischemic heart injury by regulating cardiac myocyte apoptosis and MAPK pathways. *Am J Physiol Heart C.* (2019) 316:H971–84. doi: 10.1152/ajpheart.00360.2018
16. Vergnes L, Chin R, Young SG, Reue K. Heart-type fatty acid-binding protein is essential for efficient brown adipose tissue fatty acid oxidation and cold tolerance. *J Biol Chem.* (2011) 286:380–90. doi: 10.1074/jbc.M110.184754
17. Nomura S, Satoh M, Fujita T, Higo T, Sumida T, Ko T, et al. Cardiomyocyte gene programs encoding morphological and functional signatures in cardiac hypertrophy and failure. *Nat Commun.* (2018) 9:4435. doi: 10.1038/s41467-018-06639-7
18. Goldberg IJ, Trent CM, Schulze PC. Lipid metabolism and toxicity in the heart. *Cell Metab.* (2012) 15:805–12. doi: 10.1016/j.cmet.2012.04.006
19. Barger PM, Brandt JM, Leone TC, Weinheimer CJ, Kelly DP. Deactivation of peroxisome proliferator-activated receptor-alpha during cardiac hypertrophic growth. *J Clin Invest.* (2000) 105:1723–30. doi: 10.1172/jci9056
20. Liu F, Song R, Feng Y, Guo J, Chen Y, Zhang Y, et al. Upregulation of MG53 induces diabetic cardiomyopathy through transcriptional activation of peroxisome proliferation-activated receptor α. *Circulation.* (2015) 131:795–804. doi: 10.1161/circulationaha.114.012285
21. Del Collado M, da Silveira JC, Sangalli JR, Andrade GM, Sousa L, Silva LA, et al. Fatty acid binding protein 3 and transzonal projections are involved in lipid accumulation during *in vitro* maturation of bovine oocytes. *Sci Rep.* (2017) 7:2645. doi: 10.1038/s41598-017-02467-9
22. DeLaughter DM, Bick AG, Wakimoto H, McKean D, Gorham JM, Kathiriya IS, et al. Single-cell resolution of temporal gene expression during heart development. *Dev Cell.* (2016) 39:480–90. doi: 10.1016/j.devcel.2016.10.001
23. Chen K, Chen QJ, Wang LJ, Liu ZH, Zhang Q, Yang K, et al. Increment of HFABP level in coronary artery in-stent restenosis segments in diabetic and nondiabetic minipigs: HFABP overexpression promotes multiple pathway-related inflammation, growth and migration in human vascular smooth muscle cells. *J Vasc Res.* (2016) 53:27–38. doi: 10.1159/000446652
24. Gerede DM, Gulec S, Kilickap M, Kaya CT, Vurgun VK, Ozcan OU, et al. Comparison of a qualitative measurement of heart-type fatty acid-binding protein with other cardiac markers as an early diagnostic marker in the diagnosis of non-ST-segment elevation myocardial infarction. *Cardiovasc J Afr.* (2015) 26:204–9. doi: 10.5830/cvja-2015-028
25. Jacobs LH, van Borren M, Gemen E, van Eck M, van Son B, Glatz JF, et al. Rapidly rule out acute myocardial infarction by combining copeptin and heart-type fatty acid-binding protein with cardiac troponin. *Ann Clin Biochem.* (2015) 52:550–61. doi: 10.1177/0004563215578189
26. Kagawa Y, Toyofuku M, Masaoka Y, Muraoka Y, Okimoto T, Otsuka M, et al. Comparison of heart-type fatty acid binding protein and sensitive troponin for the diagnosis of early acute myocardial infarction. *Int J Cardiol.* (2013) 166:347–51. doi: 10.1016/j.ijcard.2011.10.080
27. O'Donoghue M, de Lemos JA, Morrow DA, Murphy SA, Buros JL, Cannon CP, et al. Prognostic utility of heart-type fatty acid binding protein in patients with acute coronary syndromes. *Circulation.* (2006) 114:550–7. doi: 10.1161/CIRCULATIONAHA.106.641936
28. Kilcullen N, Viswanathan K, Das R, Morrell C, Farrin A, Barth JH, et al. Heart-type fatty acid-binding protein predicts long-term mortality after acute coronary syndrome and identifies high-risk patients across the range of troponin values. *J Am Coll Cardiol.* (2007) 50:2061–7. doi: 10.1016/j.jacc.2007.08.021
29. Robinson E, Grieve DJ. Significance of peroxisome proliferator-activated receptors in the cardiovascular system in health and disease. *Pharmacol Ther.* (2009) 122:246–63. doi: 10.1016/j.pharmthera.2009.03.003
30. Mirza AZ, Althagafi II, Shamshad H. Role of PPAR receptor in different diseases and their ligands: physiological importance and clinical implications. *Eur J Med Chem.* (2019) 166:502–13. doi: 10.1016/j.ejmech.2019.01.067
31. Feige JN, Gelman L, Michalik L, Desvergne B, Wahli W. From molecular action to physiological outputs: peroxisome proliferator-activated receptors are nuclear receptors at the crossroads of key cellular functions. *Prog Lipid Res.* (2006) 45:120–59. doi: 10.1016/j.plipres.2005.12.002
32. Burkart EM, Sambandam N, Han X, Gross RW, Courtois M, Gierasch CM, et al. Nuclear receptors PPARbeta/delta and PPARalpha direct distinct metabolic regulatory programs in the mouse heart. *J Clin Invest.* (2007) 117:3930–9. doi: 10.1172/jci32578
33. Finck BN, Lehman JJ, Leone TC, Welch MJ, Bennett MJ, Kovacs A, et al. The cardiac phenotype induced by PPARα overexpression mimics that caused by diabetes mellitus. *J Clin Invest.* (2002) 109:121–30. doi: 10.1172/JCI14080
34. Kaimoto S, Hoshino A, Ariyoshi M, Okawa Y, Tateishi S, Ono K, et al. Activation of PPAR-alpha in the early stage of heart failure maintained myocardial function and energetics in pressure-overload heart failure. *Am J Physiol Heart Circ Physiol.* (2017) 312:H305–13. doi: 10.1152/ajpheart.00553.2016
35. Hughes ML, Liu B, Halls ML, Wagstaff KM, Patil R, Velkov T, et al. Fatty acid-binding proteins 1 and 2 differentially modulate the activation of peroxisome proliferator-activated receptor α in a ligand-selective manner. *J Biol Chem.* (2015) 290:13895–906. doi: 10.1074/jbc.M114.605998

36. Velkov T. Interactions between human liver fatty acid binding protein and peroxisome proliferator activated receptor selective drugs. *PPAR Res.* (2013) 2013:1–14. doi: 10.1155/2013/938401
37. Hostetler HA, McIntosh AL, Atshaves BP, Storey SM, Payne HR, Kier AB, et al. L-FABP directly interacts with PPARα in cultured primary hepatocytes. *J Lipid Res.* (2009) 50:1663–75. doi: 10.1194/jlr.M900058-JLR200
38. Tan NS, Shaw NS, Vinckenbosch N, Liu P, Yasmin R, Desvergne B, et al. Selective cooperation between fatty acid binding proteins and peroxisome proliferator-activated receptors in regulating transcription. *Mol Cell Biol.* (2002) 22:5114–27. doi: 10.1128/mcb.22.14.5114-5127.2002

3

Guanxin V Acts as an Antioxidant in Ventricular Remodeling

*Bo Liang[1], Rui Li[1], Yi Liang[2] and Ning Gu[3]**

[1] Nanjing University of Chinese Medicine, Nanjing, China, [2] Southwest Medical University, Luzhou, China, [3] Nanjing Hospital of Chinese Medicine Affiliated to Nanjing University of Chinese Medicine, Nanjing, China

***Correspondence:**
Ning Gu
guning@njucm.edu.cn

Background: Our previous studies have shown that Guanxin V (GXV) is safe and effective in the treatment of ventricular remodeling (VR), but its mechanism related to oxidative stress has not been studied deeply.

Methods: We applied integrating virtual screening and network pharmacology strategy to obtain the GXV-, VR-, and oxidative stress-related targets at first, and then highlighted the shared targets. We built the networks and conducted enrichment analysis. Finally, the main results were validated by molecular docking and solid experiments.

Results: We obtained 251, 11,425, and 9,727 GXV-, VR-, and oxidative stress-related targets, respectively. GXV-component-target-VR and protein–protein interaction networks showed the potential mechanism of GXV in the treatment of VR. The following enrichment analysis results gathered many biological processes and "two GXV pathways" of oxidative stress-related to VR. All our main results were validated by molecular docking and solid experiments.

Conclusion: GXV could be prescribed for VR through the mechanism, including complex interactions between related components and targets, as predicted by virtual screening and network pharmacology and validated by molecular docking and solid experiments. Our study promotes the explanation of the biological mechanism of GXV for VR.

Keywords: Guanxin V, ventricular remodeling, oxidative stress, network pharmacology, virtual screening, molecular docking, two GXV pathways, validation

INTRODUCTION

Ventricular remodeling (VR) refers to the changes at the cellular and anatomical levels that occur based on gene expression changes, mainly cardiomyocytes, non-cardiomyocytes, and extracellular matrix (1). Cell structure and function are reconstructed and finally related to arrhythmia and heart failure, which can lead to death (2). Early reversal of VR has a significant effect on reducing major adverse cardiovascular events. Nowadays, the drugs used to treat VR are mainly empirical, including angiotensin-converting enzyme inhibitor/angiotensin receptor blocker/angiotensin receptor-neprilysin inhibitor, beta-blockers, and aldosterone receptor inhibitors. Nondrug therapy, such as device-assisted therapy, cannot benefit many patients because of its high price and high requirements for technology of the surgeons. Therefore, we urgently need an alternative and complementary therapy.

Traditional Chinese medicine, mainly from the East, has been used clinically for nearly 3,000 years and has gradually received acceptance and recognition abroad and overseas in the recent years (3, 4). Guanxin V (GXV) is a mixture of traditional Chinese medication, which has been used clinically for decades. Our previous clinical studies showed that GXV could increase ejection fraction, cardiac output, and stroke volume, left ventricular end-diastolic diameter, left ventricular end-systolic diameter, and left ventricular late diastolic A peak velocity while decreasing left ventricular early diastolic E peak velocity among coronary artery disease patients with VR with no adverse reaction, indicating that GXV is a potentially safe and effective treatment for VR (5). Moreover, our subsequent animal experiments also showed that GXV could inhibit or even reverse VR in animals with acute myocardial infarction (6).

Oxidative stress is the result of the imbalance between reactive oxygen species formation and enzymatic and non-enzymatic antioxidants (7). Excessive reactive oxygen species can cause oxidative damage to lipids, proteins, and DNA (8), and is accompanied by a significant decrease in antioxidant levels and antioxidant enzyme activities (9). Therefore, increased reactive oxygen species production or impaired antioxidant system could tilt the cell redox balance to oxidative imbalance and lead to the overproduction of reactive oxygen species (10). Oxidative stress is considered to be an important component of various diseases (11), including VR (12). In recent years, the study of the mechanism of oxidative stress in VR has achieved certain results (13, 14), showing that oxidative stress may be one of the targets of anti-VR (15, 16). Our previous studies have shown that GXV can reverse VR, but its effect on oxidative stress is not particularly clear. Here, we used virtual screening and network pharmacology methods to determine the oxidative stress-related targets of GXV in the treatment of VR, and further verify it through molecular docking and robust experiments (**Figure 1**). We hope that our results can further promote our understanding of the molecular biological mechanism of anti-oxidative stress of GXV in VR, and lay an experimental foundation for the further clinical application of GXV.

METHODS

Targets Screening

We first obtained active compounds and corresponding targets for GXV from our previous study (17). In another previous study (6), we identified the effective components in GXV by ultra-performance liquid chromatography-quadrupole time-of-flight high-resolution mass spectrometry (UPLC-Q-TOF/HRMS E). In this study, we supplemented the targets of these effective components in SwissTargetPrediction by the structure of each effective component (18), as described previously (19). The targets of VR were obtained from our previous study (17). Taking "oxidative stress" as a keyword, we obtained oxidative stress-related targets from GeneCards, a searchable and integrative database that provides comprehensive information on all annotated and predicted human genes (20).

Network Construction

All targets were standardized in Universal Protein (UniProt) (21), and then taking the intersection of the targets in GXV, VR, and oxidative stress, these shared targets were considered as key therapeutic targets related to GXV against oxidative stress of VR, as described previously (22), and were visualized by Venn diagram. We also constructed a GXV-component-target-VR (G-C-T-V) network to visualize the relationships of targets between GXV and VR. Moreover, the cytoHubba plugin (23) in Cytoscape (24) was applied to evaluate the multiple centralities. A protein–protein interaction (PPI) network of all shared targets was then constructed with all genes as the background (25). The network diagram was completed in the string database (26) with the organism option was set to *Homo sapiens* (Human) and medium confidence was more than 0.400. Then, we used the MCODE plugin (27) in Cytoscape (24) to cluster the PPI network based on the topology to find densely connected regions.

Functional Enrichment

DAVID Bioinformatics Resources (28) was utilized to conduct functional enrichment analysis {including Gene Ontology [GO] terms (29) and Kyoto Encyclopedia of Genes and Genomes [KEGG] pathways (30)} of all shared targets. We also used *Homo sapiens* (Human) as the background. To avoid over counting duplicated genes, based on corresponding DAVID gene IDs, we calculated the Fisher Exact statistics to remove all redundancies in original IDs. The threshold of EASE score, a modified Fisher Exact *P* value, was applied for the evaluation of gene-enrichment analysis. Fisher Exact *P* value range from 0 to 1, $\leq$0.05 was considered strongly enriched, and equal to 0 were considered perfect enrichment. All results had to pass the thresholds (EASE $\leq$ 0.05 and the number of genes annotated with a GO term or KEGG pathway was more than or equal to 5) to ensure only significant enrichment terms were displayed. The top 20 results were visualized by the *ggplot2* package in R (31). KEGG Mapper is a collection of tools for KEGG mapping, which could realize the visualization of the situation of the certain gene set in the corresponding signaling pathways or other, high-level enrichment features (32). We used this tool to mapper specific signaling pathways.

In addition, the ClueGO plugin (33) in Cytoscape (24) was used to create and visualize a functionally grouped network of terms in cluster networks from the PPI network.

Computational Validation

Refer to our previous research results (17), we selected two key targets from established "two GXV pathways" (TGF-β1 and Caspase-3) and their corresponding compounds from the established G-C-T-V network (MOL000358 [Beta-Sitosterol], MOL000006 [Luteolin], MOL007154 [Tanshinone IIA], MOL002714 [Baicalein]) to validate computationally by molecular docking. Detailly, we used receptor-ligand molecular docking to assess these interactions. The structures of protein crystal and compound were obtained from Protein Data Bank (34) and PubChem (35), respectively. The binding energy was calculated by AutoDockTools (36) and the docking was visualized by Discovery Studio.

Experimental Validation

H9c2(2-1) cells were incubated with H_2O_2 (300 μM) for 24 h to establish the oxidative stress model and then treated

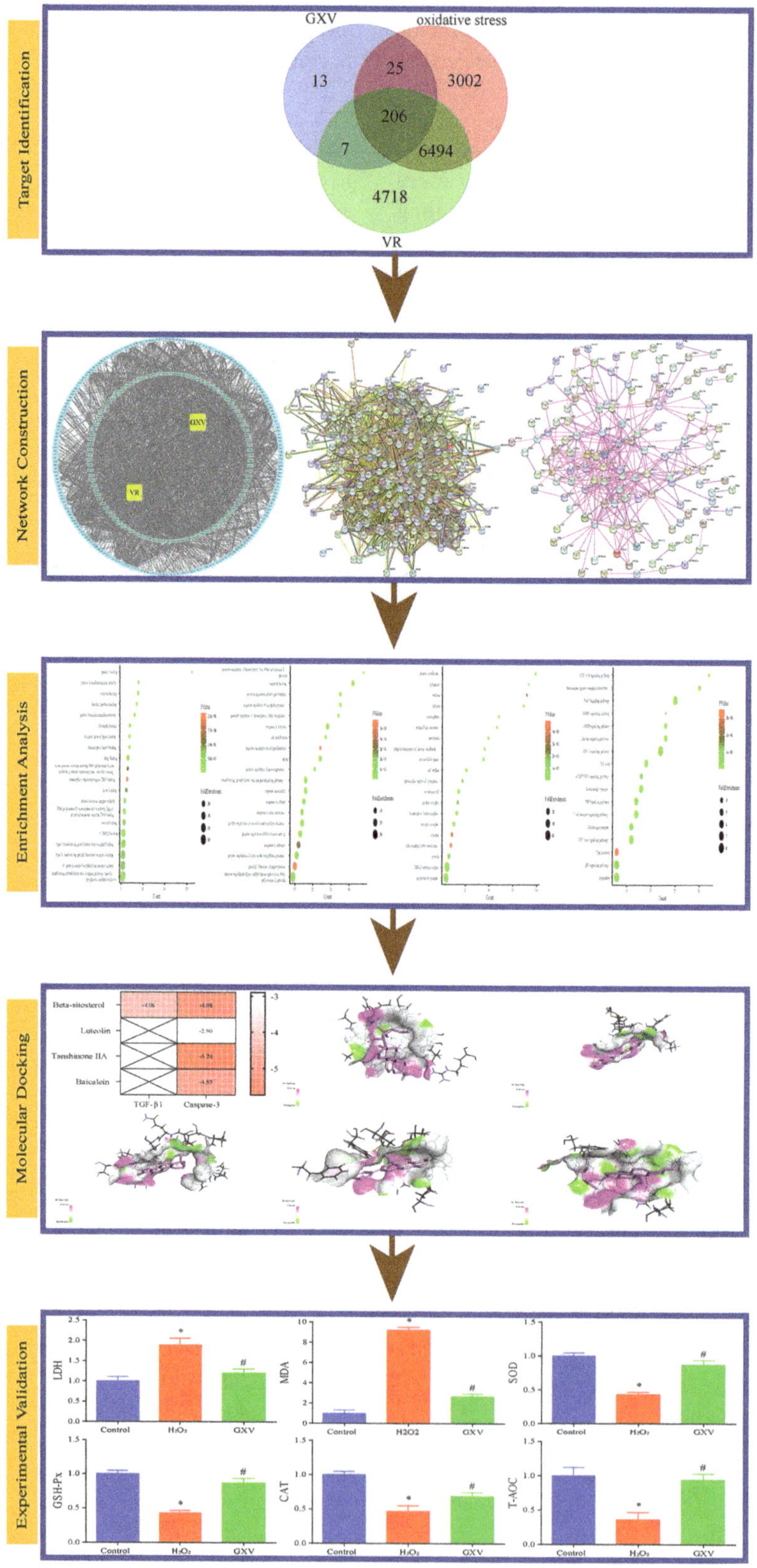

FIGURE 1 | The overall workflow of this study.

with GXV (1 g/L) for another 24 h (17). Supernatants and cells were harvested and the antioxidant activities were investigated *via* malondialdehyde (MDA, NJJCBIO, Nanjing, China), superoxide dismutase (SOD, mlbio, Shanghai Enzyme-linked Biotechnology Co., Ltd., Shanghai, China), lactate dehydrogenase (LDH, NJJCBIO, Nanjing, China), catalase (CAT, Jiangsu Meimian Industrial Co., Ltd., Yancheng, China), total antioxidant capacity (T-AOC, Beyotime, Shanghai, China), and glutathione peroxidase (GSH-PX, NJJCBIO, Nanjing, China) according to the instructions of the manufacturers.

RESULTS

Identification of the Targets of GXV, VR, and Oxidative Stress

We obtained 119 active compounds and corresponding 196 targets for GXV from our previous study (17). Moreover, we supplemented 77 targets for 15 effective components in GXV. After integrating all the targets, we obtained 251 GXV-related targets. We got 11,425 known therapeutic targets for VR from our previous study (17). A total of 9,727 targets were identified as stress-related oxidative.

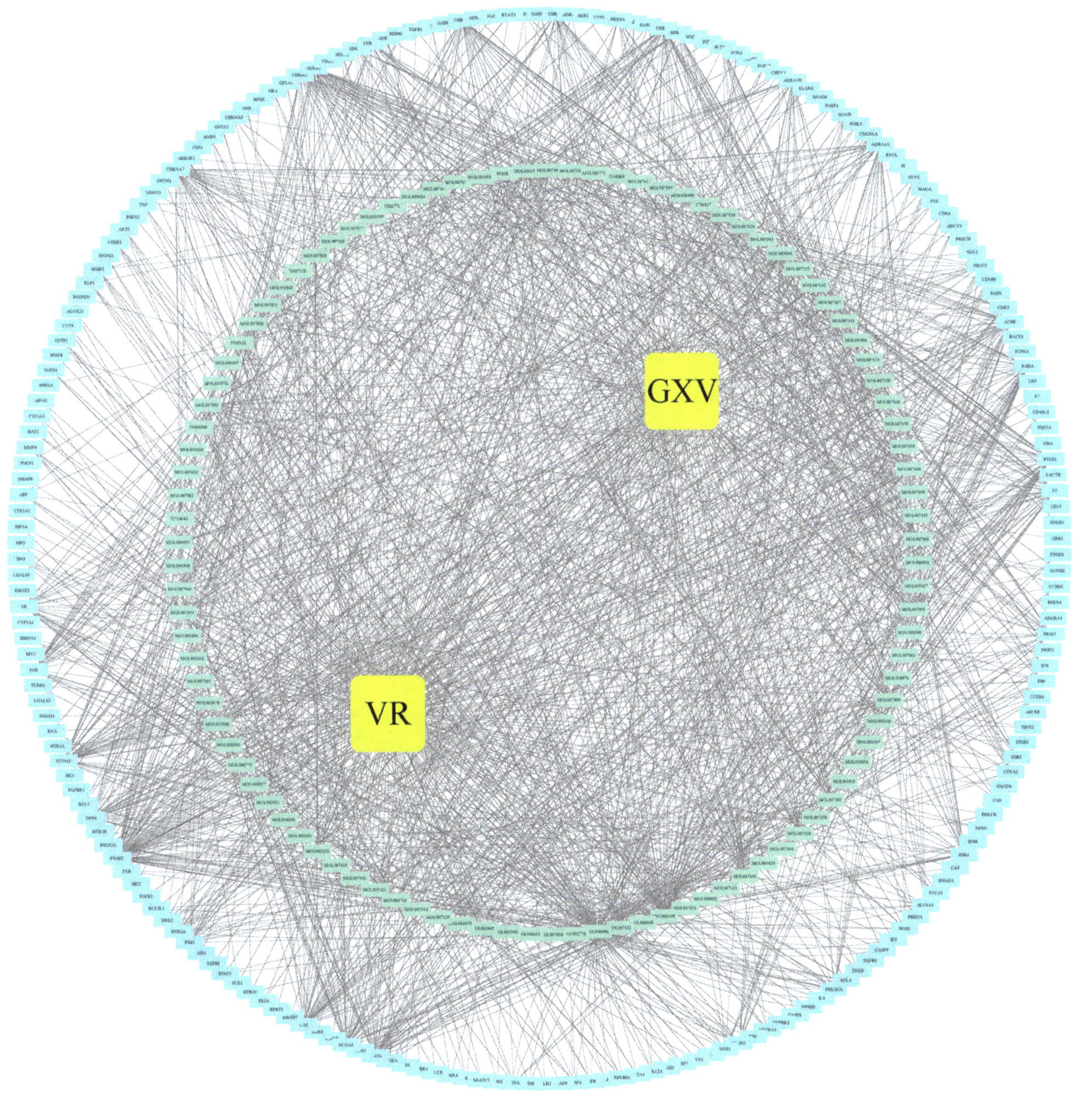

FIGURE 2 | The G-C-T-V network.

TABLE 1 | Multiple centralities of compounds in the G-C-T-V network (MCC ≥ 30).

Node	Annotation	Local-based method				Global-based method						
		MCC	DMNC	MNC	Degree	EPC	Bottle Neck	EcCentricity	Closeness	Radiality	Betweenness	Stress
MOL000006	Luteolin	55	0	1	109	22.320	1	0.33333	158.0000	3.69649	9101.1310	192292
MOL003896	7-Methoxy-2-Methyl Isoflavone	38	0	1	38	20.399	1	0.33333	146.6667	3.58786	1058.2190	51582
MOL007154	Tanshinone IIA	38	0	1	38	17.247	2	0.33333	146.6667	3.58786	2350.5920	46280
5705531	Dihydrocatalpol	32	0	1	32	7.3510	24	0.33333	142.6667	3.54952	10983.5200	209800
MOL007100	Dihydrotanshinlactone	32	0	1	32	19.210	1	0.33333	142.6667	3.54952	618.3010	43020
MOL000358	Beta-Sitosterol	32	0	1	32	16.302	1	0.33333	142.6667	3.54952	1458.1340	37480
MOL002714	Baicalein	32	0	1	32	12.111	1	0.33333	142.6667	3.54952	1900.3660	30926

MCC, maximal clique centrality; DMNC, density of maximum neighborhood Component; MNC, maximum neighborhood component; EPC, edge percolated component.

TABLE 2 | Multiple centralities of targets in G-C-T-V network (MCC ≥ 30).

Node	Annotation	Local-based method				Global-based method						
		MCC	DMNC	MNC	Degree	EPC	Bottle Neck	Ec Centricity	Closeness	Radiality	Betweenness	Stress
PTGS2	Prostaglandin-Endoperoxide Synthase 2	62	0	1	66	27.172	1	0.25	170.4167	3.82428	4497.1270	148412
NCOA1	Nuclear Receptor Coactivator 1	36	0	1	39	21.072	1	0.25	153.0833	3.65815	1082.7710	52242
SCN5A	Sodium Voltage-Gated Channel A Subunit 5	36	0	1	38	22.735	1	0.25	153.0833	3.65815	879.1755	49214
ADRB2	Adrenoceptor B 2	35	0	1	38	22.861	1	0.25	152.4167	3.65176	724.7611	48948
NCOA2	Nuclear Receptor Coactivator 2	33	0	1	38	18.692	1	0.25	151.0833	3.63898	2341.6570	62710
PTGS1	Prostaglandin-Endoperoxide Synthase 1	33	0	1	36	21.744	1	0.25	151.0833	3.63898	1046.6570	59386
CHRM1	Cholinergic Receptor Muscarinic 1	32	0	1	35	21.879	1	0.25	150.4167	3.63259	633.7786	43362
CHRNA7	Cholinergic Receptor Nicotinic A 7 Subunit	31	0	1	34	21.611	1	0.25	149.7500	3.62620	534.4842	40906
F2	Coagulation Factor II, Thrombin	31	0	1	32	16.676	1	0.25	149.7500	3.62620	853.0783	29594
RXRA	Retinoid X Receptor A	30	0	1	33	19.255	1	0.25	149.0833	3.61981	647.0734	40368
ACHE	Acetylcholinesterase	30	0	1	31	16.274	1	0.25	149.0833	3.61981	873.2213	28376
CA2	Carbonic Anhydrase 2	30	0	1	31	17.575	15	0.25	155.0833	3.77316	2965.7050	65226

MCC, maximal clique centrality; DMNC, density of maximum neighborhood component; MNC, maximum neighborhood component; EPC, edge percolated component.

Network Construction

The Venn diagram showed that there were 206 shared targets among 251 GXV-related targets, 11,425 VR-related targets, and 9,727 oxidative stress-related targets (**Supplementary Figure S1**). These 206 shared targets were considered as key therapeutic targets related to GXV against oxidative stress of VR. Subsequently, we built the G-C-T-V network to illustrate the potential mechanism of GXV acting on VR. To simplify the network, we only used the shared targets and their related compounds to construct the G-C-T-V network, which is composed of 314 nodes and 1,503 edges (**Figure 2**). Moreover, we revealed the most important nodes in this network. Multiple centralities demonstrated that MOL000006 (Luteolin), MOL003896 (7-Methoxy-2-Methyl Isoflavone), MOL007154 (Tanshinone IIA), 5705531 (Dihydrocatalpol), MOL007100 (Dihydrotanshinlactone), MOL000358 (Beta-Sitosterol), and MOL002714 (Baicalein) were the most important compounds in our G-C-T-V network (**Table 1**); while PTGS2, NCOA1, SCN5A, ADRB2, NCOA2, PTGS1, CHRM1, CHRNA7, F2, RXRA, ACHE, and CA2 were the most important targets in

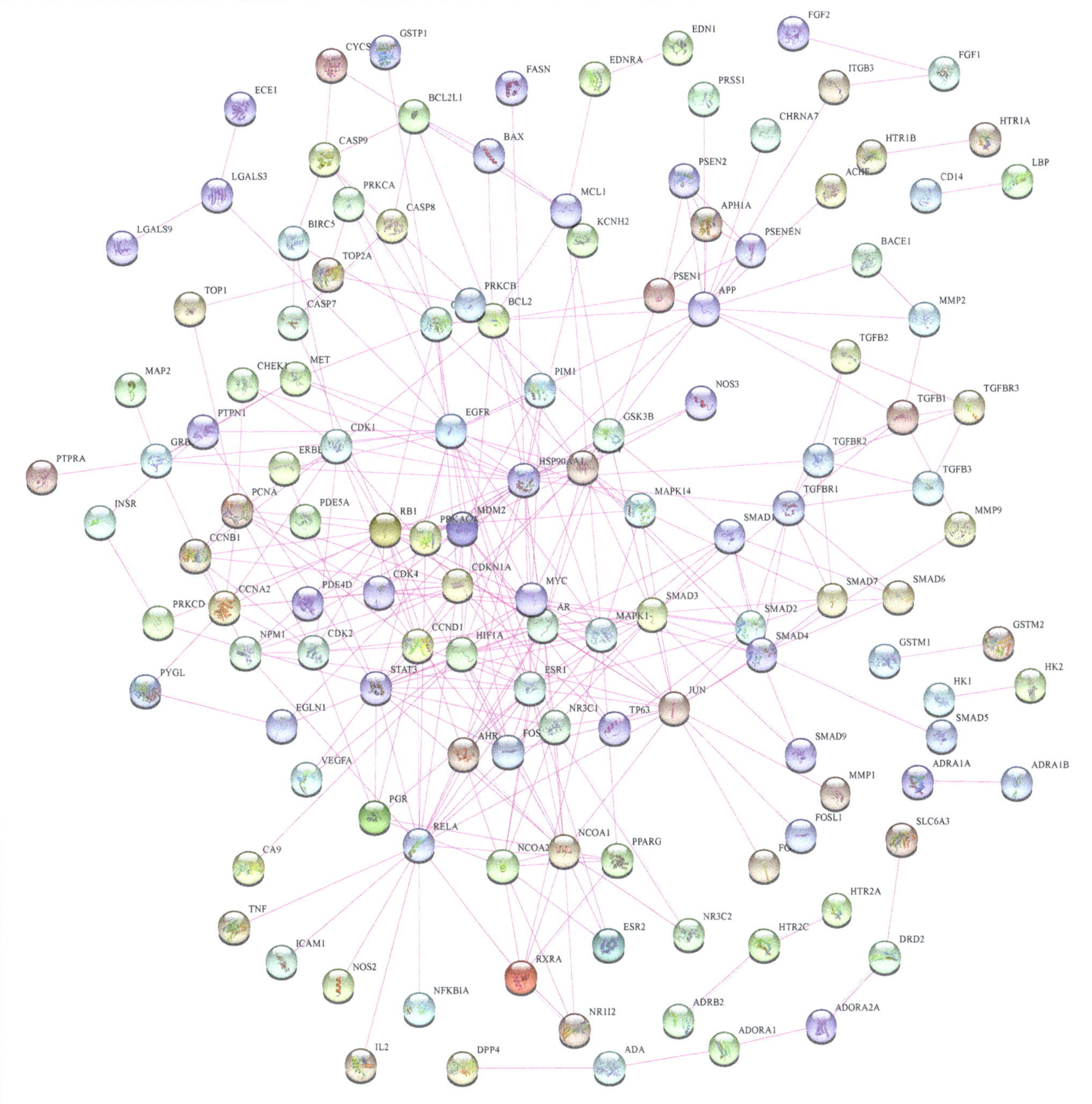

FIGURE 3 | The protein–protein interaction (PPI) network with known interactions comes from experimentally determined evidence.

TABLE 3 | Four cluster networks with the highest clustering scores.

Cluster	Score	Nodes	Edges	Node IDs
1	6.333	7	38	CDK2, CDKN1A, PCNA, RB1, CDK1, CCNA2, CCNB1
2	5.000	5	20	PSEN1, APP, PSEN2, PSENEN, APH1A
3	4.750	9	38	SMAD2, MYC, SMAD4, TGFBR1, SMAD7, MAPK1, STAT3, ESR1, JUN
4	3.412	18	58	GRB2, RXRA, CDK4, MCL1, HSP90AA1, MET, BAX, NCOA1, BCL2, BCL2L1, PTPN1, CASP3, PPARG, CASP8, RELA, SMAD3, NR1I2, NR3C1

our G-C-T-V network (**Table 2**). We have reasons to believe that these compounds and targets played key roles in GXV for treating VR.

Moreover, in this study, we also constructed a PPI network of the 206 shared targets, which consisted of 206 nodes and 6,116 edges (**Supplementary Figure S2**). This means that the proteins have more interactions among themselves than a random set of proteins of similar size drawn from the genome. Such an enrichment indicates that the proteins are at least partially biologically connected as a group and the network highlights the complexity of interactions among proteins. We later applied the PPI network with known interactions supported by the experimentally determined evidence hiding disconnected nodes in the PPI network

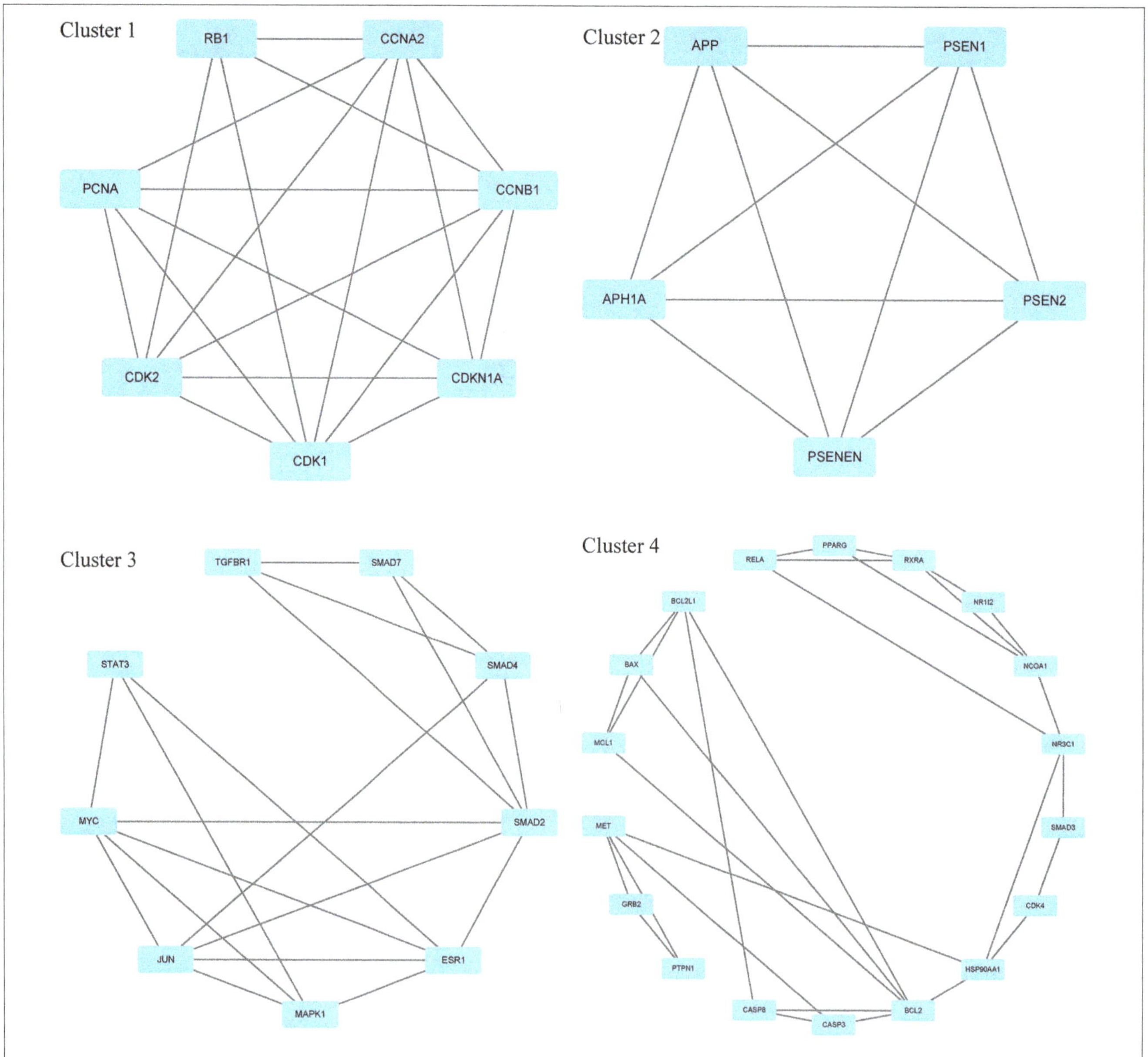

FIGURE 4 | Four cluster networks are divided from the PPI network.

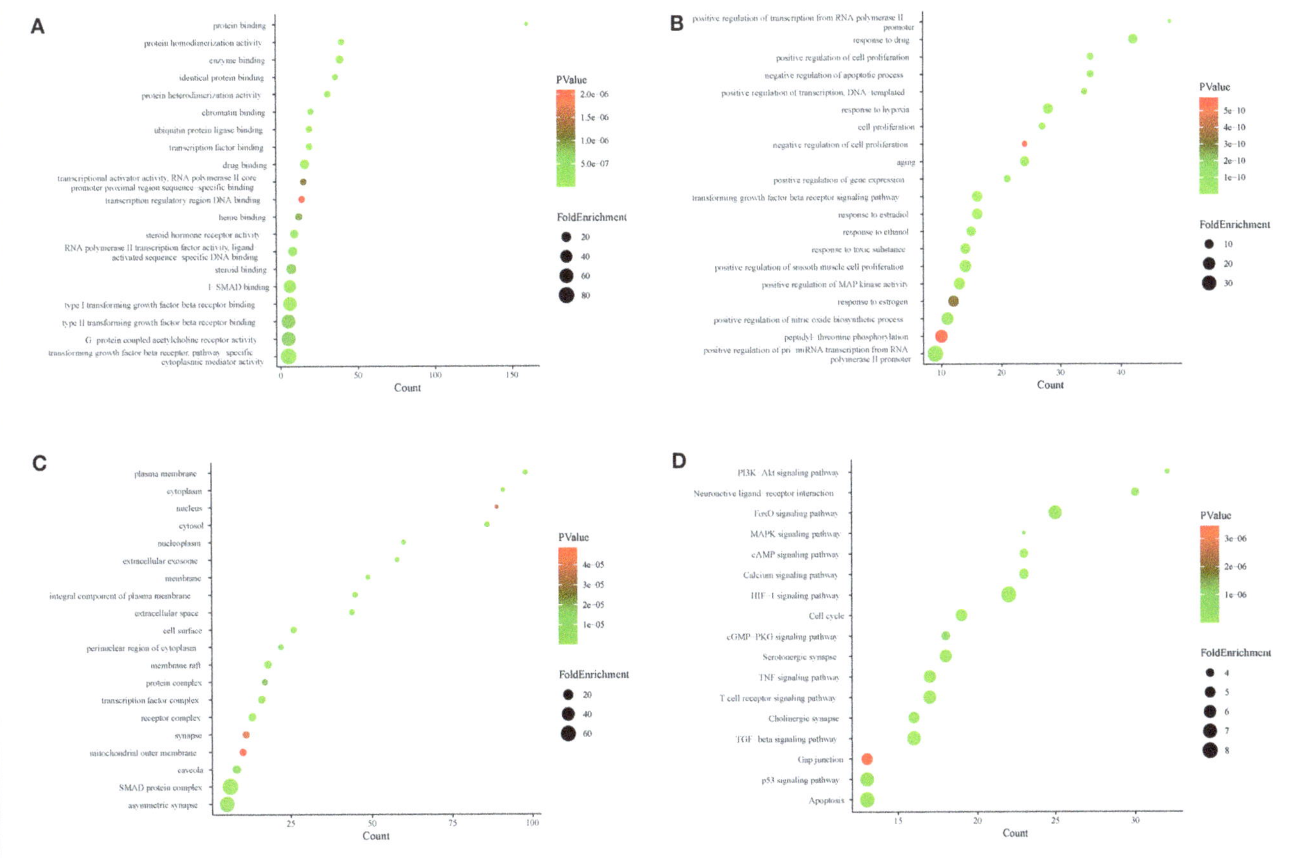

FIGURE 5 | Functional enrichment analysis. **(A)** Top 20 MF of GO analysis colored by *P* value. **(B)** Top 20 BP of GO analysis colored by *P* value. **(C)** Top 20 CC of GO analysis colored by *P* value. **(D)** Kyoto Encyclopedia of Genes and Genomes (KEGG) pathway enrichment analysis colored by *P* value. The X-axis represents the significant enrichment counts of these terms, while the Y-axis represents the corresponding terms of the target genes.

(**Figure 3**). Through the MCODE plugin, we obtained 4 cluster networks with the highest clustering scores (**Table 3**, **Figure 4**).

Functional Enrichment Analysis

To clarify the oxidative stress mechanism of GXV in treating VR, we conducted GO and KEGG functional enrichment analysis for 206 shared targets. GO enrichment items were classified into three functional groups: molecular function (**Figure 5A**), biological process (**Figure 5B**), and cellular component (**Figure 5C**). The results indicated that numerous molecular functions were involved in enzyme binding, protein homodimerization activity, drug binding, protein binding, protein heterodimerization activity, identical protein binding, transcription factor binding, ubiquitin-protein ligase binding, type I transforming growth factor beta receptor binding, and transforming growth factor beta receptor, pathway-specific cytoplasmic mediator activity (**Figure 5A**). The results indicated that numerous biological processes were related to the treatment of VR, including response to the drug, response to hypoxia, aging, negative regulation of the apoptotic process, positive regulation of cell proliferation, positive regulation of transcription from RNA polymerase II promoter, positive regulation of transcription, DNA-templated, positive regulation of smooth muscle cell proliferation, transforming growth factor beta receptor signaling pathway, and cell proliferation (**Figure 5B**). The results indicated that numerous cellular components were involved in the plasma membrane, cytosol, membrane raft, extracellular space, an integral component of the plasma membrane, cell surface, transcription factor complex, SMAD protein complex, receptor complex, and nucleoplasm (**Figure 5C**). The top 20 enriched KEGG pathways for the 206 shared targets are shown in **Figure 5D**. Among these pathways, the HIF-1 signaling pathway, FoxO signaling pathway, neuroactive ligand-receptor interaction, calcium-signaling pathway, PI3K-Akt-signaling pathway, cell cycle, and TGF-β signaling pathway were involved in the development and pathogenesis of VR. In a word, these enrichment findings support the potential pharmacological mechanism of GXV in the treatment of VR. Importantly, the "two GXV pathways" (TGF-β signaling pathway and apoptosis pathway) we obtained before (17) have been verified here. We reconstructed the PPI network diagram of the targets related to the "two GXV pathways" and visualized the pathways (**Supplementary Figure S3**).

Through GO biological process enrichment of 4 cluster networks from the PPI network, we found that cluster 1 enriched in negative regulation of G1/S transition of the

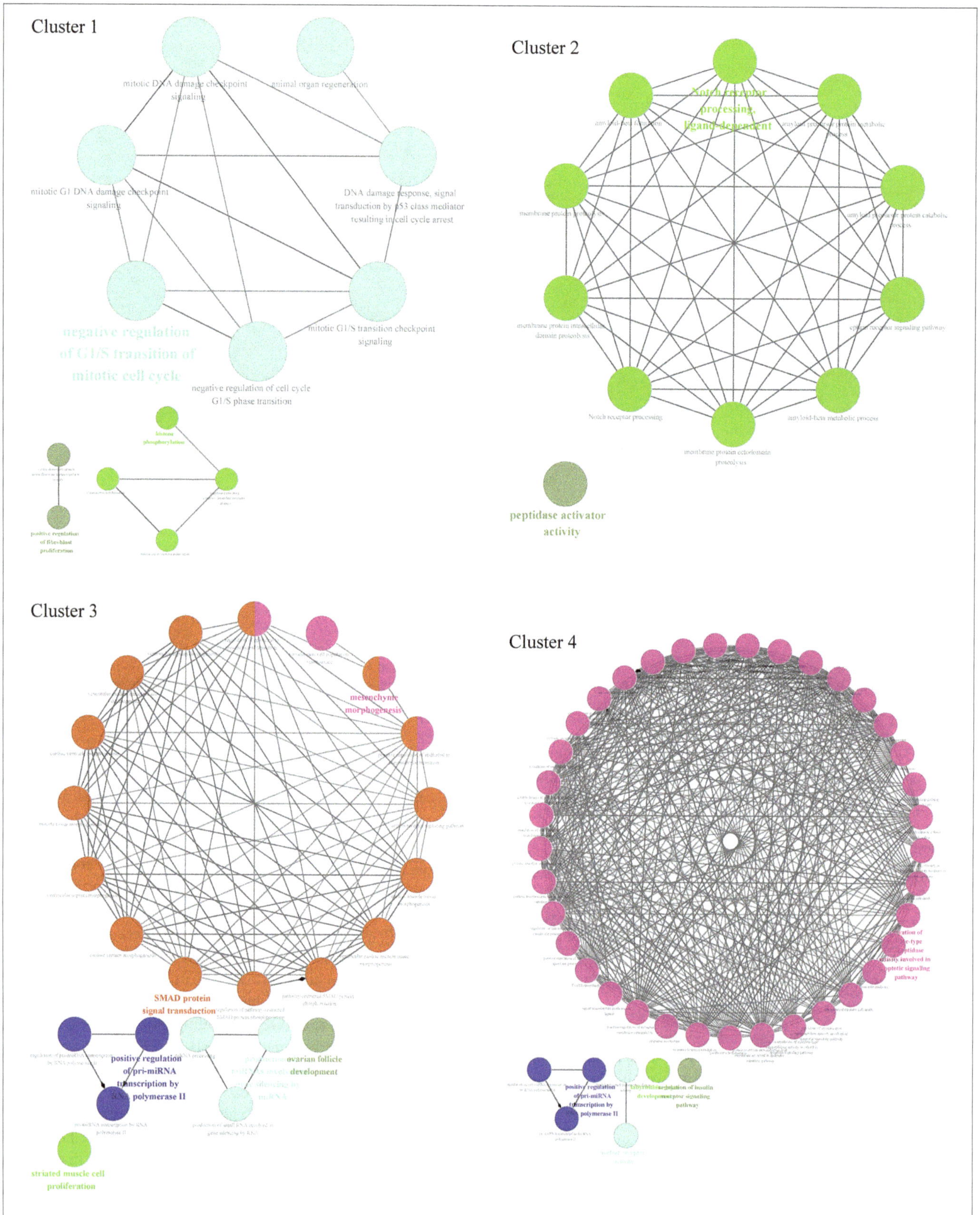

FIGURE 6 | Functional enrichment analysis of 4 cluster networks divided from the PPI network.

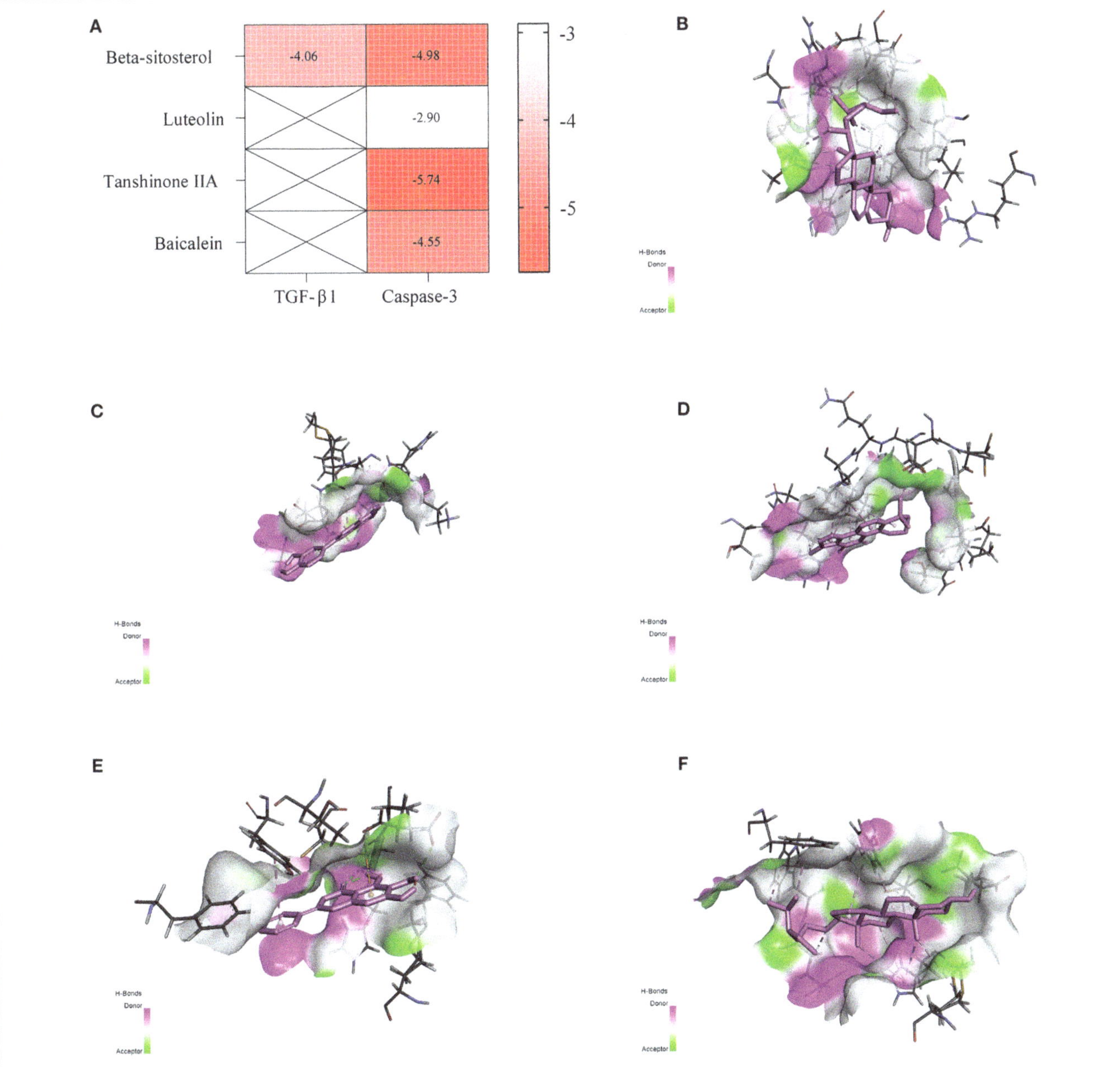

FIGURE 7 | Molecular docking. **(A)** Heatmap of binding energy. **(B)** Transforming growth factor (TGF)-β1 and Beta-Sitosterol. **(C)** Caspase-3 and Luteolin. **(D)** Caspase-3 and Tanshinone IIA. **(E)** Caspase-3 and Baicalein. **(F)** Caspase-3 and Beta-Sitosterol.

mitotic cell cycle, positive regulation of fibroblast proliferation, and histone phosphorylation; cluster 2 enriched in Notch receptor processing and peptidase activator activity; cluster 3 enriched in SMAD protein signal transduction, mesenchyme morphogenesis, striated muscle cell proliferation, positive regulation of pri-miRNA transcription by RNA polymerase II, and production of miRNAs involved in gene silencing by miRNA; and cluster 4 enriched in activation of cysteine-type endopeptidase activity involved in the apoptotic signaling pathway, positive regulation of pri-miRNA transcription by RNA polymerase II, nuclear receptor activity, and regulation of insulin receptor signaling pathway (**Figure 6, Supplementary Table S1**).

Computational Validation

The PDB entry codes for TGF-β1 and Caspase-3 are 6P7J (37) and 5I9B (38), respectively, and the PubChem IDs of Beta-Sitosterol, Luteolin, Tanshinone IIA, and Baicalein are 222284, 5280445, 164676, and 5281605, respectively. The compounds from GXV likely interacted strongly with the identified key targets (**Figure 7A**). The three-dimensional structural diagrams of molecular docking are shown in **Figures 7B–F**.

Experimental Validation

H9c2(2-1) cells incubated with 300 μM H_2O_2 had increased LDH and MDA and decreased SOD, GSH-Px, CAT, and T-AOC (**Figure 8**) indicating that the level of

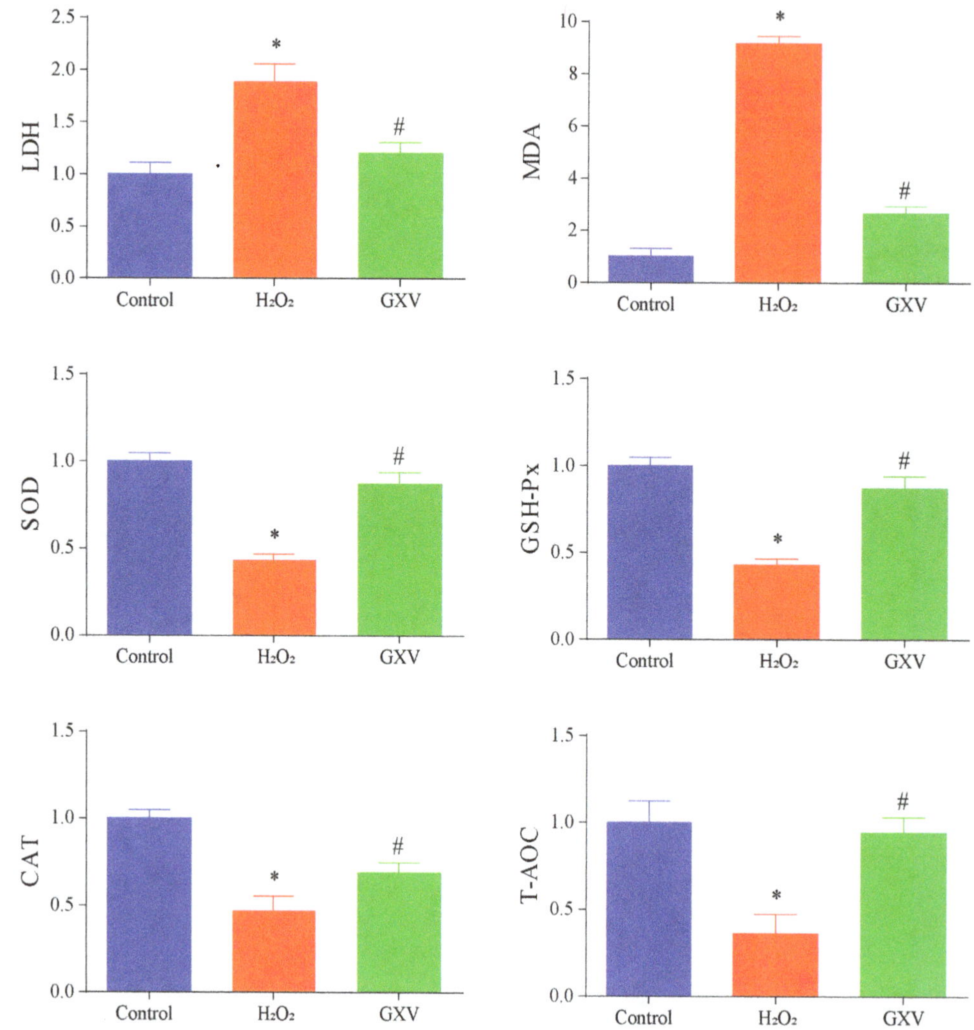

FIGURE 8 | Guanxin V (GXV) alleviates H_2O_2-induced oxidative stress. There were at least 3 independent biological replicates in each group of each experiment. $^{*}P < 0.05$ compared with the Control group, $^{\#}P < 0.05$ compared with the H_2O_2 group.

oxidative stress was elevated. Administration of GXV could reverse the elevated oxidative stress (**Figure 8**). Together, we concluded that GXV could consider as an antioxidant.

DISCUSSION

VR is an important factor leading to the poor prognosis of many cardiovascular diseases in the middle and late stages (39). Therefore, delaying VR is of great significance for improving the quality of life. Our previous studies have shown that GXV has great potential for delaying or even reversing VR (5, 6), here, we aim to detect the oxidative stress-related mechanism of GXV in treating VR through virtual screening and network pharmacology integration strategy and molecular docking, and robust experiments verification strategy to provide evidence of traditional Chinese medicine for VR.

Different from the previous method of obtaining the effective ingredients and targets of drugs directly from the database (25), we identified the effective components of GXV by UPLC-Q-TOF/HRMS E and then obtained the corresponding targets through its structure as a supplement, which can well avoid the bias of target selection. After screening the related datasets, we identified 251 GXV-related targets, 11,425 VR-related targets, and 9,727 oxidative stress-related targets, respectively. Then, we converted these targets data to the G-C-T-V network. From the established G-C-T-V network, we identified several key components and targets through multiple centrality assessments. Luteolin, a widely distributed flavonoid found in many herbal extracts (12), is known to be a potent antioxidant and is demonstrated to have protective actions against Ang II-induced VR, which could be mediated through attenuation of oxidative stress (40). Meanwhile, luteolin improved monocrotaline-induced right VR at least partly through suppressing HIPPO-YAP/PI3K/AKT signaling pathway (41). Tanshinone IIA may alleviate VR in rats by reducing oxidative stress, inflammatory response, and cardiomyocyte apoptosis (42, 43), and enhanced autophagy (44) *via* the inhibition of TLR4/MyD88/NF-κB signaling pathway (45) and activation of SIRT1 signaling pathway (43). Ongoing STAMP-REMODELING trial, a randomized controlled trial, will provide important clinical evidence on the efficacy of Tanshinone IIA in patients with STEMI that might significantly reduce adverse left VR and potentially improve clinical outcomes (46). Baicalein can significantly ameliorate Ang II-induced VR *via* the inhibition of inflammation, oxidative stress, and multiple signaling pathways (AKT/mTOR, ERK1/2, NF-κB, and calcineurin) (47), and monocrotaline-induced vascular remodeling *via* the MAPK and NF-κB pathways (48) and Akt/Erk1/2/GSK3β/β-catenin/ET-1/ET_AR signaling (49). Besides, we used the shared targets to build the PPI network and simplified the 4 cluster networks. The GO biological processes were enriched proliferation, apoptosis, and TGF-β, which are consistent with our previous research results (6, 17). We also enriched TGF-β signaling pathway and apoptosis pathway that were considered "two GXV pathways" in our previous study (17), in KEGG functional analysis. The enrichment analysis of 4 cluster networks also focused on various biological processes related to VR, which reflects the mechanism related to oxidative stress of GXV in the treatment of VR. More importantly, we computationally validated the interaction between components from GXV and shared targets, and experimentally validated that GXV can indeed alleviate oxidative stress.

There are some limitations that should be considered in our further study. First, traditional Chinese medicine generally has the characteristics of multitarget and multieffect, which means that it is not enough to determine only two pathways, although this is confirmed by our previous research results. Moreover, although we verified the results obtained from virtual screening and network pharmacology through molecular docking and solid experiments, more experiments are still required to further verify our reliable findings. Finally, some important targets of GXV, VR, and oxidative stress might be ignored and missed that is the inevitable bias of network pharmacology (22), so we not only enriched our components acquisition with UPLC-Q-TOF/HRMS E, but also searched as many available databases as possible.

CONCLUSIONS

Our study predicts the targets of the synergistic pharmacological mechanism of GXV and explores the potential mechanism involved in alleviating and even reversing VR through integrating virtual screening and network pharmacology strategy and molecular docking and experimental validation, which provide a complementary and alternative medication for VR.

AUTHOR CONTRIBUTIONS

BL and NG conceived, designed, and planned the study. BL and YL acquired and analyzed the data. BL and RL completed the *in vitro* experiments. All authors interpreted the results. BL drafted the manuscript. NG contributed to the critical revision of the manuscript. All authors read and approved the final manuscript.

ACKNOWLEDGMENTS

We thank all individuals involved in GXV and VR. We are also grateful to all research scientists who participated in the aforementioned databases. We thank Nanjing Hospital of Chinese Medicine Affiliated to Nanjing University of Chinese Medicine (Nanjing, China) for the support in GXV and Zhong-Ren Xu from Nanjing University of Chinese Medicine (Nanjing, China) for his support in H_2O_2. The experimental validation is mainly completed in Biological Technology Center for Innovation in Chinese Medicine, Medical Research Center of First College of Chinese Medicine, Nanjing University of Chinese Medicine (Nanjing, China), we thank all colleagues and teachers for their help and support.

SUPPLEMENTARY MATERIAL

Supplementary Table S1 | Functional enrichment analysis of 4 cluster networks divided from the protein-protein interaction (PPI) network.

Supplementary Figure S1 | Venn diagram.

Supplementary Figure S2 | The PPI network with all interactions.

Supplementary Figure S3 | PPI networks and Kyoto Encyclopedia of Genes and Genomes (KEGG) pathways of "two GXV pathways". **(A)** The PPI network with all interactions of "two GXV pathways". The red nodes represent the transforming growth factor (TGF)-β signaling pathway, and the blue nodes represent apoptosis. **(B)** The PPI network with known interactions comes from experimentally determined evidence. The red nodes represent the TGF-β signaling pathway, and the blue nodes represent apoptosis. **(C)** KEGG pathway map of TGF-β signaling pathway. The red pentagrams indicate the genes shared by GXV and ventricular remodeling. **(D)** KEGG pathway map of apoptosis. The red pentagrams indicate the shared targets.

REFERENCES

1. Uriel N, Sayer G, Annamalai S, Kapur NK, Burkhoff D. Mechanical unloading in heart failure. *J Am Coll Cardiol.* (2018) 72:569–80. doi: 10.1016/j.jacc.2018.05.038
2. Pezel T, Viallon M, Croisille P, Sebbag L, Bochaton T, Garot J, et al. Imaging interstitial fibrosis, left ventricular remodeling, and function in stage A and B heart failure. *JACC Cardiovasc Imaging.* (2021) 14:1038–52. doi: 10.1016/j.jcmg.2020.05.036
3. Liang B, Zhou Y, Fu L, Liao HL. Antiarrhythmic mechanisms of Chinese herbal medicine Dingji Fumai Decoction. *Evid Based Complement Alternat Med.* (2020) 2020:9185707. doi: 10.1155/2020/9185707
4. Liang B, Zou FH, Fu L, Liao HL. Chinese Herbal Medicine Dingji Fumai Decoction for ventricular premature contraction: a real-world trial. *Biomed Res Int.* (2020) 2020:5358467. doi: 10.1155/2020/5358467
5. Liang B, Qu Y, Zhao QF, Gu N. Guanxin V for coronary artery disease: a retrospective study. *Biomed Pharmacother.* (2020) 128:110280. doi: 10.1016/j.biopha.2020.110280

6. Zhang XX, Shao CL, Cheng SY, Zhu Y, Liang B, Gu N. Effect of Guanxin V in animal model of acute myocardial infarction. *BMC Complement Med Ther.* (2021) 21:72. doi: 10.1186/s12906-021-03211-7
7. Marrocco I, Altieri F, Peluso I. Measurement and clinical significance of biomarkers of oxidative stress in humans. *Oxid Med Cell Longev.* (2017) 2017:6501046. doi: 10.1155/2017/6501046
8. Yang S, Feskanich D, Willett WC, Eliassen AH, Wu T. Association between global biomarkers of oxidative stress and hip fracture in postmenopausal women: a prospective study. *J Bone Miner Res.* (2014) 29:2577–83. doi: 10.1002/jbmr.2302
9. Zhou Q, Zhu L, Zhang D, Li N, Li Q, Dai P, et al. Oxidative stress-related biomarkers in postmenopausal osteoporosis: a systematic review and meta-analyses. *Dis Markers.* (2016) 2016:7067984. doi: 10.1155/2016/7067984
10. Flatow J, Buckley P, Miller BJ. Meta-analysis of oxidative stress in schizophrenia. *Biol Psychiatry.* (2013) 74:400–9. doi: 10.1016/j.biopsych.2013.03.018
11. Frijhoff J, Winyard PG, Zarkovic N, Davies SS, Stocker R, Cheng D, et al. Clinical relevance of biomarkers of oxidative stress. *Antioxid Redox Signal.* (2015) 23:1144–70. doi: 10.1089/ars.2015.6317
12. Liang B, Zhu YC, Lu J, Gu N. Effects of traditional Chinese medication-based bioactive compounds on cellular and molecular mechanisms of oxidative stress. *Oxid Med Cell Longev.* (2021) 2021:3617498. doi: 10.1155/2021/3617498
13. Münzel T, Camici GG, Maack C, Bonetti NR, Fuster V, Kovacic JC. Impact of oxidative stress on the heart and vasculature: part 2 of a 3-part series. *J Am Coll Cardiol.* (2017) 70:212–29. doi: 10.1016/j.jacc.2017.05.035
14. Mikhael M, Makar C, Wissa A, Le T, Eghbali M, Umar S. Oxidative stress and its implications in the right ventricular remodeling secondary to pulmonary hypertension. *Front Physiol.* (2019) 10:1233. doi: 10.3389/fphys.2019.01233
15. Pena E, Brito J, El Alam S, Siques P. Oxidative stress, kinase activity and inflammatory implications in right ventricular hypertrophy and heart failure under hypobaric hypoxia. *Int J Mol Sci.* (2020) 21:6421. doi: 10.3390/ijms21176421
16. Tsutsui H, Kinugawa S, Matsushima S. Oxidative stress and heart failure. *Am J Physiol Heart Circ Physiol.* (2011) 301:H2181–H90. doi: 10.1152/ajpheart.00554.2011
17. Liang B, Liang Y, Li R, Zhang H, Gu N. Integrating systematic pharmacology-based strategy and experimental validation to explore the synergistic pharmacological mechanisms of Guanxin V in treating ventricular remodeling. *Bioorg Chem.* (2021) 115:105187. doi: 10.1016/j.bioorg.2021.105187
18. Daina A, Michielin O, Zoete V. SwissTargetPrediction: updated data and new features for efficient prediction of protein targets of small molecules. *Nucleic Acids Res.* (2019) 47:W357–W64. doi: 10.1093/nar/gkz382
19. Liang Y, Liang B, Chen W, Wu XR, Liu-Huo WS, Zhao LZ. Potential mechanism of Dingji Fumai Decoction against atrial fibrillation based on network pharmacology, molecular docking, and experimental verification integration strategy. *Front Cardiovasc Med.* (2021) 8:712398. doi: 10.3389/fcvm.2021.712398
20. Stelzer G, Rosen N, Plaschkes I, Zimmerman S, Twik M, Fishilevich S, et al. The genecards suite: from gene data mining to disease genome sequence analyses. *Curr Protoc Bioinformatics.* (2016) 54:1.30.1–1.30.3. doi: 10.1002/cpbi.5
21. Consortium TU. UniProt: a worldwide hub of protein knowledge. *Nucleic Acids Res.* (2018) 47:D506–D15. doi: 10.1093/nar/gky1049
22. Liang Y, Liang B, Wu XR, Chen W, Zhao LZ. Network pharmacology-based systematic analysis of molecular mechanisms of Dingji Fumai Decoction for ventricular arrhythmia. *Evid Based Complement Alternat Med.* (2021) 2021:5535480. doi: 10.1155/2021/5535480
23. Chin CH, Chen SH, Wu HH, Ho CW, Ko MT, Lin CY. cytoHubba: identifying hub objects and sub-networks from complex interactome. *BMC Syst Biol.* (2014) 8 Suppl 4:S11. doi: 10.1186/1752-0509-8-S4-S11
24. Shannon P, Markiel A, Ozier O, Baliga NS, Wang JT, Ramage D, et al. Cytoscape: a software environment for integrated models of biomolecular interaction networks. *Genome Res.* (2003) 13:2498–504. doi: 10.1101/gr.1239303
25. Liang B, Zhang XX, Gu N. Virtual screening and network pharmacology-based synergistic mechanism identification of multiple components contained in Guanxin V against coronary artery disease. *BMC Complement Med Ther.* (2020) 20:345. doi: 10.1186/s12906-020-03133-w
26. Szklarczyk D, Gable AL, Lyon D, Junge A, Wyder S, Huerta-Cepas J, et al. STRING v11: protein-protein association networks with increased coverage, supporting functional discovery in genome-wide experimental datasets. *Nucleic Acids Res.* (2019) 47:D607–D13. doi: 10.1093/nar/gky1131
27. Bader GD, Hogue CWV. An automated method for finding molecular complexes in large protein interaction networks. *BMC Bioinformatics.* (2003) 4:2. doi: 10.1186/1471-2105-4-2
28. Huang DW, Sherman BT, Lempicki RA. Systematic and integrative analysis of large gene lists using DAVID bioinformatics resources. *Nat Protoc.* (2009) 4:44–57. doi: 10.1038/nprot.2008.211
29. Ashburner M, Ball CA, Blake JA, Botstein D, Butler H, Cherry JM, et al. Gene ontology: tool for the unification of biology. The gene ontology consortium. *Nat Genet.* (2000) 25:25–8. doi: 10.1038/75556
30. Kanehisa M, Goto S. KEGG Kyoto encyclopaedia of genes and genomes. *Nucleic Acids Res.* (2000) 28:27–30. doi: 10.1093/nar/28.1.27
31. Zhou JG, Liang B, Jin SH, Liao HL, Du GB, Cheng L, et al. Development and validation of an RNA-Seq-Based prognostic signature in neuroblastoma. *Front Oncol.* (2019) 9:1361. doi: 10.3389/fonc.2019.01361
32. Kanehisa M, Sato Y. KEGG Mapper for inferring cellular functions from protein sequences. *Protein Sci.* (2020) 29:28–35. doi: 10.1002/pro.3711
33. Bindea G, Mlecnik B, Hackl H, Charoentong P, Tosolini M, Kirilovsky A, et al. ClueGO: a Cytoscape plug-in to decipher functionally grouped gene ontology and pathway annotation networks. *Bioinformatics.* (2009) 25:1091–3. doi: 10.1093/bioinformatics/btp101
34. Goodsell DS, Zardecki C, Di Costanzo L, Duarte JM, Hudson BP, Persikova I, et al. RCSB Protein Data Bank: enabling biomedical research and drug discovery. *Protein Sci.* (2020) 29:52–65. doi: 10.1002/pro.3730
35. Kim S, Chen J, Cheng T, Gindulyte A, He J, He S, et al. PubChem in 2021: new data content and improved web interfaces. *Nucleic Acids Res.* (2021) 49:D1388–D95. doi: 10.1093/nar/gkaa971
36. Morris GM, Huey R, Lindstrom W, Sanner MF, Belew RK, Goodsell DS, et al. AutoDock4 and AutoDockTools4: automated docking with selective receptor flexibility. *J Comput Chem.* (2009) 30:2785–91. doi: 10.1002/jcc.21256
37. Stachowski TR, Snell ME, Snell EH. Structural insights into conformational switching in latency-associated peptide between transforming growth factor β-1 bound and unbound states. *IUCrJ.* (2020) 7(Pt 2):238–52. doi: 10.1107/S205225251901707X
38. Maciag JJ, Mackenzie SH, Tucker MB, Schipper JL, Swartz P, Clark AC. Tunable allosteric library of caspase-3 identifies coupling between conserved water molecules and conformational selection. *Proc Natl Acad Sci U S A.* (2016) 113:E6080–E8. doi: 10.1073/pnas.1603549113
39. Yan Z, Qi Z, Yang X, Ji N, Wang Y, Shi Q, et al. The NLRP3 inflammasome: Multiple activation pathways and its role in primary cells during ventricular remodeling. *J Cell Physiol.* (2021) 236:5547–63. doi: 10.1002/jcp.30285
40. Nakayama A, Morita H, Nakao T, Yamaguchi T, Sumida T, Ikeda Y, et al. A food-derived flavonoid luteolin protects against angiotensin II-Induced cardiac remodeling. *PLoS ONE.* (2015) 10:e0137106. doi: 10.1371/journal.pone.0137106
41. Zuo W, Liu N, Zeng Y, Xiao Z, Wu K, Yang F, et al. Luteolin ameliorates experimental pulmonary arterial hypertension via suppressing hippo-YAP/PI3K/AKT signaling pathway. *Front Pharmacol.* (2021) 12:663551. doi: 10.3389/fphar.2021.663551
42. Li X, Xiang D, Shu Y, Zeng X, Li Y. Mitigating effect of tanshinone IIA on ventricular remodeling in rats with pressure overload-induced heart failure. *Acta Cir Bras.* (2019) 34:e201900807. doi: 10.1590/s0102-865020190080000007
43. Feng J, Li S, Chen H. Tanshinone IIA inhibits myocardial remodeling induced by pressure overload via suppressing oxidative stress and inflammation: possible role of silent information regulator 1. *Eur J Pharmacol.* (2016) 791:632–9. doi: 10.1016/j.ejphar.2016.09.041
44. Mao S, Vincent M, Chen M, Zhang M, Hinek A. Exploration of multiple signaling pathways through which sodium tanshinone IIA sulfonate attenuates pathologic remodeling experimental infarction. *Front Pharmacol.* (2019) 10:779. doi: 10.3389/fphar.2019.00779
45. Wu DM, Wang YJ, Han XR, Wen X, Li L, Xu L, et al. Tanshinone IIA prevents left ventricular remodelling via the TLR4/MyD88/NF-κB signalling

pathway in rats with myocardial infarction. *J Cell Mol Med.* (2018) 22:3058–72. doi: 10.1111/jcmm.13557

46. Mao S, Li X, Wang L, Yang PC, Zhang M. Rationale and design of sodium tanshinone IIA sulfonate in left ventricular remodeling secondary to acute myocardial infarction (STAMP-REMODELING) trial: a randomized controlled study. *Cardiovasc Drugs Ther.* (2015) 29:535–42. doi: 10.1007/s10557-015-6625-2
47. Wang AW, Song L, Miao J, Wang HX, Tian C, Jiang X, et al. Baicalein attenuates angiotensin II-induced cardiac remodeling via inhibition of AKT/mTOR, ERK1/2, NF-κB, and calcineurin signaling pathways in mice. *Am J Hypertens.* (2015) 28:518–26. doi: 10.1093/ajh/hpu194
48. Shi R, Wei Z, Zhu D, Fu N, Wang C, Yin S, et al. Baicalein attenuates monocrotaline-induced pulmonary arterial hypertension by inhibiting vascular remodeling in rats. *Pulm Pharmacol Ther.* (2018) 48:124–35. doi: 10.1016/j.pupt.2017.11.003
49. Hsu WL, Lin YC, Jeng JR, Chang HY, Chou TC. Baicalein ameliorates pulmonary arterial hypertension caused by monocrotaline through downregulation of ET-1 and ETR in pneumonectomized rats. *Am J Chin Med.* (2018) 46:769–83. doi: 10.1142/S0192415X18500404

4

Organelle Crosstalk Regulators are Regulated in Diseases, Tumors and Regulatory T Cells: Novel Classification of Organelle Crosstalk Regulators

Ming Liu[1,2], Na Wu[3†], Keman Xu[1†], Fatma Saaoud[1†], Eleni Vasilopoulos[1†], Ying Shao[1†], Ruijing Zhang[1,4†], Jirong Wang[1,5†], Haitao Shen[3†], William Y. Yang[6†], Yifan Lu[1], Yu Sun[1], Charles Drummer IV[1], Lu Liu[7], Li Li[2], Wenhui Hu[7], Jun Yu[7], Domenico Praticò[8], Jianxin Sun[9], Xiaohua Jiang[1,7], Hong Wang[7] and Xiaofeng Yang[1,7]*

[1] Centers for Cardiovascular Research, Lewis Katz School of Medicine at Temple University, Philadelphia, PA, United States, [2] Department of Cell Biology and Genetics, School of Basic Medical Science, Shanxi Medical University, Taiyuan, China, [3] Departments of Endocrinology and Emergency Medicine, Shengjing Hospital of China Medical University, Shenyang, China, [4] Department of Nephrology, The Affiliated People's Hospital of Shanxi Medical University, Taiyuan, China, [5] Department of Cardiology, The Affiliated People's Hospital of Shanxi Medical University, Taiyuan, China, [6] Rutgers University, New Brunswick, NJ, United States, [7] Metabolic Disease Research, Inflammation, Translational & Clinical Lung Research, Thrombosis Research, Lewis Katz School of Medicine at Temple University, Philadelphia, PA, United States, [8] Alzheimer's Center, Lewis Katz School of Medicine at Temple University, Philadelphia, PA, United States, [9] Department of Medicine, Center for Translational Medicine, Thomas Jefferson University, Philadelphia, PA, United States

***Correspondence:**
Xiaofeng Yang
xfyang@temple.edu

[†] These authors have contributed equally to this work

To examine whether the expressions of 260 organelle crosstalk regulators (OCRGs) in 16 functional groups are modulated in 23 diseases and 28 tumors, we performed extensive -omics data mining analyses and made a set of significant findings: (1) the ratios of upregulated vs. downregulated OCRGs are 1:2.8 in acute inflammations, 1:1 in metabolic diseases, 1:1.2 in autoimmune diseases, and 1:3.8 in organ failures; (2) sepsis and trauma-upregulated OCRG groups such as vesicle, mitochondrial (MT) fission, and mitophagy but not others, are termed as the cell crisis-handling OCRGs. Similarly, sepsis and trauma plus organ failures upregulated seven OCRG groups including vesicle, MT fission, mitophagy, sarcoplasmic reticulum–MT, MT fusion, autophagosome–lysosome fusion, and autophagosome/endosome–lysosome fusion, classified as the cell failure-handling OCRGs; (3) suppression of autophagosome–lysosome fusion in endothelial and epithelial cells is required for viral replications, which classify this decreased group as the viral replication-suppressed OCRGs; (4) pro-atherogenic damage-associated molecular patterns (DAMPs) such as oxidized low-density lipoprotein (oxLDL), lipopolysaccharide (LPS), oxidized-1-palmitoyl-2-arachidonoyl-sn-glycero-3-phosphocholine (oxPAPC), and interferons (IFNs) totally upregulated 33 OCRGs in endothelial cells (ECs) including vesicle, MT fission, mitophagy, MT fusion, endoplasmic reticulum (ER)–MT contact, ER–plasma membrane (PM) junction, autophagosome/endosome–lysosome fusion, sarcoplasmic reticulum–MT, autophagosome–endosome/lysosome fusion, and ER–Golgi complex (GC) interaction as the 10 EC-activation/inflammation-promoting OCRG groups; (5) the expression of OCRGs is upregulated more than downregulated in regulatory T cells (Tregs) from the lymph nodes, spleen, peripheral blood, intestine, and brown adipose tissue in comparison with that of $CD4^{+}CD25^{-}$ T effector controls; (6) toll-like receptors (TLRs), reactive oxygen species (ROS) regulator nuclear factor erythroid 2-related factor 2 (Nrf2), and inflammasome-activated regulator caspase-1 regulated the expressions of OCRGs in diseases, virus-infected cells, and pro-atherogenic DAMP-treated ECs; (7) OCRG expressions are significantly modulated in all the 28 cancer datasets, and the upregulated OCRGs are correlated with tumor immune infiltrates in some tumors; (8) tumor promoter factor IKK2 and tumor suppressor Tp53 significantly modulate the expressions of OCRGs. Our findings provide novel insights on the roles of upregulated OCRGs in the pathogenesis of inflammatory diseases and cancers, and novel pathways for the future therapeutic interventions for inflammations, sepsis, trauma, organ failures, autoimmune diseases, metabolic cardiovascular diseases (CVDs), and cancers.

Keywords: organelle crosstalk, inflammation, cancers and tumors, viral infections, endothelial cell activation, Treg

INTRODUCTION

Cardiovascular diseases (CVDs), such as coronary heart disease, hypertension, stroke, and peripheral artery disease, have become the number 1 cause of death globally (1, 2). We and others recently reported that CVD stressors and risk factors such as hyperlipidemia (3, 4), hyperglycemia (5), hyperhomocysteinemia (6, 7), and chronic kidney disease (8–10) promote atherosclerosis and vascular inflammation via several mechanisms. These mechanisms include innate immune activation (11) of endothelial cells (ECs) (3, 12–15) promoting EC injury (16); Ly6Chigh inflammatory mouse monocyte and $CD40^{+}$ human monocyte differentiation (7, 17–19); disease reprogrammed macrophages (20–22); cytokine and secretome regulation (23–30); decreased/transdifferentiated $CD4^{+}Foxp3^{+}$ regulatory T cells (Treg) (24, 31–34); and impaired vascular repairability of bone marrow-derived progenitor cells (35, 36). In addition, we recently proposed new models such as intracellular organelle dangers (37) and reactive oxygen species (ROS) as an integrated sensing system for metabolic homeostasis and alarming (38), which indicated that metabolic reprogramming and dysfunction trigger mitochondrial (MT) ROS (4, 39–42); caspase-1/inflammasome activation (8, 10) downregulated histone modification enzymes (43) and increased expressions of trained immunity pathway enzymes (22, 39, 44–47). These reports have clearly demonstrated that mitochondria play significant roles in connecting metabolic reprogramming and dysfunction to inflammation initiation and gene transcription. However, the question of how organelle crosstalk regulates the progression of various diseases remains poorly characterized.

With progress of super-multiplexed optical imaging and barcoding (48) and other system-level spectral imaging and analyses (49, 50), it has been recognized that the crosstalk between mitochondria and other organelles, such as lysosomes, peroxisomes, and the endoplasmic reticulum (ER) (51), is mediated by transcriptional programs and other signaling mechanisms (52). Organelle exchange materials including lipids, ions, and proteins at the membrane contact sites (MCSs), which may be different from membrane trafficking between organelles by vesiculotubular carriers regulated by Rab GTPase (53). Organelle interactions also likely mediate organelle dysfunction downstream of MT impairments (54). In addition, external or internal stress activates several well-orchestrated processes aimed at either restoring cellular homeostasis or committing cell death (55). These processes include unfolded protein response (UPR) in ER and mitochondria (56), autophagy, hypoxia, and MT function, which underlie the ER stress response (57), suggesting that cellular pathological responses may be mediated in organelle crosstalk mechanisms (58). Accordingly, alterations to these networks, such as impaired ER–mitochondria MCSs, have been linked to several diseases such as neurodegeneration (59, 60), CVD (61), diabetes (62), kidney diseases (63, 64), and cancers (65, 66).

Regardless of significant progress in the field, the following questions remained poorly understood: (1) how many regulators (regulatomes) participate in organelle crosstalk; (2) whether the expressions of organelle crosstalk regulatomes are modulated in various disease conditions such as acute inflammation (AI) and injuries, chronic inflammations, autoimmune diseases (ADs), metabolic diseases (MDs), and cancers; (3) whether the expressions of organelle crosstalk regulatomes are differentially modulated in various cell types in response to pathological stimuli; and (4) what are the potential mechanisms regulating expression of organelle crosstalk regulators (OCRGs). To address these important questions, we examined our novel hypothesis that pathological conditions and various DAMPs significantly modulate the expressions of organelle crosstalk regulators in disease-specific and cell type-specific manner. To test this hypothesis, we collected 260 organelle crosstalk regulators as the regulatomes that participate in 16 organelle crosstalk processes including (1) MT biogenesis, (2) MT fission, (3) MT fusion, (4) MT fission and fusion, (5) mitophagy, (6) MT protein translocation, (7) MT contact site, (8) ER (67)–MT contact (68), (9) sarcoplasmic reticulum–MT

(69), (10) ER–plasma conjunctions (70, 71), (11) ER–Golgi interaction, (12) ER–endosome, (13) autophagosome–lysosome fusion, (14) autophagosome–endosome/lysosome fusion (68), (15) endosome–Golgi trafficking, and (16) vesicle (**Table 1**). We performed an extensive -omics database mining and determined the expressions of 260 organelle crosstalk regulators in more than 50 microarrays from more than 20 diseases and 28 cancers/tumors. Corresponding mechanisms were explored, such as the regulation of (a) (TLRs); (b) caspase-1; (c) ROS; and (d) oncogenes/tumor suppressors and made a set of significant findings. Our findings have provided novel insights on pathophysiological roles of OCRGs in various inflammations, diseases, and cancers and provide novel therapeutic targets and strategies for various inflammations, CVD, MDs, and cancers.

METHODS

Expression Profile of Organelle Crosstalk Regulator Genes in Microarray Data From Patients With Various Inflammatory Diseases and Cancers

The 25 microarray datasets of AI and injuries, ADs, MDs, and CVDs (**Table 2**); one microarray dataset of Middle East respiratory syndrome coronavirus (MERS-CoV)-infected human microvascular ECs; one microarray dataset of severe respiratory syndrome coronavirus (SARS-CoV)-infected human airway epithelial cells; two microarray datasets of influenza virus-infected lung epithelial cells, Calu-3 cells (non-small-cell lung cancer cell line), and human umbilical vein ECs (HUVECs); one microarray of Kaposi sarcoma-associated herpes virus-infected primary human dermal ECs (**Table 3**); six microarrays of ECs treated by pro-atherogenic DAMPs (**Table 4**); six microarray datasets of Treg cells (**Table 5**); 15 microarrays of Treg regulator deficiency (**Table 6**); six microarrays of TLR deficiencies (**Table 7**); one microarray of ROS negative regulator nuclear factor erythroid 2-related factor 2 (Nrf2) deficiency (**Table 8**); and two microarrays of caspase-1 deficiency (**Table 9**) were collected from National Institutes of Health (NIH)–National Center for Biotechnology Information (NCBI)–Gene Expression Omnibus (GEO) databases (https://www.ncbi.nlm.nih.gov/gds/) and analyzed with an online software GEO2R (https://www.ncbi.nlm.nih.gov/geo/geo2r/). In addition, gene expression data from 28 cancers were analyzed with the Gene Expression Profiling Interactive Analysis (GEPIA2) database (http://gepia2.cancer-pku.cn/#index), in which dataset sources were from The Cancer Genome Atlas (TCGA)/Genotype-Tissue Expression (GTEx) data (**Table 10**). Furthermore, 19 microarray datasets of oncogene and tumor suppressor deficiencies were collected from NCBI–GEO and analyzed with GEO2R (**Table 11**). The differentially expressed OCRGs and their changes in all microarrays and TCGA datasets are listed in **Supplementary Tables 1, 2**. The original microarray experiments used different cells, which prevented us from comparing the effects of disease conditions in regulating OCRGs in the same cell types. Of note, our approach was well-justified. For example, as a common practice, we (23) and others (72) often studied gene expression in non-ideal heterogeneous peripheral blood mononuclear cell (PBMC) populations in pathophysiological conditions, which are actually composed of many cell types (also see the Discussion section).

Metascape Pathway Analysis

We utilized Metascape Pathway Analysis (MPA; http://metascape.org/gp/index.html#/main/step1) (73) to characterize molecular and cellular functions related to the identified genes in our microarray analysis. Differentially expressed genes were identified and uploaded into MPA for analysis. The core and pathways analysis was used to identify molecular and cellular pathways, as we have previously reported (23).

Protein–Protein Interaction Analysis

Protein–protein interaction (PPI) networks were generated from STRING database (https://string-db.org/). Enrichment analysis results of the shared gene and top 10 connected proteins were downloaded and visualized by using Cytoscape software 3.7.2 (https://cytoscape.org/) (74).

Immune Infiltrate Analyses

TISIDB database (75) (http://cis.hku.hk/TISIDB/index.php) and Gene Set Cancer Analysis (GSCA) database (http://bioinfo.life.hust.edu.cn/GSCA/#/immune) (76) were used in the immune cell infiltrate analyses.

Statistical Analysis of Microarray Data

Twelve housekeeping genes including CHMP2A, EMC7, GPI, PSMB2, PSMB4, RAB7A, SNRPD3, VPS29, VCP, ACTB, RPL27, and OAZ1 (**Supplementary Table 3** of Housekeeping Genes) in all 85 GEO datasets regardless of species were chosen for this study. The housekeeping gene list was extracted from the list provided by Eisenberg and de Jonge (77, 78). Briefly, the mean fold change (FC) of housekeeping genes between treatment and control groups varies from 0.72 to 1.55. As this variation was out of the range of FC < 0.5 or FC > 2 ($|\log2FC| > 1$), we concluded that the datasets were of high quality. The target genes with expression changes more than 2-fold in microarrays were defined as the upregulated genes, while genes with their expression decreased more than 2-fold in microarrays were defined as downregulated genes ($p < 0.05$, $|\log2FC| > 1$).

RESULTS

The Ratios of Upregulated vs. Downregulated Organelle Crosstalk Regulators in Diseases Are Different, and Differentially Expressed Organelle Crosstalk Regulators Are Shared in Diseases

We hypothesized that pathological conditions significantly modulate the expressions of organelle crosstalk regulators in disease-specific and cell type-specific manner. To examine this hypothesis, we collected 260 organelle crosstalk regulators (regulatomic genes and OCRGs) in 16 groups (**Figure 1**) and

TABLE 1 | Two hundred sixty organelle crosstalk regulators (OCRGs) were searched from three databases such as National Center for Biotechnology Information (NCBI), Gene Set Enrichment Analysis (GSEA), and the Human Protein Atlas (HPA) website.

Classification of OCRGs	No.	Gene symbol	Source
Mitochondrial biogenesis	5	POLG, VCP, HSPD1, HSPA4, LONP1	PMID: 28094012, 24784582, 22298039, 22424226, 21659532
Mitochondrial fission	28	COX10, DCN, DDHD1, DDHD2, DHODH, DNM1, DNM2, DNM3, GGNBP1, INF2, KDR, LRRK2, MAPT, MIEF1, MIEF2, MTFP1, MTFR1, MTFR1L, MTFR2, MX1, MX2, MYO19, PINK1, PPARGC1A, SLC25A46, STAT2, TMEM135, VPS35	Gene Set Enrichment Analysis (GSEA) (https://www.gsea-msigdb.org/gsea/index.jsp)
Mitochondrial fusion	15	ADCK1, AFG3L2, BAK1, BAX, CHCHD3, MFN1, MFN2, MIGA1, MIGA2, OMA1, PID1, PLD6, STOML2, USP30, VAT1	GSEA (https://www.gsea-msigdb.org/gsea/index.jsp)
Mitochondrial fission and fusion	7	BNIP3, DNM1L, FIS1, GDAP1, MFF, MUL1, OPA1	GSEA (https://www.gsea-msigdb.org/gsea/index.jsp)
Mitophagy	28	PINK1, OPTN, SQSTM1, PARL, USP30, RING1, RNF2, ATG9a, VMP1, CALCOCO2, ATG4a, ATG7, ATG3, ATG12, ATG5, ATG10, ATG13, OMA1, TBK1, GABARAP, MAP1LC3A, VDAC1, BNIP3L, BNIP3, FUNDC1, BCL2L13, FKBP8,	PMID: 27291334, 25479550, 29358684, 29370689, 30540226
Mitochondrial protein translocation	7	TOMM5, TOMM6, TOMM7, TOMM20, TOMM22, TOMM40, TOMM70	PMID: 28301740
Mitochondrial contact site	4	CHCHD3, CHCHD6, APOO, APOOL, IMMT	PMID: 24687277
Endoplasmic reticulum–mitochondria contact	13	RMDN3, VAPB, VAPA, BCAP31, MCU, ITPR1, HSPA9, BAK1, DAPK1, MFN1, MFN2, VDAC1, FIS1	PMID: 28301744, 26627931
Sarcoplasmic reticulum–mitochondria contact	9	VDAC1, HSPA9, ITPR1, SIGMAR1, ATP2A1, VAPB, RMDN3, OSBPL8, OSBPL5	PMID: 28275246
Endoplasmic reticulum–plasma membrane junctions	10	ORAI1, STIM1, SEC61B, JPH1, JPH2, JPH3, JPH4, PTPN1, STX1A, SEC22B	PMID: 26322679, 22914293, 28554772, 28301744
Endoplasmic reticulum–Golgi interaction	6	VAPA, VAPB, PLEKHA8, PITPNM1, OSBP, STX5	PMID: 32065234, 23913272, 24209621, 31357511
Endoplasmic reticulum–endosome	7	STARD3, PTPN1, EGFR, OSBPL1A, STARD3NL, RAB7A, NPC1	PMID: 26627931
Autophagosome–lysosome fusion	4	OCRL, MCOLN1, TLR9, TIRAP	PMID: 27398910
Autophagosome–endosome/lysosome fusion	9	VAMP8, RAB7A, PLEKHM1, RILP, ATG14, VPS39, VPS41, SNAP29, STX17	PMID: 27283760
Endosome–Golgi trafficking	4	TBC1D23, GOLGA1, GOLGA4, FAM91A1	PMID: 29084197
Vesicle	125	AASS, ABCD3, ABHD14A, ACAA1, ACBD5, ADCYAP1R1, AGPS, AKAP9, ANKFY1, ANKRD2, ANKRD6, AP1B1, AP1G1, ARCN1, ATP11A, ATP23, AZU1, BMP2, C7orf43, CAT, CCDC93, CCZ1, CCZ1B, CD24, CDKL1, CHGB, CHIC2, CLIP4, CLOCK, CLTA, CLTC, CNNM2, CSF2, CSTF2T, CTAG2, CTSA, CYB5A, CYP27C1, DAB1, DAB, DBH, DNAJA3, DPP7, DRAM2, DYRK4, ECI2, EDA, EIF4ENIF1, EPS15, ERGIC1, FAF2, FYCO1, GPRC5A, GRN, GTPBP2, HDHD3, HEXIM1, HGS, HIP1, HSD17B4, HSD3B7, IGF2R, ITCH, ITM2B, KLRG1, LAMP3, MBD1, MEF2D, MIA3, MITD1, NACC1, NMRK2, NOV, NSDHL, OSBPL5, P4HA2, PDCD6IP, PDXDC1, PEX14, PICALM, PLCH1, PLIN3, PLIN4, PNPLA2, POU2F2, PPARG, PPOX, PUSL1, RAB11A, RAB11FIP1, RAB11FIP5, RAB20, RAB30, RAB5C, RALY, RANBP2, RANGAP1, RC3H2, RPS6KC1, RPTOR, RUNX1, SAMD9, SEC23IP, SERPINA1, SERTM1, SET, SNX1, SPINK5, SQSTM1, STK11IP, STX16, SYNDIG1, SYNPO2, TBK1, TMEM63A, TNPO3, TYR, VAC14, VPS26A, VTI1B, ZDHHC13, ZFYVE16, ZFYVE9, ZNF266, ZNF326	The human protein atlas (HPA) (https://www.proteinatlas.org/humanproteome/cell/vesicles)

were effectively detected (**Table 1**). Among the OCRGs, 19 genes can be classified into two groups, and one gene can be classified into three groups (**Supplementary Figure 1**), so that a total of 281 genes were calculated when using a donut chart to show percentages of the gene classifications. The OCRGs included (1) five genes in MT biogenesis (2%), (2) 28 genes in MT fission (10%), (3) 15 genes in MT fusion (5%), (4) seven genes in MT fission and fusion (2%), (5) 28 genes in mitophagy (10%), (6) seven genes in MT protein translocation (2%), (7) four genes in MT contact site (1%), (8) 13 genes in ER–MT contact (5%), (9) nine genes in sarcoplasmic reticulum–MT (3%), (10) 10 genes in ER–plasma conjunctions (3%), (11) six genes in ER–Golgi interaction (2%), (12) seven genes in ER–endosome (2%), (13) four genes in autophagosome–lysosome fusion (1%), (14) nine genes in autophagosome–endosome/lysosome fusion (3%), (15) four genes in endosome–Golgi trafficking

TABLE 2 | Twenty-five microarray datasets including acute inflammations, metabolic diseases, autoimmune diseases, and organ failure diseases in the National Institutes of Health (NIH)–National Center for Biotechnology Information (NCBI)–Gene Expression Omnibus (GEO) dataset database (https://www.ncbi.nlm.nih.gov/gds/) were collected to analyze the expression changes of organelle crosstalk regulators (OCRGs).

GEO ID	Disease/phenotype	Tissue	Comparison	Upregulated	Downregulated	PMID
Acute inflammation						
GSE32707	Lung injury	Whole blood	Sepsis day 0 vs. without sepsis	4	8	22461369
	Lung injury	Whole blood	Sepsis day 7 vs. without sepsis	6	2	22461369
	Lung injury	Whole blood	Sepsis ARDS day 0 vs. without sepsis ARDS	2	10	22461369
	Lung injury	Whole blood	Sepsis ARDS day 7 vs. without Sepsis ARDS	7	5	22461369
GSE13904	Septic shock	Whole blood	Sepsis day 1 vs. normal	13	6	19325468
	Septic shock	Whole blood	Sepsis day 3 vs. normal	3	1	19325468
	Septic shock	Whole blood	Sepsis shock day 1 vs. normal	9	9	19325468
	Septic shock	Whole blood	Sepsis shock day 3 vs. normal	12	13	19325468
GSE5580	Severe trauma	Monocytes	Severe trauma vs. health	4	20	17032758
	Severe trauma	Leukocytes	Severe trauma vs. health	3	21	17032758
	Severe trauma	T cells	Severe trauma vs. health	8	23	17032758
Metabolic disease						
GSE2508	Obese	Adipocytes	Non-diabetic obese vs. non-diabetic lean	1	2	16059715
GSE48964	Obese	Adipose stem cells	Morbidly obese vs. nonobese	0	1	24040759
GSE55200	MHO	Subcutaneous adipose	MHO vs. LH	0	1	24933025
	MUO	Subcutaneous adipose	MUO vs. LH	1	1	24933025
GSE94752	Obese IR	Adipocytes	Obese IR vs. lean	2	0	28570579
	Obese IS	Adipocytes	Obese IS vs. lean	0	0	28570579
GSE23343	T2D	Liver	T2D vs. normal glucose tolerance	7	7	21035759
GSE29221	T2D	Skeletal muscle	T2D vs. non-diabetes	10	22	23308243
GSE29226	T2D	Subcutaneous adipose	T2D vs. non-diabetes	6	6	23308243
GSE29231	T2D	Visceral adipose	T2D vs. non-diabetes	17	5	23308243
GSE28829	Atherosclerosis	Carotid artery	Advanced plaque vs. early plaque	3	0	22388324
GSE41571	Atherosclerosis	Macrophages from plaques	Ruptured plaques vs. stable plaque	14	11	23122912
GSE6054	FHC and atherosclerosis	Monocytes	FHC homozygote vs. control	5	9	19040724
GSE6088	FHC and atherosclerosis	T cell	FHC homozygote vs. control	4	7	19040724
GSE1010	FCH	Lymphoblastic cells	FCH vs. normal	1	2	15388524
Autoimmune disease						
GSE10500	RA	Macrophages*	RA vs. normal	18	31	18345002
GSE97779	RA	Macrophages*	RA vs. normal	25	40	28813657
GSE109248	ACLE	Skin	ACL vs. normal	15	9	29889098
	CCLE	Skin	CCL vs. normal	15	5	29889098
	Psoriasis	Skin	Psoriasis vs. normal	39	20	29889098
	SCLE	Skin	SCL vs. normal	22	24	29889098
GSE38713	UC	Sigmoid colon or rectum	UC active involved vs. normal	13	13	23135761
GSE3365	UC	PBMC	UC vs. normal	1	4	16436634
	CD	PBMC	CD vs. normal	2	1	16436634
Organ failure						
GSE76701	Heart failure	Left ventricle	Failing heart vs. non-failing heart	1	2	26756417
GSE38941	HBV-ALF	Liver	HBV-ALF vs. normal	24	25	23185381
GSE37171	ESRF	Whole blood	Chronic renal failure vs. healthy controls	0	38	23809614
GSE15072	CKD hemodialysis	PBMC	Hemodialysis vs. healthy controls	16	63	19698090

Expression of OCRGs was examined in a total of 39 comparison datasets. There are significantly expressed OCRGs in 38 datasets (except GSE94752 obese IS vs. lean) ($p < 0.05$, $|logFC| > 1$).

Macrophages, macrophages from synovial fluids for RA and blood-derived macrophages for control. All the studies and samples are from humans.*

ARDS, acute respiratory distress syndrome; ALI, acute liver injury; ALF, acute liver failure; PBMC, peripheral blood mononuclear cell; IS, insulin sensitive; IR, insulin resistance; MHO, metabolically healthy obese; MUO, metabolically unhealthy obese; LH, lean health; T2D, type 2 diabetes; FCH, familial combined hyperlipidemia; FHC, familial hypercholesterolemia; RA, rheumatoid arthritis; ACLE, acute cutaneous lupus; CCLE, chronic cutaneous lupus; SCLE, subacute cutaneous lupus; UC, ulcerative colitis; CD, Crohn's Disease; HBV-ALF, hepatitis B virus-associated acute liver failure; ESRF, end-stage renal failure; CKD, chronic kidney disease.

TABLE 3 | Three microarray datasets of time course including MERS coronavirus, SARS coronavirus, avian influenza virus, one dataset of influenza virus infected human umbilical vein endothelial cells and one dataset of Kaposi sarcoma-associated herpes virus infection in the National Institutes of Health (NIH)–National Center for Biotechnology Information (NCBI)–Gene Expression Omnibus (GEO) datasets database (https://www.ncbi.nlm.nih.gov/gds/) were collected to analyze the expression changes of genes that we are interested in.

GEO ID	Comparison	Cell/tissue	Upregulated	Downregulated	PMID
GSE79218	icMERS-inoculated vs. mock-inoculated (0 h)	Human microvascular endothelial cells	0	1	28830941
	icMERS-inoculated vs. mock-inoculated (12 h)	Human microvascular endothelial cells	20	16	28830941
	icMERS-inoculated vs. mock-inoculated (24 h)	Human microvascular endothelial cells	41	44	28830941
	icMERS-inoculated vs. mock-inoculated (36 h)	Human microvascular endothelial cells	39	46	28830941
	icMERS-inoculated vs. mock-inoculated (48 h)	Human microvascular endothelial cells	25	24	28830941
GSE47960	SARS-CoV-infected vs. mock-infected (0 h)	Human airway epithelium cells	3	0	23935999
	SARS-CoV-infected vs. mock-infected (12 h)	Human airway epithelium cells	0	0	23935999
	SARS-CoV-infected vs. mock-infected (24 h)	Human airway epithelium cells	2	1	23935999
	SARS-CoV-infected vs. mock-infected (36 h)	Human airway epithelium cells	1	0	23935999
	SARS-CoV-infected vs. mock-infected (48 h)	Human airway epithelium cells	3	0	23935999
	SARS-CoV-infected vs. mock-infected (60 h)	Human airway epithelium cells	15	0	23935999
	SARS-CoV-infected vs. mock-infected (72 h)	Human airway epithelium cells	4	2	23935999
	SARS-CoV-infected vs. mock-infected (84 h)	Human airway epithelium cells	5	0	23935999
	SARS-CoV-infected vs. mock-infected (96 h)	Human airway epithelium cells	7	1	23935999
	H1N1-infected vs. mock-infected (0 h)	Human airway epithelium cells	1	0	23935999
	H1N1-infected vs. mock-infected (6 h)	Human airway epithelium cells	6	0	23935999
	H1N1-infected vs. mock-infected (12 h)	Human airway epithelium cells	11	6	23935999
	H1N1-infected vs. mock-infected (18 h)	Human airway epithelium cells	20	21	23935999
	H1N1-infected vs. mock-infected (24 h)	Human airway epithelium cells	22	29	23935999
	H1N1-infected vs. mock-infected (36 h)	Human airway epithelium cells	27	30	23935999
	H1N1-infected vs. mock-infected (48 h)	Human airway epithelium cells	18	16	23935999
GSE49840	H7N9-infected vs. mock-infected (3 h)	Calu-3 cells	1	2	24496798
	H7N9-infected vs. mock-infected (7 h)	Calu-3 cells	3	0	24496798
	H7N9-infected vs. mock-infected (12 h)	Calu-3 cells	8	3	24496798
	H7N9-infected vs. mock-infected (24 h)	Calu-3 cells	30	70	24496798
	H7N7-infected vs. mock-infected (3 h)	Calu-3 cells	1	0	24496798
	H7N7-infected vs. mock-infected (7 h)	Calu-3 cells	0	0	24496798
	H7N7-infected vs. mock-infected (12 h)	Calu-3 cells	5	4	24496798
	H7N7-infected vs. mock-infected (24 h)	Calu-3 cells	38	109	24496798
	H5N1-infected vs. mock-infected (3 h)	Calu-3 cells	1	2	24496798
	H5N1-infected vs. mock-infected (7 h)	Calu-3 cells	2	0	24496798
	H5N1-infected vs. mock-infected (12 h)	Calu-3 cells	6	0	24496798
	H5N1-infected vs. mock-infected (24 h)	Calu-3 cells	40	92	24496798
	H3N2-infected vs. mock-infected (3 h)	Calu-3 cells	1	3	24496798
	H3N2-infected vs. mock-infected (7 h)	Calu-3 cells	3	0	24496798
	H3N2-infected vs. mock-infected (12 h)	Calu-3 cells	12	16	24496798
	H3N2-infected vs. mock-infected (24 h)	Calu-3 cells	19	42	24496798
GSE59226	Influenza virus (H9N2)-infected vs. inactivate virus-infected	Human umbilical vein endothelial cells	27	137	25863179
GSE1377	Kaposi sarcoma-associated herpes virus-infected for 7 days vs. uninfected control	Primary human dermal endothelial cells	6	10	15220917

MERS-CoV, Middle East respiratory syndrome coronavirus; SARS-CoV, severe acute respiratory syndrome coronavirus; H1N1, H7N9, H7N7, H5N1, H3N2, and H9N2, influenza viruses.

(1%), and (16) 125 genes in vesicle (44%). To confirm the functional focuses of the OCRGs, we performed the MPA using the database (http://metascape.org/gp/index.html#/main/step1) (73). Our analysis showed that 260 OCRGs were indeed enriched in MT organization, MT fission, autophagy, vesicle organization, and organelle organization, which can be viewed in **Supplementary Figure 2**. As shown in **Table 2**, the expressions of 260 OCRGs were examined in four major categories of diseases, in a total of 23 types of diseases. These diseases and cell types were (a) three types of AIs such as lung injury (whole blood), septic shock (whole blood), and severe trauma (monocytes, leukocytes, and T cells); (b) nine types of MDs including obesity (adipocytes and adipose stem cells) and metabolically healthy obesity (MHO; subcutaneous adipose). Based on the criteria,

TABLE 4 | Six microarray datasets about endothelial cells in pro-atherogenic damage-associated molecular patterns (DAMPs) such as oxLDL, LPS, oxPAPC, and IFN treated conditions in the National Institutes of Health (NIH)–National Center for Biotechnology Information (NCBI)–Gene Expression Omnibus (GEO) datasets database (https://www.ncbi.nlm.nih.gov/gds/) were collected to analyze the changes of organelle interactions and vesicle-related gene.

GEO ID	Comparison	Cell/tissue	Upregulated	Downregulated	PMID
GSE5883	10-ng LPS stimulation for 4 h vs. without LPS stimulation	Human lung microvascular endothelial cells	8	7	NA
	10-ng LPS stimulation for 8 h vs. without LPS stimulation	Human lung microvascular endothelial cells	17	15	NA
	10-ng LPS stimulation for 24 h vs. without LPS stimulation	Human lung microvascular endothelial cells	9	14	NA
GSE3920	1,000 IU IFNα treated for 5 h vs. untreated control	Human umbilical vein endothelial cells	7	0	17202376, 19553003
	1,000 IU IFNβ treated for 5 h vs. untreated control	Human umbilical vein endothelial cells	11	0	17202376, 19553003
	1,000 IU IFNγ treated for 5 h vs. untreated control	Human umbilical vein endothelial cells	6	0	17202376, 19553003
GSE85987	Scrambled control siRNA vs. NOTCH1 siRNA	Human umbilical vein endothelial cells	0	0	29449332
	NOTCH1 siRNA + IL-1β treated for 24 h vs. scrambled siRNA	Human umbilical vein endothelial cells	0	1	29449332
GSE72633	NOTCH1 siRNA vs. scrambled control siRNA	Human aortic endothelial cells	3	6	26552708
	oxPAPC treated vs. scrambled control siRNA	Human aortic endothelial cells	8	6	26552708
GSE26953	Oscillatory shear vs. laminar shear (fibrosa)	Human aortic valvular endothelial cells	0	0	21705672
	Oscillatory shear vs. laminar shear (ventricularis)	Human aortic valvular endothelial cells	0	0	21705672
GSE39264	ApoE KO vs. WT	Mouse aortic endothelial cells	0	0	23990205
	LPS treated for 4 h vs. DMEM treated for 4 h	Mouse aortic endothelial cells	3	5	23990205
	oxLDL treated for 4 h vs. DMEM treated for 4 h	Mouse aortic endothelial cells	0	6	23990205
	oxPAPC treated for 4 h vs. DMEM treated for 4 h	Mouse aortic endothelial cells	7	7	23990205

LPS, lipopolysaccharide; IFN, interferon; oxPAPC, oxidized 1-palmitoyl-2-arachidonoyl-sn-glycero-3-phosphocholine (inflammatory lipids); oxLDL, oxidized low-density lipoprotein; KO, knockout; WT, wild type; DMEM, Dulbecco's minimum essential medium.

TABLE 5 | Six microarray datasets about Treg cells in the National Institutes of Health (NIH)–National Center for Biotechnology Information (NCBI)–Gene Expression Omnibus (GEO) datasets database (https://www.ncbi.nlm.nih.gov/gds/) were collected to analyze the changes of organelle interactions and vesicle-related gene ($p < 0.05$, $|\log FC| > 1$).

GEO ID	Comparison	Tissue	Upregulated	Downregulated	PMID
GSE37532	$CD3^+CD4^+CD25^+$ Treg cells vs. $CD3^+CD4^+CD25^-$ Tconv cells	LN	3	0	25550516
	$CD3^+CD4^+CD25^+$ Treg cells vs. $CD3^+CD4^+CD25^-$ Tconv cells	Visceral adipose tissue	12	0	25550516
GSE64909	$CD4^+CD25^+Foxp3^+$ Treg vs. $CD4^+Foxp3^-$ Tconv (cold)	Brown adipose tissue	2	0	25714366
	$CD4^+CD25^+Foxp3^+$ Treg vs. $CD4^+Foxp3^-$ Tconv (warm)	Brown adipose tissue	3	0	25714366
	$CD4^+CD25^+Foxp3^+$ Treg vs. $CD4^+Foxp3^-$ Tconv (warm)	Spleen	3	1	25714366
GSE50096	$CD4^+$ $Foxp3^+$ Treg cells vs. $CD4^+$ $Foxp3^-$ Tconv cells (injured 4d)	Skeletal muscle	4	4	24315098
	$CD4^+$ $Foxp3^+$ Treg cells vs. $CD4^+$ $Foxp3^-$ Tconv cells (injured 14d)	Skeletal muscle	7	2	24315098
	$CD4^+$ $Foxp3^+$ Treg cells vs. $CD4^+$ $Foxp3^-$ Tconv cells (injured 4d)	Spleen	3	0	24315098
	$CD4^+$ $Foxp3^+$ Treg cells vs. $CD4^+$ $Foxp3^-$ Tconv cells (injured 14d)	Spleen	3	0	24315098
GSE119169	$CD4^+CD25^+Foxp3^+$ Treg cells vs. $CD4^+CD25^+Foxp3^-$ Tconv cells (Female)	Spleen	0	0	30962454
	$CD4^+CD25^+Foxp3^+$ Treg cells vs. $CD4^+CD25^+Foxp3^-$ Tconv cells (Male)	Spleen	1	0	
GSE20366	$CD4^+Foxp3^-GFP^+$ T cells vs. $CD4^+Foxp3^-GFP^-$ T cells	Small intestinal lamina propria	4	1	25550516
GSE15390	$CD4^+CD25^+$ Treg cells and $CD4^+CD25^-$ cells	Peripheral blood	1	1	21841785

patients with MHO have no metabolic syndrome (MetS) and insulin resistance (IR) (20) and are metabolically unhealthy obese (MUO; subcutaneous adipose). The difference between MUO and MHO can be found as cited (79), obese with IR (adipocytes), obese with insulin sensitivity (IS) (adipocytes), type 2 diabetes (T2D; liver, skeletal muscle, subcutaneous adipose,

TABLE 6 | Fifteen microarrays of regulatory T cell regulator deficiency in the National Institutes of Health (NIH)–National Center for Biotechnology Information (NCBI)–Gene Expression Omnibus (GEO) datasets database (https://www.ncbi.nlm.nih.gov/gds/) were collected to analyze the expression changes of OCRGs ($p < 0.05$, $|logFC| > 1$).

GEO ID	Comparison	Source	Cell	Upregulated	Downregulated	PMID
GSE39864	Gata3 knockout vs. wild type	Spleen and LN	$CD4^+CD25^+$ Treg	0	0	22922362
GSE40493	Bcl6 knockout vs. wild type	Spleen and LN	$FoxP3^+$ Treg	7	0	23053511
GSE27896	Hdac6 knockout vs. wild type	Lymphoid tissues	$CD4^+CD25^+$ Treg	1	0	21444725
GSE36095	Hdac9 knockout vs. wild type	Spleen and LN	$CD4^+CD25^+$ Treg	0	0	22715468
GSE11818	Dicer knockout vs. wild type/heterozygote	LN	$CD4^+$ T cells	5	1	18725525
GSE14350	IL-2R defective vs. normal	Spleen	$CD4^+CD25^+$ Treg	1	3	19185518
GSE27143	Blimp1 gfp/gfp vs. +/gfp	Bone marrow	$CD4^+CD25^+$ Treg	3	6	21378976
GSE37532	Pparg– vs. Pparg+	LN	$CD4^+$ T cells	0	0	22722857, 25550516
	Pparg– vs. Pparg+	VAT	$CD4^+$ T cells	1	3	22722857, 25550516
GSE40273	Eos knockout vs. wild type	Spleen	$CD4^+$CD25hi Treg	0	0	22961053
GSE40657	Foxo1 knockout vs. wild type	thymus, Spleen and LN	$CD4^+$ T cells	6	1	23135404
GSE47989	Ep300–/– vs. wild type	Spleen	$CD4^+CD25^+$ Treg	0	1	23955711
GSE60318	deletion of p300 vs. wild type	Spleen and LN	$CD4^+CD25^+$ Treg	0	1	25154413
GSE18148	Cbfb-deficient vs. control	Peripheral $CD4^+$CD25hi cells	$FoxP3^+$ Treg	2	0	19800266
GSE32224	Trim28 knockout vs. wild type	Spleen and LN	$CD4^+CD62^+CD25^+$ Treg	3	5	22544392
GSE61077	TCR knockout vs. wild type	spleen and LN	CD44 high Treg	1	1	25263123

KO, knockout; WT, wild type; LN, lymph node; VAT, visceral adipose tissue.

TABLE 7 | Six microarrays of toll-like receptor deficiencies in the National Institutes of Health (NIH)–National Center for Biotechnology Information (NCBI)–Gene Expression Omnibus (GEO) datasets database (https://www.ncbi.nlm.nih.gov/gds/) were collected to analyze the expression changes of organelle crosstalk regulators (OCRGs) ($p < 0.05$, $|logFC| > 1$).

GEO ID	Comparison	Cell/tissue	Upregulated	Downregulated	PMID
GSE24935	Tlr2 KO+infection of SA vs. WT+infection of SA (6 h)	Glial	6	0	21901759
	Tlr2 KO+infection of SA vs. WT+infection of SA (12 h)	Glial	2	14	21901759
GSE56426	Tlr2 KO+injection of MTX vs. WT+injection of MTX	Proximal jejunum	24	23	25589072
GSE45861	Tlr2 KO+infection of European strain (P1/7) of *Streptococcus suis* vs. WT+infection of European strain (P1/7) of *S. suis*	Spleen	5	1	23724118
	Tlr2 KO+infection of Chinese strain (SC84) of *S. suis* vs. WT+infection of Chinese strain (SC84) of *S. suis*	Spleen	4	6	23724118
GSE31066	Tlr4 KO+LPS treatment vs. WT+LPS treatment	Macrophage	4	10	21865549
	Tlr4 KO+lipid A treatment vs. WT+lipid A treatment	Macrophage	4	10	21865549
GSE103750	Tlr7 KO+infection of STM vs. WT+infection of STM	Macrophage	1	1	29616197
GSE92358	Tlr3/7/9 KO+injection with MOPC cells vs. WT+injection with MOPC cells (day 4)	Tumor tissues	5	7	28300057
	Tlr3/7/9 KO+injection with MOPC cells vs. WT+injection with MOPC cells (day 6)	Tumor tissues	7	8	28300057

KO, knockout; WT, wild type; SA, Staphylococcus aureus; MTX, methotrexate; STM, Salmonella enterica serovar Typhimurium; MOPC, murine oropharyngeal carcinoma cell.

TABLE 8 | Reactive oxygen species (ROS) negative regulator Nrf2 deficiency microarray (GSE7810) in the National Institutes of Health (NIH)–National Center for Biotechnology Information (NCBI)–Gene Expression Omnibus (GEO) datasets database (https://www.ncbi.nlm.nih.gov/gds/) was collected to analyze the expression changes of organelle interactions and vesicle-related genes ($p < 0.05$, $|logFC| > 1$).

GEO ID	Comparison	Cell	Upregulated	Downregulated	PMID
GSE7810	Nrf2–/– vs. Nrf2+/+	Mouse type II cells	14	7	17895394

TABLE 9 | Caspase-1 deficiency microarrays in the National Institutes of Health (NIH)–National Center for Biotechnology Information (NCBI)–Gene Expression Omnibus (GEO) datasets database (https://www.ncbi.nlm.nih.gov/gds/) were collected to analyze the expression changes of organelle crosstalk regulators (OCRGs) ($p < 0.05$, $|logFC| > 1$).

GEO ID	Comparison	Cell/tissue	Upregulated	Downregulated	PMID
GSE25205	Casp1 KO vs. WT	Epididymal white adipose tissue	2	3	21876127
GSE32515	Casp1 KO vs. WT	Duodenum	1	1	23160218
	Casp1 KO vs. WT	Jejunum	2	1	23160218
	Casp1 KO vs. WT	Ileum	1	0	23160218
	Casp1 KO vs. WT	Liver	2	1	23160218

KO, knockout; WT, wild type.

TABLE 10 | Organelle crosstalk regulators (OCRGs) were examined in 28 types of cancers.

Cancer in TCGA	Detail	No. of OCRGs (a)		No. of total differently expressed genes (b)		Ratio (a/b)%	
		Up	Down	Up	Down	Up	Down
ACC	Adrenocortical carcinoma	4	28	545	2,544	0.73	1.10
BLCA	Bladder urothelial carcinoma	6	20	855	1,888	0.70	1.06
BRCA	Breast invasive carcinoma	19	19	1,418	2,137	1.34	0.89
CESC	Cervical squamous cell carcinoma and endocervical adenocarcinoma	18	44	1,851	3,907	0.97	1.13
COAD	Colon adenocarcinoma	33	25	2,649	2,671	1.25	0.94
DLBC	Lymphoid neoplasm diffuse large B-cell lymphoma	133	12	8,804	945	1.51	1.27
ESCA	Esophageal carcinoma	40	12	2,633	1,412	1.52	0.85
GBM	Glioblastoma multiforme	71	24	5,208	2,436	1.36	0.99
HNSC	Head and neck squamous cell carcinoma	17	9	1,488	589	1.14	1.53
KICH	Kidney chromophobe	6	38	741	3,451	0.81	1.10
KIRC	Kidney renal clear cell carcinoma	18	10	1,626	1,322	1.11	0.76
KIRP	Kidney renal papillary cell carcinoma	13	12	986	1,421	1.32	0.84
LAML	Acute myeloid leukemia	30	49	4,706	3,254	0.64	1.51
LGG	Brain lower grade glioma	63	18	3,977	1,762	1.58	1.02
LIHC	Liver hepatocellular carcinoma	19	5	1,475	722	1.29	0.69
LUAD	Lung adenocarcinoma	1	32	1,109	3,130	0.09	1.02
LUSC	Lung squamous cell carcinoma	14	47	1,920	4,035	0.73	1.16
OV	Ovarian serous cystadenocarcinoma	24	54	2,618	5,014	0.92	1.08
PAAD	Pancreatic adenocarcinoma	150	**3**	8,730	478	1.72	0.63
PRAD	Prostate adenocarcinoma	5	20	681	2,324	0.73	0.86
READ	Rectum adenocarcinoma	37	29	2,829	2,935	1.31	0.99
SKCM	Skin cutaneous melanoma	34	33	2,543	3,907	1.34	0.84
STAD	Stomach adenocarcinoma	55	7	3,745	896	1.47	0.78
TGCT	Testicular germ cell tumors	31	65	2,528	11,265	1.23	0.58
THCA	Thyroid carcinoma	6	38	659	3,402	0.91	1.12
THYM	Thymoma	166	10	11,809	934	1.41	1.07
UCEC	Uterine corpus endometrial carcinoma	20	49	2,036	5,088	0.98	0.96
UCS	Uterine carcinosarcoma	19	51	1,916	4,692	0.99	1.09

Differentially expressed gene lists of these 28 subtypes of cancers were downloaded from EGPIA2 database (http://gepia2.cancer-pku.cn/#index), in which the dataset sources were from The Cancer Genome Atlas (TCGA)/Genotype-Tissue Expression (GTEx) data (adjp < 0.05, $|logFC| > 1$).
Up, upregulated OCRGs; Down, downregulated OCRGs.

and visceral adipose), atherosclerosis (carotid artery plaques, macrophages, and T cells), atherosclerosis and familial combined hyperlipidemia (FCH; plaques and monocytes), and familial hypercholesterolemia (FHC; lymphoblastic cells); (c) seven types of ADs including rheumatoid arthritis (RA; macrophages), acute cutaneous lupus (ACLE; skin), chronic cutaneous lupus

TABLE 11 | Nineteen microarrays of deficiencies of oncogene and tumor suppressor in the National Institutes of Health (NIH)–National Center for Biotechnology Information (NCBI)–Gene Expression Omnibus (GEO) datasets database (https://www.ncbi.nlm.nih.gov/gds/) were collected to analyze the expression changes of organelle crosstalk regulators (OCRGs) ($p < 0.05$, $|\log FC| > 1$).

GEO ID	Comparison	Organism	Cells/tissue	Upregulated	Downregulated	PMID
GSE30049	IKK2 knockout vs. wild type	*Mus musculus*	Lung tumor cell lines	5	5	22327365
	IKK2 knockout vs. wild type	*M. musculus*	Lung tumor nodules	1	0	22327365
GSE46250	IKK complex inhibition vs. control	*M. musculus*	Leukemia cells	1	0	24054986
GSE46251	IKK complex inhibition vs. control	*Homo sapiens*	Leukemia cells	0	1	24054986
GSE71444	IKK2 knockdown vs. scramble control	*H. sapiens*	Human MDA-MD-231 cells	0	0	29662632
	RELA knockdown vs. scramble control	*H. sapiens*	Human MDA-MD-231 cells	1	2	29662632
GSE36568	Rela knockout vs. wild type	*M. musculus*	Lung carcinoma cells	5	2	NA
GSE54645	JAK2 knockdown vs. control	*H. sapiens*	AML cell line	0	1	24740812
GSE44652	STAT1 knockdown vs. control	*H. sapiens*	Human T-All cell line	1	5	23471820
GSE75325	Stat3 knockout vs. wild type	*M. musculus*	Mouse mammary tumors	2	1	26719528
GSE48124	STAT3 knockdown vs. control	*H. sapiens*	Urothelial cancer cell line	0	1	24525232
GSE34760	Tp53 knockout vs. wild type	*M. musculus*	Liver tumors	23	48	22342966
	Tp53 knockout vs. wild type	*M. musculus*	Liver	6	13	22342966
GSE40545	Tp53, Rb double knockout vs. wild type	*M. musculus*	Mammary epithelial cells	7	1	25602521
	Tp53 knockout vs. wild type	*M. musculus*	Mammary epithelial cells	15	4	25602521
GSE62694	Mutant Tp53 vs. control	*M. musculus*	Oviductal cells	4	1	25810107
GSE76296	Mutant Tp53 vs. wild type	*M. musculus*	Neural stem cells	0	1	26984279
GSE70262	Tp53 knockout vs. wild type	*M. musculus*	Small intestine	0	0	18533991
	APC knockout vs. wild type	*M. musculus*	Small intestine	6	3	18533991
GSE39955	Tp53 knockout vs. control	*M. musculus*	Neu primary tumor	6	4	25330770
	PTEN knockout vs. control	*M. musculus*	Neu primary tumor	7	4	25330770
GSE54265	PTEN knockdown vs. control	*H. sapiens*	Breast cells lines	5	1	24553445
GSE68869	PTEN knockdown vs. control	*H. sapiens*	Lung adenocarcinoma cells	1	0	25995385
GSE120478	PTEN null vs. wild type	*M. musculus*	Mouse embryonic fibroblasts	1	0	31169889
GSE121217	PTEN knockdown vs. control	*H. sapiens*	Lung adenocarcinoma cells	0	2	31461649

(CCLE; skin), psoriasis (skin), subacute cutaneous lupus (SCLE; skin), ulcerative colitis (UC; colon/rectum and PBMCs), and Crohn's disease (CD; PBMC); and (d) *four* types of organ failures (OFs) such as heart failure (left ventricle), hepatitis B virus-associated acute liver failure (liver), end-stage renal failure (ESRF; whole blood), and chronic kidney disease (CKD) hemodialysis (PBMC). In a total of 39 comparison datasets, we made the following findings: (i) the expressions of OCRGs were modulated except obese with IS; (ii) the expressions of OCRGs in AIs such as septic shock, trauma, ADs, and OFs except heart failure were changed more than those in MDs; (iii) among 38 datasets (except obese IS vs. lean), the downregulations of OCRGs were more than the upregulations of OCRGs in 21 datasets; (iv) the most significant downregulation of OCRGs was found in monocytes, leukocytes, and T cells in severe trauma, skeletal muscle in T2D, and whole blood and PBMC in end-stage renal disease and CKD hemodialysis; (v) the expression changes of OCRGs in T cells in severe trauma were much more than those in T cells in atherosclerosis, suggesting that OCRG expression changes were more disease-dependent rather than cell type-dependent; and (vi) adipocytes had less OCRG expression changes than other cell types.

To determine whether among 260 OCRGs upregulated and downregulated regulators were shared in disease categories, we performed a Venn diagram analysis. As shown in **Figures 2A–D**, in 26 upregulated OCRGs in AIs, the upregulation of two regulators, SERPINA1 and AZU1, was shared among acute respiratory distress syndrome (ARDS), sepsis, and trauma; upregulation of CD24 and FKBP8 was shared among ARDS and trauma; and upregulation of GRN was shared between sepsis and trauma. In 46 upregulated OCRGs in MDs, upregulation of two regulators VAMP8 and SERPINA1 was shared between obese and atherosclerosis; and two upregulated regulators DNM2 and MTFP1 were shared between T2D and atherosclerosis. In 80 upregulated OCRGs in ADs, three regulators (i.e., GPRC5A, LAMP3, and MX2) were shared among RA, autoimmune skin disease (ASD), and inflammatory bowel disease (IBD); three regulators (i.e., OSBPL8, SERPINA1, and MX1) were shared between RA and IBD; seven regulators (i.e., PPARG, MYO19, MAP1LC3A, TLR9, NACC1, P4HA2, and SAMD9) were shared between RA and ASD; and four regulators (i.e., POU2F2, VMP1, ATP11A, and KDR) were shared between ASD and IBD. In 39 upregulated OCRGs in OFs, two regulators (i.e., BAX and GRN) were shared between CKD hemodialysis and hepatitis B virus liver failure. These results have demonstrated that first, the

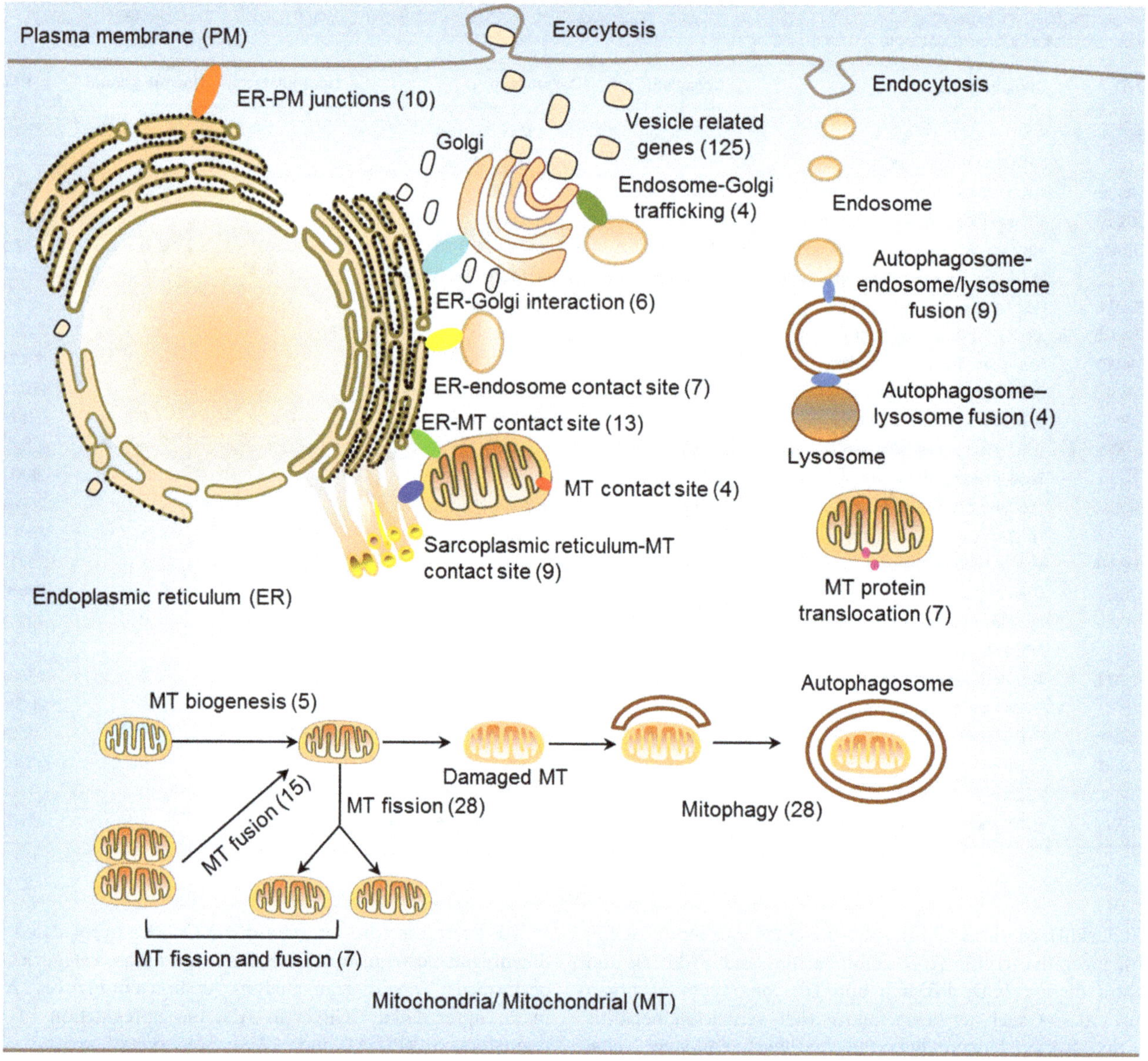

FIGURE 1 | Two hundred sixty organelle crosstalk regulators (OCRGs) in 16 groups were analyzed. There are 16 classification or function of these genes, including nine mitochondria (MT)-related gene populations: MT biogenesis (five genes), MT fusion (15 genes), MT fission (28 genes), MT fission and fusion (seven genes), mitophagy (28 genes), ER–MT contact site (13 genes), MT contact site (four genes), sarcoplasmic reticulum–MT contact site (nine genes), and MT protein translocation (seven genes); three endoplasmic reticulum (ER)-related populations except ER–MT contact site: ER–endosome contact site (seven genes), ER–Golgi interact genes (6), and ER–PM junctions (10 genes); endosome–Golgi trafficking (four genes); autophagosome–lysosome fusion (four genes); autophagosome–endosome/lysosome fusion (nine genes); vesicle-related (125 genes) coded proteins are enhanced by the Human Protein Atlas. Because some genes have more than one function, the final selection is 260 non-repetitive genes. The detailed gene list is in **Table 1**.

majority of the upregulated OCRGs was disease-specific; second, ADs shared more upregulated OCRGs than other diseases; and third, the ratios of upregulated OCRGs vs. downregulated OCRGs were 1:2.8 in AIs, 1:1 in MDs, 1:1.2 in ADs, and 1:3.8 in OFs, suggesting that AIs and OFs had downregulated OCRGs much more than those of upregulated in comparison with those of others. We then used a Venn diagram to analyze the overlapping OCRGs and their classifications among AIs, MDs, ADs, and OFs (**Figure 2E**) and listed the exclusively expressed OCRGs upregulated and downregulated in these four types of diseases in **Supplementary Tables 4A,B**. The results showed that a total of 24 upregulated OCRGs were shared by two or three different diseases. AIs and MDs, and AIs and ADs shared three and one OCRGs, respectively. MDs and ADs, and MDs and OFs shared five and three OCRGs, respectively. ADs and OFs shared six OCRGs. AIs, MDs, and ADs shared three OCRGs. AIs, MDs, and OFs shared one OCRG. MDs, ADs, and OFs shared one OCRG. There were 12, 17, 43, and

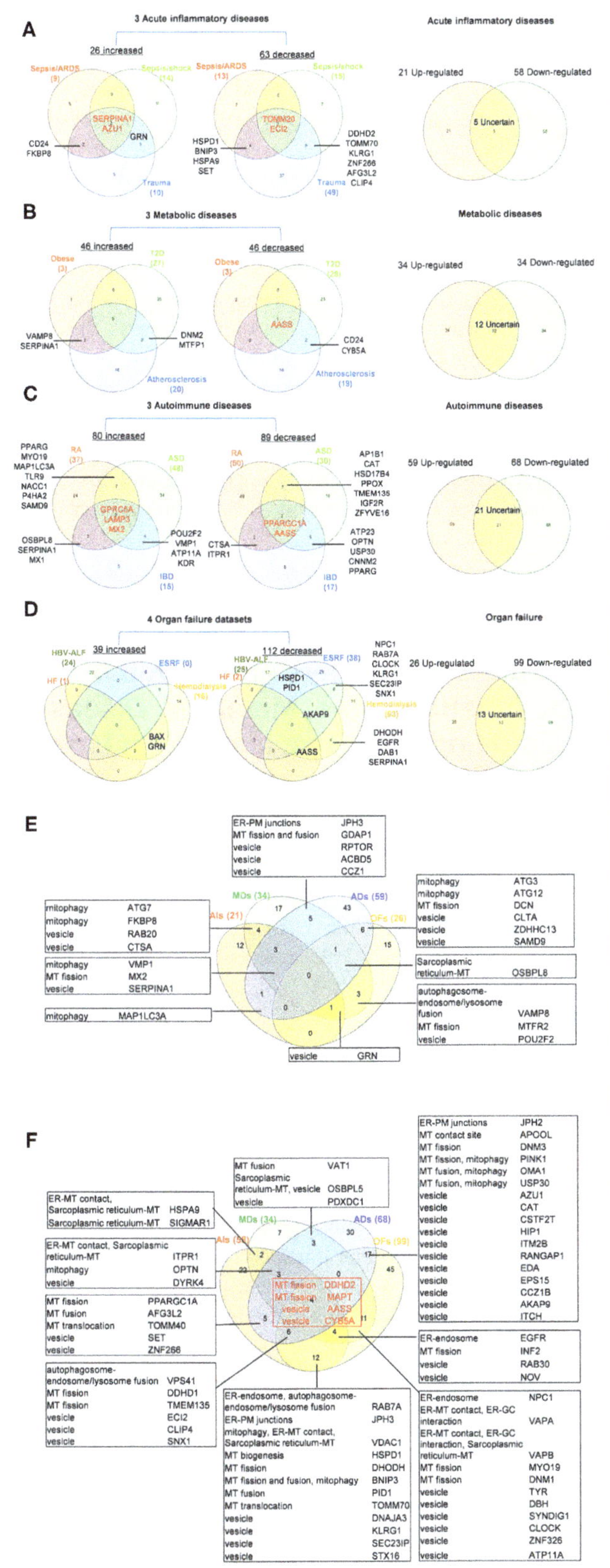

FIGURE 2 | Venn diagram shows that there are several shared OCRGs in acute inflammations (AIs), metabolic diseases (MDs), autoimmune diseases (ADs), and organ failures (OFs). **(A)** Venn diagram shows 17 genes are shared

(Continued)

FIGURE 2 | among acute inflammatory diseases (AIs). SERPINA1 and AZU1 are shared upregulated genes; TOMM20 and ECI2 are shared downregulated genes by sepsis/ARDS, sepsis/shock, and trauma. CD24, FKBP8, and GRN are shared upregulated genes by sepsis and trauma. HSPD1, BNIP3, HSPA9, SET, DDHD2, TOMM70, KLRG1, ZNF266, AFG3L2, and CLIP4 are 10 genes that are commonly downregulated in sepsis and trauma groups. After removing five uncertain genes (upregulated in one type of disease and downregulated in another type of disease), 21 genes are upregulated and 58 genes are downregulated in AIs. **(B)** Venn diagram shows seven genes are shared among metabolic diseases (MDs). VAMP8 and SERPINA1 are shared upregulated genes by obese and atherosclerosis; DNM2 and MTFP1 are shared upregulated genes by type 2 diabetes (T2D) and atherosclerosis. AASS is shared a downregulated gene by three metabolic diseases, and CD24 and CYB5A are shared downregulated genes by T2D and atherosclerosis. After removal of 12 uncertain genes, 34 genes are upregulated and 34 genes are downregulated in MDs. **(C)** Venn diagram shows 33 genes are shared among autoimmune diseases. GPRC5A, LAMP3, and MX2 are shared upregulated genes; PPARGC1A and AASS are shared downregulated genes by rheumatoid arthritis (RA), autoimmune skin disease (ASD), and inflammatory bowel disease (IBD). Other 28 genes are common genes between two autoimmune diseases. After removal of 21 uncertain genes, 59 genes are upregulated, and 68 genes are downregulated in ADs. **(D)** Venn diagram shows 16 genes are shared in organ failure datasets. BAX and GRN are shared upregulated genes by hepatitis B virus-associated acute liver failure (HBV-ALF). AKAP9 is the common downregulated gene in HBV-ALF, end-stage renal failure (ESRF), and hemodialysis; NPC1, RAB7A, CLOCK, KLRG1, SEC23IP, and SNX1 are the common downregulated genes in ESRF and hemodialysis. After removal of 13 uncertain genes, 26 genes are upregulated and 99 genes are downregulated in OFs. **(E)** Venn diagram shows the shared and exclusive upregulated and downregulated OCRGs in these four diseases. In upregulated OCRGs, a total of 24 genes were shared by two or three different diseases. AIs and MDs shared four genes, two vesicle-related genes (RAB20 and CTSA), and two mitophagy genes (FKBP8 and ATG7). AIs and ADs shared mitophagy gene (MAP1LC3A). AIs, MDs, and OFs shared vesicle genes (GRN). MDs and OFs shared three genes autophagosome–endosome/lysosome fusion regulator (VAMP8), MT fission gene (MTFR2), and vesicle gene (POU2F2). AIs, MD, and ADs shared mitophagy (VMP1), MT fission (MX2), and vesicle (SERPINA1) genes. MDs, ADs, and OFs shared sarcoplasmic reticulum–MT gene (OSBPL8). ADs and OFs shared two mitophagy genes (ATG3 and ATG12), one MT fission gene (DCN), and three vesicle genes (CLTA, ZDHHC13, and SAMD9). MDs and ADs shared five genes including one ER–PM junctions gene (JPH3), one MT fission and fusion regulator (GDAP1), and three vesicle genes (RPTOR, ACBD5, and CCZ1). Other exclusive upregulated genes in these four diseases are listed in **Supplementary Table 4A**. **(F)** In downregulated OCRGs, a total of 67 genes were shared by two or more than two different diseases. Two MT fission genes (DDHD2 and MAPT) and two vesicle genes (AASS and CYB5A), were shared by four types of diseases (red box). ADs and OFs shared 17 OCRGs, including one ER–PM junction regulator (JPH2) and one MT contact site gene (APOOL), two MT fission regulators (DNM3 and PINK1) (also mitophagy regulator), two genes with MT fusion and mitophagy function (OMA1 and USP30), and 11 vesicle genes. AIs and OFs shared 12 OCRGs, RAB7A (ER–endosome and autophagosome–endosome/lysosome fusion), JPH3 (ER–PM junctions), VDAC1 (mitophagy, ER–MT contact, and sarcoplasmic reticulum–MT), HSPD1 (MT biogenesis), DHODH (MT fission), BNIP3 (MT fission and fusion, and mitophagy), PID1 (MT fusion), TOMM70 (MT translocation), and four vesicle genes (DNAJA3, KLRG1, SEC23IP, and STX16). MDs and OFs shared 11 OCRGs including ER–endosome genes (NPC1), ER–MT contact and ER–GC interaction regulator VAPA, ER–MT contact, ER–GC interaction and sarcoplasmic reticulum–MT regulator VAPB, two MT fission genes MYO19 and DNM1, and six vesicle genes. AIs and MDs, AIs and ADs, and MDs and ADs shared two, five, and three downregulated OCRGs, respectively. AIs, MDs, and ADs shared three downregulated OCRGs, ITPR1 (ER–MT contact, sarcoplasmic reticulum–MT), OPTN (mitophagy), and DYRK4 (vesicle gene). AIs, MDs, and OFs shared four OCRGs (EGFR, INF2, RAB30, and NOV). AIs, ADs, and OFs shared six OCRGs, VPS41 (autophagosome–endosome/lysosome fusion), two MT fission regulators

(Continued)

FIGURE 2 | DDHD1 and TMEM135, and three vesicle regulators (ECI2, CLIP4, and SNX1). Other exclusive downregulated genes in these four diseases are listed in **Supplementary Table 4B**. Abbreviations: AIs, acute inflammations; MDs, metabolic diseases; ADs, autoimmune diseases; OFs, organ failures; ARDS, acute respiratory distress syndrome; T2D, type 2 diabetes; HF, heart failure; HBV-ALF, hepatitis B virus-associated acute liver failure; ESRF, end-stage renal failure.

15 exclusively upregulated OCRGs in AIs, MDs, ADs, and OF diseases, respectively (**Supplementary Table 4A**). A total of 67 downregulated OCRGs were shared by two or more than two different diseases (**Figure 2F**). The four OCRGs including two MT fission genes (i.e., DDHD2 and MAPT) and two vesicle genes (i.e., AASS and CYB5A) were downregulated by four types of diseases. OFs and other diseases (AIs, MDs, and ADs) shared more downregulated OCRGs (12, 11, and 17, respectively). There were 22, 7, 30, and 45 downregulated OCRGs in AIs, MDs, ADs, and OFs, respectively (**Supplementary Table 4B**). These results showed that differentially classified OCRGs were shared in different diseases.

Sepsis and Trauma-Upregulated Organelle Crosstalk Regulator Groups Are Classified as the Acute Crisis-Handling Organelle Crosstalk Regulators; and Organ Failure-Upregulated Organelle Crosstalk Regulators Groups Are Classified as the Cell Failure-Handling Organelle Crosstalk Regulators

We then hypothesized that every major disease group modulates differentially 16 OCRG groups. We used the donut chart analysis. As shown in **Figure 3**, the 21 upregulated OCRGs in AIs were distributed in three categories including vesicle (64%), mitophagy (23%), and MT fission (14%). The 26 upregulated OCRGs in OFs were distributed in seven groups including vesicle (50%), MT fusion (12%), mitophagy (12%), MT fission (8%), sarcoplasmic reticulum–MT (8%), autophagosome–endosome/lysosome fusion (8%), and autophagosome–lysosome fusion (4%). The 34 upregulated OCRGs in MDs were distributed in 12 groups, including vesicle (43%), MT fission (11%), mitophagy (11%), ER–PM junctions (9%), and MT fusion (6%), and in the rest of the seven groups (3% of each). The 59 upregulated OCRGs in ADs were distributed in 14 groups, including vesicle (41%), MT fission (13%), mitophagy (11%), ER–PM junctions (8%), ER–MT contact (5%), and sarcoplasmic reticulum–MT (5%), and in the rest of other groups (2–3% of each). However, the downregulated OCRGs in AIs, OFs, MDs, and ADs were distributed in 15, 15, 9, and 14 groups, respectively. These results have demonstrated that *first*, vesicle, MT fission, and mitophagy were three top groups of organelle crosstalk regulators upregulated in all four major diseases. Since these three groups of OCRGs are only upregulated in AIs, sepsis, and trauma, we also classify those three groups including vesicle, MT fission, and mitophagy as the cell crisis-handling OCRGs, at least in the partial functions of the three groups, which were well-correlated with a previous report that mitophagy regulator PINK1 is an MT quality control gate keeper (80); *second*, ER crosstalk regulators were only upregulated in MD and AD groups but not in AIs and OFs; *third*, a few groups of OCRGs were upregulated in AIs (three groups) and OFs (seven groups), but the other two disease groups had more groups of OCRGs upregulated (MDs had 12 groups and ADs had 14 groups). Therefore, similar to the cell crisis-handling OCRGs that we defined, we also classify vesicle, MT fission, mitophagy, sarcoplasmic reticulum–MT, MT fusion, autophagosome–lysosome fusion, and autophagosome/endosome–lysosome fusion as the cellular failure-handling OCRGs, at least in the partial functions of seven groups; *fourth*, MT fusion regulators and sarcoplasmic reticulum–MT regulators were upregulated in MDs, ADs, and OFs; and *fifth*, AIs, MDs, ADs, and OFs downregulated 15, 9, 14, and 15 OCRG groups, respectively, suggesting that AIs and OFs upregulate less OCRG groups but downregulate more OCRG groups than MDs and ADs.

The Majority of Upregulated Pathways Are Disease Group-Specific, and Some Upregulated Pathways Are Shared by Acute Inflammations, Metabolic Diseases, Autoimmune Diseases, and Organ Failures

To determine the functions of upregulated OCRGs, we performed MPAs. As shown in **Figures 4A–D**, AIs upregulated the top pathways including vacuole organization, lysosomal transport, neutrophil degranulation, regulation of endocytosis, positive regulation of peptidase activity, protein transfer within lipid bilayer, MT fission, vesicle organization, response to acid chemical, lysosomal organization, and receptor-mediated endocytosis. MDs upregulated the top pathways including MT organization, organelle fusion, macroautophagy, vesicle organization, response to anesthesia, myeloid leukocyte activation, protein localization, positive regulation of transmembrane transport, and endosomal transport. ADs upregulated the top pathways including MT fission, protein localization, membrane fusion, organelle fusion, neurodegeneration with brain iron accumulation (NBIA) subtype pathway, insertion of tail-anchored proteins, calcium ion transmembrane transport, vesicle fusion, Fragile X syndrome, MT localization, response to inorganic substance, regulation of NIK/NF-kB signaling, bile acid metabolic process, cholesterol metabolism, lung fibrosis, and protein targeting. OFs upregulated the top pathways including macroautophagy, organelle fusion, autophagosome maturation, cytosolic calcium ion transport, negative regulation of neuron apoptotic process, antigen processing and presentation, and negative regulation of cellular component organization. In **Figures 5A–D**, AIs downregulated the top 10 pathways including mitochondrion organization, autophagy, MT fission, protein localization, MT fusion, autophagy–animal, selective autophagy, response to nutrient levels, MT calcium ion homeostasis, and frataxin complex. MDs downregulated the top pathways including MT fission, autophagy, Golgi vesicle transport, mitochondrion

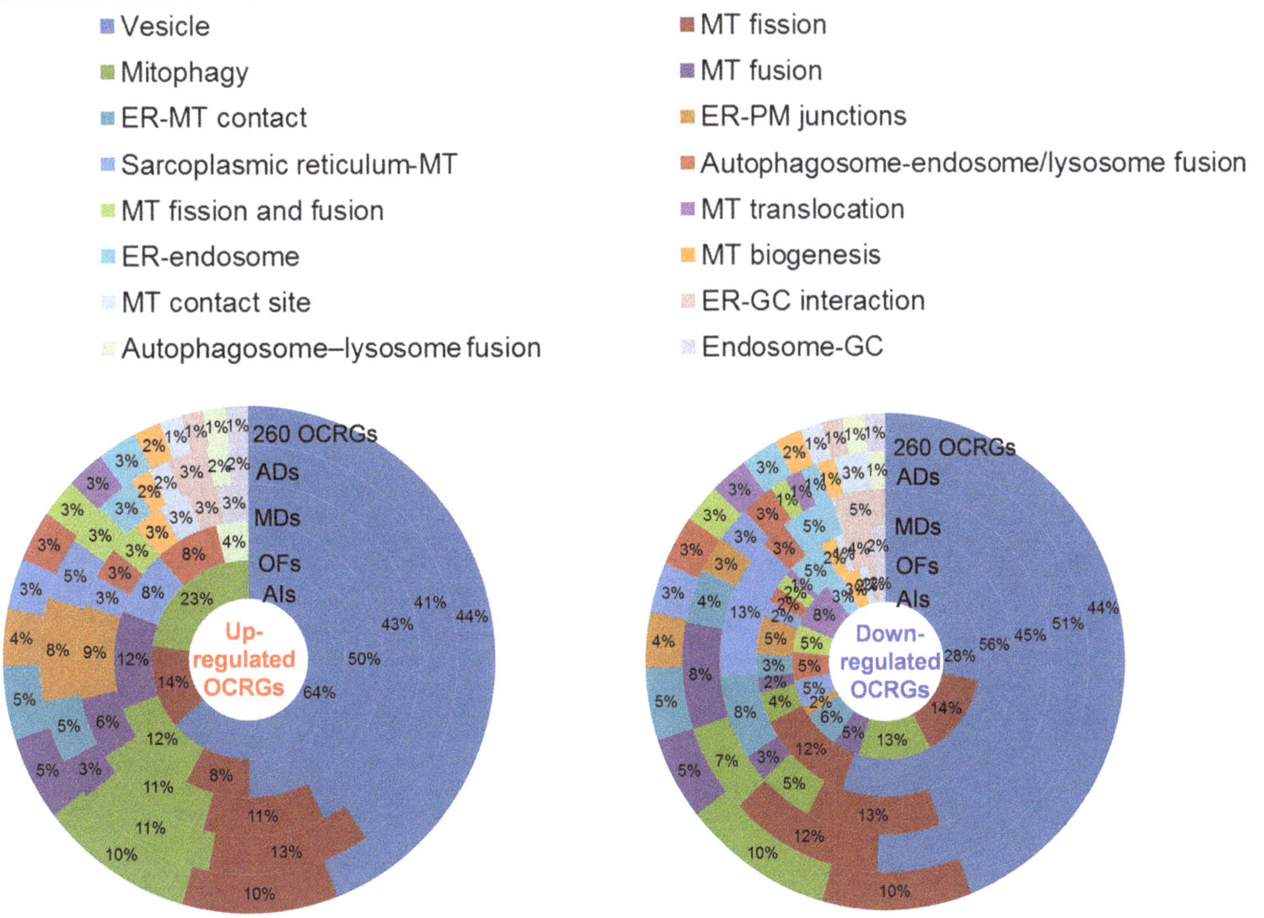

FIGURE 3 | Donut chart shows the different classification/function ratios of upregulated and downregulated OCRGs in acute inflammations (AIs), metabolic diseases (MDs), autoimmune diseases (ADs), and organ failures (OFs). From the center to the outside of the donut chart, the circle represents the ratios of OCRGs in acute inflammations (AIs), organ failures (OFs), metabolic diseases (MD), autoimmune diseases (ADs), and all 260 OCRGs in turn. Groups of upregulated OCRGs in AIs (3) and OFs (7) are less than in MDs (12) and OFs (14) (left). In the 21 upregulated genes in AIs, vesicle-related genes account for 64%, and mitophagy and mitochondrial (MT) fission genes account for 14 and 23%, respectively. In the 26 upregulated genes in OFs, the top 3 high-number genes are vesicle- (50%), mitophagy- (12%), and MT fusion-related (12%) OCRGs. In the 34 upregulated genes in MDs, vesicle- (43%), MT fission- (11%), and mitophagy-related (11%) genes are the top 3 genes with high proportion. In the 59 upregulated genes of ADs, vesicle-related genes account for 41%, MT fission genes account for 13%, and mitophagy genes account for 11%. The downregulated OCRGs distributed in AIs, OFs, MDs, and ADs are 15, 15, nine, and 14 groups, respectively (right). In the 58 downregulated genes in AIs, the top 3 high-number genes are vesicle- (28%), MT fission- (14%), and mitophagy-related (13%) genes. In the 99 downregulated genes in OFs, the proportions of vesicle (56%), MT fission (12%), and ER–plasma membrane (PM) junctions (5%) genes are higher than those of others. In the 34 downregulated genes in MDs, the numbers of vesicle (45%), MT fission (13%), and endoplasmic reticulum (ER)–MT contact genes (13%) are higher. In ADs, vesicle (51%), MT fission (12%), and MT fusion genes (8%) are the top 3. These results show that different diseases have different expression patterns of OCRGs and that the classification proportion of upregulated and downregulated genes in the same type of diseases is different, which may explain the different functions of OCRGs in the occurrence and development of diseases. Abbreviations: ER, endoplasmic reticulum; GC, Golgi complex; MT, mitochondria; PM, ER–plasma membrane.

localization, response to light stimulus, response to cadmium ion, positive regulation of blood circulation, regulation of peptide hormone secretion, L1CAM interactions, and cellular response to unfolded protein. ADs downregulated the top pathways including mitochondrion organization, autophagy, organelle fusion, MT membrane organization, endocytosis, positive regulation of apoptotic process, establishment of protein localization to organelle, negative regulation of MT fission, vesicle organization, and lysosomal transport. OFs downregulated the top pathways including MT fission, vesicle organization, protein localization, organelle fusion, Golgi vesicle transport, regulation of vesicle-mediated transport, MT fusion, negative regulation of mitochondrion organization, lysosomal transport, ROS metabolic process, endocytosis, and response to hyperoxia.

A Venn diagram was used to analyze the overlapping pathways of upregulated and downregulated OCRGs among these four major types of diseases. As shown in **Figure 4E**, for upregulated OCRGs, vesicle organization was shared by AIs and MDs; MT fission was shared by AIs and ADs; macroautophagy was shared by MDs and OFs; organelle fusion was shared by MDs, ADs, and OFs. **Figure 4F** lists the exclusively enriched upregulated pathways in these four diseases. In **Figure 5E**, for downregulated OCRGs, MT fragmentation involved in the

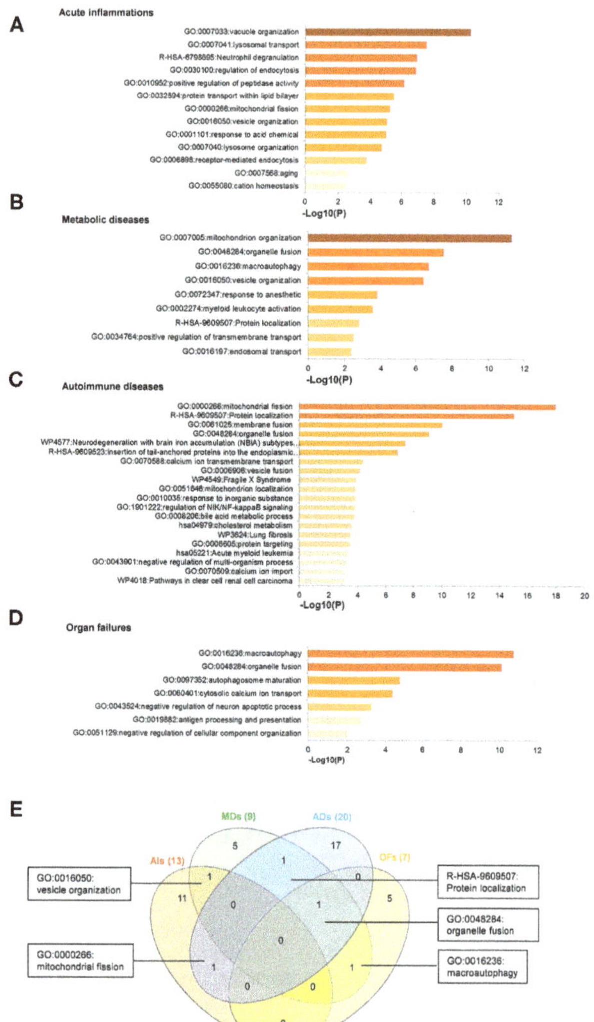

F

Diseases (Number of pathways)	Exclusively enriched pathways
Acute inflammatory diseases (AIs) (11)	GO:0055080:cation homeostasis
	GO:0007568:aging
	GO:0006898:receptor-mediated endocytosis
	GO:0007040:lysosome organization
	GO:0001101:response to acid chemical
	GO:0032594:protein transport within lipid bilayer
	GO:0010952:positive regulation of peptidase activity
	GO:0030100:regulation of endocytosis
	R-HSA-6798695:Neutrophil degranulation
	GO:0007041:lysosomal transport
	GO:0007033:vacuole organization
Metabolic diseases (MDs) (5)	GO:0016197:endosomal transport
	GO:0034764:positive regulation of transmembrane transport
	GO:0002274:myeloid leukocyte activation
	GO:0072347:response to anesthetic
	GO:0007005:mitochondrion organization
Autoimmune diseases (ADs) (17)	WP4018:Pathways in clear cell renal cell carcinoma
	GO:0070509:calcium ion import
	GO:0043901:negative regulation of multi-organism process
	hsa05221:Acute myeloid leukemia
	GO:0006605:protein targeting
	WP3624:Lung fibrosis
	hsa04979:cholesterol metabolism
	GO:0008206:bile acid metabolic process
	GO:1901222:regulation of NIK/NF-kappaB signaling
	GO:0010035:response to inorganic substance
	GO:0051646:mitochondrion localization
	WP4549:Fragile X Syndrome
	GO:0006906:vesicle fusion
	GO:0070588:calcium ion transmembrane transport
	R-HSA-9609523:Insertion of tail-anchored proteins into the endoplasmic reticulum membrane
	WP4577:Neurodegeneration with brain iron accumulation (NBIA) subtypes pathway
	GO:0061025:membrane fusion
Organ failure diseases (OFs) (5)	GO:0051129:negative regulation of cellular component organization
	GO:0019882:antigen processing and presentation
	GO:0043524:negative regulation of neuron apoptotic process
	GO:0060401:cytosolic calcium ion transport
	GO:0097352:autophagosome maturation

FIGURE 4 | Enrichment analysis results show that several pathways of upregulated OCRGs were involved in acute inflammations (AIs), metabolic diseases (MDs), autoimmune diseases (ADs), and organ failures (OFs). Gene *(Continued)*

FIGURE 4 | Ontology (GO)-based enrichment of significant upregulated OCRGs in different types of diseases was analyzed using Metascape software (http://metascape.org/gp/index.html#/main/step1; PMID: 30944313). **(A)** There are 14 significant GO enrichment results in 21 upregulated OCRGs in acute inflammations (AIs). The top 3 GO enrichments of OCRGs are vacuole organization, lysosomal transport, and neutrophil degranulation. Except for neutrophil degranulation, relative to acute inflammatory diseases, regulation of endocytosis and receptor-mediated endocytosis are significant GO enrichment results, which show that endocytosis is increased in AIs. **(B)** There are nine significant GO enrichment results in 34 upregulated OCRGs in metabolic diseases (MDs). The top 3 GO enrichments of OCRGs are mitochondrion organization, organelle fusion, and macroautophagy. Some genes are enriched in myeloid leukocyte activation, which suggested that these genes are involved in chronic low-grade inflammation. **(C)** There are 20 significant GO enrichment results in 60 upregulated OCRGs in autoimmune diseases (ADs). Mitochondrial fission, protein localization, and macroautophagy are the top 3 GO enrichments. Additionally, calcium ion transmembrane transport and regulation of NIK/NF-kappaB signaling are the significant GO enrichment results. **(D)** There are seven significant GO enrichment results in 26 upregulated OCRGs in organ failures (OFs). The upregulated genes are enriched in macroautophagy organelle fusion, autophagosome maturation, cytosolic calcium ion transport, negative regulation of neuron apoptotic process, antigen processing and presentation, and negative regulation of cellular component organization. **(E)** There are shared and exclusive pathways in four types of diseases in upregulated OCRGs. Venn diagram shows that there were five significant pathways shared by acute inflammations (AIs), metabolic diseases (MDs), autoimmune diseases (ADs), and organ failures (OFs). One pathway vesicle organization was shared by AIs and MDs. Mitochondrial fission pathway was shared by AIs and ADs. Macroautophagy pathway was shared by MDs and OFs. Organelle fusion was shared by MDs, ADs, and OFs. **(F)** The exclusive upregulated pathways in AIs, MDs, ADs, and OFs were 11, five, 17, and five, respectively.

apoptotic process and mitochondrion organization was shared by AIs and ADs; autophagy signaling was shared by AIs, MDs, and ADs; MT fusion was shared by AIs and OFs; response to nutrient levels was shared by AIs, ADs, and OFs; regulated exocytosis, lysosomal transport, vesicle organization, and organelle fusion were shared by ADs and OFs; response to light stimulus and Golgi vesicle transport were shared by MDs and OFs; protein localization and MT fission were shared by AIs, MDs, and OFs. **Figure 5F** lists the exclusively enriched downregulated pathways in these four diseases. These results have demonstrated that (1) the majority of signal pathways for upregulated OCRGs are the major disease group-specific; (2) upregulated pathway organelle fusion is shared by three disease groups such as MDs, ADs, and OFs; (3) upregulated MT fission is shared by AIs and ADs; (4) upregulated vesicle organization is shared by AIs and MDs; (5) upregulated protein localization is shared by MDs and ADs; and (6) more downregulated pathways are shared than upregulated pathways among diseases.

Decreased Autophagosome–Lysosome Fusion Is Required for Viral Replications, Which Classify This Decreased Group as the Viral Replication-Suppressed Organelle Crosstalk Regulators

It has been reported that using single organelle multispectral flow cytometry identified altered energy metabolism, changes in MT size, and MT membrane potential in viral infected cells

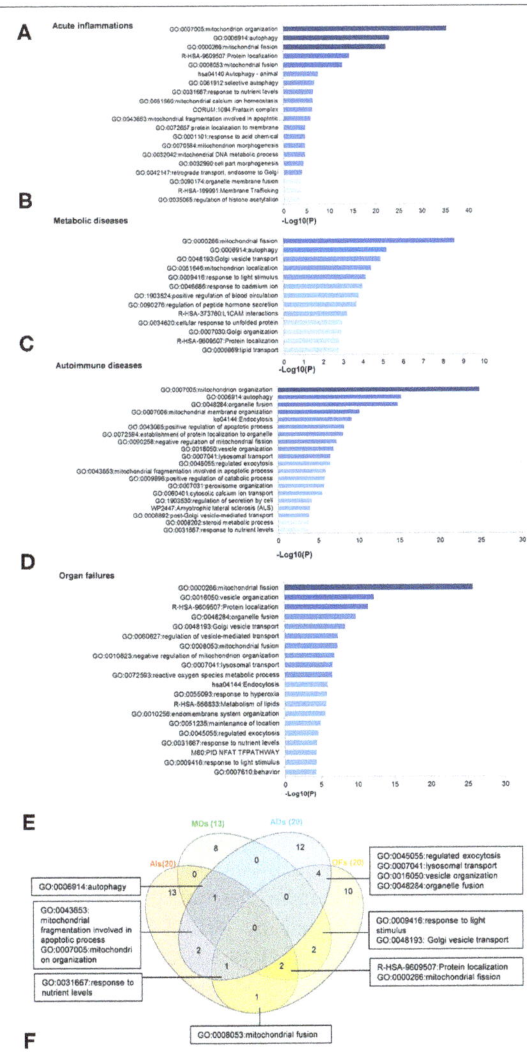

F

Diseases (Number of pathways)	Exclusively enriched pathways
Acute inflammatory diseases (AIs) (13)	GO:0035065:regulation of histone acetylation
	R-HSA-199991:Membrane Trafficking
	GO:0090174:organelle membrane fusion
	GO:0042147:retrograde transport, endosome to Golgi
	GO:0032990:cell part morphogenesis
	GO:0032042:mitochondrial DNA metabolic process
	GO:0070584:mitochondrion morphogenesis
	GO:0001101:response to acid chemical
	GO:0072657:protein localization to membrane
	CORUM:1094:Frataxin complex
	GO:0051560:mitochondrial calcium ion homeostasis
	GO:0061912:selective autophagy
	GO:0007005:mitochondrion organization
Metabolic diseases (MDs) (8)	GO:0006869:lipid transport
	GO:0007030:Golgi organization
	GO:0034620:cellular response to unfolded protein
	R-HSA-373760:L1CAM interactions
	GO:0090276:regulation of peptide hormone secretion
	GO:1903524:positive regulation of blood circulation
	GO:0046686:response to cadmium ion
	GO:0051646:mitochondrion localization
Autoimmune diseases (ADs) (12)	GO:0008202:steroid metabolic process
	GO:0006892:post-Golgi vesicle-mediated transport
	WP2447:Amyotrophic lateral sclerosis (ALS)
	GO:1903530:regulation of secretion by cell
	GO:0060401:cytosolic calcium ion transport
	GO:0007031:peroxisome organization
	GO:0009896:positive regulation of catabolic process
	GO:0090258:negative regulation of mitochondrial fission
	GO:0072594:establishment of protein localization to organelle
	GO:0043065:positive regulation of apoptotic process
	ko04144:Endocytosis
	GO:0007006:mitochondrial membrane organization
Organ failure diseases (OFs) (10)	GO:0007610:behavior
	M80:PID NFAT TFPATHWAY
	GO:0051235:maintenance of location
	GO:0010256:endomembrane system organization
	R-HSA-556833:Metabolism of lipids
	GO:0055093:response to hyperoxia
	hsa04144:Endocytosis
	GO:0072593:reactive oxygen species metabolic process
	GO:0010823:negative regulation of mitochondrion organization
	GO:0060627:regulation of vesicle-mediated transport

FIGURE 5 | Enrichment analysis results show that several pathways of downregulated OCRGs were involved in acute inflammations (AIs), metabolic diseases (MDs), autoimmune diseases (ADs), and organ failures (OFs). Gene

(Continued)

FIGURE 5 | Ontology-based enrichment of significant downregulated OCRGs in different types of diseases was analyzed by using Metascape software (http://metascape.org/gp/index.html#/main/step1; PMID: 30944313). **(A)** In the 20 significant GO enrichment results of 58 downregulated OCRGs in acute inflammations (AIs), the top 3 of downregulated OCRGs are enriched in mitochondrion organization, autophagy, and mitochondrial fission. Mitochondrial calcium ion homeostasis is downregulated in acute inflammation diseases. **(B)** There are 13 significant GO enrichment results in 34 downregulated OCRGs in metabolic disease (MDs). Mitochondrial fission, autophagy, and Golgi vesicle transport are the top 3 downregulated signaling that enriched downregulated OCRGs. Additionally, lipid transport is suppressed. **(C)** In the 20 significant GO enrichment results of 67 downregulated OCRGs in autoimmune diseases (ADs), regulation of mitochondrion organization, organelle fusion, and autophagy are the top 3 downregulated enrichment signaling. Cytosolic calcium ion transport is suppressed, while calcium ion transmembrane transport is active in ADs (**Figure 5**). That is, calcium transporting between membrane-bounded organelles is active. **(D)** The 20 significant GO enrichment results of 99 downregulated OCRGs in organ failures (OFs). Top 3 GO enrichments of OCRGs are mitochondrial fission, vesicle organization, and protein localization. Reactive oxygen species metabolic process and metabolism of lipids were suppressed in organ failure diseases. **(E)** There are shared and exclusive pathways in four types of diseases in downregulated OCRGs. Venn diagram shows 13 significant pathways shared by acute inflammations (AIs), metabolic diseases (MDs), autoimmune diseases (ADs), and organ failures (OFs). Mitochondrial fragmentation involved in apoptotic process and mitochondrion organization pathways are downregulated in AIs and ADs. Autophagy signaling is decreased in AIs, MDs, and ADs. Mitochondrial fusion pathway is shared by AIs and OFs. Response to nutrient levels is downregulated in AIs, ADs, and OFs. Four pathways regulated exocytosis, lysosomal transport, vesicle organization, and organelle fusion and are downregulated in ADs and OFs. Response to light stimulus and Golgi vesicle transport are downregulated in MDs and OFs. Downregulation of R-HSA-9609507:Protein localization and mitochondrial fission are shared by AIs, MDs, and OFs. **(F)** The exclusive downregulated pathways in AIs, MDs, ADs, and OFs are 13, eight, 12 and 10, respectively.

(81). We hypothesized that organelle crosstalk is modulated in cells infected by viruses. We collected 38 microarray datasets for comparison with seven groups of virus-infected cells including MERS-CoV infected human microvascular ECs (82) (0, 12, 24, 36, and 48 h post infection), SARS-CoV-infected human airway epithelium cells (83) (0, 12, 24, 36, 48, 60, 72, 84, and 96 h post infection), human influenza virus H1N1 infected human airway epithelium cells (83) (0, 6, 12, 18, 24, 36, and 48 h post infection), avian influenza virus A H7N9-infected Calu-3 human lung epithelium cells (84) (3, 7, 12, and 24 h post infection), avian influenza virus H7N7 infected Calu-3 human lung epithelium cells (84) (3, 7, 12, and 24 h post infection), avian influenza virus H5N1-infected Calu-3 human lung epithelium cells (84) (3, 7, 12, and 24 h post infection), human influenza virus H3N2-infected Calu-3 human lung epithelium cells (84) (3, 7, 12, and 24 h post infection), and H9N2-infected HUVECs (24 h). As shown in **Table 3**, our results indicated that (1) MERS-CoV infection in human microvascular ECs gradually modulated OCRG expressions in 12, 24, 36, and 48 h post infection with the peaks at 24 and 36 h (upregulated 41 and downregulated 44 OCRGs at 24 h and upregulated 39 and downregulated 46 OCRGs, respectively); (2) SARS-CoV infection slightly modulated OCRG expressions in human airway epithelial cells in 0, 24, 36, 48, 60, 72, 84, and 96 h post infection with the peak at 60 h post infection (upregulated 15 OCRGs and downregulated zero OCRG); (3)

human influenza virus H1N1 infection significantly modulated OCRG expressions in human airway epithelial cells in 0, 6, 12, 18, 24, 36, and 48 h post infection with the peaks at 18, 24, 36, and 48 h post infection (upregulated 20, 22, 27, and 18 OCRGs and downregulated 21, 29, 30, and 16 OCRGs, respectively); (4) infections of avian influenza virus strains H7N9, H7N7, and H5N1 in human lung Calu-3 epithelium cells and strain H9N2 in HUVECs significantly modulated OCRG expressions at 24 h post infection with upregulation of 30, 38, 40, and 27 OCRGs and downregulation of 70, 109, 92, and 137 OCRGs, respectively; and (5) infection of human influenza virus strains H3N2 in human lung Calu-3 epithelium cells significantly modulated OCRG expressions at 12 and 24 h post infection with upregulation of 12 and 19 OCRGs and downregulation of 16 and 42 OCRGs, respectively.

Infections of avian influenza virus strains at 24 h significantly modulated OCRG expressions. We used a Venn diagram and MPA to examine avian influenza virus modulation of OCRGs. The result showed that 87 OCRGs were upregulated and 190 OCRGs were downregulated in influenza virus strains H1N1-, H7N9-, H7N7-, H5N1-, H3N2-, and H9N2-infected cells. MX1 and SYNPO2 were the commonly upregulated OCRGs shared by these six strains of influenza virus-infected cells; there were no commonly downregulated OCRGs by these six influenza virus-infected cells. Besides the overlapped 47 OCRGs, 40 OCRGs were upregulated (**Supplementary Table 5A**) and were from 12 functional groups except MT fusion, MT biogenesis, autophagosome–lysosome fusion, and endosome–Golgi complex (GC) groups; 143 OCRGs were downregulated and were from all the 16 functional groups (**Figures 6A,C**). The significant pathways for upregulated OCRGs included protein localization, mitochondrion organization, membrane fusion, organelle fusion, regulation of calcium ion transmembrane transporter activity, regulation of viral process, endomembrane system organization, metabolism of steroids, regulation of organelle assembly, and leukocyte chemotaxis. The top 10 pathways for downregulated OCRGs included mitochondrion organization, autophagy, MT fusion, MT transport, negative regulation of mitochondrion organization, lysosomal transport, organelle localization, endosomal transport, endocytosis, and protein localization (**Supplementary Figures 3A,B**).

Since MERS-CoV infection in human microvascular ECs induced significant modulation of OCRGs, we further used a Venn diagram and MPA to examine MERS-CoV modulation of OCRGs. As shown in **Figure 6B**, MERS-CoV infection resulted in upregulation of 62 OCRGs and downregulation of 65 OCRGs. The majority of upregulated OCRGs in 12, 24, 36, and 48 h post infections were shared in at least two time points; four OCRGs were shared in all four time points such as HSPD1, MX1, STX1A, and GTPBP2. Seven downregulated OCRGs such as OPTN, BNIP3L, VAMP8, VPS41, AASS, EPS15, and PDCD6IP were shared in all four time points. Besides the overlapped three genes, the upregulated 59 OCRGs were from 15 functional groups, except autophagosome–lysosome fusion; and the downregulated 62 OCRGs were from 11 functional groups, except ER–PM junctions, sarcoplasmic reticulum–MT, MT biogenesis, ER–GC interaction, and endosome–GC groups (**Figure 6C**). As shown in **Supplementary Table 5B**, downregulation of five including VAMP8, VPS41, ATG14, STX17, and RILP out of nine regulators were in autophagosome–endosome/lysosome fusion; and downregulation of one out of four regulators, TIRAP, was in the autophagosome–lysosome fusion group. The top 10 pathways for upregulated OCRGs included mitochondrion organization, synaptic vesicle budding from presynaptic endocytic zone membrane, regulation of mitochondrion organization, autophagy, protein localization, response to unfolded protein, cargo recognition for clathrin-mediated endocytosis, divalent metal ion transport, MT DNA metabolic process, and tissue remodeling. The top 10 pathways for downregulated OCRGs included macroautophagy, organelle fusion, autophagosome maturation, protein localization, vacuolar transport, regulation of MT fission, membrane trafficking, autophagosome membrane docking, endocytosis, and MT transport. The Venn diagram indicated that MT transport, endocytosis, regulated exocytosis, and autophagosome maturation pathways were commonly downregulated in influenza virus- and MERS infectious clone (icMERS)-inoculated cells (**Supplementary Figures 3C,D**). Taken together, our results have demonstrated that (1) virus infection in ECs and lung epithelial cells significantly modulate OCRGs in all the functional groups; (2) decreased one group autophagosome–lysosome fusion and four signaling pathways including MT transport, endocytosis, regulated exocytosis, and autophagosome maturation are the significant organelle crosstalk features of viral infections. The significant modulation of OCRGs by MERS-CoV in human microvascular ECs may be the underlying mechanism for much higher (41–50%) acute kidney injuries caused by MERS-CoV than that of SARS-CoV (6.7%) and COVID-19 (3%) (85). These results suggest that increased organelle crosstalk in all 15 functional groups (except autophagosome–lysosome fusion) but decreased lysosome degradation are required for viral replication; and significant modulation of organelle crosstalk in human microvascular ECs in coronavirus family infection represented by MERS-CoV may be the important underlying mechanism for COVID-19 (caused by SARS-CoV 2)-induced cardiovascular complications (86, 87).

Organelle Crosstalk Regulators Upregulated by Pro-atherogenic Damage-Associated Molecular Patterns in Endothelial Cells Are Classified Endothelial Cell-Activation/Inflammation-Promoting Organelle Crosstalk Regulator Groups

Our previous reports showed that sterile inflammatory stimuli can cause intracellular organelle stress that occurs not only in cancer cells but also in vascular ECs (37). We reported that lysolipids are capable of transdifferentiating human aortic ECs (HAECs) into innate immune cells, including induction of potent DAMP receptors, such as CD36 molecule (14). CD36 pathways are activated by several distinct ligands, which converged on these pathways and results in inflammatory responses and endothelial dysfunction. CD36 pathway may be an underlying

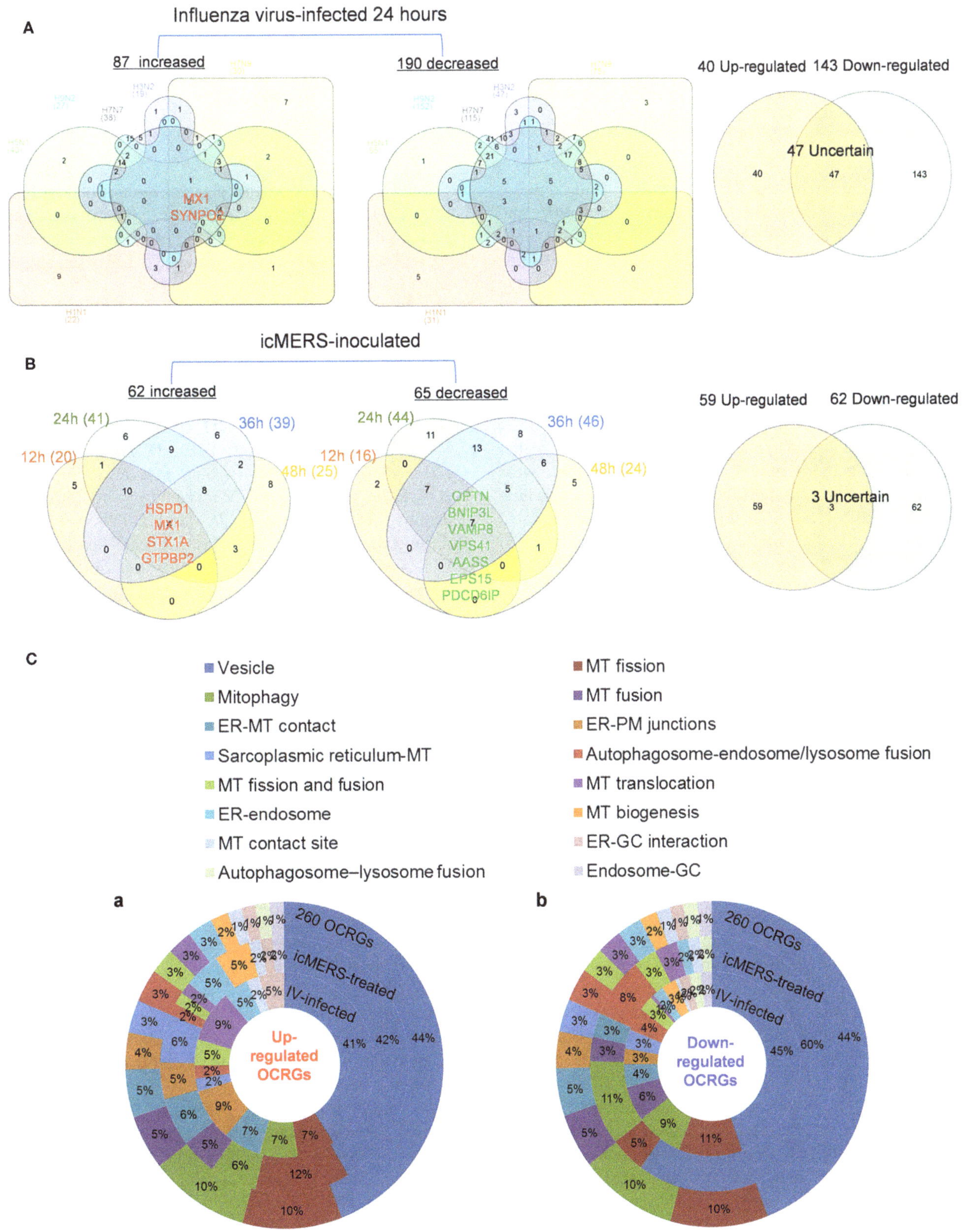

FIGURE 6 | More OCRGs were significantly expressed in influenza virus- and icMERS-inoculated cells. **(A)** In H1N1-infected human microvascular endothelial cells, H7N9-, H7N7-, H5N1-, and H3N2-infected Calu-3 cells and H9N2-infected human umbilical vein endothelial cells, MX1 and SYNPO2 were the common upregulated OCRGs shared by these six types of flu virus-treated cells; no common downregulated genes were shared by these six flu virus-treated cells. When the overlapped 47

(Continued)

FIGURE 6 | genes were removed, 40 genes are upregulated and 143 genes are downregulated in these five influenza virus-infected cells. **(B)** In time course, MERS coronavirus-inoculated human microvascular endothelial cells, HSPD1, MX1, STX1A, and GTPBP2 were the common upregulated OCRGs; and OPTN, BNIP3L, VAMP8, VPS41, AASS, EPS15, and PDCD6IP were the common downregulated OCRGs. When the overlapped three genes were removed, 59 genes are upregulated and 62 genes are downregulated in MERS coronavirus-inoculated cells. **(C)** Donut chart shows the ratio of classification of upregulated OCRGs **(A)** and downregulated OCRGs **(B)** in virus-treated cells. Classifications of upregulated OCRGs in icMERS- and influenza virus-inoculated cells are 15 and 12, respectively. Classifications of downregulated OCRGs in icMERS- and influenza virus-inoculated cells are 11 and 16, respectively.

cause of CVDs and cerebrovascular diseases (88). Oxidized lipids upregulated by CD36 can modulate endothelial properties and may contribute to atherogenesis (89). However, how DAMP receptor signaling modulates expression of organelle crosstalking in ECs remains poorly understood. We examined the expression changes of OCRGs in ECs under stimulations of various pathogen-associated molecular patterns (PAMPs)/DAMPs (90–92). As shown in **Table 3**, influenza virus infection in HUVECs upregulated 27 OCRGs and downregulated 137 OCRGs. Kaposi sarcoma-associated herpes virus infection in human dermal ECs upregulated six OCRGs and downregulated 10 OCRGs, suggesting that acute inflammatory virus infection has higher OCRG expression modulation than chronic tumorigenic virus infection. Lipopolysaccharide (LPS) stimulation of human lung microvascular ECs (HLMECs) for 4, 8, and 24 h upregulated 8, 17, and 9 OCRGs, respectively, and downregulated 7, 15, and 14 OCRGs, respectively. LPS stimulation of mouse aortic ECs (MAECs) for 4 h upregulated three OCRGs and downregulated five OCRGs, which were similar to those found in HLMECs. It has been reported that Notch1 signaling is involved in regulating MT biogenesis (93). On the other hand, organelle crosstalking also regulates Notch1 signaling. For example, the endocytic trafficking of Notch receptor leads to either transportation to lysosomes for degradation via multi-vesicular bodies (MVBs) and late endosomes or recycling back to the plasma membrane for ligand binding activation (94). However, how modulation of Notch signaling regulates organelle crosstalking in ECs remains poorly characterized. Inhibition of endothelial NOTCH1 (inflammation promoting) signaling with siRNA in the absence or presence of inflammatory cytokine interleukin-1β (IL-1β) stimulation for 24 h in HUVECs resulted in no modulation or one OCRG downregulation (with IL-1β) (95). However, another report showed that reduction of NOTCH1 expression in HAECs by siRNA, in the absence of stimulations with inflammatory lipids or cytokines, increased inflammatory molecules and binding of monocytes (96). In the datasets of this paper, we found that inhibition of NOTCH1 expression with siRNA in HAECs upregulated three OCRGs and downregulated six OCRGs. In addition, interferon-α (IFNα), IFNβ and IFNγ treatment of HUVECs led to upregulation of 7, 11, and 6 OCRGs, respectively, but no downregulation of OCRGs. Of note, oscillatory shear vs. laminar shear (fibrosa), oscillatory shear vs. laminar shear (ventricularis) (97), and MAECs from atherogenic apolipoprotein E (ApoE)-deficient mice vs. MAECs from wild-type control mice had no modulation of OCRG expressions potentially due to a long-term chronic adaptation process in response to shear stress or hyperlipidemia. Pro-atherogenic DAMP stimuli oxidized low-density lipoprotein (oxLDL) (98) and proinflammatory oxidized 1-palmitoyl-2-arachidonoyl-sn-glycerol-3-phosphatidylcholine (oxPAPC) stimulation of MAECs presumably via transient receptor potential ankyrin 1 (TRPA1) (99) upregulated three, zero, and seven OCRGs and downregulated five, six, and seven OCRGs (**Table 4**).

As shown in **Figures 7A,B** (**Supplementary Table 6** showed the detailed differentially expressed OCRGs), the 33 upregulated OCRGs in ECs included 10 out of 16 functional groups of OCRGs (except MT fission and fusion, MT translocation, MT biogenesis, MT contact site, autophagosome–lysosome fusion, and endosome–GC groups): (1) six MT fission regulators, DNM2, INF2, TMEM135, COX10, DDHD1, and LRRK2; (2) two mitophagy regulators, SQSTM1 (also vesicle group) and OPTN; (3) two ER–MT contact and sarcoplasmic reticulum–MT regulators, HSPA9 and ITPR1; (4) one ER–PM junction regulator, JPH2; (5) one MT fusion regulator, BAK1 (also ER–MT contact group); (6) one autophagosome–endosome/lysosome fusion regulator, STX17; and (7) the rest of the 17 vesicle regulators including BMP2, CD24, CSF2, POU2F2, ATP23, CLTC, P4HA2, VPS26A, ATP11A, CCZ1, EIF4ENIF1, RPS6KC1, GTPBP2, NOV, PICALM, PNPLA2, and RUNX1. The 36 downregulated OCRGs in ECs also included 10 out of 16 functional groups of OCRGs (except MT fusion, sarcoplasmic reticulum–MT, autophagosome–endosome/lysosome fusion, MT biogenesis, MT contact site, and endosome–GC groups). The upregulated top 5 pathways involved in DAMP-stimulated ECs included MT fission, autophagy, membrane trafficking, Golgi organization, and WNT pathway (**Figure 7C**). The downregulated top 5 pathways included MT fission, autophagy, synthesis of bile acids and bile salts, endocytosis, and RAB geranylgeranylation (**Figure 7D**). By comparison, 20 OCRGs were upregulated and were classified into five groups (**Supplementary Figures 5A,B**); the top pathways involved in upregulating OCRGs in LPS-stimulated ECs included MT fission, endosomal transport, receptor internalization, cytokine signaling in immune system, and ZNF410 TARGET GENES (**Supplementary Figure 5C**), latter four top pathways of which were different from those in DAMP-stimulated upregulation of OCRGs in ECs. The top pathways involved in downregulating OCRGs in LPS-stimulated ECs included MT fission, regulation of calcium ion transmembrane transporter activity, negative regulation of transferase activity, receptor metabolic process, and establishment of organelle localization, also latter four top pathways of which were different from those in DAMP-stimulated upregulation of OCRGs in ECs (**Supplementary Figure 5D**). Taken together, our results have demonstrated that (1) acute inflammatory (influenza) virus infection has higher OCRG modulation than in chronic tumorigenic (herpes) virus infection in ECs; (2) EC activation

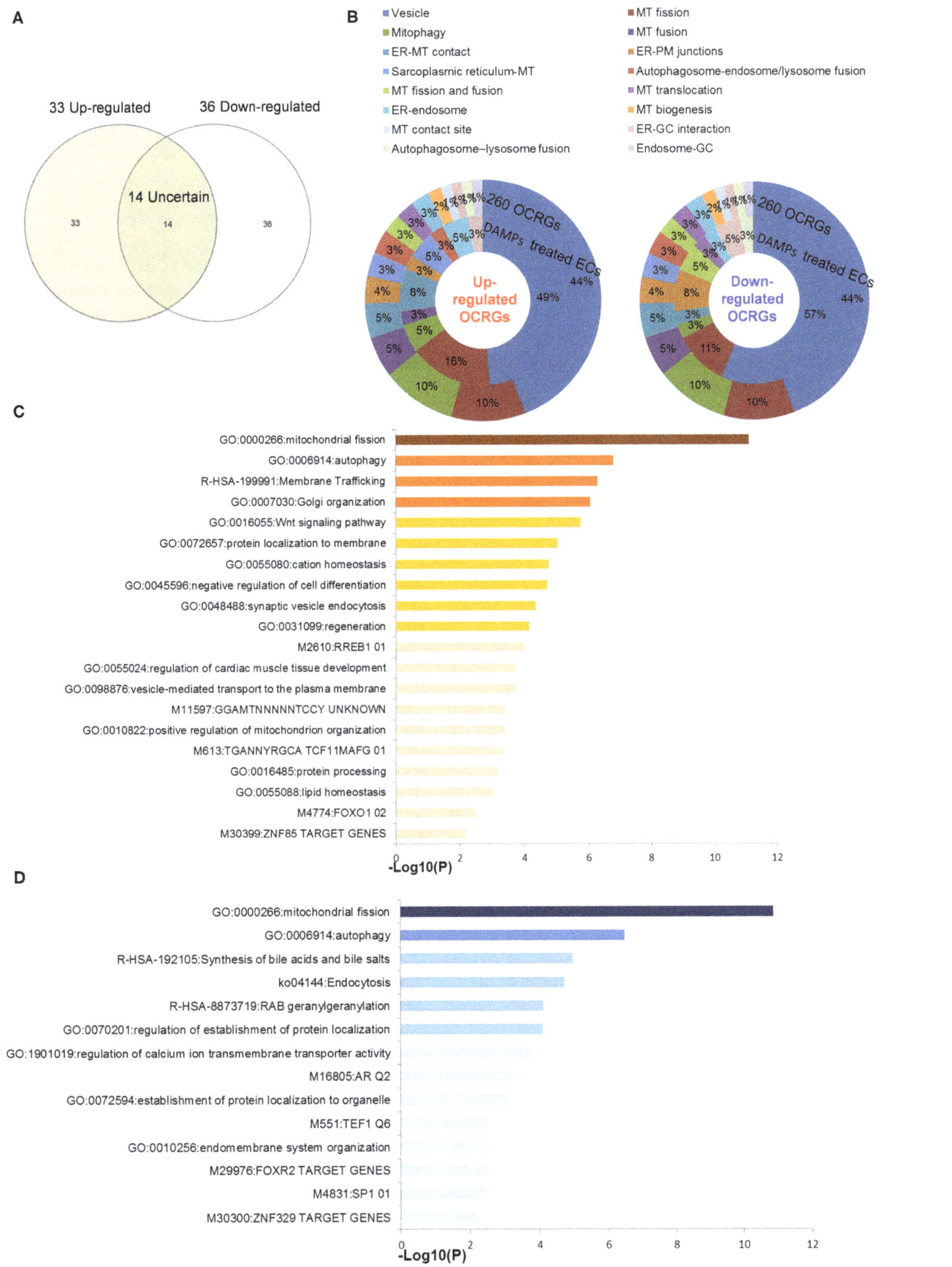

FIGURE 7 | Classifications of OCRGs differentially expressed in endothelial cells treated with pro-atherogenic DAMPs such as oxLDL, LPS, oxPAPC, and IFNs treated. **(A)** When the overlapped genes in all upregulated OCRGs and in all downregulated OCRGs were removed, 33 genes are upregulated and 36 genes are downregulated exclusively in inflammatory factor-treated endothelial cells. **(B)** Donut chart shows the ratio of classification of upregulated OCRGs (left) and

(Continued)

FIGURE 7 | downregulated OCRGs (right) in pro-atherogenic DAMP-treated endothelial cells. There are 10 classifications in 33 upregulated and 36 downregulated OCRGs, respectively. There are no MT fission and fusion, MT translocation, MT biogenesis, MT contact site, autophagosome–lysosome fusion, and endosome–GC OCRGs in upregulated genes and not MT fusion, sarcoplasmic reticulum–MT, autophagosome–endosome/lysosome fusion, MT biogenesis, MT contact site, and endosome–GC OCRGs in downregulated genes. **(C)** There are 20 significant GO enrichment results in 33 upregulated OCRGs of pro-atherogenic DAMP-treated endothelial cells. Top 3 GO enrichments of OCRGs are membrane trafficking, autophagy, and mitochondrial fission. Wnt signaling pathway is upregulated, and this change suggests inflammatory factors may be via Wnt signaling pathway, promoting inflammation induced by OCRGs. **(D)** There are 14 significant GO enrichment results in 36 downregulated OCRGs in inflammatory factor-treated endothelial cells. Calcium ion transmembrane transporter activity signaling is downregulated, and this change suggests that inflammatory factors can change calcium ion transmembrane transporter activity via OCRGs in endothelial cells. Enrichment analysis was performed by using Metascape software (http://metascape.org/gp/index.html#/main/step1; PMID: 30944313).

stimuli such as TLR4 stimulation by LPS and oxLDL result in modulation of OCRGs in HAECs and MAECs; (3) modulation of OCRGs by inhibition of NOTCH1 in HAEC is associated with increased inflammatory status and increased atherosclerosis in endothelial NOTCH1 heterozygous mice; (4) proinflammatory cytokines type 1 IFN (α, β, and probably ω, κ, and ε) signaling and type II IFN (γ) (100) modulated OCRG expression in ECs; and (5) oscillatory shear vs. laminar shear vs. laminar shear and ApoE KO MAECs have no modulation of OCRGs, potentially due to adaptation of ApoE KO MAECs and interplays of multiple pathways bone morphogenetic protein (BMP)-transforming growth factor-β (TGFβ), Wingless and Int-1 (WNT), Notch membrane receptors (NOTCH), hypoxia inducible factor-α (HIF1α a transcription factor), Twist family basic helix-loop-helix (BHLH) transcription factor 1 (TWIST1), and a subset of homeobox genes (HOX family) (101).

The Expressions of Organelle Crosstalk Regulators Are Modulated in Regulatory T Cells in Comparison With Those of CD4$^+$CD25$^-$ T Effector Controls; Upregulated Organelle Crosstalk Regulators Are More Than Downregulated Organelle Crosstalk Regulators in Regulatory T Cells

Recent reports showed that the MT membrane potential and the proliferation inhibition function of CD4$^+$Foxp3$^+$ Treg from patients with myasthenia gravis are enhanced by autophagy inducing agent rapamycin and suppressed by phosphoinositide 3-kinase (PI3 kinase) and autophagy inhibitor 3-methyladenine (3-MA) (102) and that during autoimmune conditions, Treg function alterations associate with MT oxidative stress, dysfunctional mitophagy, and enhanced DNA damage and cell death (103, 104). We hypothesized that the expressions of OCRGs are modulated in CD4$^+$CD25^{high}FOXP3$^+$ Treg in comparison with those of CD4$^+$CD25$^-$ T effector cell controls. As shown in **Table 5**, Treg from eight different tissues including lymph nodes (LNs), visceral adipose tissue, brown adipose tissue (cold), brown adipose tissue (warm), spleen from mice with skeletal muscle injury for 4 days, spleen from mice with skeletal muscle injury for 14 days, and spleen from male and female mice had no downregulated OCRGs. In addition, Treg from five tissues such as warm spleen, skeletal muscle from mice with skeletal muscle injury for 4 days, skeletal muscle from mice with skeletal muscle injury for 14 days, intestine, and peripheral blood had one, four, two, one, and one downregulated OCRGs, respectively. Moreover, Treg in spleen from female mice had no upregulated OCRGs; and Treg from the rest of the 12 groups had one to 12 upregulated OCRGs (**Supplementary Table 7** listed, in detail, the significant expressed OCRGs in Treg compared with conventional T cells). To examine a hypothesis that the expressions of OCRGs are required for the suppressive functions of Treg, we determined this hypothesis with Treg signature gene deficient microarray datasets. The 15 microarrays of Treg regulator deficiency datasets were collected to analyze the expression changes of OCRGs (**Table 6**). In the deficiency datasets of Treg signature genes GATA binding protein 3 (Gata3), histone deacetylase 9 (Hdac9), and peroxisome proliferator activated receptor gamma (Pparg) in LNs, there were no significant expression changes of OCRGs. There were seven significantly upregulated OCRGs and no downregulated OCRGs in Treg signature transcription factor B-cell lymphoma 6 (Bcl6) knockout Treg from spleen and LN. There were six significantly upregulated OCRGs and one downregulated OCRG in Foxo1 knockout Treg from the thymus, spleen, and LNs. In Dicer 1 (ribonuclease III, microRNA-maturation enzyme) knockout CD4$^+$ T cells, there were five upregulated OCRGs and one downregulated OCRG. In tripartite motif containing 28 [E3 small ubiquitin-like modifier (SUMO)-protein ligase Trim28] knockout Treg, there were three upregulated OCRGs and five downregulated OCRGs. In B lymphocyte-induced maturation protein 1 (Blimp1) deficiency Treg, there were three upregulated OCRGs and six downregulated OCRGs.

As shown in **Figure 8A**, when combining all the upregulated and downregulated OCRGs in the Treg, besides the overlapping genes, four OCRGs downregulated in Treg included sarcoplasmic reticulum–mitochondria contact regulator OSBP-related protein 8 (Osbpl8) (105), MT fission regulators MX1 and MX2, and one vesicle regulator Hexim1 (**Supplementary Table 8**). There were no significant pathways of the upregulated OCRGs from MPA. The 19 upregulated OCRGs included one autophagosome–lysosome fusion regulator Tirap, one mitophagy regulator Vmp1, one MT fission gene Dcn, one MT translocation Tomm7, Vdac1 with more function (mitophagy, ER–MT contact, sarcoplasmic reticulum–MT), MT fission and fusion, mitophagy regulator Bnip3, and the other 13 vesicle regulators (**Supplementary Table 8** and **Figure 8B**). The top signaling pathways of these upregulated OCRGs from the MPA included positive regulation of macroautophagy, regeneration, regulation of protein stability, positive regulation of apoptotic process,

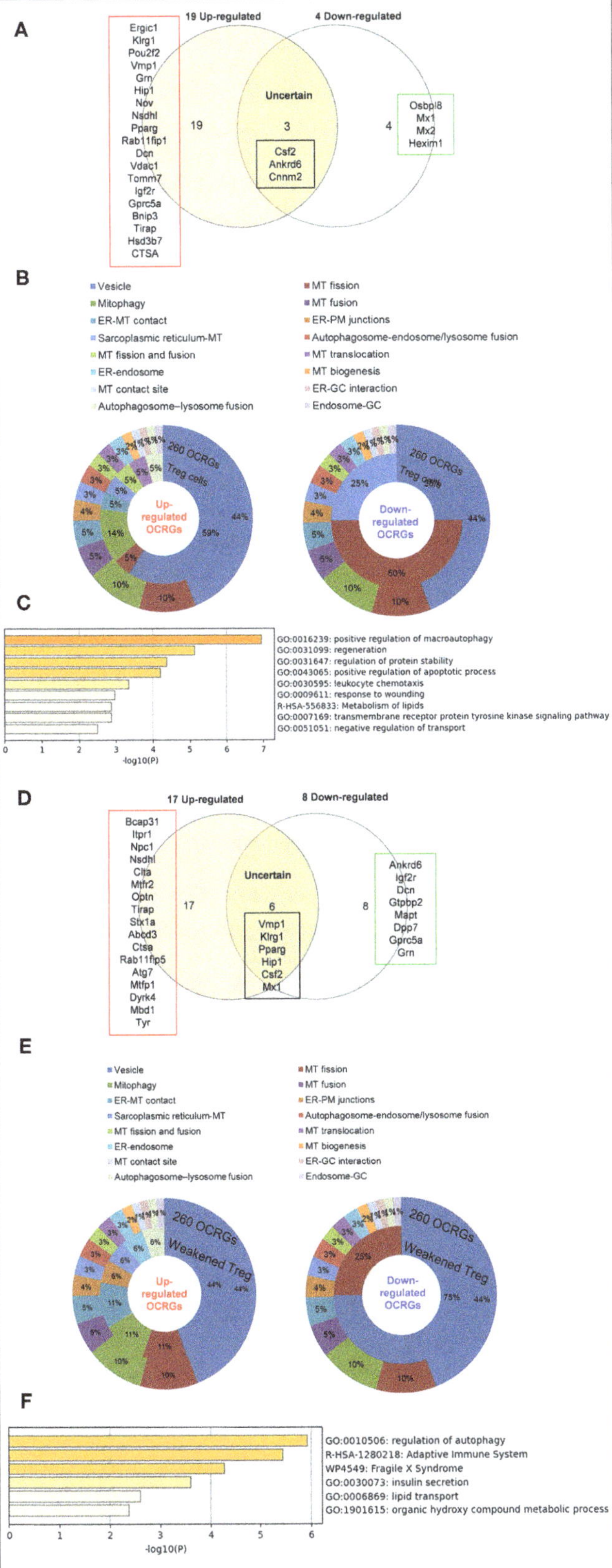

FIGURE 8 | Less classification of OCRGs differentially expressed in regulatory T cells and weakened Treg cells. **(A)** When the overlapped three genes in all upregulated OCRGs and in all downregulated OCRGs were removed, 19

(Continued)

FIGURE 8 | genes are upregulated and four genes are downregulated exclusively in regulatory T cells. **(B)** Donut chart shows the ratio of classification of upregulated OCRGs (left) and downregulated OCRGs (right) in regulatory T cells. There are eight classifications in 19 upregulated OCRGs and three classifications in four downregulated OCRGs. **(C)** Enrichment analysis results of 19 upregulated genes show signaling pathways of positive regulation of macroautophagy, regeneration, regulation of protein stability, positive regulation of apoptotic process, leukocyte chemotaxis, response to wounding, metabolism of lipids, transmembrane receptor protein tyrosine kinase signaling pathway, and negative regulation of transport were upregulated. **(D)** When the overlapped five genes in all upregulated genes and in all downregulated genes were removed, 17 genes are upregulated and eight genes are downregulated exclusively in regulatory T-cell signature gene deficiency (weakened regulatory T cells). **(E)** Donut chart shows the ratio of classification of upregulated OCRGs (left) and downregulated OCRGs (right) in weakened regulatory T cells. There are eight classifications (vesicle, MT fission, Mitophagy, ER–MT contact, ER–PM junctions, sarcoplasmic reticulum–MT, ER–endosome, and autophagosome–lysosome fusion) in 17 upregulated OCRGs and two classifications (vesicle and MT fission) in eight downregulated OCRGs, respectively. **(F)** Enrichment analysis results of 17 upregulated genes show signaling pathways of regulation of autophagy, adaptive immune system, Fragile X syndrome, insulin secretion, lipid transport, and organic hydroxy compound metabolic process.

and leukocyte chemotaxis (**Figure 8C**). These results have demonstrated for the first time that Treg from various tissues and mice with injured skeletal muscle have upregulation of OCRGs compared with those of $CD4^{+}CD25^{-}$ T effector controls; and Treg slightly upregulate a few OCRGs in Treg from visceral adipose tissue, skeletal muscle, and intestine. The results of weakened Treg cells from 11 microarrays (Treg signature gene knockout datasets) showed that the upregulated OCRGs were more than downregulated OCRGs (**Table 6** and **Supplementary Table 9** list in detail differentially expressed OCRGs). As shown in **Figure 8D**, the 17 upregulated OCRGs included one autophagosome–lysosome fusion gene Tirap, one ER–endosome contact gene Npc1, two ER–MT contact genes Bcap31 and Itpr1 (also sarcoplasmic reticulum-MT group), one ER–PM junctions Stx1a, two mitophagy genes Optn and Atg7, two MT fission genes Mtfr2 and Mtfp1, and the other eight vesicle regulators (Nsdhl, Clta, Abcd3, Ctsa, Rab11fip5, Dyrk4, Mbd1, and Tyr). The eight downregulated OCRGs included two MT fission regulators Dcn and Mapt and six vesicle regulators (Ankrd6, Igf2r, Gtpbp2, Dpp7, Gprc5a, and Grn) (**Supplementary Table 9** and **Figure 8E**). There were no significant pathways in the downregulated OCRGs from MPA. The signaling pathways of these upregulated OCRGs included regulation of autophagy, adaptive immune system, Fragile X syndrome, insulin secretion lipid transport, and organic hydroxy compound metabolic process (**Figure 8F**). Taken together, our results have demonstrated that (1) the expression of OCRGs are modulated in $CD4^{+}FOXP3^{+}$ Treg and Treg cells with signature genes deficiencies; and (2) upregulated OCRGs in Treg are more than downregulated OCRGs. In weakened Treg when Treg signature genes are deficient, upregulated OCRGs are more than downregulated OCRGs; and (3) positive regulation of macroautophagy, regeneration, regulation of protein stability, positive regulation of apoptotic process, and leukocyte chemotaxis signaling are upregulated in Treg; and regulation of autophagy, adaptive immune system, Fragile X syndrome, insulin secretion, lipid transport, and organic hydroxy compound metabolic process are upregulated in weakened Treg.

Toll-Like Receptors, Reactive Oxygen Species Regulator Nuclear Factor Erythroid 2-Related Factor 2, and Inflammasome-Activated Caspase-1 Regulate the Expressions of Organelle Crosstalk Regulators

In order to determine the mechanisms underlying the expression changes of OCRGs in diseases, virus-infected cells, and pro-atherogenic DAMP-treated ECs, we examined expressions of OCRGs in nine microarrays including six TLRs (106), one ROS regulator Nrf2 (23), and two caspase-1-deficient microarrays. Caspase-1 is activated in the DAMP/PAMP-sensing protein complexes termed inflammasomes (3, 11, 16, 36, 39, 90, 106–110) (**Tables 7–9**). The results showed that TLR2, TLR4, and TLR3/7/9 deficiencies upregulated 29, seven, and nine OCRGs and downregulated 37, 12, and 12 OCRGs, respectively (**Supplementary Figure 6**). In addition, ROS negative regulator Nrf2 deficiency upregulated 14 and downregulated seven OCRGs. Moreover, caspase-1 deficiency upregulated seven and downregulated five OCRGs. Then we proposed two models to explore the mechanisms underlying the expression changes of OCRGs regulated by DAMP/PAMP sensing TLRs and caspase-1/inflammasomes (**Figures 9A,B**). A Venn diagram was used to identify the regulated OCRGs in diseases, virus infections, and cells stimulated by pro-atherogenic DAMPs (**Supplementary Figures 7–11**). As shown in **Figure 9C** and **Supplementary Table 10**, TLRs, caspase-1, and ROS regulators play significant roles in upregulating a total of 46 OCRGs (17.7%) from 14 groups (except for MT fission and fusion and ER–MT contact OCRGs) in different diseases, virus, and pro-atherogenic factor-treated cells. Of note, the signaling pathways in upregulating 12 OCRGs (i.e., CSF2, MX1, ABCD3, ATP2A1, APOOL, PDXDC1, MX2, CSF2, POU2F2, MCOLN1, NPC1, RUNX1, and BMP2) are shared by two groups of upstream regulators. These findings suggest that these 12 OCRGs may play important roles in pathophysiologies upregulated by DAMP/PAMP signaling.

Organelle Crosstalk Regulators Are Significantly Modulated in Cancer; Upregulations of Organelle Crosstalk Regulators in Liver Hepatocellular Carcinoma and Lung Squamous Cell Carcinoma Are Correlated With Immune Infiltrates; Mitochondrial Import Machine Is Upregulated in Cancers and Is Associated With Immune Infiltrates

It has been reported that mitophagy pathways are intricately linked to the metabolic rewiring of cancer cells to support the high bioenergetic demand of the tumors (111); autophagy, acting as a cancer-suppressive function, is inclined to hinder metastasis by selectively downregulating critical transcription factors of the epithelial–mesenchymal transition (EMT) in the early phases (112). The molecular mechanisms underlying fusion, with either lysosomes or plasma membrane, are key determinants to maintain cell homeostasis upon stressing stimuli. The accumulation of undigested substrates leads to cancer and other diseases such as lysosomal storage disorders and age-related neurodegenerative diseases (113). We hypothesized that carcinogenesis modulates the expressions of OCRGs. To examine this hypothesis, we collected the expression data of 260 OCRGs in 28 cancer datasets in the NIH-NCI TCGA (https://www.cancer.gov/about-nci/organization/ccg/research/structural-genomics/tcga/using-tcga)/GTEx database (GTEx Portal, https://www.gtexportal.org/home/) from EGPIA2 (http://gepia2.cancer-pku.cn/#index). As shown in **Table 10**, all the 28 cancers from the gastrointestinal, respiratory, brain, genitourinary, hematopoietic, and digestive systems significantly modulated the expressions of OCRGs. The upregulated OCRGs range from one OCRG in lung adenocarcinoma (LUAD) to 166 OCRGs in thymoma; and downregulated OCRGs range from three in pancreatic adenocarcinoma (PAAD) to 65 in testicular germ cell tumor.

To identify the common features of OCRG modulation in cancers, we calculated the percentage (a/b%) of upregulated OCRGs (a) over total upregulated expressed genes and (b) in the cancer microarrays, and the ratios of downregulated OCRGs over total downregulated genes. We noticed that 16 cancers had upregulated OCRG percentage >1% and 12 cancers had upregulated OCRGs percentages <1%. Cancers were roughly classified into eight systems to explore the expression changes of OCRGs. The numbers of upregulated OCRGs were more than those of downregulated genes in tumors of the immune system, digestive system, and nervous system. The numbers of downregulated OCRGs were more than those of the upregulated OCRGs in tumors of the endocrine system, respiratory system, and circulation system and most tumors of the reproductive system and urinary system. In breast invasive carcinoma (BRCA) and skin cutaneous melanoma (SKCM), the numbers of upregulated OCRGs were more than those of downregulated OCRGs. In head and neck squamous cell carcinoma (HNSC), the numbers of upregulated OCRGs were less than those of downregulated OCRGs (**Figures 10A,B**). We then examined a hypothesis that upregulations of OCRGs are correlated with increased immune cell infiltration. To examine this hypothesis, GSCA database (http://bioinfo.life.hust.edu.cn/GSCA/#/immune) (76) was used to analyze the correlation of upregulated OCRGs with immune infiltrates. Liver hepatocellular carcinoma (LIHC) and lung squamous cell carcinoma (LUSC) were studied for the details as an example. The result in **Figure 10C** shows that almost 19 upregulated OCRGs in LIHC were positively correlated with B cells, natural killer (NK) cells, effector-memory T cells, naturally occurring Treg (nTreg), CD8 T cells, dendritic cells (DCs), type 1 Treg (Tr1), and type 1 T helper cells (Th1) infiltration but negatively correlated with macrophages, neutrophils, CD4 T cells, inducible Treg (iTreg), central memory T cells, monocytes, Th17, and

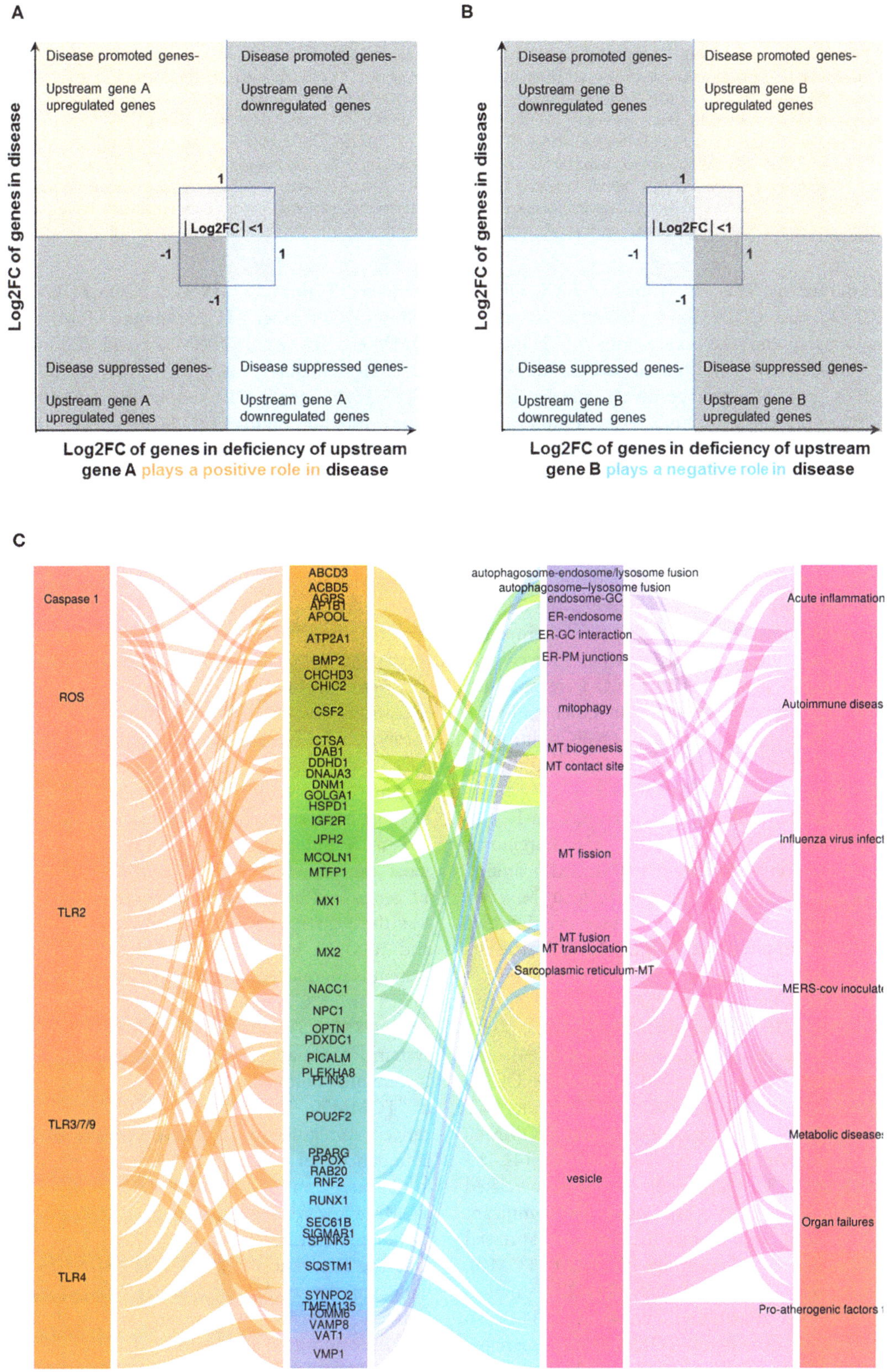

FIGURE 9 | Three types of regulators (TLRs, caspase-1, and ROS regulators) upregulated a total of 46 OCRGs in different diseases, and virus- and pro-atherogenic factor-treated cells. **(A)** Two models were used to explore the mechanisms of expression changes of OCRGs in the upstream gene-deficient microarrays. When the

(Continued)

FIGURE 9 | upstream gene A plays a positive role (promote disease) in disease (or in virus, pro-atherogenic DAMP-treated cells), OCRGs upregulated in the disease will be downregulated in deficiency of upstream gene A (upper left box). OCRGs downregulated in the disease will be upregulated in deficiency of upstream gene A (bottom right box). **(B)** When the upstream gene B plays a negative role (suppress disease) in disease (or in virus, pro-atherogenic DAMP-treated cells), OCRGs upregulated in the disease will be upregulated in deficiency of upstream gene B (upper right box). OCRGs downregulated in the disease will be downregulated in deficiency of upstream gene B (bottom left box). **(C)** Alluvial plot shows the regulated 46 OCRGs by TLR2, TLR4, TLR3/7/9, caspase-1, and ROS regulator Nrf2; and these 46 OCRGs classified 14 groups of all 16 groups (except for MT fission and fusion, and ER–MT contact OCRGs), and vesicle, MT fission, and mitophagy are the top 3 groups. TLR2 regulated 24 OCRGs and caspase-1 regulated five OCRGs. Twelve OCRGs (i.e., CSF2, MX1, ABCD3, ATP2A1, APOOL, PDXDC1, MX2, CSF2, POU2F2, MCOLN1, NPC1, RUNX1, and BMP2) were regulated by two upstream regulators; other OCRGs were regulated by one upstream regulator. The regulated OCRGs were more in autoimmune diseases and virus-infected cells than in other diseases. Alluvial plot was plotted by http://www.bioinformatics.com.cn, an online platform for data analysis and visualization. The detailed relation between OCRGs and upstream regulators is listed in **Supplementary Table 10**.

CD4 naïve cell infiltrations. The expressions of BAX, OPTN, GRN, CTSA, CLTA, and CD24 were positively correlated with infiltration scores; and the expressions of TOMM20 were negatively correlated with infiltration scores. Almost 14 upregulated OCRGs in LUSC were positively correlated with CD8 T cells, nTreg, and effector-memory T-cell infiltrations and were negatively correlated with CD4 T cells, gamma-delta T cells, NK cells, mucosal-associated invariant T cells (MAIT), cytotoxic macrophages, NK cells, and follicular T helper (Tfh) cells infiltrations. The expressions of all 14 OCRGs were negatively correlated with immune cell infiltration scores (**Figure 10D**). Therefore, our findings have demonstrated that the expression modulations of OCRGs can predict the degrees of tumor immune infiltrations and serve as potential therapeutic targets. The GO (Gene Ontology) chord analysis showed that more upregulated OCRGs in LIHC and LUSC were enriched in mitochondrion organization pathway than other pathways (**Figures 10E,F**). In fact, the upregulated OCRGs in most tumors can be enriched in mitochondrion organization pathways (**Supplementary Figure 12**).

We further examined five digestive cancers such as PAAD, stomach adenocarcinoma (STAD), rectal adenocarcinoma (READ), LIHC, and colon adenocarcinoma (COAD) among the cancer groups with >1% OCRGs and performed the Venn diagram analysis on upregulated OCRGs of these five digestive cancers. As shown in **Supplementary Figure 13A**, the results showed that PAAD had 80 specific OCRGs (54.8%) out of 146 upregulated OCRGs. In contrast, the other cancers had much lower specific OCRGs. For example, STAD, READ, LIHC, and COAD had three (5.6%), one (2.8%), two (11.1%), and zero (0%) specific OCRGs, respectively. Of note, one OCRG shared by all five cancer groups was translocase of outer MT membrane 40 (TOMM40). We also found that TOMM40 was upregulated in 14 out of 33 types of cancers (42.4%) (**Supplementary Figure 13B**). Our results are well-correlated with previous reports that TOMM40 (TOM40) and significant numbers of MT protein import machineries overexpressed in cancers such as the TOM complex (TOM20, TOM40, TOM7, and TOM70), TIM23 complex, TIM22 complex, small Tim chaperons and Mia40, and Tim 44 (111, 114). To elucidate the functional aspects of TOMM40, we searched the PPI network database in the STRING database (https://string-db.org/). As shown in **Supplementary Figure 13C**, the top 10 proteins functionally interacted with TOMM40 including translocase of outer MT membrane (TOM) complex members TOMM7, TOMM20, TOMM70A, and TOMM22; translocase of inner MT membrane (TIM) complex members TIMM50, TIMM44, TIMM13, and TIMM10; sorting and assembly machinery complex (SAM) member SAMM50; and CYC1 (cytochrome C1, complex III subunit 4). As shown in **Supplementary Figures 13D,E**, the most relative top 10 genes to TOMM40 were localized in two types of protein complexes, the translocase of outer MT membrane complexes (TOMs) and translocase of inner MT membrane complexes (TIMs), and were mainly enriched in protein targeting to mitochondria, protein transporter activity and MT protein complex in biology process, molecular function and cell component (115, 116). The enriched pathways of these 11 genes were MT protein import, Pink/Parkin-mediated mitophagy, and Ub-specific processing proteases (117). We further determined whether increased expressions of TOMM40 and 10 interaction proteins in cancers lead to better prognosis by analyzing the overall survival map of hazard ratio (HR) and disease-free survival map [relapse-free survival (RFS)] of TOMM40 and 10 interaction proteins. The result showed that overall survival of patients in most cancers were positively related to these 11 genes (red box in **Supplementary Figure 13F**); and RFS of patients in most cancers was positively related to upregulation of these 11 genes (red box in **Supplementary Figure 13G**; the blue box was the negative correlation between the expression of genes and RFS). It has been reported that MT protein transport system is modulated in cancers (118). A previous report showed that TOMM70 acts as receptor of the MT antiviral-signaling protein (MAVS) and thereby participates in the corresponding system of innate immunity against viral infections (119). It remains unknown whether this innate immune function of TOMM70 is correlated with the better prognosis of cancers upregulating TOMM40 complexes. Relations between abundance of tumor-infiltrating lymphocytes, immuno-inhibitors, immuno-stimulators, MHCs, and expression of TOMM40 were explored by using TISIDB database (http://cis.hku.hk/TISIDB/index.php) (75). The results indicated that the expressions of TOMM40 were positively correlated with abundance of act CD8, act CD4, CD56, and monocyte cells in most of the cancers and that immuno-inhibitor PVRL2; immuno-stimulators CD276, PVR, TNFRSF18, TNFRSF25, and TNFRSF4; and HLA-A, HLA-B, HLA-C, HLA-F, TAP1, TAP2, and TAPBP molecules were positively correlated with expression of TOMM40 in most of cancers (**Supplementary Figure 14**). We speculate that upregulation of

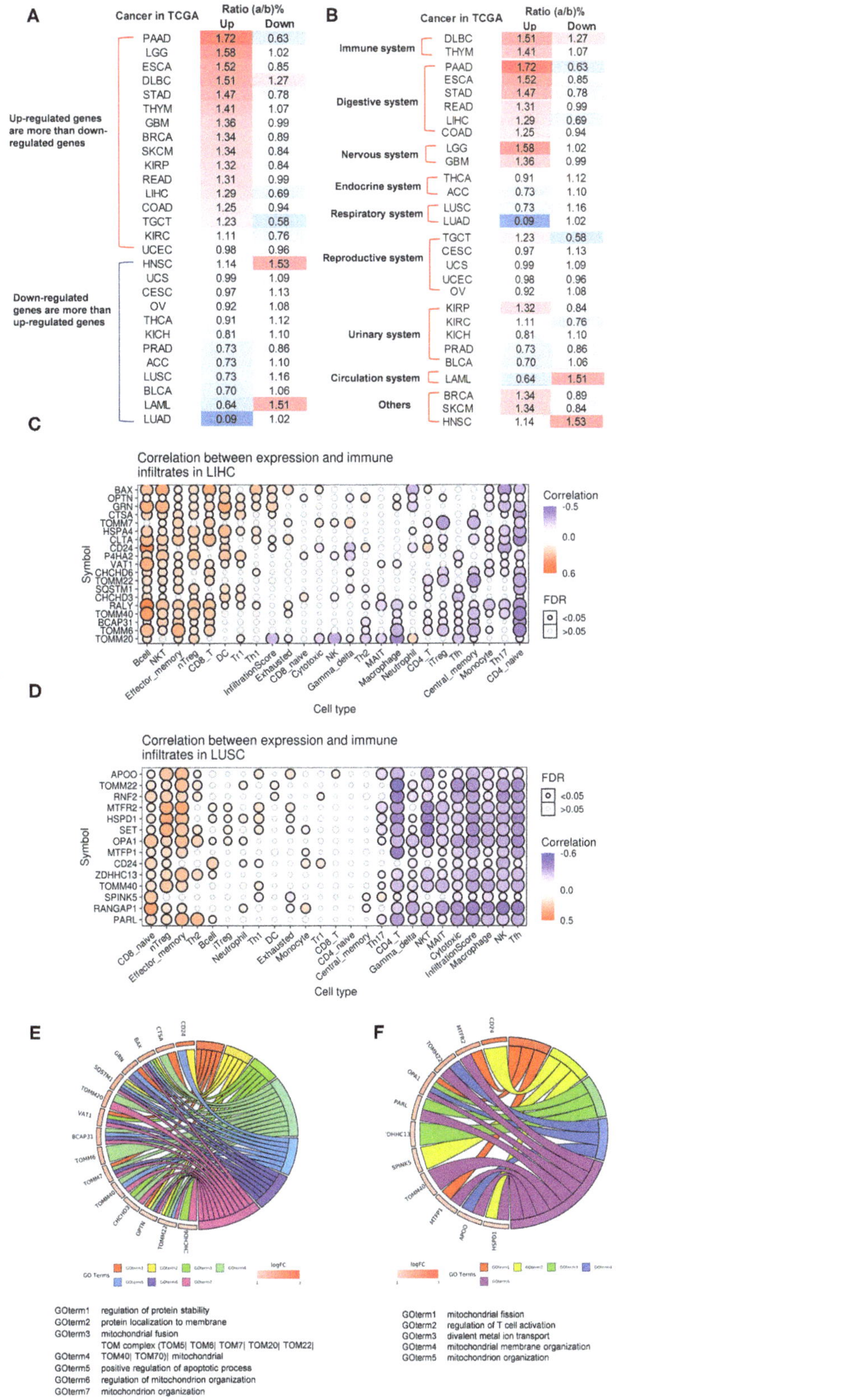

FIGURE 10 | The ratio of upregulated and downregulated OCRGs has different dominance in tumors of different systems, and differentially expressed OCRGs are correlated with immune infiltrates in liver hepatocellular carcinoma (LIHC) and lung squamous cell carcinoma (LUSC). **(A)** Tumors are listed according to the ratio of

(Continued)

FIGURE 10 | upregulated and downregulated OCRGs. The results show that in pancreatic adenocarcinoma (PAAD), brain lower-grade glioma (LCC), and esophageal carcinoma (ESCA), these 15 cancers [from PAAD to uterine corpus endometrial carcinoma (UCEC)] upregulated OCRGs more than the downregulated OCRGs; in lung adenocarcinoma (LUAD), adrenocortical carcinoma (ACC), and acute myeloid leukemia (LAML), these 13 cancers (from HNSC to LUAD) downregulated OCRGs more than the upregulated genes. In order to rule out the influence of the overall expression profile on our interest OCRGs, we take the ratio of number of OCRGs and number of total differently expressed genes as the comparison criteria for the number of upregulated and downregulated genes. Result show that 16 cancers have upregulated OCRG percentage >1% and that 12 cancers have upregulated OCRGs percentages <1%. **(B)** Expression of OCRGs in tumors was roughly classified according to the system. The numbers of upregulated OCRGs are more than downregulated genes in tumors of immune system, digestive system, and nervous system. The numbers of downregulated OCRGs are more than upregulated OCRGs in tumors of the endocrine system, respiratory system, and circulation system and most tumors of the reproductive system and urinary system. In breast invasive carcinoma (BRCA) and skin cutaneous melanoma (SKCM), the numbers of upregulated OCRGs are more than those of downregulated OCRGs. In head and neck squamous cell carcinoma (HNSC), the numbers of upregulated OCRGs are less than those of downregulated OCRGs. **(C)** Almost 19 upregulated OCRGs in LIHC are positively correlated with B cell, NKT, effector memory, nTreg, CD8 T, DC, Tr1, and Th1 infiltration but negatively correlated with macrophage, neutrophil, CD4 T, iTreg, central memory, monocyte, Th17, and CD4 naïve cell infiltration. Expressions of BAX, OPTN, GRN, CTSA, CLTA, and CD24 are positively correlated with infiltration score, and expression of TOMM20 is negatively correlated with infiltration score. **(D)** Fourteen upregulated OCRGs in LUSC are positively correlated with CD8 T, nTreg, and effector-memory cell infiltration and negatively correlated with CD4 T, gamma-delta, NKT, MAIT, cytotoxic macrophage, NK, and Tfh cell infiltration. Expressions of all 14 OCRGs are negatively correlated with infiltration score. Correlations between expression of upregulated OCRGs and immune infiltrates were analyzed in LIHC and LUSC in Gene Set Cancer Analysis (GSCA) database (http://bioinfo.life.hust.edu.cn/GSCA/#/immune). **(E)** Fifteen out 19 upregulated OCRGs in LIHC enriched in seven significant pathways including regulation of protein stability, protein localization to membrane, mitochondrial fusion, TOM mitochondrial, positive regulation of apoptotic process, regulation of mitochondrion organization, and mitochondrion organization. More OCRGs enriched in TOM complex mitochondrial and mitochondrion organization (GOterm4 and GOterm7). **(F)** Eleven out of 14 OCRGs in LUSC enriched in five significant pathways including mitochondrial fission, regulation of T cell activation, divalent metal ion transport, mitochondrial membrane organization, and mitochondrion organization. More OCRGs (TOMM40, APOO, PARL, HSPD1, MTFP1, TOMM22, OPA1, and MTFR2) enriched mitochondrion organization pathway (GOterm5). GO (Gene Ontology) chord was generated by http://www.bioinformatics.com.cn, an online platform for data analysis and visualization.

TOMM40 may improve the prognosis of patients by promoting tumor immunity.

Tumor Promoter Factor and Tumor Suppressor Significantly Modulate the Expressions of Organelle Crosstalk Regulators; Vesicle Regulators May Attenuate or Increase Tumorigenesis When Tumor Promoter Factor or Tumor Suppressor Is Deficient

We then hypothesized that oncogenes and tumor suppressors play important roles in regulating the expressions of OCRGs in cancer cells. To test this hypothesis, we collected a total of 19 microarrays from the deficiencies of oncogenes and tumor suppressors in NIH–NCBI–GEO dataset database (https://www.ncbi.nlm.nih.gov/gds/). Since NF-kB and inflammation have been linked to Kras mutations and cancer development, inhibitor of NF-kB kinase subunit b (IKK2) depletion in lung tumor cells significantly attenuates tumor proliferation and prolongs mouse survival (120). As shown in **Table 11**, IKK2 KO vs. wild-type control upregulated five OCRG and downregulated five OCRGs in mouse lung tumor lines. Four additional IKK and IKK2 knockout (KO) in mouse lung tumor nodules, mouse and human leukemia cells, and human MDA-MB-231 breast cancer epithelial cells did not significantly modulate OCRGs. Deficiencies of NF-kB subunit Rela in mouse lung carcinoma cells and human MDA-MD-231 cells upregulated one and five OCRGs and downregulated two OCRGs. In addition, the Janus kinases (JAKs)/signal transducer and activator of transcription proteins (STATs) signaling pathway provide important roles in contributing to oncogenesis in hematological malignancies and solid tumors (121). JAK2 knockdown (KD) in human acute myelogenous leukemia (AML) cell line, STAT1 KD in human T cell acute lymphocytic leukemia cells, Stat3 KD in mouse mammary tumor, and STAT3 KD in human urothelial cancer cells resulted in zero to two OCRG upregulation and one to five OCRG downregulations. Moreover, tumor suppressor and transcription factor Tp53 KO in mouse liver tumor (122), mouse mammary epithelial cells, oviductal cells, neural stem cells, small intestine, and neu primary tumor led to upregulation of zero up to 23 OCRGs and downregulation of zero up to 48 OCRGs, respectively. Of note, adenomatous polyposis coli (APC) is a multi-functional tumor suppressor gene (123); and a limited role for Tp53 is found in modulating early tumor progression induced by APC loss in mouse intestine (124). APC KO led to six OCRG upregulation and three OCRG downregulation compared with that of wild-type controls, respectively. Furthermore, phosphatidylinositol 3-kinase (PI3-kinase) and phosphatase and tensin homolog deleted on chromosome 10 (PTEN) are major positive and negative regulators of PI3 kinase pathway in regulating cell growth, survival, and proliferation and are two of the most frequently mutated proteins in human cancers (125). PTEN is a tumor suppressor (126); and PTEN KD and KO resulted in zero to seven OCRG upregulation and zero to four OCRG downregulation. In all the significantly modulated OCRGs, there were 13 upregulated and 16 downregulated OCRGs in the oncogene deficiency databases examined and 47 upregulated and 50 downregulated OCRGs in tumor suppressors deficiency databases (**Supplementary Figures 15A,B**, **Supplementary Tables 11, 12** listed, in detail, the modulated OCRGs). These results have demonstrated that in tumor conditions, upregulated oncogenes positively increased the expressions of 16 upregulated OCRGs and 13 downregulated OCRGs. In contrast, tumor suppressors deficiencies upregulated 47 OCRGs in these datasets. Upregulated and downregulated OCRGs were classified into seven groups in oncogene deficiencies and were classified into 12 and 14 groups in tumor suppressors deficiencies (**Supplementary Figure 15C**).

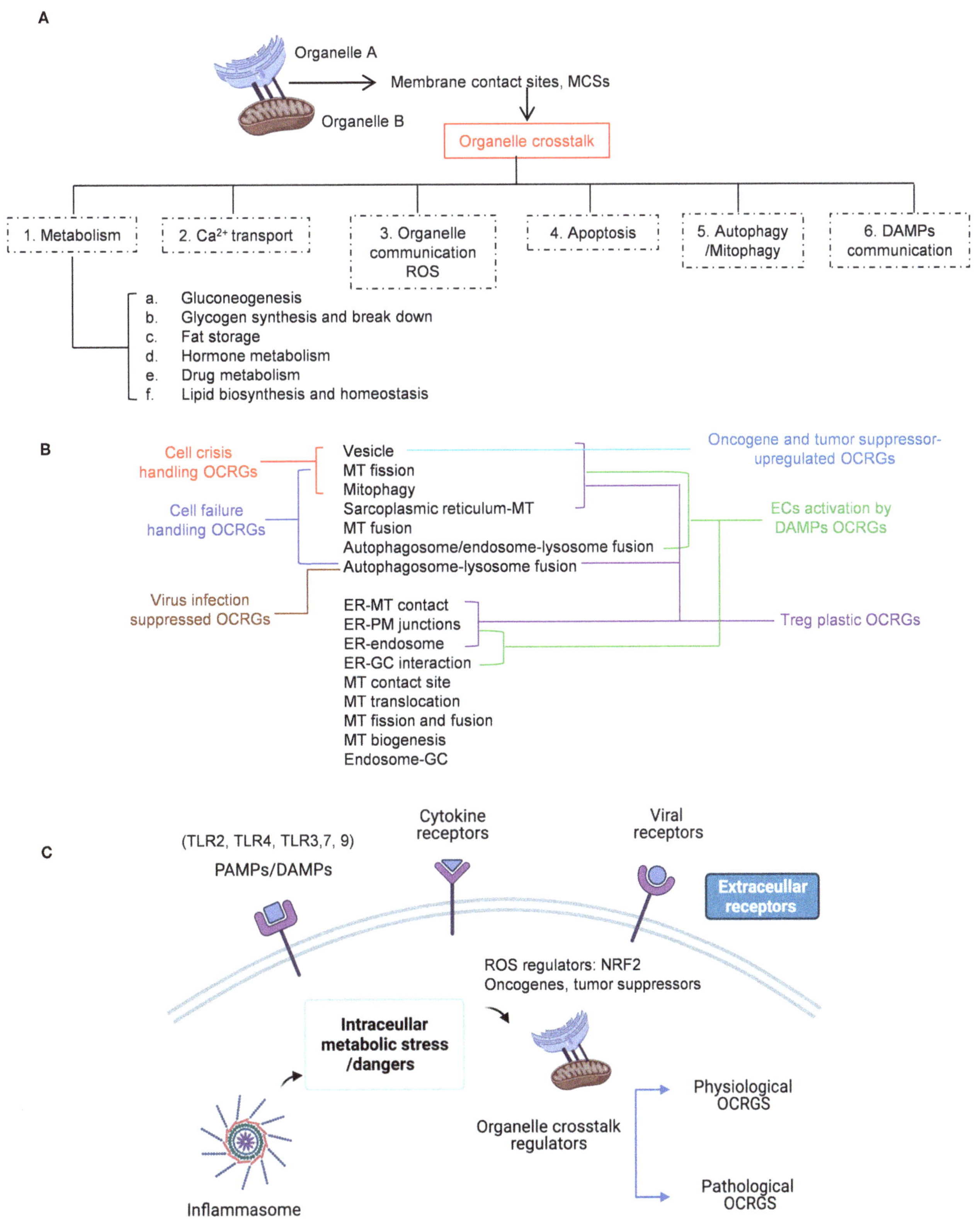

FIGURE 11 | A novel working model shows the function, classification, and regulated mechanisms of OCRGs in diseases, and DAMP- and virus-treated cells. **(A)** The membrane contact sites between two organelles, at least between ER and mitochondria (Mito, MT), have been found to play several significant functions from previous

(Continued)

FIGURE 11 | reports and our study, such as in metabolism (including gluconeogenesis, glycogen synthesis and breakdown, fat storage, hormone metabolism, drug metabolism, lipid biosynthesis, and homeostasis), Ca^{2+} transport, organelle communication ROS, apoptosis, autophagy/mitophagy, and DAMP communication. **(B)** Thirteen of 16 functional groups of OCRGs are differently modulated in various diseases and cancers. Three groups of OCRGs such as vesicle, mitochondrial fission, and mitophagy were identified as the cell crisis-handling OCRGs (red line pointed). Seven groups of OCRGs including three cell crisis-handling OCRGs plus sarcoplasmic reticulum-mito, mitochondrial fusion, autophagosome–lysosome fusion, and autophagosome/endosome–lysosome fusion were identified as the cell failure-handling OCRGs (blue line pointed). Autophagosome–lysosome fusion OCRGs can be regarded as virus infection-suppressed OCRGs (brown line pointed). Eight classification groups (i.e., vesicle, MT fission, mitophagy, sarcoplasmic reticulum–MT, autophagosome–lysosome fusion, ER–MT contact, ER–PM junctions, and ER–endosome) are Treg plastic OCRGs (purple line pointed). Ten groups of ECs activation by DAMP OCRGs include seven Treg plastic OCRGs (except autophagosome–lysosome fusion) and add MT fusion, autophagosome/endosome–lysosome fusion, and ER–GC interaction OCRGs (green line pointed). Vesicle regulators can be regarded as oncogenes and tumor suppressor-promoted OCRGs (light blue line pointed). **(C)** Extracellular pathogen-associated molecular patterns (PAMPs)/damage-associated molecular patterns (DAMPs), cytokines, and viruses act via their receptors including TLRs on the cell membrane and intracellular locations (Nod-like receptors and inflammasomes) to activate OCRGs directly or indirectly by activating intracellular organelle dangers first and then OCRGs. And ROS regulator NRF2 oncogenes and tumor suppressors also regulate the expression of OCRGs in diseases and tumors. A new concept that the organelle crosstalk serves as both new DAMP sensing and communicating network and new cell crisis and cell failure-handling network to fulfill both physiological functions and pathological functions. *Created with BioRender.com.

Our data in **Table 11** show that IKK2 depletion upregulated five OCRGs in lung tumor cells, which were well-correlated with the finding that IKK2 depletion attenuated tumor proliferation and prolonged mouse survival. We then tested a hypothesis that IKK2 depletion upregulated OCRGs may partially overlap with LUAD-downregulated OCRGs. As shown in **Supplementary Figure 16A**, the Venn diagram indicated that vesicle regulator perilipin 4 (PLIN4) was overlapped between the LUAD-downregulated OCRGs and the IKK2 KO-upregulated OCRGs. As shown in **Supplementary Figure 16B**, the expression profile analysis using cancer and normal gene expression database GEPIA (http://gepia.cancer-pku.cn/index.html) (127) showed that the expression of PLIN4 was decreased in 23 out of 33 tumor types compared with controls. Our data in **Table 8** show that tumor suppressor Tp53 KO in liver tumors upregulated 23 OCRGs and downregulated 48 OCRGs, which were associated with induction of carcinomas in Tp53 KO mice (122, 126). Similarly, we then tested a hypothesis that Tp53 KO upregulated OCRGs may partially overlap with that liver tumor (LIHC)-upregulated OCRGs; and Tp53 KO downregulated OCRGs may partially overlap with liver tumor (LIHC)-downregulated OCRGs. As shown in **Supplementary Figure 16C**, the Venn diagram indicated that prolyl 4-hydroxylase subunit alpha 2 (P4HA2) was shared between the Tp53 KO upregulated OCRGs and the liver tumor (LIHC)-upregulated OCRGs; and alpha-aminoadipic semialdehyde synthase (AASS) was shared between the Tp53 KO downregulated OCRGs and the liver tumor (LIHC)-downregulated OCRGs. The cancer gene expression database analysis showed that the expressions of vesicle regulator P4HA2 were increased in seven out of 33 tumor types compared with controls (**Supplementary Figure 16D**); and the expression of vesicle regulator AASS in seven out of 33 tumor types was decreased compared with that of controls (**Supplementary Figure 16E**). Taken together, our results have demonstrated that *first*, tumor promoter IKK2 and tumor suppressor Tp53 significantly modulate the expressions of OCRGs; *second*, lung tumor LUAD-downregulated vesicle regulator PLIN4 may contribute to IKK2 KO-promoted tumor formation; *third*, liver tumor (LIHC)-upregulated vesicle regulator P4HA2 may increase Tp53 KO-promoted liver tumorigenesis; and *fourth*, LIHC-downregulated vesicle regulator AASS may contribute to Tp53 suppression of liver tumorigenesis.

DISCUSSION

Although alterations to these networks, such as impaired ER–mitochondria MCSs, have been linked to several diseases such as neurodegeneration (59, 60), CVD (61), diabetes (62), kidney diseases (63, 64), and cancers (65, 66), an important question remains poorly characterized how the expressions of organelle crosstalk regulator genes are modulated in various diseases. To examine whether the expressions of 260 OCRGs in 16 functional groups are modulated in 23 diseases and 28 tumors, we performed extensive -omics data mining analyses in a panoramic manner with the method that we pioneered in 2004 (23, 26, 29, 91, 107, 109, 128) and made a set of significant findings: (1) the ratios of upregulated vs. downregulated OCRGs are 1:2.8 in AIs, 1:1 in MDs, 1:1.1 in ADs, and 1:3.8 in OFs; and AIs and OFs upregulate less OCRG groups (three to seven out of 16) than metabolic and ADs (11 to 13 out of 16); (2) sepsis and trauma-upregulated OCRG groups including vesicle, MT fission, and mitophagy but not other groups of OCRGs; thus, the three groups of OCRGs are classified as the acute crisis-handling OCRGs; and similarly, sepsis and trauma plus OFs-upregulated seven OCRG groups including vesicle, MT fission, mitophagy, sarcoplasmic reticulum–MT, MT fusion, autophagosome–lysosome fusion, and autophagosome/endosome–lysosome fusion are classified as the cell failure-handling OCRGs; (3) the majority of upregulated pathways are disease group-specific; upregulated organelle fusion and macroautophagy are shared by MDs, ADs, and OFs; upregulated MT fission is shared by AIs, MDs, and ADs; upregulated vesicle organization is shared by AI and MDs; and upregulated protein localization is shared by MDs and ADs; (4) increased OCRG expressions in all the 15 functional groups except autophagosome–lysosome fusion but decreased autophagosome–lysosome fusion are required for viral replications, which classify this decreased group as the viral replication-suppressed OCRGs. (5) PAMPs from influenza virus and Kaposi sarcoma-associated herpes virus infections and pro-atherogenic DAMPs such as oxLDL, LPS, oxPAPC, and IFNs totally upregulated 33 OCRGs in ECs, which classify vesicle, MT fission, mitophagy, MT fusion, ER–MT contact, ER–PT junction, and autophagosome/endosome–lysosome fusion as the seven EC-activation/inflammation-promoting OCRG groups; (6) the expression of OCRGs is modulated in Treg from the LNs, spleen, peripheral blood, intestine, and brown adipose tissue in comparison with that of $CD4^{+}CD25^{-}$ T effector controls; (7) TLR2, TLR4, TLR3/7/9, caspase-1, and ROS regulator Nrf2 can upregulate 46 OCRGs from 14 groups out of all 16 groups (except for MT fission and fusion, and ER–MT contact OCRGs), suggesting that DAMP/PAMP-sensing systems play significant roles in modulating the expressions of OCRGs; (8) OCRG expressions are significantly modulated in all the 28 cancer datasets; upregulated OCRGs in LIHC and LUSC are correlated with immune cell infiltrations, suggesting that upregulation of certain OCRGs may promote immune cell infiltration; MT protein translocase TOMM40 and MT import machine are upregulated in cancers and are positively associated with better prognosis; and TOMM40 is correlated with some immune infiltration signature genes, suggesting that increase of protein transport into mitochondria may facilitate the immune cell infiltration; and (9) tumor promoter factor IKK2 and tumor suppressor Tp53 significantly modulate the expressions of OCRGs; lung tumor-downregulated vesicle regulator PLIN4 may contribute to IKK2 KO-attenuated tumor formation; liver tumor-upregulated vesicle regulator P4HA2 may increase Tp53 deficiency-promoted liver tumorigenesis; and liver tumor-downregulated vesicle regulator AASS may contribute to Tp53 suppression of liver tumorigenesis.

The original microarray experiments we analyzed used different cells, which prevented us from comparing the effects of various regulators in regulating the expressions of OCRGs in the same cell types, although our database mining method was not ideal. However, to fill in the important knowledge gaps, our approach was justified. Actually, this approach has been a common practice that we (23) and others (72, 129) often use in studying gene expression in non-ideal, heterogeneous PBMC populations in disease conditions vs. healthy conditions, and PBMCs are actually composed of many cell types, such as B cells (~15%), T cells (~70%), monocytes (~5%), and NK cells (~10%) (130).

To summarize our findings from a panoramic analysis on the expression changes of 260 OCRGs in 51 diseases and cancers presented here, we propose a novel working model to integrate these results, as follows, in **Figure 11A**: *first*, the MCSs between two organelles, at least between ER and mitochondria (Mito, MT), have been found to play several significant functions such as metabolism and Ca^{2+} transport as we reported (4); organelle communicating ROS as we recently reported (4, 38, 40–42, 131); apoptosis as we have reported (132, 133); and autophagy, mitophagy, and DAMP communication as we have reported (37). The metabolism regulatory functions between ER–MT contact sites include gluconeogenesis, glycogen synthesis and breakdown, fat storage, hormone metabolism, drug metabolism, lipid biosynthesis, and homeostasis (134); *second*, since our study analyzed the 260 OCRGs in 51 major diseases and cancers and many other master regulator deficient transcriptomic data, we have demonstrated for the first time that 16 functional groups of OCRGs are not equally modulated in various diseases and cancers. As shown in **Figure 11B**, we identified three groups of OCRGs such as vesicle, MT fission, and mitophagy as the cell crisis-handling OCRGs, at least in partial functions of the three groups; seven groups of OCRGs including three cell crisis-handling OCRGs plus sarcoplasmic reticulum–MT, MT fusion, autophagosome–lysosome fusion, and autophagosome/endosome–lysosome fusion as the cell failure-handling OCRGs; and autophagosome–lysosome fusion as virus-suppressed OCRGs. Previous reports showed that growing numbers of viruses are found to weaponize the ubiquitin modification system to suppress anti-viral type I IFN pathways (135). Similarly, we found that virus infections weaponize the suppression of autophagosome–lysosome fusion group potentially for virus replication. Since most viruses use endocytosis to enter the host cell, 11 clinically approved generic drugs are identified as potential candidates for repurposing as blockers of several potential routes for severe acute SARS-CoV-2 endocytosis (136), which needs to be further re-considered since we found that coronavirus and other virus infections in ECs and epithelial cells suppress endocytosis–lysosome pathways (**Supplementary Figure 4**); 10 groups of OCRGs activated by DAMPs in ECs including vesicle (137), MT fission, mitophagy, autophagosome/endosome–lysosome fusion, ER–MT contact, ER–PM junctions, sarcoplasmic reticulum–MT, MT fusion, ER–endosome, and ER–GC interaction. Treg plastic OCRGs, and oncogenes and tumor suppressors promoted vesicle regulators; and *third*, extracellular PAMPs/DAMPs, cytokines, and viruses act via their receptors including TLRs on the cell membrane and intracellular locations (Nod-like receptors and inflammasomes) (90) to activate OCRGs directly or indirectly by activating intracellular organelle dangers first and then OCRGs. Therefore, similar to our recently proposed new concept that ROS are an integrated system for sensing and alarming organelle metabolic homeostasis and dysfunction (38), here, we propose a new concept that the organelle crosstalk serves as both new DAMPs sensing and communicating network and new cell crisis and cell failure-handling network (37) to fulfill both physiological functions and pathological functions (**Figure 11C**).

One limitation of the current study is that due to the low throughput nature of verification techniques in every laboratory including ours, we could not verify every result we identified with the analyses of high-throughput data, which are similar to all the papers with RNA-Seq, single-cell RNA-Seq, and other -omics data. We acknowledge that carefully designed *in vitro* and *in vivo* experimental models will be needed in the future to verify regulator gene deficiency-upregulated OCRGs further and the underlying mechanisms we report here. Nevertheless, our findings provide novel insights on the roles of upregulated OCRGs in the pathogenesis of inflammatory diseases and cancers, novel pathways for the future therapeutic interventions for inflammations, sepsis, trauma, OFs, ADs, metabolic CVDs, and cancers.

AUTHOR CONTRIBUTIONS

ML carried out the data gathering and data analysis and prepared the tables and figures. NW, KX, FS, EV, YS, RZ, JW, HS, WY, YL, YS, CD, LLiu, LLi, WH, JY, DP, JS, XJ, and HW aided with analysis of the data. XY supervised the experimental design, data analysis, and manuscript writing. All authors read and approved the final manuscript.

ACKNOWLEDGMENTS

ML was supported by a fellowship from the School of Basic Medical Science, Shanxi Medical University.

REFERENCES

1. Benjamin EJ, Blaha MJ, Chiuve SE, Cushman M, Das SR, Deo R, et al. Heart disease and stroke statistics-2017 update: a report from the American Heart Association. *Circulation.* (2017) 135:e146–603. doi: 10.1161/CIR.0000000000000491
2. Libby P, Buring JE, Badimon L, Hansson GK, Deanfield J, Bittencourt MS, et al. Atherosclerosis. *Nat Rev Dis Primers.* (2019) 5:56. doi: 10.1038/s41572-019-0106-z
3. Yin Y, Li X, Sha X, Xi H, Li YF, Shao Y, et al. Early hyperlipidemia promotes endothelial activation via a caspase-1-sirtuin 1 pathway. *Arterioscler Thromb Vasc Biol.* (2015) 35:804–16. doi: 10.1161/ATVBAHA.115.305282
4. Li X, Fang P, Li Y, Kuo YM, Andrews AJ, Nanayakkara G, et al. Mitochondrial reactive oxygen species mediate lysophosphatidylcholine-induced endothelial cell activation. *arterioscler Thromb Vasc Biol.* (2016) 36:1090–100. doi: 10.1161/ATVBAHA.115.306964
5. Fang P, Zhang D, Cheng Z, Yan C, Jiang X, Kruger WD, et al. Hyperhomocysteinemia potentiates hyperglycemia-induced inflammatory monocyte differentiation and atherosclerosis. *Diabetes.* (2014) 63:4275–90. doi: 10.2337/db14-0809
6. Xi H, Zhang Y, Xu Y, Yang WY, Jiang X, Sha X, et al. Caspase-1 inflammasome activation mediates homocysteine-induced pyrop-apoptosis in endothelial cells. *Circ Res.* (2016) 118:1525–39. doi: 10.1161/CIRCRESAHA.116.308501
7. Yang J, Fang P, Yu D, Zhang L, Zhang D, Jiang X, et al. Chronic kidney disease induces inflammatory CD40+ monocyte differentiation via homocysteine elevation and DNA hypomethylation. *Circ Res.* (2016) 119:1226–41. doi: 10.1161/CIRCRESAHA.116.308750
8. Ferrer LM, Monroy AM, Lopez-Pastrana J, Nanayakkara G, Cueto R, Li YF, et al. Caspase-1 plays a critical role in accelerating chronic kidney disease-promoted neointimal hyperplasia in the carotid artery. *J Cardiovasc Transl Res.* (2016) 9:135–44. doi: 10.1007/s12265-016-9683-3
9. Monroy MA, Fang J, Li S, Ferrer L, Birkenbach MP, Lee IJ, et al. Chronic kidney disease alters vascular smooth muscle cell phenotype. *Front Biosci.* (2015) 20:784–95. doi: 10.2741/4337
10. Sun Y, Johnson C, Zhou J, Wang L, Li YF, Lu Y, et al. Uremic toxins are conditional danger- or homeostasis-associated molecular patterns. *Front Biosci.* (2018) 23:348–87. doi: 10.2741/4595
11. Shao Y, Saredy J, Yang WY, Sun Y, Lu Y, Saaoud F, et al. Vascular endothelial cells and innate immunity. *Arterioscler Thromb Vasc Biol.* (2020) 40:e138–52. doi: 10.1161/ATVBAHA.120.314330
12. Sha X, Meng S, Li X, Xi H, Maddaloni M, Pascual DW, et al. Interleukin-35 inhibits endothelial cell activation by suppressing MAPK-AP-1 pathway. *J Biol Chem.* (2015) 290:19307–18. doi: 10.1074/jbc.M115.663286
13. Shao Y, Cheng Z, Li X, Chernaya V, Wang H, Yang XF. Immunosuppressive/anti-inflammatory cytokines directly and indirectly inhibit endothelial dysfunction–a novel mechanism for maintaining vascular function. *J Hematol Oncol.* (2014) 7:80. doi: 10.1186/s13045-014-0080-6
14. Li X, Wang L, Fang P, Sun Y, Jiang X, Wang H, et al. Lysophospholipids induce innate immune transdifferentiation of endothelial cells, resulting in prolonged endothelial activation. *J Biol Chem.* (2018) 293:11033–45. doi: 10.1074/jbc.RA118.002752
15. Li A, Sun Y. Drummer Ct, Lu Y, Yu D, Zhou Y, et al. Increasing upstream chromatin long-range interactions may favor induction of circular RNAs in LysoPC-activated human aortic endothelial cells. *Front Physiol.* (2019) 10:433. doi: 10.3389/fphys.2019.00433
16. Lopez-Pastrana J, Ferrer LM Li YF, Xiong X, Xi H, Cueto R, et al. Inhibition of caspase-1 activation in endothelial cells improves angiogenesis: a novel therapeutic potential for ischemia. *J Biol Chem.* (2015) 290:17485–94. doi: 10.1074/jbc.M115.641191
17. Zhang CE, Wei W, Liu YH, Peng JH, Tian Q, Liu GP, et al. Hyperhomocysteinemia increases beta-amyloid by enhancing expression of gamma-secretase and phosphorylation of amyloid precursor protein in rat brain. *Am J Pathol.* (2009) 174:1481–91. doi: 10.2353/ajpath.2009.081036
18. Zhang D, Fang P, Jiang X, Nelson J, Moore JK, Kruger WD, et al. Severe hyperhomocysteinemia promotes bone marrow-derived and resident inflammatory monocyte differentiation and atherosclerosis in LDLr/CBS-deficient mice. *Circ Res.* (2012) 111:37–49. doi: 10.1161/CIRCRESAHA.112.269472
19. Fang P, Li X, Shan H, Saredy JJ, Cueto R, Xia J, et al. Ly6C(+) inflammatory monocyte differentiation partially mediates hyperhomocysteinemia-induced vascular dysfunction in type 2 diabetic db/db mice. *Arterioscler Thromb Vasc Biol.* (2019) 39:2097–119. doi: 10.1161/ATVBAHA.119.313138
20. Johnson C, Drummer C IV, Shan H, Shao Y, Sun Y, Lu Y, et al. A novel subset of CD95(+) pro-inflammatory macrophages overcome miR155 deficiency and may serve as a switch from metabolically healthy obesity to metabolically unhealthy obesity. *Front Immunol.* (2020) 11:619951. doi: 10.3389/fimmu.2020.619951
21. Lai B, Wang J, Fagenson A, Sun Y, Saredy J, Lu Y, et al. Twenty novel disease group-specific and 12 new shared macrophage pathways in eight groups of 34 diseases including 24 inflammatory organ diseases and 10 types of tumors. *Front Immunol.* (2019) 10:2612. doi: 10.3389/fimmu.2019.02612
22. Drummer CT, Saaoud F, Shao Y, Sun Y, Xu K, Lu Y, et al. Trained immunity and reactivity of macrophages and endothelial cells. *Arterioscler Thromb Vasc Biol.* (2021) 41:1032–46. doi: 10.1161/ATVBAHA.120.315452
23. Zhang R, Saredy J, Shao Y, Yao T, Liu L, Saaoud F, et al. End-stage renal disease is different from chronic kidney disease in upregulating ROS-modulated proinflammatory secretome in PBMCs - A novel multiple-hit model for disease progression. *Redox Biol.* (2020) 34:101460. doi: 10.1016/j.redox.2020.101460
24. Zhang R, Xu K, Shao Y, Sun Y, Saredy J, Cutler E, et al. Tissue Treg secretomes and transcription factors shared with stem cells contribute to a Treg niche to maintain Treg-ness with 80% innate immune pathways, and functions of immunosuppression and tissue repair. *Front Immunol.* (2020) 11:632239. doi: 10.3389/fimmu.2020.632239
25. Li X, Fang P, Yang WY, Wang H, Yang X. IL-35, as a newly proposed homeostasis-associated molecular pattern, plays three major functions including anti-inflammatory initiator, effector, and blocker in cardiovascular diseases. *Cytokine.* (2019) 122:154076. doi: 10.1016/j.cyto.2017.06.003
26. Li X, Mai J, Virtue A, Yin Y, Gong R, Sha X, et al. IL-35 is a novel responsive anti-inflammatory cytokine–a new system of categorizing anti-inflammatory cytokines. *PLoS ONE.* (2012) 7:e33628. doi: 10.1371/journal.pone.0033628
27. Li X, Shao Y, Sha X, Fang P, Kuo YM, Andrews AJ, et al. IL-35 (Interleukin-35) suppresses endothelial cell activation by inhibiting mitochondrial reactive oxygen species-mediated site-specific acetylation of H3K14 (Histone 3 Lysine 14). *Arterioscler Thromb Vasc Biol.* (2018) 38:599–609. doi: 10.1161/ATVBAHA.117.310626

28. Mai J, Nanayakkara G, Lopez-Pastrana J, Li X, Li YF, Wang X, et al. Interleukin-17A promotes aortic endothelial cell activation via transcriptionally and post-translationally activating p38 mitogen-activated Protein Kinase (MAPK) pathway. *J Biol Chem.* (2016) 291:4939–54. doi: 10.1074/jbc.M115.690081
29. Liu M, Saredy J, Zhang R, Shao Y, Sun Y, Yang WY, et al. Approaching inflammation paradoxes-proinflammatory cytokine blockages induce inflammatory regulators. *Front Immunol.* (2020) 11:554301. doi: 10.3389/fimmu.2020.554301
30. Fu H, Sun Y, Shao Y, Saredy J, Cueto R, Liu L, et al. Interleukin 35 delays hindlimb ischemia-induced angiogenesis through regulating ROS-extracellular matrix but spares later regenerative angiogenesis. *Front Immunol.* (2020) 11:595813. doi: 10.3389/fimmu.2020.595813
31. Xiong Z, Song J, Yan Y, Huang Y, Cowan A, Wang H, et al. Higher expression of Bax in regulatory T cells increases vascular inflammation. *Front Biosci.* (2008) 13:7143–55. doi: 10.2741/3217
32. Xiong Z, Yan Y, Song J, Fang P, Yin Y, Yang Y, et al. Expression of TCTP antisense in CD25(high) regulatory T cells aggravates cuff-injured vascular inflammation. *Atherosclerosis.* (2009) 203:401–8. doi: 10.1016/j.atherosclerosis.2008.07.041
33. Yang WY, Shao Y, Lopez-Pastrana J, Mai J, Wang H, Yang XF. Pathological conditions re-shape physiological Tregs into pathological Tregs. *Burns Trauma.* (2015) 3:1. doi: 10.1186/s41038-015-0001-0
34. Xu K, Yang WY, Nanayakkara GK, Shao Y, Yang F, Hu W, et al. GATA3, HDAC6, and BCL6 regulate FOXP3+ Treg plasticity and determine Treg conversion into either novel antigen-presenting cell-like Treg or Th1-Treg. *Front Immunol.* (2018) 9:45. doi: 10.3389/fimmu.2018.00045
35. Nelson J, Wu Y, Jiang X, Berretta R, Houser S, Choi E, et al. Hyperhomocysteinemia suppresses bone marrow CD34+/VEGF receptor 2+ cells and inhibits progenitor cell mobilization and homing to injured vasculature-a role of beta1-integrin in progenitor cell migration and adhesion. *FASEB J.* (2015) 29:3085–99. doi: 10.1096/fj.14-267989
36. Li YF, Huang X, Li X, Gong R, Yin Y, Nelson J, et al. Caspase-1 mediates hyperlipidemia-weakened progenitor cell vessel repair. *Front Biosci.* (2016) 21:178–91. doi: 10.2741/4383
37. Zeng H, Nanayakkara GK, Shao Y, Fu H, Sun Y, Cueto R, et al. DNA checkpoint and repair factors are nuclear sensors for intracellular organelle stresses-inflammations and cancers can have high genomic risks. *Front Physiol.* (2018) 9:516. doi: 10.3389/fphys.2018.00516
38. Sun Y, Lu Y, Saredy J, Wang X, Drummer Iv C, Shao Y, et al. ROS systems are a new integrated network for sensing homeostasis and alarming stresses in organelle metabolic processes. *Redox Biol.* (2020) 37:101696. doi: 10.1016/j.redox.2020.101696
39. Fagenson AM, Xu K, Saaoud F, Nanayakkara G, Jhala NC, Liu L, et al. Liver ischemia reperfusion injury, enhanced by trained immunity, is attenuated in caspase 1/caspase 11 double gene knockout mice. Pathogens. (2020) 9:879. doi: 10.3390/pathogens9110879
40. Li X, Fang P, Mai J, Choi ET, Wang H, Yang XF. Targeting mitochondrial reactive oxygen species as novel therapy for inflammatory diseases and cancers. *J Hematol Oncol.* (2013) 6:19. doi: 10.1186/1756-8722-6-19
41. Nanayakkara GK, Wang H, Yang X. Proton leak regulates mitochondrial reactive oxygen species generation in endothelial cell activation and inflammation - A novel concept. *Arch Biochem Biophys.* (2019) 662:68–74. doi: 10.1016/j.abb.2018.12.002
42. Cheng J, Nanayakkara G, Shao Y, Cueto R, Wang L, Yang WY, et al. Mitochondrial proton leak plays a critical role in pathogenesis of cardiovascular diseases. *Adv Exp Med Biol.* (2017) 982:359–70. doi: 10.1007/978-3-319-55330-6_20
43. Shao Y, Chernaya V, Johnson C, Yang WY, Cueto R, Sha X, et al. Metabolic diseases downregulate the majority of histone modification enzymes, making a few upregulated enzymes novel therapeutic targets–"sand out and gold stays". *J Cardiovasc Transl Res.* (2016) 9:49–66. doi: 10.1007/s12265-015-9664-y
44. Zhong C, Yang X, Feng Y, Yu J. Trained immunity: an underlying driver of inflammatory atherosclerosis. *Front Immunol.* (2020) 11:284. doi: 10.3389/fimmu.2020.00284
45. Lu Y, Sun Y. Drummer Ct, Nanayakkara GK, Shao Y, Saaoud F, et al. Increased acetylation of H3K14 in the genomic regions that encode trained immunity enzymes in lysophosphatidylcholine-activated human aortic endothelial cells - Novel qualification markers for chronic disease risk factors and conditional DAMPs. *Redox Biol.* (2019) 24:101221. doi: 10.1016/j.redox.2019.101221
46. Li X, Fang P, Sun Y, Shao Y, Yang WY, Jiang X, et al. Anti-inflammatory cytokines IL-35 and IL-10 block atherogenic lysophosphatidylcholine-induced, mitochondrial ROS-mediated innate immune activation, but spare innate immune memory signature in endothelial cells. *Redox Biol.* (2020) 28:101373. doi: 10.1016/j.redox.2019.101373
47. Yang Q, Zhang R, Tang P, Sun Y, Johnson C, Saredy J, et al. Ultrasound may suppress tumor growth, inhibit inflammation, and establish tolerogenesis by remodeling innatome via pathways of ROS, immune checkpoints, cytokines, and trained immunity/tolerance. *J Immunol Res.* (2021) 2021:6664453. doi: 10.1155/2021/6664453
48. Hu F, Zeng C, Long R, Miao Y, Wei L, Xu Q, et al. Supermultiplexed optical imaging and barcoding with engineered polyynes. *Nat Methods.* (2018) 15:194–200. doi: 10.1038/nmeth.4578
49. Valm AM, Cohen S, Legant WR, Melunis J, Hershberg U, Wait E, et al. Applying systems-level spectral imaging and analysis to reveal the organelle interactome. *Nature.* (2017) 546:162–7. doi: 10.1038/nature22369
50. Shai N, Yifrach E, van Roermund CWT, Cohen N, Bibi C. L IJ, et al. Systematic mapping of contact sites reveals tethers and a function for the peroxisome-mitochondria contact. *Nat Commun.* (2018) 9:1761. doi: 10.1038/s41467-018-03957-8
51. Salvador-Gallego R, Hoyer MJ, Voeltz GK. SnapShot: functions of endoplasmic reticulum membrane contact sites. *Cell.* (2017) 171:1224–e1. doi: 10.1016/j.cell.2017.11.005
52. Bohnert M, Schuldiner M. Stepping outside the comfort zone of membrane contact site research. *Nat Rev Mol Cell Biol.* (2018) 19:483–4. doi: 10.1038/s41580-018-0022-1
53. Stenmark H. Rab GTPases as coordinators of vesicle traffic. *Nat Rev Mol Cell Biol.* (2009) 10:513–25. doi: 10.1038/nrm2728
54. Diogo CV, Yambire KF, Fernandez Mosquera L, Branco FT, Raimundo N. Mitochondrial adventures at the organelle society. *Biochem Biophys Res Commun.* (2018) 500:87–93. doi: 10.1016/j.bbrc.2017.04.124
55. Quiros PM, Mottis A, Auwerx J. Mitonuclear communication in homeostasis and stress. *Nat Rev Mol Cell Biol.* (2016) 17:213–26. doi: 10.1038/nrm.2016.23
56. Shpilka T, Haynes CM. The mitochondrial UPR: mechanisms, physiological functions and implications in ageing. *Nat Rev Mol Cell Biol.* (2018) 19:109–20. doi: 10.1038/nrm.2017.110
57. Senft D, Ronai ZA, UPR. autophagy, and mitochondria crosstalk underlies the ER stress response. *Trends Biochem Sci.* (2015) 40:141–8. doi: 10.1016/j.tibs.2015.01.002
58. Fransen M, Lismont C, Walton P. The peroxisome-mitochondria connection: how and why? *Int J Mol Sci.* (2017) 18:1126. doi: 10.3390/ijms18061126
59. Area-Gomez E, Schon EA. Mitochondria-associated ER membranes and Alzheimer disease. *Curr Opin Genet Dev.* (2016) 38:90–6. doi: 10.1016/j.gde.2016.04.006
60. Deus CM, Yambire KF, Oliveira PJ, Raimundo N. Mitochondria-lysosome crosstalk: from physiology to neurodegeneration. *Trends Mol Med.* (2020) 26:71–88. doi: 10.1016/j.molmed.2019.10.009
61. Kaasik A, Veksler V, Boehm E, Novotova M, Minajeva A, Ventura-Clapier R. Energetic crosstalk between organelles: architectural integration of energy production and utilization. *Circ Res.* (2001) 89:153–9. doi: 10.1161/hh1401.093440
62. Castano C, Novials A, Parrizas M. Exosomes and diabetes. *Diabetes Metab Res Rev.* (2019) 35:e3107. doi: 10.1002/dmrr.3107
63. Inoue T, Maekawa H, Inagi R. Organelle crosstalk in the kidney. *Kidney Int.* (2019) 95:1318–25. doi: 10.1016/j.kint.2018.11.035
64. Inagi R. The Implication of organelle cross talk in AKI. *Nephron.* (2020) 144:634–7. doi: 10.1159/000508639
65. Bebelman MP, Smit MJ, Pegtel DM, Baglio SR. Biogenesis and function of extracellular vesicles in cancer. *Pharmacol Ther.* (2018) 188:1–11. doi: 10.1016/j.pharmthera.2018.02.013
66. Xu J, Camfield R, Gorski SM. The interplay between exosomes and

autophagy - partners in crime. J Cell Sci. (2018) 131:jcs.215210. doi: 10.1242/jcs.215210
67. Joshi AS, Zhang H, Prinz WA. Organelle biogenesis in the endoplasmic reticulum. *Nat Cell Biol.* (2017) 19:876–82. doi: 10.1038/ncb3579
68. Soto-Heredero G, Baixauli F, Mittelbrunn M. Interorganelle communication between mitochondria and the endolysosomal system. *Front Cell Dev Biol.* (2017) 5:95. doi: 10.3389/fcell.2017.00095
69. Lopez-Crisosto C, Pennanen C, Vasquez-Trincado C, Morales PE, Bravo-Sagua R, Quest AFG, et al. Sarcoplasmic reticulum-mitochondria communication in cardiovascular pathophysiology. *Nat Rev Cardiol.* (2017) 14:342–60. doi: 10.1038/nrcardio.2017.23
70. Besprozvannaya M, Dickson E, Li H, Ginburg KS, Bers DM, Auwerx J, et al. GRAM domain proteins specialize functionally distinct ER-PM contact sites in human cells. *Elife.* (2018) 7:e31019. doi: 10.7554/eLife.31019
71. Lees JA, Messa M, Sun EW, Wheeler H, Torta F, Wenk MR, et al. Lipid transport by TMEM24 at ER-plasma membrane contacts regulates pulsatile insulin secretion. *Science.* (2017) 355:eaah6171. doi: 10.1126/science.aah6171
72. Li Y, Oosting M, Smeekens SP, Jaeger M, Aguirre-Gamboa R, Le KTT, et al. A functional genomics approach to understand variation in cytokine production in humans. *Cell.* (2016) 167:1099–110 e14. doi: 10.1016/j.cell.2016.10.017
73. Zhou Y, Zhou B, Pache L, Chang M, Khodabakhshi AH, Tanaseichuk O, et al. Metascape provides a biologist-oriented resource for the analysis of systems-level datasets. *Nat Commun.* (2019) 10:1523. doi: 10.1038/s41467-019-09234-6
74. Shannon P, Markiel A, Ozier O, Baliga NS, Wang JT, Ramage D, et al. Cytoscape: a software environment for integrated models of biomolecular interaction networks. *Genome Res.* (2003) 13:2498–504. doi: 10.1101/gr.1239303
75. Ru B, Wong CN, Tong Y, Zhong JY, Zhong SSW, Wu WC, et al. TISIDB: an integrated repository portal for tumor-immune system interactions. *Bioinformatics.* (2019) 35:4200–2. doi: 10.1093/bioinformatics/btz210
76. Liu CJ, Hu FF, Xia MX, Han L, Zhang Q, Guo AY. GSCALite: a web server for gene set cancer analysis. *Bioinformatics.* (2018) 34:3771–2. doi: 10.1093/bioinformatics/bty411
77. Eisenberg E, Levanon EY. Human housekeeping genes, revisited. *Trends Genet.* (2013) 29:569–74. doi: 10.1016/j.tig.2013.05.010
78. de Jonge HJ, Fehrmann RS, de Bont ES, Hofstra RM, Gerbens F, Kamps WA, et al. Evidence based selection of housekeeping genes. *PLoS ONE.* (2007) 2:e898. doi: 10.1371/journal.pone.0000898
79. Targher G, Byrne CD. Obesity: Metabolically healthy obesity and NAFLD. *Nat Rev Gastroenterol Hepatol.* (2016) 13:442–4. doi: 10.1038/nrgastro.2016.104
80. Leites EP, Morais VA. Mitochondrial quality control pathways: PINK1 acts as a gatekeeper. *Biochem Biophys Res Commun.* (2018) 500:45–50. doi: 10.1016/j.bbrc.2017.06.096
81. Schneider A, Kurz S, Manske K, Janas M, Heikenwalder M, Misgeld T, et al. Single organelle analysis to characterize mitochondrial function and crosstalk during viral infection. *Sci Rep.* (2019) 9:8492. doi: 10.1038/s41598-019-44922-9
82. Menachery VD, Mitchell HD, Cockrell AS, Gralinski LE, Yount BL Jr, Graham RL, et al. MERS-CoV accessory ORFs play key role for infection and pathogenesis. *mBio.* (2017) 8:e00665-17. doi: 10.1128/mBio.00665-17
83. Mitchell HD, Eisfeld AJ, Sims AC, McDermott JE, Matzke MM, Webb-Robertson BJ, et al. A network integration approach to predict conserved regulators related to pathogenicity of influenza and SARS-CoV respiratory viruses. *PLoS ONE.* (2013) 8:e69374. doi: 10.1371/journal.pone.0069374
84. Josset L, Zeng H, Kelly SM, Tumpey TM, Katze MG. Transcriptomic characterization of the novel avian-origin influenza A (H7N9) virus: specific host response and responses intermediate between avian (H5N1 and H7N7) and human (H3N2) viruses and implications for treatment options. *MBio.* (2014) 5:e01102-13. doi: 10.1128/mBio.01102-13
85. Zhu Z, Lian X, Su X, Wu W, Marraro GA, Zeng Y. From SARS and MERS to COVID-19: a brief summary and comparison of severe acute respiratory infections caused by three highly pathogenic human coronaviruses. *Respir Res.* (2020) 21:224. doi: 10.1186/s12931-020-01479-w
86. Evans PC, Rainger GE, Mason JC, Guzik TJ, Osto E, Stamataki Z, et al. Endothelial dysfunction in COVID-19: a position paper of the ESC Working Group for Atherosclerosis and Vascular Biology, and the ESC Council of Basic Cardiovascular Science. *Cardiovasc Res.* (2020) 116:2177–84. doi: 10.1093/cvr/cvaa230
87. Gustafson D, Raju S, Wu R, Ching C, Veitch S, Rathnakumar K, et al. Overcoming barriers: the endothelium as a linchpin of coronavirus disease 2019 pathogenesis? *Arterioscler Thromb Vasc Biol.* (2020) 40:1818–29. doi: 10.1161/ATVBAHA.120.314558
88. Cho S. CD36 as a therapeutic target for endothelial dysfunction in stroke. *Curr Pharm Des.* (2012) 18:3721–30. doi: 10.2174/138161212802002760
89. Silverstein RL. Oxidized Lipid Uptake by Scavenger Receptor CD36 (Cluster of Differentiation 36) modulates endothelial surface properties and may contribute to atherogenesis. *Arterioscler Thromb Vasc Biol.* (2018) 38:4–5. doi: 10.1161/ATVBAHA.117.310351
90. Yin Y, Pastrana JL Li X, Huang X, Mallilankaraman K, Choi ET, et al. Inflammasomes: sensors of metabolic stresses for vascular inflammation. *Front Biosci.* (2013) 18:638–49. doi: 10.2741/4127
91. Wang X, Li YF, Nanayakkara G, Shao Y, Liang B, Cole L, et al. Lysophospholipid receptors, as novel conditional danger receptors and homeostatic receptors modulate inflammation-novel paradigm and therapeutic potential. *J Cardiovasc Transl Res.* (2016) 9:343–59. doi: 10.1007/s12265-016-9700-6
92. Shao Y, Nanayakkara G, Cheng J, Cueto R, Yang WY, Park JY, et al. Lysophospholipids and their receptors serve as conditional DAMPs and DAMP receptors in tissue oxidative and inflammatory injury. *Antioxid Redox Signal.* (2018) 28:973–86. doi: 10.1089/ars.2017.7069
93. Chandel NS. Mitochondria as signaling organelles. *BMC Biol.* (2014) 12:34. doi: 10.1186/1741-7007-12-34
94. Zhou W, He Q, Zhang C, He X, Cui Z, Liu F, et al. BLOS2 negatively regulates Notch signaling during neural and hematopoietic stem and progenitor cell development. *Elife.* (2016) 5:e18108. doi: 10.7554/eLife.18108
95. Poulsen LC, Edelmann RJ, Kruger S, Dieguez-Hurtado R, Shah A, Stav-Noraas TE, et al. Inhibition of endothelial NOTCH1 signaling attenuates inflammation by reducing cytokine-mediated histone acetylation at inflammatory enhancers. *Arterioscler Thromb Vasc Biol.* (2018) 38:854–69. doi: 10.1161/ATVBAHA.117.310388
96. Briot A, Civelek M, Seki A, Hoi K, Mack JJ, Lee SD, et al. Endothelial NOTCH1 is suppressed by circulating lipids and antagonizes inflammation during atherosclerosis. *J Exp Med.* (2015) 212:2147–63. doi: 10.1084/jem.20150603
97. Holliday CJ, Ankeny RF, Jo H, Nerem RM. Discovery of shear- and side-specific mRNAs and miRNAs in human aortic valvular endothelial cells. *Am J Physiol Heart Circ Physiol.* (2011) 301:H856–67. doi: 10.1152/ajpheart.00117.2011
98. Erbilgin A, Siemers N, Kayne P, Yang WP, Berliner J, Lusis AJ. Gene expression analyses of mouse aortic endothelium in response to atherogenic stimuli. *Arterioscler Thromb Vasc Biol.* (2013) 33:2509–17. doi: 10.1161/ATVBAHA.113.301989
99. Liu B, Tai Y, Caceres AI, Achanta S, Balakrishna S, Shao X, et al. Oxidized phospholipid OxPAPC activates TRPA1 and contributes to chronic inflammatory pain in mice. *PLoS ONE.* (2016) 11:e0165200. doi: 10.1371/journal.pone.0165200
100. Nallar SC, Kalvakolanu DV. Interferons, signal transduction pathways, and the central nervous system. *J Interferon Cytokine Res.* (2014) 34:559–76. doi: 10.1089/jir.2014.0021
101. Souilhol C, Serbanovic-Canic J, Fragiadaki M, Chico TJ, Ridger V, Roddie H, et al. Endothelial responses to shear stress in atherosclerosis: a novel role for developmental genes. *Nat Rev Cardiol.* (2020) 17:52–63. doi: 10.1038/s41569-019-0239-5
102. Wang N, Yuan J, Karim MR, Zhong P, Sun YP, Zhang HY, et al. Effects of mitophagy on regulatory T cell function in patients with myasthenia gravis. *Front Neurol.* (2020) 11:238. doi: 10.3389/fneur.2020.00238
103. Procaccini C, Matarese G. Where mitochondria meet autoimmunity: the Treg Cell link. *Cell Metab.* (2020) 32:507–9. doi: 10.1016/j.cmet.2020.08.006
104. Alissafi T, Kalafati L, Lazari M, Filia A, Kloukina I, Manifava M, et al. Mitochondrial oxidative damage underlies regulatory T

cell defects in autoimmunity. *Cell Metab.* (2020) 32:591–604 e7. doi: 10.1016/j.cmet.2020.07.001

105. Beaslas O, Metso J, Nissila E, Laurila PP, Kaiharju E, Batchu KC, et al. Osbpl8 deficiency in mouse causes an elevation of high-density lipoproteins and gender-specific alterations of lipid metabolism. *PLoS ONE.* (2013) 8:e58856. doi: 10.1371/journal.pone.0058856
106. Yang XF, Yin Y, Wang H. Vascular inflammation and atherogenesis are activated via receptors for PAMPs and suppressed by regulatory T Cells. *Drug Discov Today Ther Strateg.* (2008) 5:125–42. doi: 10.1016/j.ddstr.2008.11.003
107. Yin Y, Yan Y, Jiang X, Mai J, Chen NC, Wang H, et al. Inflammasomes are differentially expressed in cardiovascular and other tissues. *Int J Immunopathol Pharmacol.* (2009) 22:311–22. doi: 10.1177/039463200902200208
108. Shen J, Yin Y, Mai J, Xiong X, Pansuria M, Liu J, et al. Caspase-1 recognizes extended cleavage sites in its natural substrates. *Atherosclerosis.* (2010) 210:422–9. doi: 10.1016/j.atherosclerosis.2009.12.017
109. Wang L, Fu H, Nanayakkara G, Li Y, Shao Y, Johnson C, et al. Novel extracellular and nuclear caspase-1 and inflammasomes propagate inflammation and regulate gene expression: a comprehensive database mining study. *J Hematol Oncol.* (2016) 9:122. doi: 10.1186/s13045-016-0351-5
110. Li YF, Nanayakkara G, Sun Y, Li X, Wang L, Cueto R, et al. Analyses of caspase-1-regulated transcriptomes in various tissues lead to identification of novel IL-1beta-, IL-18- and sirtuin-1-independent pathways. *J Hematol Oncol.* (2017) 10:40. doi: 10.1186/s13045-017-0406-2
111. Vara-Perez M, Felipe-Abrio B, Agostinis P. Mitophagy in cancer: a tale of adaptation. *Cells.* (2019) 8:493. doi: 10.3390/cells8050493
112. Chen HT, Liu H, Mao MJ, Tan Y, Mo XQ, Meng XJ, et al. Crosstalk between autophagy and epithelial-mesenchymal transition and its application in cancer therapy. *Mol Cancer.* (2019) 18:101. doi: 10.1186/s12943-019-1030-2
113. Buratta S, Tancini B, Sagini K, Delo F, Chiaradia E, Urbanelli L, et al. Lysosomal exocytosis, exosome release and secretory autophagy: the autophagic- and endo-lysosomal systems go extracellular. *Int J Mol Sci.* (2020) 21:2576. doi: 10.3390/ijms21072576
114. Palmer CS, Anderson AJ, Stojanovski D. Mitochondrial protein import dysfunction: mitochondrial disease, neurodegenerative disease and cancer. *FEBS Lett.* (2021) 595:1107–31. doi: 10.1002/1873-3468.14022
115. Wiedemann N, Pfanner N. Mitochondrial machineries for protein import and assembly. *Annu Rev Biochem.* (2017) 86:685–714. doi: 10.1146/annurev-biochem-060815-014352
116. Hansen KG, Herrmann JM. Transport of proteins into mitochondria. *Protein J.* (2019) 38:330–42. doi: 10.1007/s10930-019-09819-6
117. Jadiya P, Tomar D. Mitochondrial protein quality control mechanisms. *Genes.* (2020) 11:563. doi: 10.3390/genes11050563
118. Lytovchenko O, Kunji ERS. Expression and putative role of mitochondrial transport proteins in cancer. *Biochim Biophys Acta.* (2017) 1858:641–54. doi: 10.1016/j.bbabio.2017.03.006
119. Kreimendahl S, Rassow J. The mitochondrial outer membrane protein Tom70-mediator in protein traffic, membrane contact sites and innate immunity. Int J Mol Sci. (2020) 21:7262. doi: 10.3390/ijms21197262
120. Xia Y, Yeddula N, Leblanc M, Ke E, Zhang Y, Oldfield E, et al. Reduced cell proliferation by IKK2 depletion in a mouse lung-cancer model. *Nat Cell Biol.* (2015) 17:532. doi: 10.1038/ncb3145
121. Thomas SJ, Snowden JA, Zeidler MP, Danson SJ. The role of JAK/STAT signalling in the pathogenesis, prognosis and treatment of solid tumours. *Br J Cancer.* (2015) 113:365–71. doi: 10.1038/bjc.2015.233
122. Katz SF, Lechel A, Obenauf AC, Begus-Nahrmann Y, Kraus JM, Hoffmann EM, et al. Disruption of Trp53 in livers of mice induces formation of carcinomas with bilineal differentiation. *Gastroenterology.* (2012) 142:1229–39 e3. doi: 10.1053/j.gastro.2012.02.009
123. Aoki K, Taketo MM. Adenomatous polyposis coli (APC): a multi-functional tumor suppressor gene. *J Cell Sci.* (2007) 120:3327–35. doi: 10.1242/jcs.03485
124. Reed KR, Meniel VS, Marsh V, Cole A, Sansom OJ, Clarke AR, et al. limited role for p53 in modulating the immediate phenotype of Apc loss in the intestine. *BMC Cancer.* (2008) 8:162. doi: 10.1186/1471-2407-8-162
125. Chalhoub N, Baker SJ, PTEN. and the PI3-kinase pathway in cancer. *Annu Rev Pathol.* (2009) 4:127–50. doi: 10.1146/annurev.pathol.4.110807.092311
126. Chatterjee N, Pazarentzos E, Mayekar MK, Gui P, Allegakoen DV, Hrustanovic G, et al. Synthetic essentiality of metabolic regulator PDHK1 in PTEN-deficient cells and cancers. *Cell Rep.* (2019) 28:2317–30 e8. doi: 10.1016/j.celrep.2019.07.063
127. Tang Z, Li C, Kang B, Gao G, Li C, Zhang Z, et al. a web server for cancer and normal gene expression profiling and interactive analyses. *Nucleic Acids Res.* (2017) 45:W98–102. doi: 10.1093/nar/gkx247
128. Ng B, Yang F, Huston DP, Yan Y, Yang Y, Xiong Z, et al. Increased noncanonical splicing of autoantigen transcripts provides the structural basis for expression of untolerized epitopes. *J Allergy Clin Immunol.* (2004) 114:1463–70. doi: 10.1016/j.jaci.2004.09.006
129. Zemmour D, Zilionis R, Kiner E, Klein AM, Mathis D, Benoist C. Single-cell gene expression reveals a landscape of regulatory T cell phenotypes shaped by the TCR. *Nat Immunol.* (2018) 19:291–301. doi: 10.1038/s41590-018-0051-0
130. Corkum CP, Ings DP, Burgess C, Karwowska S, Kroll W, Michalak TI. Immune cell subsets and their gene expression profiles from human PBMC isolated by Vacutainer Cell Preparation Tube (CPT) and standard density gradient. *BMC Immunol.* (2015) 16:48. doi: 10.1186/s12865-015-0113-0
131. Li X, Fang P, Yang WY, Chan K, Lavallee M, Xu K, et al. Mitochondrial ROS, uncoupled from ATP synthesis, determine endothelial activation for both physiological recruitment of patrolling cells and pathological recruitment of inflammatory cells. *Can J Physiol Pharmacol.* (2017) 95:247–52. doi: 10.1139/cjpp-2016-0515
132. Yang XF, Weber GF, Cantor H, A. novel Bcl-x isoform connected to the T cell receptor regulates apoptosis in T cells. *Immunity.* (1997) 7:629–39. doi: 10.1016/S1074-7613(00)80384-2
133. Yang Y, Yang F, Xiong Z, Yan Y, Wang X, Nishino M, et al. An N-terminal region of translationally controlled tumor protein is required for its antiapoptotic activity. *Oncogene.* (2005) 24:4778–88. doi: 10.1038/sj.onc.1208666
134. Kumar V, Maity S. ER Stress-sensor proteins and ER-mitochondrial crosstalk-signaling beyond (ER) stress response. *Biomolecules.* (2021) 11:173. doi: 10.3390/biom11020173
135. Heaton SM, Borg NA, Dixit VM. Ubiquitin in the activation and attenuation of innate antiviral immunity. *J Exp Med.* (2016) 213:1–13. doi: 10.1084/jem.20151531
136. Glebov OO. Understanding SARS-CoV-2 endocytosis for COVID-19 drug repurposing. *FEBS J.* (2020) 287:3664–71. doi: 10.1111/febs.15369
137. Yang Q, Nanayakkara GK, Drummer C, Sun Y, Johnson C, Cueto R, et al. Low-intensity ultrasound-induced anti-inflammatory effects are mediated by several new mechanisms including gene induction, immunosuppressor cell promotion, and enhancement of exosome biogenesis and docking. *Front Physiol.* (2017) 8:818. doi: 10.3389/fphys.2017.00818

5

Comprehensive Integration of Single-Cell Transcriptional Profiling Reveals the Heterogeneities of Non-Cardiomyocytes in Healthy and Ischemic Hearts

Lingfang Zhuang[1,2], *Lin Lu*[1,2], *Ruiyan Zhang*[1,2], *Kang Chen*[1,2*] *and Xiaoxiang Yan*[1,2*]

[1] *Department of Cardiology, Ruijin Hospital, Shanghai Jiao Tong University School of Medicine, Shanghai, China,* [2] *Institute of Cardiovascular Diseases, Shanghai Jiao Tong University School of Medicine, Shanghai, China*

***Correspondence:**
Xiaoxiang Yan
cardexyanxx@hotmail.com
Kang Chen
chenkang1978@163.com

Advances in single-cell RNA sequencing (scRNA-seq) technology have recently shed light on the molecular mechanisms of the spatial and temporal changes of thousands of cells simultaneously under homeostatic and ischemic conditions. The aim of this study is to investigate whether it is possible to integrate multiple similar scRNA-seq datasets for a more comprehensive understanding of diseases. In this study, we integrated three representative scRNA-seq datasets of 27,349 non-cardiomyocytes isolated at 3 and 7 days after myocardial infarction or sham surgery. In total, seven lineages, including macrophages, fibroblasts, endothelia, and lymphocytes, were identified in this analysis with distinct dynamic and functional properties in healthy and nonhealthy hearts. Myofibroblasts and endothelia were recognized as the central hubs of cellular communication via ligand-receptor interactions. Additionally, we showed that macrophages from different origins exhibited divergent transcriptional signatures, pathways, developmental trajectories, and transcriptional regulons. It was found that myofibroblasts predominantly expand at 7 days after myocardial infarction with pro-reparative characteristics. We identified signature genes of myofibroblasts, such as Postn, Cthrc1, and Ddah1, among which Ddah1 was exclusively expressed on activated fibroblasts and exhibited concordant upregulation in bulk RNA sequencing data and *in vivo* and *in vitro* experiments. Collectively, this compendium of scRNA-seq data provides a valuable entry point for understanding the transcriptional and dynamic changes of non-cardiomyocytes in healthy and nonhealthy hearts by integrating multiple datasets.

Keywords: myocardial infarction, single-cell RNA sequencing, immune system, non-cardiomyocytes, macrophages, Ddah1

INTRODUCTION

Cardiovascular diseases such as myocardial infarction (MI) are a leading cause of morbidity and mortality worldwide. Generally, the difficulties faced while treating ischemia involve not only the poor regeneration of cardiomyocytes after MI, but also the complexity of non-cardiomyocytes (non-CMs), including macrophages, fibroblasts (FBs), and T cells, which play a pivotal role in cardiac remodeling after MI (1). In the last few years, there has been an increased interest in the dynamic changes and transcriptional reprogramming of these cells after ischemia and how these cells coordinate inflammatory and reparative processes during cardiac remodeling (2).

Recently, various studies have been dedicated to the exploration of the dynamic and functional changes of non-CMs after MI using a new method called single-cell RNA sequencing (scRNA-seq) (3), which provides a new entry point for understanding the temporal functions of different cell types in healthy and injured hearts by detecting and analyzing these cells simultaneously (4). These scRNA-seq data have been deposited in public databases, such as the GEO or ArrayExpress database, increasing the possibility of integrating similar scRNA-seq data of non-CMs in healthy and ischemic hearts for a more comprehensive understanding of their dynamics and crosstalk in different states.

In this study, we explored recently published articles on scRNA-seq investigating the functional changes of non-CMs in healthy or ischemic hearts and integrated three representative datasets containing cells collected at 0, 3, and 7 days after MI for a deeper analysis. A total of 27,349 cells, including major non-CM lineages, such as macrophages, FBs, endothelia, and smooth muscle cells (SMCs), were clustered into 20 subpopulations with distinct gene signatures. Analysis of the dynamics and intercellular communication of non-CMs revealed that FBs and endothelial cells (ECs) played a dramatic role in the cellular crosstalk via ligand-receptor interactions. Moreover, the endothelial-like macrophages (MAC-Endo) and FB-like macrophages (MAC-Fib) that exhibited a transcriptional profile of endothelia or FBs under a macrophage background were described in this study. By integrating these scRNA-seq data, we pointed to a novel marker of activated FBs, dimethylarginine dimethylaminohydrolase 1 (Ddah1), which was found to be sharply upregulated after MI in bulk RNA sequencing data and *in vivo* and *in vitro* experiments.

To our knowledge, this is the first study inquiring the possibility of integrating published scRNA-seq data to investigate the transcriptional and dynamic changes of non-CMs in healthy and nonhealthy hearts with unprecedented resolutions.

MATERIALS AND METHODS

Mice and Myocardial Infarction

Male C57BL/6 mice were purchased from the Shanghai Laboratory Animal Center (Shanghai, China) and maintained under a light/dark cycle. All animal experimental procedures were approved by the Animal Care Committee of Shanghai Jiao Tong University School of Medicine. The MI model was used to induced cardiac ischemia *in vivo* as described previously (5). Briefly, 8–10-week-old mice were anesthetized with isoflurane, intubated, and mechanically ventilated with a low concentration of isoflurane gas (1.0%). After opening chest in 3-4 intercostal and removing the pericardium, the left anterior descending artery was ligated with an 8-0 silk suture, followed by closing the chest and skin with 5-0 and 3-0 silk sutures, respectively. In the sham group, all mice underwent an identical procedure except for the artery ligation.

Analysis and Integration of scRNA-seq Data

The three datasets included in this analysis were downloaded from the GEO database (https://www.ncbi.nlm.nih.gov/geo/) or from ArrayExpress database (https://www.ebi.ac.uk/arrayexpress/) with full expression matrix and mapped Ensemble genes. Firstly, quality control of single cells was performed in every dataset by selecting single viable cells. Specifically, the percentage of mitochondria and the number of features in every cell were set as the limitations. Data on single cells were then filtered according to the source article criteria before the next analysis. After this quality-control procedure, each feature of the cells was normalized by dividing the total unique molecular identifiers and multiplying by 10,000 to obtain a value in transcripts per million, followed by logarithmic transformation using the R package Seurat (6, 7). Notably, we integrated three datasets with a "FindIntegratedanchors" function using 2,000 variable genes differentially expressed among all cells. Then, by conducting "RunPCA," "FindNeighbors," and "FindClusters" serially, we were able to partition cell populations according to their expression of marker genes. Notably, the "FindAllMarkers" function in Seurat (with parameters min.pct = 0.25 and logfc.threshold = 0.25) was used to identify specific markers of each cluster, and the results were displayed as a heatmap or uploaded as **Supplementary Tables**. Then, the "FindMarkers" function was used to identify differentially expressed genes among distinct experimental conditions or among clusters of interest for an enrichment analysis.

Enrichment Analysis

For pathway enrichment analysis, all cluster-specific markers or differentially expressed genes resulting from the "FindMarkers" function in Seurat were used for Gene Ontology (GO) analysis or Gene Set Enrichment Analysis (GSEA) (8) in RStudio. The R package clusterProfiler (9) was used in this analysis with a cutoff q-value of 0.05. The results were generated with ggplot2 as bar plots or GSEA plots and uploaded as **Supplementary Tables**, and the volcano plots used to compare the expression levels of differential genes between groups were generated using ggplot2 in R.

Cellular Crosstalk

Cell-cell communication networks were assessed according to a previously published algorithm (10). Briefly, a collection of ligand-receptor pairs generated from the STRING database (11) were further analyzed only if they expressed at least 10% of the cells in a given cell population. Notably, the communication network consisted of source populations expressing differential

Abbreviations: MI, myocardial infarction; scRNA-seq, single-cell RNA sequencing; non-CM, non-cardiomyocyte; SMC, smooth muscle cell; GSEA, gene set enrichment analysis; SCENIC, single-cell regulatory network inference and clustering; FB, fibroblast; EC, endothelial cell; TR, tissue resident; ECM, extracellular matrix.

ligands among clusters and target clusters with corresponding receptors. The weighted path connecting source populations to target clusters via a ligand-receptor pair was calculated as the sum of weights along that path. After adjusting the p-value using the Benjamini-Hochberg (BH) method, significant connections between ligands and receptors were included for other analysis at a p-value < 0.01. A crosstalk network graph was generated using the R packages circlize (12) and Gephi (https://gephi.org).

Immunofluorescence (IF) Staining

Immunostaining was performed on the hearts of mice at 0, 3, and 7 days after MI surgery as reported previously (5). After intracardiac perfusion with phosphate-buffered saline and paraformaldehyde, the hearts were fixed for 24 h in 4% paraformaldehyde and subsequently embedded in paraffin and sectioned into 5 μm slices for staining. After antigen retrieval and permeabilization, the slides were blocked with 5% bovine serum albumin buffer for 30 min and then probed overnight with primary antibodies. After washing with phosphate-buffered saline and incubation with the corresponding Alexa Fluor-conjugated secondary antibodies for 2 h and 4′,6-diamidino-2-phenylindole for 5 min. Images were taken using a fluorescence microscope. The following antibodies were used for IF staining: Ddah1 (ab180599, 1:100; Abcam, Cambridge, UK) and α-smooth muscle actin (sc-53142, 1:100; Santa Cruz Biotechnology, Inc., Dallas, TX, USA). In all quantifications of immunofluorescence images, we performed at least three individual samples for every group and acquired at least five high-resolution images for every section.

Western Blot

Total protein was extracted from the heart tissues of mice after MI or sham surgery using a sodium dodecyl sulfate lysis buffer, and then protein concentrations were measured using a BCA assay kit. Western blot analysis was performed as described previously (5). Briefly, protein samples were separated using sodium dodecyl sulfate-polyacrylamide gel electrophoresis, transferred to a polyvinylidene fluoride membrane (Millipore, Burlington, MA, USA), and incubated with 5% fat-free milk for 1 h before being incubated with primary antibodies at 4°C overnight. Antibody Ddah1 (ab180599, 1:1,000; Abcam) was used, and GAPDH was used as the control.

Pseudotime Trajectory Analysis

Pseudotime analysis was specifically performed on macrophage and FB lineages from our integrated single-cell data using the R Package Monocle (13). The unique expression matrix and cell identities were fetched from Seurat files and used as input material for further analyses. After integrating and reducing dimensions with default parameters, clusters were defined using the "cluster_cells" function with a resolution of $10^{-3.3}$, and their pseudotime trajectory was determined using the "learn_graph" function. The results were plotted in three-dimensional space. To analyze differentially expressed genes triggering a particular pseudotime distribution of cell populations, we used the "graph_test" function to investigate differential genes among cell clusters.

Transcriptional Regulon Analysis

Core regulatory transcription factors of macrophages and T cell lineages were predicted using the R package SCENIC (14). The GENIE3 package (Step 1) was used to infer gene regulatory networks from the expression matrix of the included cells on the basis of the coexpression networks. Then, a RcisTarget analysis (Step 2) was performed to investigate the DNA motif and predict regulons among cell populations on the basis of the "mm9-tss-centered-10kb" database. The activity of the regulatory networks was evaluated on the full dataset in the scoring step with AUCell (Step 3). Notably, regulons annotated as "extended" included target genes harboring motifs that have been linked to the respective transcription factor by lower confidence annotations.

Statistical Analysis

Data were presented as box-and-whisker plots or bar plots with all points, which were evaluated and organized using the commercial software GraphPad Prism (version 7.0a; GraphPad Software, San Diego, CA, USA). Statistically significant differences between every two groups were analyzed using Student's two-sided t-test. For experiments with more than two groups, after confirming normality and homogeneity of variance, one-way analysis of variance (ANOVA) followed by Tukey's post hoc test was used for comparison. For comparison between multiple experimental groups with a control group, the Dunnett's post hoc test was used in SPSS Statistics (version 23; IBM, Armonk, NY, USA). For all analyses, statistical significance was set at $p < 0.05$.

RESULTS

Integration of the Three Single-Cell RNA Sequencing Datasets Exhibits a Cell-Type-Dependent Distribution of Non-cardiomyocytes

First, to investigate the possibility of integrating similar scRNA-seq data, we collected and summarized recently published single-cell sequencing data of mouse hearts (**Supplementary Table I**). Three articles were chosen for further analysis (10, 15, 16): (1) isolating and sequencing CD45+ leukocytes from MI-operated hearts at 4 days after surgery ($n = 1{,}866$) or sham-operated hearts ($n = 703$) (15) (**Supplementary Figures 1A,B**); (2) isolating all interstitial cells from murine hearts at 3 days ($n = 4{,}067$), and 7 days ($n = 4{,}194$) after MI or sham ($n = 5{,}977$) surgery (10) (**Supplementary Figures 1C,D**); (3) collecting nonmyocyte cells from the ventricles of mouse hearts (16) under a homeostatic condition ($n = 10{,}542$; **Supplementary Figure 1E**). After a similar quality-control procedure according to their source study, each independent dataset was processed with an unsupervised clustering algorithm to identify cell lineages and visualize with t-SNE plots (6) (**Supplementary Figure 1**). Next, to find the correspondences among these datasets, we harmonized these datasets into a single reference using the "FindIntegratedanchors" function in Seurat (7) and visualized the distributions of cells with UMAP reduction plots. A total of 27,349 non-CM cells constituting nine cell lineages were partitioned into 20 subpopulations depending on their dominant expressed marker genes (**Figure 1A**). Of note, each cluster consisted of cells from all conditions without showing significant batch effects, indicating the reliability of our integration strategy (**Figure 1B**).

In this analysis, cells were clustered and designated depending on the concordant expression of well-characterized marker genes (**Supplementary Table II, Figure 1C**). Specifically, secreted phosphoprotein 1 (Spp1) (17) and arginase 1 (Arg1) (18, 19), which are dramatically upregulated on M2 macrophages, were found to be predominantly expressed in the MAC-M2 cluster, whereas periostin (Postn) (20) was found to exclusively exist in activated FBs (Fibro_Myo; **Figure 1C**). Additionally, T cells/natural killer (NK) cells (expressing Cd3g and Cd3d), B cells (expressing Cd79a and Cd79b), and SMCs (expressing Acta2) were also identified in this study (**Figure 1C**). Furthermore, the UMAP plots of curated conservative marker genes indicated well-partitioned cell lineages. Specifically, the cell-type-dependent expression of Adgre1 (marker of macrophages; **Figure 1D**), Pecam1 (marker of ECs; **Figure 1E**), Acta2 (marker of SMCs; **Figure 1F**), Col3a1 (marker of FBs; **Figure 1G**), Postn (marker of myofibroblasts; **Figures 1H,I**), Cd79a (marker of B cells; **Supplementary Figure 1F**), Cd8b1 (marker of T cells; **Supplementary Figure 1G**), and Vtn (marker of pericytes; **Supplementary Figure 1H**) confirmed the well-clustered cell populations in our integrated scRNA-seq data, providing us with an important basis to further explore the dynamics and functional changes of each cell cluster.

Taken together, these findings demonstrate that, by integrating different datasets, we were able to analyze non-CMs in healthy and injured hearts in a single-cell resolution.

Cell Dynamics and Cellular Communication Analysis Reveal Temporal and Functional Differences Between Cell Types

To delineate the composition of each cluster reflecting disease-related cell fluxes under ischemic conditions, separated UMAP plots including cells from sham, 3 or 7 days after MI (MI-3d, MI-7d, respectively) were mapped for a more directed visualization of cell composition during healing process (**Figure 2A, Supplementary Figure 2A**). We observed drastically ischemia-induced cell fluxes. For example, the expansion of the MAC_M2 population peaked at 3 days after MI surgery and the proportion of Fibro_Myo sharply increased at 7 days after MI, as previously reported (21). Besides, significantly infiltrated T/NK and B cells were observed at 7 days after MI, whereas neutrophil and dendritic cell populations dramatically expanded at 3 days (**Figure 2B**). This distinct time window of cell expansion after MI suggests varied functions of non-CMs during cardiac repair and remodeling process.

Increased cell-cell communication is a hallmark of cardiac repair and plays a pivotal role in cardiac remodeling (22). To investigate the crosstalk of non-CMs, we analyzed the expression of ligands and receptors in each cell population using a curated collection of human ligand-receptor pairs (23) and the STRING database (11). Then, after computing their weighted expression among source and target populations (cells with differentially expressed ligands referred to source clusters and cells with upregulated receptors related to target populations), a total of 636 ligand-receptor pairs were identified in our data with differential expression on total cell populations (**Supplementary Table III**). By summarizing all the weighted paths, we found that FBs possess the largest number of ligands among all cell clusters. More specifically, the Fibro_Myo, Fibro_1, Fibro_2, Fibro_3, and Fibro_5 populations were recognized as the top five clusters with dominant outbound connections. Moreover, Fibro_Myo have the most prominent number of differentially expressed ligands, suggesting their indispensable function in communicating with other cells for cardiac repair (**Figures 2C,D**). Besides, it is intriguing that ECs (Endo_1) were found to have the most weighted path as the target population, implying their crucial role in ligand binding and cell response (**Figures 2C,E**) after MI. An integrated map including cell clusters, ligands, and receptors (**Figure 2F**) confirmed our previous analysis, underscoring the centrality hub roles of Fibro_Myo and Endo_1 as source and target populations in cell-cell communication. Notably, we found that the integrin family, including integrin subunit beta 1 (Itgb1), had the largest weighted connections with ligands expressed in multiple cell populations (**Figure 2F**). Collectively, these observations emphasize the profound function of FBs and ECs in the repair process.

Macrophage/Monocyte Populations in Healthy and Injured Hearts

As macrophages constitute the largest number of immune cells in the heart and exhibit a dramatic cell flux in injured hearts (**Figures 2A,B**), it was therefore important to figure out not only the flux of macrophages, but also its functional differences under homeostatic and ischemic conditions. In this study, a total of seven subclusters of macrophages were identified (**Figure 1A**) and selected for deeper analysis (specifically IFNIC, MAC_Mo/M1, MAC_M2, MAC_TR, MAC_APC, MAC_4, and MAC_3; **Figure 3A**). In line with a previous study (24), we observed distinct tissue-resident (TR) macrophages (MAC_TR) that exhibited increased expression of Cx3cr1 and H2-Aa (**Figures 3D,E**) and downregulated expression of the proinflammatory gene Ly6c2. Among these TR macrophages, some cells displayed exclusively expressed proreparative genes, Cd163 and Mrc1 (**Figures 3B,C**), while lacking H2-Aa compared to others, suggesting that these cells assume more anti-inflammatory roles during ischemic injuries rather than antigen processing and presentation, consistent with other single-cell sequencing research on cardiac hypertrophy models (25). Besides, some proinflammatory macrophage populations with higher levels of Ly6c2 and oncostatin M (Osm; **Figures 3F,G**) were found to be far from TR macrophages, suggesting dramatic differences in cell phenotypes and molecular functions between these two types of cell populations.

Furthermore, we aligned all macrophage populations for pseudotemporal analysis to reconstruct the possible trajectory of macrophages and determine the regulators of cell fate using the R package Monocle (13, 26). A three-dimensional UMAP plot revealed 10 separate cell clusters, including MAC_Mo/M1,

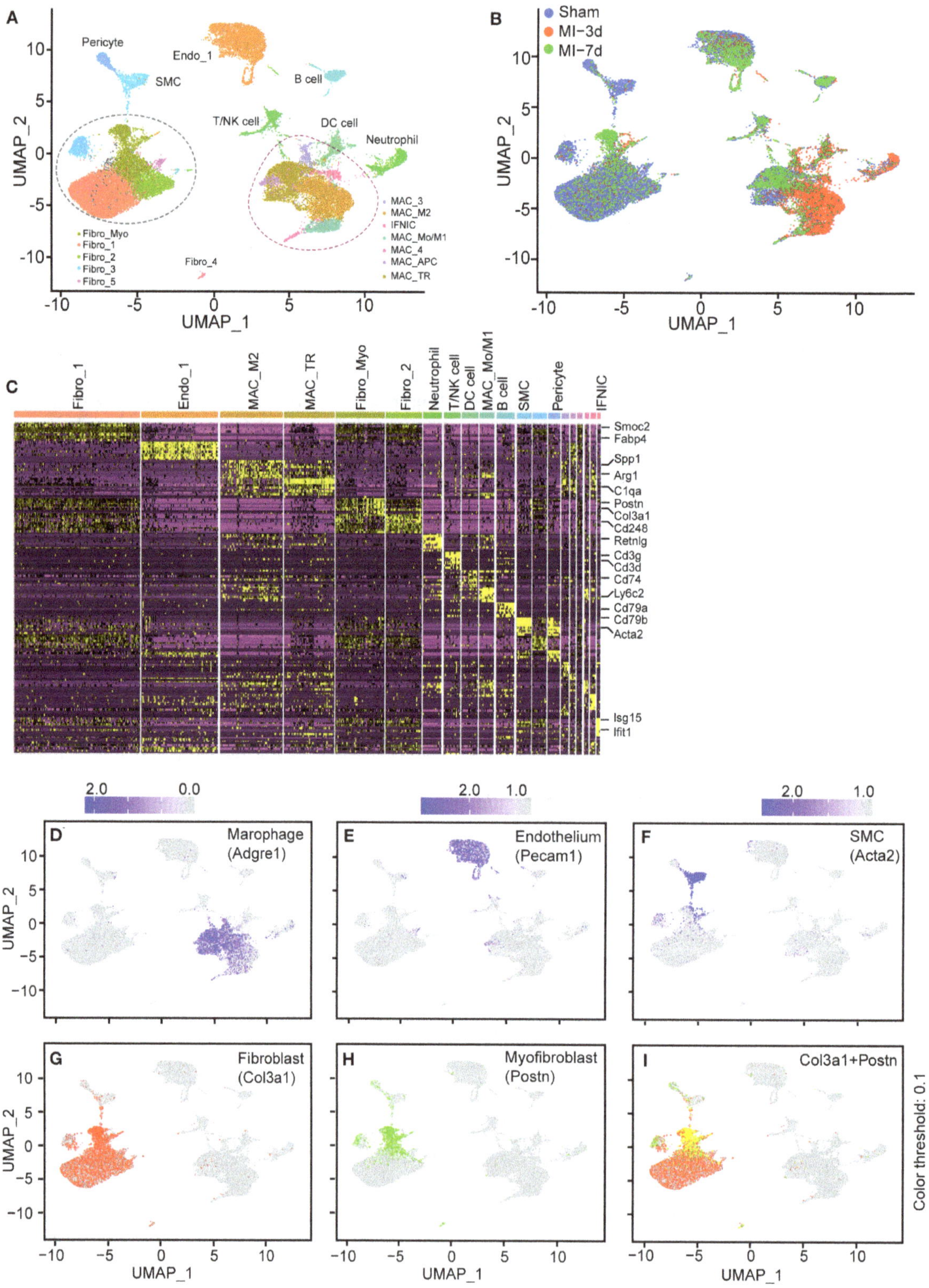

FIGURE 1 | Integration of non-cardiomyocytes (non-CMs) in healthy and nonhealthy hearts. **(A)** UMAP plot of non-CMs from the sham group or 3 and 7 days after myocardial infarction (MI), showing the construction of 20 subpopulations in different colors. **(B)** UMAP plot of integrated non-CMs under different conditions shown in different colors. **(C)** Heatmap of 20 subclusters with differentially expressed genes across cell populations for cell identification, in which the upper bars refer to subclusters. **(D–I)** UMAP visualization of all cells, combined with the expression of Adgre1 **(D)**, Pecam1 **(E)**, Acta2 **(F)**, Col3a1 **(G)**, and Postn **(H,I)**. The scaled expression of target genes were indicated in the upper portion of each panel.

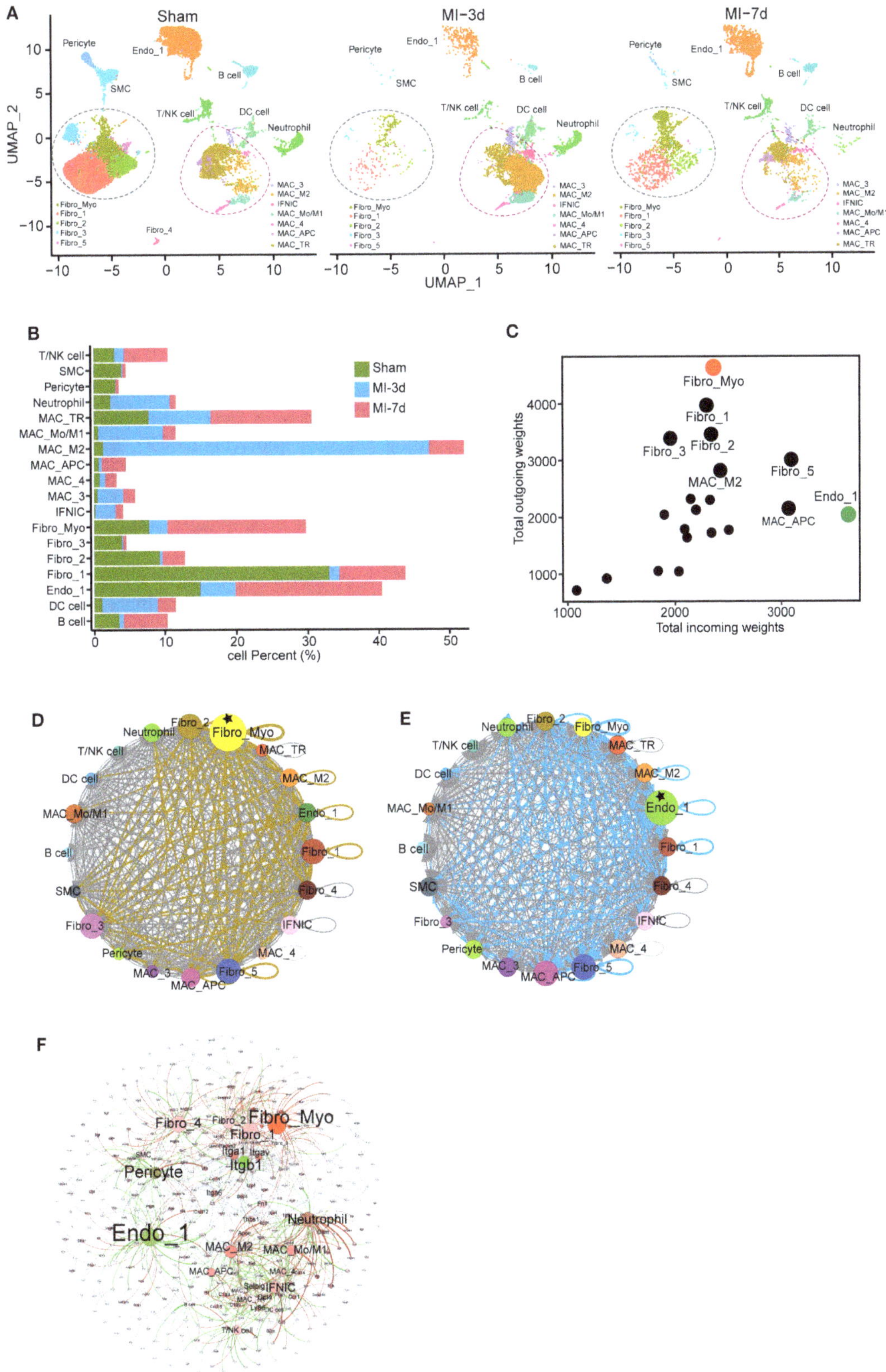

FIGURE 2 | Dynamics and cell communication of non-cardiomyocytes (non-CMs). **(A)** Separated UMAP plots showing heterogeneous non-CM populations in the sham group, 3 and 7 days after myocardial infarction (MI). Fibroblasts (FBs) and macrophages were circled with dashed lines. **(B)** Bar plot showing the dynamics of cell

(Continued)

FIGURE 2 | clusters in sham and MI hearts. **(C)** Cell communication across all subpopulations was identified with well-characterized ligand-receptor pairs. Outcoming and incoming weights refer to the weighted numbers of ligands and receptors among all cell populations. **(D,E)** Putative cell communication based on differentially expressed ligands **(D)** and receptors **(E)** including total cell clusters. Circular compartments representing subclusters with weighted sizes. **(F)** Putative cell-cell interactions, including cell types, ligands, and receptors. All interactions of ligands from source cell populations to receptors (target populations) were plotted; cell type, ligands, and receptors were filled as nodes; and interactions were shown as edges. The source data were uploaded as **Supplementary Table III**.

MAC_M2, IFNIC, and MAC_TR, which have been verified in the Seurat algorithm. Additionally, we observed the existence of FB-like (MAC_Fib) and endothelial-like (MAC_Endo) macrophages in our analysis (**Figure 3H**). These cell populations showed exclusive expression of FB markers (Col1a1) and endothelial markers (Cdh5) in macrophages (**Figure 3I**). In fact, several previous studies confirmed the possibility that macrophages would transform into FB-like cells during MI remodeling (27); however, the possibility of whether macrophages can transform into endothelia still requires further exploration. In line with the scRNA-seq results, we validated the existence of endothelial-like macrophages by costaining CD31 and CD68 using immunofluorescence technology (**Figure 3J**). Additionally, by ordering the pseudotime cell trajectory, we described a continuous stage of macrophages starting from early infiltrating monocytes and M1 macrophages to late proreparative M2 macrophages (**Figure 3K**), which is similar to what has been found in previous studies on single-cell analysis (10) or *in vivo* experiments (21). However, it was found that other macrophage subpopulations, such as MAC_TR, MAC_Fib, and MAC_Endo, are hard to merge into the trajectory of blood-derived macrophages, suggesting a divergent origin and transcriptional profile of these two cell types.

Next, we performed single-cell regulatory network inference and clustering (SCENIC) analysis (14) to investigate the core transcriptional regulons driving the differentiation of distinct macrophage subpopulations. Intriguingly, we discovered that blood-derived macrophages, such as MAC_Mo/M1 and IFNIC, exhibit activated proinflammatory regulons, for instance, signal transducer and activator of transcription 1 (Stat1) and interferon regulatory factor 7 (Irf7). In line with previous researches, it was found that excessive Irf3 activation and interferon production trigger the overproduction of cytokines and infiltration of immune cells after MI (15). Besides, early growth response 1 (Egr1) and Jund regulons were predominantly enriched in TR macrophages, such as MAC_TR, MAC_Fib, and MAC_Endo. Corroborating our findings, previous studies confirmed that the zinc finger transcription factor Egr1 is essential for the activation and differentiation of macrophages (**Figure 3L**) (28, 29). Taken together, these data provide new insights into the heterogenous transcriptional profile and regulons of macrophages.

Transcriptional Differences of Tissue-Resident and Blood-Derived Macrophages

In our previous work, we observed that macrophages with varied origin exhibit divergent developmental trajectory and distinct transcriptional regulons. To explore the differences of gene signatures and pathways among TR and blood-derived macrophages, we compared the expression patterns of Ccr2, a well-known marker that distinguishes TR macrophages from blood-derived macrophages. Markedly downregulated expression of Ccr2 was observed in MAC-TR, MAC_Endo, and MAC_Fib clusters, compared to other cell populations (**Figure 4A**). Next, to more specifically determine the underlying expression patterns of TR macrophages, we reassigned the three aforementioned cell clusters as a Ccr2-low cluster (Ccr2_lo) and the others as a Ccr2-high cluster (Ccr2_hi) and mapped using a UMAP plot (**Figure 4B**). By comparing differentially expressed genes among these two groups, Ccr2_lo cells showed lower expression of Ccr2 and Ly6c2, whereas the marker gene of proreparative macrophages Mrc1 was upregulated. Moreover, lymphatic vessel endothelial hyaluronan receptor 1 (Lyve1) and Cx3cr1, which have been recognized as markers of TR macrophages, were found to be highly expressed in the Ccr2_lo group (**Figure 4C**) (30). We also performed GSEA (8) on the basis of biological process terms and observed prominent differences in the activated pathway patterns between these two groups (**Figure 4D**, **Supplementary Table IV**). Specifically, the Ccr2_lo group was found to exhibit significantly enriched gene sets involved in the regulation of cell proliferation (**Figure 4E**) and cellular response to growth factors or transforming growth factor beta (TGF-β) (**Figure 4F**), in agreement with the activation of Egr1 transcriptional regulons in TR macrophages. However, it was found that myeloid cell activation, which is involved in immune responses and exocytosis, two key pathways associated with proinjury macrophages, is positively correlated with Ccr2_hi macrophages (**Figure 4G**). Overall, functional comparative analysis of Ccr2_lo and Ccr2_hi macrophages supported the protective role of TR macrophages by exerting self-renewing and anti-inflammatory effects after MI.

Flux of Fibroblasts and Activated Fibroblasts in Ischemic Hearts

As FBs constitute the largest number of non-CMs under homeostatic conditions and play an indispensable role in fibrotic scar formation and cardiac remodeling after MI, our next aim was to explore the functional changes of FBs in healthy and MI-operated hearts. In total, six FB clusters were identified (**Figures 1A**, **5A**) in this study: Fibro_1, Fibro_2, Fibro_3, Fibro_4, Fibro_5, and Fibro_Myo. Comparison of marker genes among these clusters indicated that myofibroblast markers (31), such as Col1a1, Col3a1, and Postn, are significantly upregulated in Fibro_Myo clusters (**Figure 5B**). Further exploring the flux of FBs after MI, we found that, compared with the sham surgery, the proportions of FBs were reduced at 3 days after MI, which may have resulted from a sharp ischemic condition and

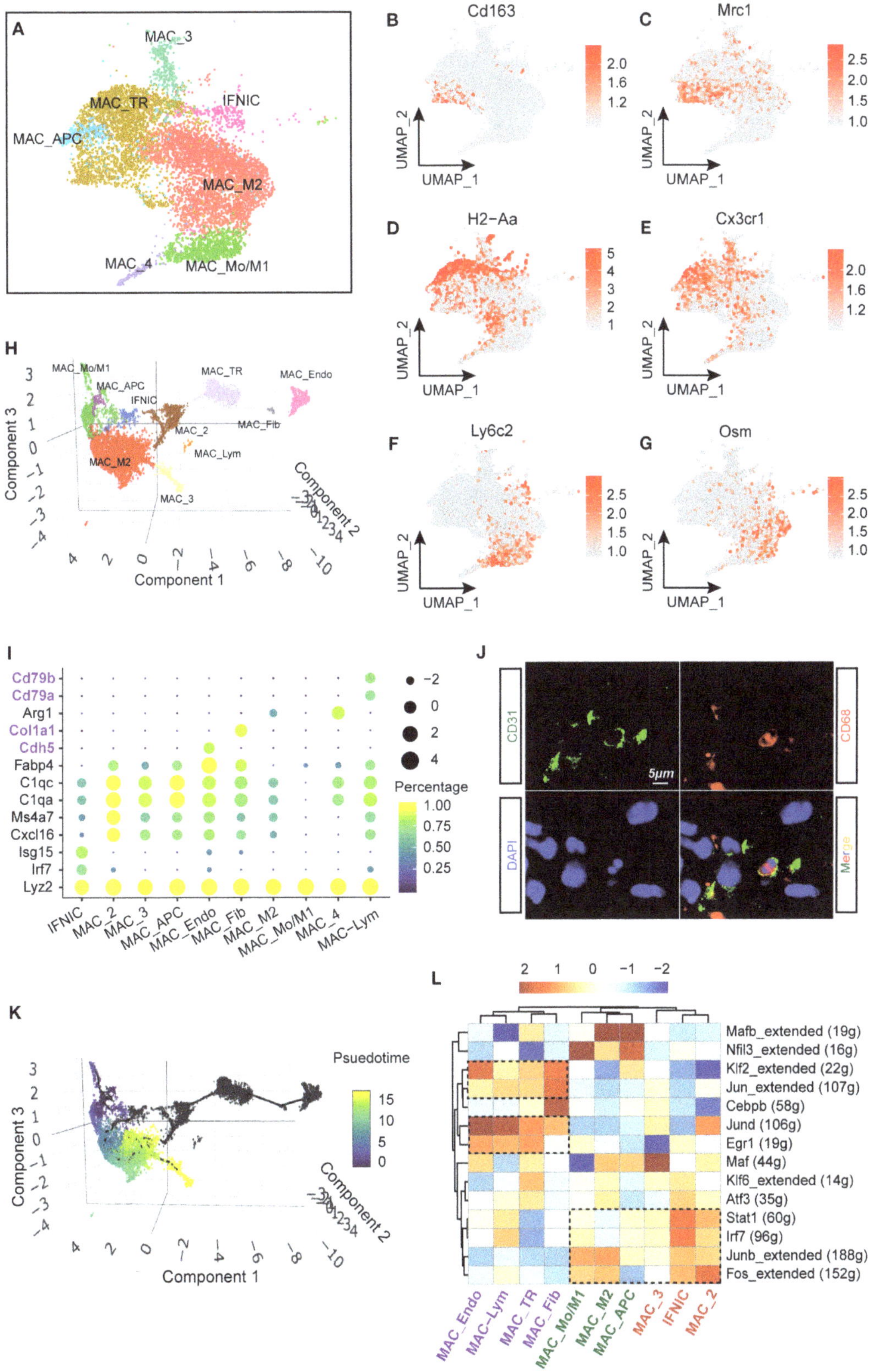

FIGURE 3 | Heterogenous gene signatures, transcriptional regulons of cardiac macrophages. **(A)** UMAP plot with all macrophage subclusters were visualized with different colors corresponding to their identity. **(B–G)** Gene expression of Cd163 **(B)**, Mrc1 **(C)**, H2-Aa **(D)**, Cx3cr1 **(E)**, Ly6c2 **(F)**, and Osm **(G)** within macrophage lineages

(Continued)

FIGURE 3 | were visualized with UMAP plots. The right bar indicated the scaled expression of each gene in macrophage subpopulations. **(H)** Reconstruction of macrophage clusters in Monocle showing the heterogeneity of cell populations. **(I)** Dot plot showing the expression of cell-type-specific signatures in identified cell clusters in Monocle. The dot size and color represented the mean expression and proportion of each cell population expressing genes, respectively. **(J)** Immunofluorescent costaining of CD31 and CD68 in mouse heart sections. **(K)** Developmental trajectory analysis including all macrophage clusters showing the pseudotemporal development of included cells. On the right, the scale going from dark to light color represented the process of maturity. **(L)** Single-cell regulatory network inference and clustering (SCENIC) analysis of macrophage clusters to investigate differentially regulated transcriptional factors, were showed as a heatmap. The dashed rectangles indicated enriched regulons among specific clusters.

loss of FBs. Notably, myofibroblasts (Fibro_Myo) prominently increased at 7 days after MI compared with other FB clusters, suggesting an important role of Fibro_Myo in ischemic responses and healing processes (**Figure 5C**). Additionally, GO analysis of Fibro_Myo with other FB clusters showed significant enrichment of prohealing pathways, such as actin filament organization, extracellular matrix (ECM) organization, and wound healing (**Figure 5D**).

We then compared differentially expressed genes between Fibro_Myo and five other clusters and observed dramatic upregulation of Cthrc1, which has been confirmed to be a marker of myofibroblasts (32), and Ddah1 (**Figure 5E**). Some previous studies confirmed that Ddah1 plays a crucial role in the clearance of asymmetric dimethylarginine and monomethyl arginine, which are strongly associated with premature cardiovascular disease and death (33). By combining the expression of Cthrc1 and Ddah1, we found exclusively co-expressed Cthrc1 and Ddah1 in myofibroblasts rather than in other FB clusters (**Figure 5F**), suggesting that Ddah1 may serve as another marker of myofibroblasts.

Next, to investigate the trajectory development of FBs and myofibroblasts, we reclustered the FB populations in the Monocle package for pseudotime analysis (**Figure 5G**). Intriguingly, we found a continuous cell development from Fibro_1 to activated FBs (Fibro_Myo), consistent with their dynamic changes after MI (**Figure 5H**). As myofibroblasts exist in the final stage of cell trajectory, we next analyzed a pattern of gene expression that triggers this developmental trajectory using the "graph autocorrelation analysis" function embedded in Monocle. Unexpectedly, we found that Cthrc1 and Ddah1 are positively correlated with the development of myofibroblasts, suggesting their crucial effect on the activation of FBs (**Figure 5I**). Taken together, these observations indicate that the heterogeneities and dynamic changes of FBs during healing process and Ddah1 exclusively expressed in myofibroblasts may represent another marker of activated FBs.

Verifying the Expression and Location of Ddah1 After Myocardial Infarction

It has been confirmed in a previous analysis that Ddah1 has a distinct function in the development and activation of FBs (**Figure 5**). To investigate and verify the expression of Ddah1 in ischemic hearts, we first recalculated the expression of Ddah1 in two curated articles in which bulk RNA sequencing was performed: (1) Transcriptome analysis of remote, border, and infarcted zones in mice at 3, 7, and 14 days after MI or sham surgery (PMID: 31259610) (34); (2) Transcriptome analysis of cardiomyocytes, FBs, leukocytes, and ECs from sham- or MI-operated neonatal (P1) and adult (8W) mouse hearts at 3 days after surgery (PMID: 28733351) (35). From the first dataset, we discovered that ischemia induced robust upregulation of Ddah1 in the border zone at 3, 7, and 14 days after surgery, whereas its expression peaked at 7 days in the infarcted zones (**Figure 6A**). Moreover, the second article, which analyzed the transcriptional expression of four cell types, indicated that upregulated Ddah1 after MI surgery exclusively existed in FBs and ECs, while lacking any significance in CMs and leukocytes (Leu; **Figure 6B**). Consistent with the first RNA-seq results, immunoblotting of Ddah1 in the sham group and at 1, 3, 7, 14, and 28 days after MI showed a drastic increase of Ddah1 in the infarcted zone at 7 and 14 days after MI operations (**Figures 6C,D, Supplementary Figure 5A**).

Next, double immunofluorescence staining of Ddah1 and fibroblasts marker, vimentin, was conducted to evaluate the expression and location of Ddah1 *in vivo* and *in vitro*. Consistent with boosted Ddah1 protein level at 7-days after MI, we showed increased Ddah1^{+}vimentin^{+} cells at 7-days after MI surgery compared with sham hearts (**Supplementary Figures 3A,B**). Furthermore, fibroblasts were isolated from neonatal rat hearts and treated with or without TGF-β before immunofluorescence analysis, the results revealed that TGF-β stimulation dramatically upregulated Ddah1 protein level in fibroblasts *in vitro* (**Supplementary Figures 3C,D**).

Next, we examined the functional role of Ddah1 in the activation of fibroblasts into myofibroblasts. First, isolated cardiac fibroblasts were treated with TGF-β and co-stained with Ddah1 and α-SMA, the results revealed that activated fibroblasts expressed more Ddah1 in response to TGF-β stimulation *in vitro* (**Supplementary Figures 3E,F**). Consistently, increased Ddah1^{+}α-SMA^{+} cells were identified in the infarcted (INF) and border zones at 3-days after MI operations vs. sham group, and these cells were significantly expanded at 7-days post-surgery (**Figures 6E,F, Supplementary Figure 4A**). Finally, isolated cardiac fibroblasts were treated with TGF-β or Ddah1 inhibitors (PD 404182) to explore its role on activation of fibroblasts. The myofibroblasts activation, as evaluated by α-SMA expression, was strongly increased in response to TGF-β stimulation and reduced when Ddah1 was inhibited by PD 404182 (**Figures 6G,H, Supplementary Figure 5B**). Thus, these findings suggest that Ddah1 is upregulated in FBs after MI stimulation and may participate in cardiac remodeling after MI by modulating the activation of myofibroblasts.

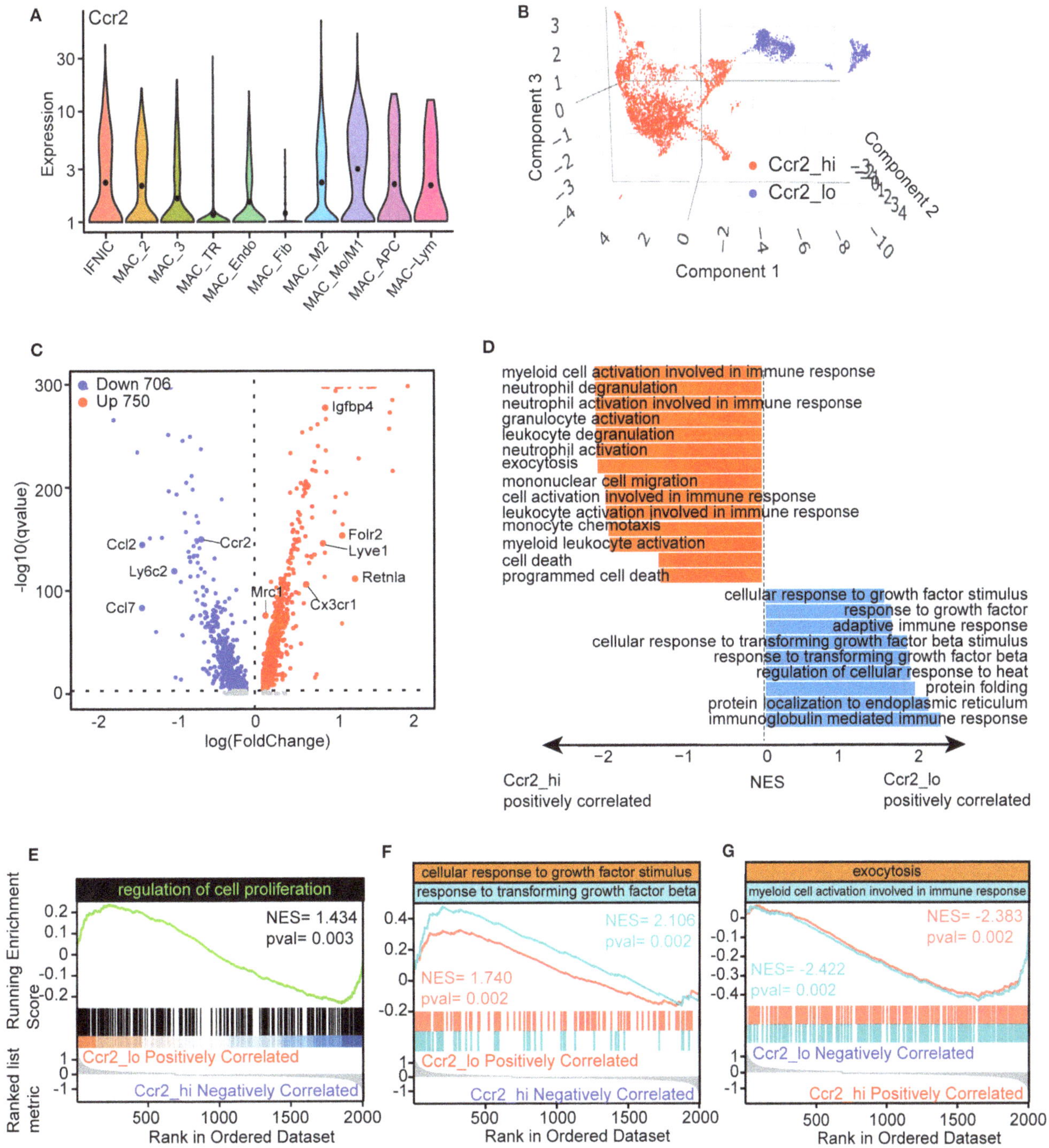

FIGURE 4 | Divergent function of tissue-resident (TR) and blood-derived macrophages. **(A)** Violin plots showing the expression of Ccr2 in macrophage clusters. **(B)** 3D UMAP plot with reassigned cell identities according to the level of Ccr2 in the macrophage populations. Specifically, MAC_TR, MAC_Endo, and MAC_Fib were renamed as Ccr2_lo, whereas others were denoted as Ccr2_hi. **(C)** Volcano plots comparing differentially expressed genes between Ccr2_lo and Ccr2_hi clusters, with each dot representing one gene. **(D)** Gene set enrichment analysis (GSEA) of differentially expressed genes between Ccr2_lo and Ccr2_hi clusters using ClusterProfiler. The results were displayed as normalized enrichment score (NES) between Ccr2_lo and Ccr2_hi group. **(E–G)** Visualization of gene sets including the regulation of cell proliferation **(E)**, cellular responses to growth factor stimulation and response to transforming growth factor-β (TGF-β) **(F)**, and exocytosis and myeloid cell activation involved in immune responses **(G)** comparing Ccr2_lo macrophages with Ccr2_hi clusters.

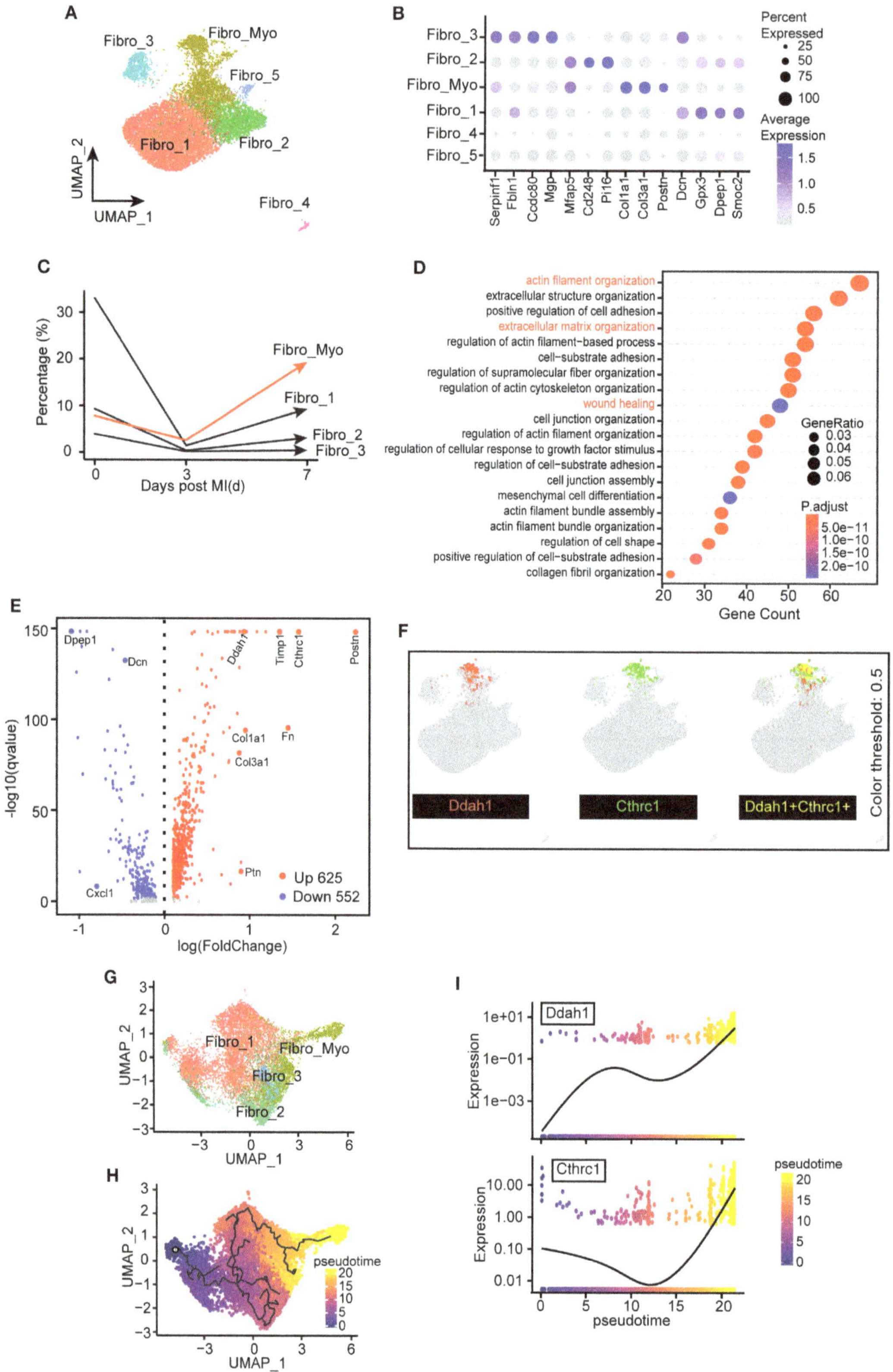

FIGURE 5 | Identification of the distinct transcriptional diversity of myofibroblasts in ischemic responses. **(A)** Subclustering of fibroblast (FB) populations for the next analysis. UMAP plot including all cell clusters with different colors. **(B)** Dot plot of selected marker genes corresponding to their cell identity. The dot size and scale

(Continued)

FIGURE 5 | colored represented the percentage of expressed genes and the mean expression of each cell population, respectively. **(C)** Percentages of different FB clusters (Fibro_Myo, Fibro_1, Fibro_2, and Fibro_3) at 0, 3, and 7 days after myocardial infarction (MI) surgery. **(D)** Hallmark gene ontology (GO) analysis between myofibroblasts (Fibro_Myo) and all other clusters based on biological process terms. **(E)** Volcano plot of differentially expressed genes between myofibroblasts and others clusters. The red dots indicated upregulated genes, whereas the blue dots indicated decreased genes. **(F)** UMAP plots showing the coexpression of myofibroblast marker genes (Ddah1, Cthrc1) in all FB populations. **(G)** Repartitioning of all FBs based on the Monocle algorithm. **(H)** Pseudotime trajectory analysis of all FBs according to highly variable genes. UMAP plot showing pseudotime score from dark to light yellow, representing the early to terminal transition. **(I)** Pseudotime expression of Ddah1 and Cthrc1, indicating their continuously upregulated expression during the healing process.

Gene Reprogramming and Dynamic Changes of Endothelial and T Cells

As shown in a previous analysis, ECs are placed at the center hub of cellular crosstalk by expressing abundant receptors during the healing process (**Figure 2C**). Hence, it is important to understand the functional changes of ECs after MI. We first identified an EC population in our integrated data with predominantly expressed EC markers, such as Pecam1 and Cdh5 (**Figures 7A,B**). Investigating the dynamics of endothelia, we found that ECs shrank at 3 days and further expanded at 7 days after MI (**Figures 2B**, **7C**). Additionally, the ECs in the sham group and at 3 days were found to be unbiasedly clustered together compared with what has been found at 7 days, suggesting distinct gene programming of ECs at 7 days. Intriguingly, by analyzing differentially expressed genes, we found a distinct transcriptional profile of ECs at 7 days compared with what has been found at 3 days. Specifically, ECs at 3 days after surgery expressed higher levels of cytokines and chemokines, for instance, Ccl9, Cxcl2, which is consistent with the activated pathways involved in myeloid leukocyte migration (**Figures 7D,E**). Enriching of the profibrotic gene Col3a1, pro-proliferating gene Tpt1, and ribosomal proteins Rpl9 and Rps12 at 7 days, fitting its positively correlated pathway of DNA packing, indicated an active transition of proinflammatory to proreparative ECs from 3 to 7 days after MI (**Figures 7D,E**). Overall, these observations confirmed the differentially expressed profile of ECs during the healing process.

Notably, a growing body of literature has emphasized the crucial functions of lymphocytes, especially T cells, in cardiac remodeling after MI on the basis of their important role in initiating and regulating immune responses (36). To uncover the underlying subtypes of T cells, we collected T cell clusters for the next analysis. Dynamic analysis of T cells among sham, MI-3d, and MI-7d indicated the occurrence of significantly extravasated T cells at 7 days after MI (**Figure 7F**). To reveal their heterogenous response after MI stimulation, T cells were repartitioned into four clusters: naïve T cells, effector T cells, regulated T cells, and NK cells (**Figure 7G**). Cells belonging to the naïve T cell cluster specifically express "naïve" marker genes, such as Tcf7 and CCR7 (37). On the other hand, the effector T cell cluster is characterized by upregulated expression of Ccl6 and Il1b, in line with positively enriched pathways about cell activation and regulation of immune system process in GSEA (**Figures 7H,I**). Conversely, negatively correlated inflammatory pathways were observed in the regulated T cell cluster (**Figure 7J**), for example, humoral immune response and myeloid leukocyte differentiation, indicating that divergent T cell clusters assume distinct anti-inflammatory and proinflammatory functions after MI. Regarding the particular differences in T cell subclusters during the healing process, a deeper understanding of the transcriptional factors inducing the transition of these cells would be important for the intervention of inflammatory responses after MI. Here, we performed a SCENIC regulon analysis and observed unique transcriptional regulons among these T cell clusters. Specifically, the effector T cells showed activated proinflammatory regulons, such as Irf5 and Fosb, whereas significantly activated Sp1 regulons in regulated T cells and Eomes regulons in NK cells were observed (**Figure 7K**). In conclusion, we discovered time-dependent and cell-cluster-dependent transcriptional programming of ECs and T cells and revealed their heterogeneous responses during the healing.

DISCUSSION

In this study, we integrated three single-cell sequencing datasets at 0, 3, and 7 days after MI surgery to obtain a more comprehensive understanding of the complex dynamics and gene programming of non-CMs under physiological and ischemic conditions. We demonstrated that activated FBs (Fibro_Myo) secrete predominant ligands for cell communication, whereas ECs possess a large number of receptors. Among all ligands and receptor pairs, the integrin family (e.g., Itgb1, Itga1, and Itgav) was identified as a pivotal interactive regulator during cardiac remodeling. Additionally, distinct functions of blood-derived and TR macrophages exhibiting altered gene profiles, regulons, and pathways were documented, allowing deeper understanding of the molecular mechanism of macrophages with different origins in response to ischemic stimulation. In addition, we showed that activated FBs (myofibroblasts) are characterized by a predominant level of Postn and Cthrc1. We also identified Ddah1, which is exclusively expressed in myofibroblasts in this study and was further confirmed using bulk RNA-seq, western blot, and immunofluorescence *in vivo* under normal and ischemic conditions. Collectively, this study provides a promising method to investigate the dynamics and cell transcriptional signature of different cell types simultaneously by integrating multiple single-cell sequencing data.

Notably, MI leads to sudden death of CMs, accompanied with the extravasation of leukocytes and lymphocytes from the blood vessels for clearance of necrotic debris, followed by replenishing of reparative cells, such as myofibroblasts, ECs, and anti-inflammatory macrophages (M2 macrophages) (2, 38). It is very important to understand the mechanism

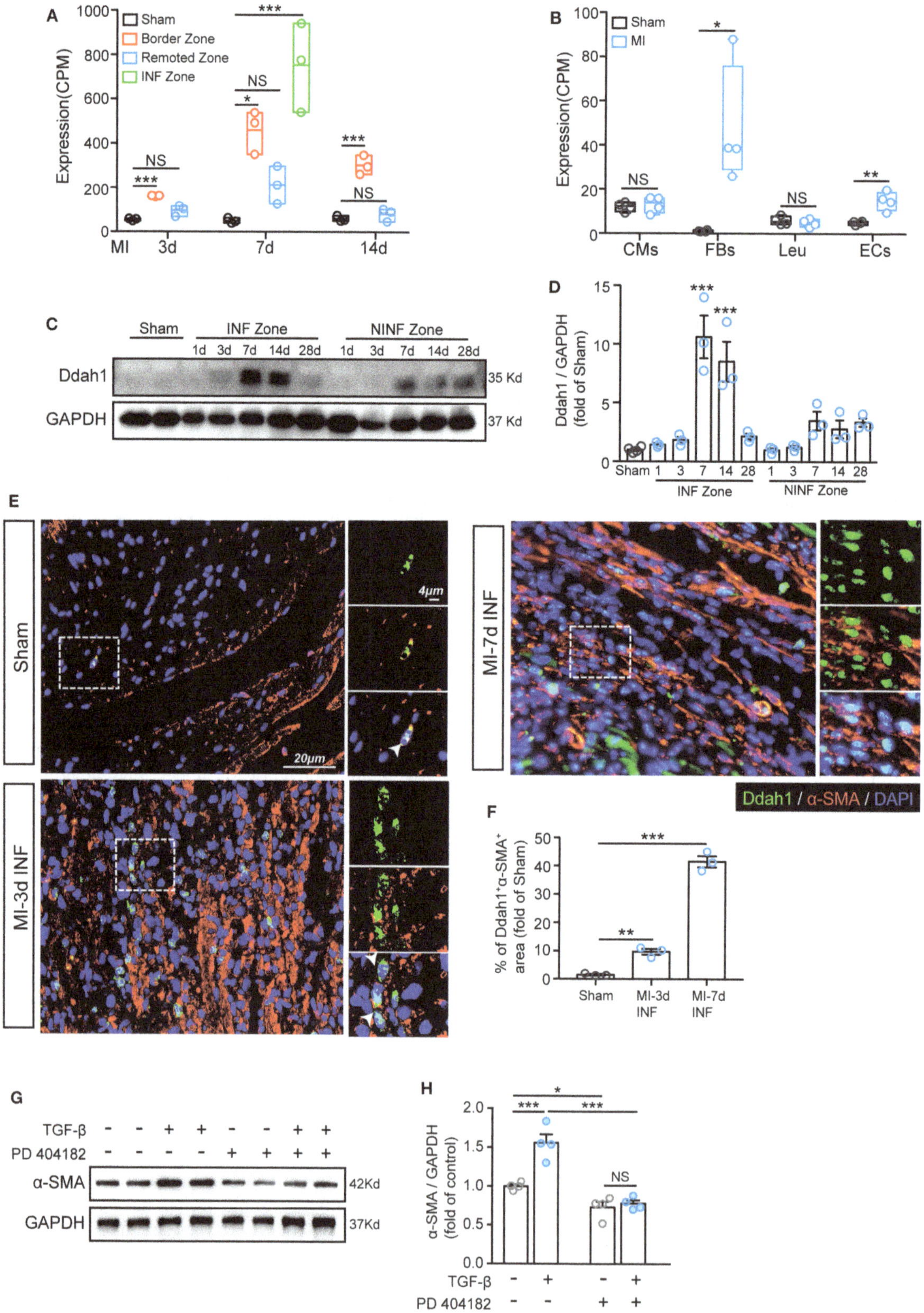

FIGURE 6 | Upregulation of Ddah1 after myocardial infarction (MI). **(A)** Recalculation the expression of Ddah1 in bulk RNA sequencing data from border, remoted, and infarcted (INF) zones at 3, 7, and 14 days after MI or sham surgery. **(B)** Recalculation the expression of Ddah1 in bulk RNA sequencing data from cardiomyocytes

(Continued)

FIGURE 6 | (CMs), fibroblasts (FBs), leukocytes (Leu), and endothelial cells (ECs) at 3 days after MI or sham surgery. **(C)** Immunostaining of Ddah1 in the INF zone and non-INF (NINF) zone from MI-operated hearts at 0, 1, 3, 7, 14, and 28 days. GAPDH was used as the control. **(D)** The quantification results of C. The data were expressed as the mean ± SEM. **(E)** Immunofluorescence co-staining of Ddah1 (green) and α-smooth muscle actin (α-SMA, red) in the sham group and the infarcted zone (INF) at 3 and 7 days after MI surgery. Nuclei were stained using 4′,6-diamidino-2-phenylindole (DAPI, blue). On the right, high-magnification images were shown, corresponding to the dashed rectangle in the images on the left. **(F)** The quantification results of panel **E**. **(G)** Western blot analysis showed the expression of α-SMA in fibroblasts in response to TGF-β or Ddah1 inhibitor, PD 404182. GAPDH was used as the control. **(H)** The quantification results of G. The data were expressed as the mean ± SEM, NS, not significant; $^{*}p < 0.05$, $^{**}p < 0.01$, $^{***}p < 0.001$. (**A**, $n = 3$, Tukey post hoc test; **B**, $n = 4$, Student's *t* test; **D,F**, $n = 3$, Dunnett *post hoc* test; **H**, $n = 4$, Tukey post hoc test).

by which these cells finely orchestrate these proinflammatory and proreparative processes during cardiac remodeling via ligand and receptor interactions. In line with a previous study (10), the crosstalk among all subpopulations revealed that myofibroblasts and ECs are the key cell types involved in cellular communication, highlighting their pivotal role in remodeling processes. Moreover, the integrin family (e.g., Itgb1, Itga1, and Itgav) was found to be the most profound protein family participating in cellular crosstalk in our analysis.

Previous researches have confirmed that integrins contribute to myofibroblast differentiation by interacting with ECM or cytoskeleton proteins and activating the transcriptional expression of TGF-β in the heart, lungs, liver, and kidneys (39–42). Consistent with this effector, block or genetic-modulating their expression would attenuate the degree of fibrosis in these organs. Furthermore, a growing body of evidence has demonstrated that integrin-ECM interaction is indispensable for the growth, maturation, and integrity of great vessels during the development of the heart (43). In addition, under hypoxic stimulation, upregulated integrins promote angiogenesis by increasing EC migration and vascular-like tube formation (44). Notably, our results underscored the important role of myofibroblasts, endothelia, and integrins in cell-cell communication during cardiac remodeling after MI. However, the mechanism by which integrins participate in fibrosis and angiogenesis, which integrin are more weighted in this process, warrants deeper investigation in future studies.

Besides FBs, recent studies have emphasized the important role of immune cells, especially macrophages, in cardiac functional modulation under hemostatic and perturbed conditions (45). In this single-cell analysis, macrophages were found to constitute the largest proportion of immune cells in sham or post-ischemic hearts, highlighting their pivotal role in immune responses and cardiac remodeling. Emerging literatures have described the heterogenous effects of macrophages with different origins on immune responses and wound healing after MI, underscoring the urgent need to understand the function and transcriptional differences of TR and blood-derived macrophages (46). Notably, we partitioned all macrophages into seven subpopulations in this study. Incongruous expressed marker genes were observed among these clusters. Specifically, Cx3cr1 were found to be predominantly upregulated in TR macrophages, whereas Osm, which contribute to the production of cytokines, were found to be exclusively expressed in blood-derived macrophages. Differentially expressed Ccr2 has been previously described to be a hallmark for distinguishing TR and blood-derived macrophages using genetic lineage tracing (24). Macrophages with a low level of Ccr2 represent a TR population in human and mouse hearts and retain their quantity via self-proliferation, whereas macrophages with a high level of Ccr2 derived from monocytes are maintained via monocyte-dependent recruitment (47, 48). To determine the differences of transcriptional signature and pathways within these two cell clusters, by assigning all macrophages into Ccr2-high and Ccr2-low clusters, we discovered high levels of proreparative genes (e.g., Lyve1 and Mrc1) on Ccr2-low macrophages, consistent with the positively enriched pathways of cell proliferation and response to TGF-β. On the other hand, macrophages with a high level of Ccr2 were found to exhibit upregulated cytokines, such as Ccl2, Ccl7, and Ly6c2, matching the active pathways of exocytosis and myeloid cell activation. These findings indicate the divergent functions and gene signatures of these two cell types. Additionally, we explored the transcriptional regulons of all macrophage clusters, revealing several distinct transcription regulatory factors among TR and blood-derived macrophages. Specifically, Egr1 and Jund were found to be dramatically activated in Ccr2-low macrophages, whereas Ccr2-high macrophages were found to exhibit increased activity of Stat1 and Irf7. Intriguingly, evidence from several studies demonstrated that Egr1, the immediate early gene, participates in the differentiation of myeloid cell precursors along macrophage lineages (29). This phenomenon indicates the important role that Egr1 plays in the maintenance of TR macrophages. Notably, in this study, we not only confirmed the distinct gene profiles and pathways of TR and monocyte-derived macrophages in a single-cell resolution but also provided insights into their differentially activated transcript regulons that may contribute to these divergent functions. However, how TR and blood-derived macrophages orchestrate these complex proinflammatory and anti-inflammatory effects in a fine sequential manner under ischemic conditions and which regulons account for this transition remain elusive and need to be urgently explored in the future.

To our knowledge, this is the first study raising the question of whether it is effective to have a comprehensive understanding of non-CM flux as well as cellular crosstalk and functions under homeostatic and ischemic conditions by integrating multiple single-cell datasets. We believe that single-cell sequencing analysis of multiple cell populations in a cell-type- and disease-dependent manner would provide new opportunities for discovering novel drugs and intervention targets for the repair processes of the heart.

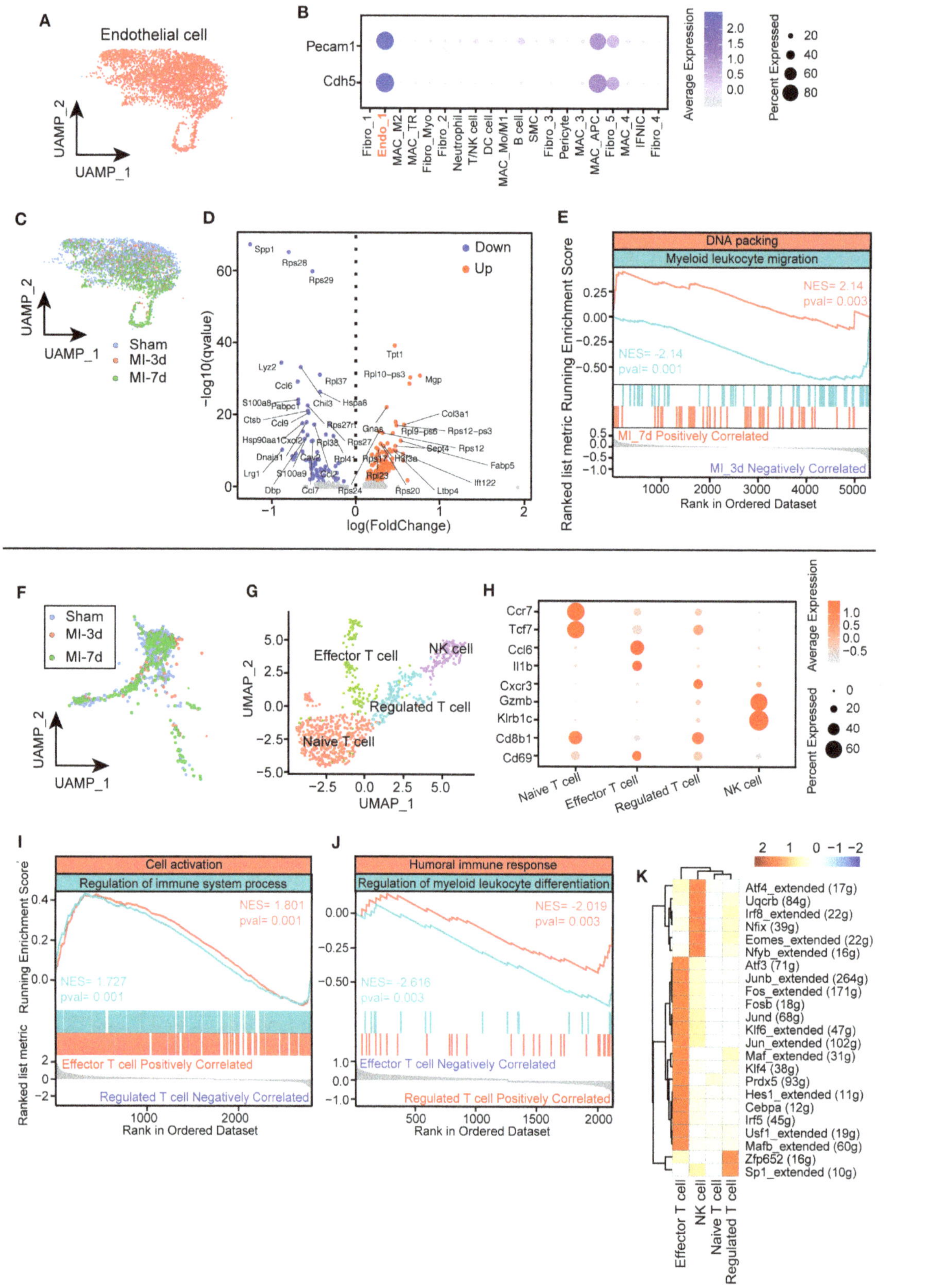

FIGURE 7 | Characterization of endothelial cells (ECs) and T cells after myocardial infarction (MI). **(A)** UMAP plots of ECs in this study selected from all integrated cells. **(B)** Dot plot showing exclusively expressed marker genes (Pecam1 and Cdh5) in ECs across all the identified cell populations. **(C)** UMAP plot showing the distribution

(Continued)

FIGURE 7 | of ECs in sham group, 3, 7 days after MI. **(D)** Volcano plot showing differentially expressed genes of ECs at 7 days after MI compared with ECs at 3 days. **(E)** Hallmark GSEA analysis of differentially expressed genes 7 days after MI compared with cells at 3 days showing that ECs at 7 days were positively correlated with DNA packing and negatively correlated with myeloid leukocyte migration. **(F)** UMAP plot of T cells from integrated data in sham group, 3, 7 days after MI surgery. **(G)** T cells were repartitioned and renamed before further analysis and showed with the UMAP plot. **(H)** Dot plot with specific marker genes of T cell clusters showing heterogeneous expression of T cells. The dot size and scale color represented the percentage of expressed genes and the mean expression of each cell population, respectively. **(I,J)** GSEA of effector T cells with regulated T cells, indicating that effector T cells were positively correlated with cell activation and immune system processes **(I)** and negatively correlated with humoral immune responses and myeloid leukocyte differentiation **(J)**. **(K)** Single-cell regulatory network inference and clustering (SCENIC) analysis showing distinct regulons cross T cell clusters.

AUTHOR CONTRIBUTIONS

LZ performed the study, analyzed the data, and wrote the manuscript. LL and RZ contributed to manuscript preparation and revision. KC and XY participated in the experimental design, data interpretation, manuscript preparation, and revision. All authors contributed to the article and approved the submitted version.

FUNDING

This study was supported by the National Natural Science Foundation of China (81400362, 81670457, 81922007, and 91939103 to XY), Shanghai Municipal Education Commission-Gaofeng Clinical Medicine Grant Support (20191803 to XY), Shanghai Rising-Star Program Grant (17QA1402300 to XY), Municipal Human Resources Development Program for Outstanding Young Talents in Medical and Health Sciences in Shanghai (2017YQ017 to XY), Shanghai Science and Technology Supporting Project (19411963400 to XY), and Natural Science Research Funding from Shanghai Jiao Tong University School of Medicine (19XJ11002 to XY).

REFERENCES

1. Pinto AR, Ilinykh A, Ivey MJ, Kuwabara JT, D'Antoni ML, Debuque R, et al. Revisiting cardiac cellular composition. *Circ Res.* (2016) 118:400–9. doi: 10.1161/CIRCRESAHA.115.307778
2. Prabhu SD, Frangogiannis NG. The biological basis for cardiac repair after myocardial infarction: from inflammation to fibrosis. *Circ Res.* (2016) 119:91–112. doi: 10.1161/CIRCRESAHA.116.303577
3. Grun D, van Oudenaarden A. Design and analysis of single-cell sequencing experiments. *Cell.* (2015) 163:799–810. doi: 10.1016/j.cell.2015.10.039
4. Ackers-Johnson M, Tan WLW, Foo RS. Following hearts, one cell at a time: recent applications of single-cell RNA sequencing to the understanding of heart disease. *Nat Commun.* (2018) 9:4434. doi: 10.1038/s41467-018-06894-8
5. Zhuang LF, Li CN, Chen QJ, Jin Q, Wu LQ, Lu L, et al. Fatty acid-binding protein 3 contributes to ischemic heart injury by regulating cardiac myocyte apoptosis and MAPK pathways. *Am J Physiol-Heart C.* (2019) 316:H971–84. doi: 10.1152/ajpheart.00360.2018
6. Butler A, Hoffman P, Smibert P, Papalexi E, Satija R. Integrating single-cell transcriptomic data across different conditions, technologies, and species. *Nat Biotechnol.* (2018) 36:411–20. doi: 10.1038/nbt.4096
7. Stuart T, Butler A, Hoffman P, Hafemeister C, Papalexi E, Mauck WM, et al. Comprehensive integration of single-cell data. *Cell.* (2019) 177:1888–902.e21. doi: 10.1016/j.cell.2019.05.031
8. Subramanian A, Tamayo P, Mootha VK, Mukherjee S, Ebert BL, Gillette MA, et al. Gene set enrichment analysis: a knowledge-based approach for interpreting genome-wide expression profiles. *Proc Natl Acad Sci USA.* (2005) 102:15545–50. doi: 10.1073/pnas.0506580102
9. Yu G, Wang LG, Han Y, He QY. clusterProfiler: an R package for comparing biological themes among gene clusters. *OMICS.* (2012) 16:284–7. doi: 10.1089/omi.2011.0118
10. Farbehi N, Patrick R, Dorison A, Xaymardan M, Janbandhu V, Wystub-Lis K, et al. Single-cell expression profiling reveals dynamic flux of cardiac stromal, vascular and immune cells in health and injury. *Elife.* (2019) 8:e43882. doi: 10.7554/eLife.43882.061
11. Szklarczyk D, Morris JH, Cook H, Kuhn M, Wyder S, Simonovic M, et al. The STRING database in 2017: quality-controlled protein-protein association networks, made broadly accessible. *Nucleic Acids Res.* (2017) 45:D362–8. doi: 10.1093/nar/gkw937
12. Gu Z, Gu L, Eils R, Schlesner M, Brors B. circlize implements and enhances circular visualization in R. *Bioinformatics.* (2014) 30:2811–2. doi: 10.1093/bioinformatics/btu393
13. Trapnell C, Cacchiarelli D, Grimsby J, Pokharel P, Li S, Morse M, et al. The dynamics and regulators of cell fate decisions are revealed by pseudotemporal ordering of single cells. *Nat Biotechnol.* (2014) 32:381–6. doi: 10.1038/nbt.2859
14. Aibar S, Gonzalez-Blas CB, Moerman T, Huynh-Thu VA, Imrichova H, Hulselmans G, et al. SCENIC: single-cell regulatory network inference and clustering. *Nat methods.* (2017) 14:1083–6. doi: 10.1038/nmeth.4463
15. King KR, Aguirre AD, Ye YX, Sun Y, Roh JD, Ng RP, et al. IRF3 and type I interferons fuel a fatal response to myocardial infarction. *Nat Med.* (2017) 23:1481–7. doi: 10.1038/nm.4428
16. Skelly DA, Squiers GT, McLellan MA, Bolisetty MT, Robson P, Rosenthal NA, et al. Single-cell transcriptional profiling reveals cellular diversity and intercommunication in the mouse heart. *Cell Rep.* (2018) 22:600–10. doi: 10.1016/j.celrep.2017.12.072
17. Shirakawa K, Endo J, Kataoka M, Katsumata Y, Yoshida N, Yamamoto T, et al. IL (interleukin)-10-STAT3-galectin-3 axis is essential for osteopontin-producing reparative macrophage polarization after myocardial infarction. *Circulation.* (2018) 138:2021–35. doi: 10.1161/CIRCULATIONAHA.118.035047
18. Jung M, Ma Y, Iyer RP, DeLeon-Pennell KY, Yabluchanskiy A, Garrett MR, et al. IL-10 improves cardiac remodeling after myocardial infarction by stimulating M2 macrophage polarization and fibroblast activation. *Basic Res Cardiol.* (2017) 112:33. doi: 10.1007/s00395-017-0622-5
19. Zhu M, Goetsch SC, Wang Z, Luo R, Hill JA, Schneider J, et al. FoxO4 promotes early inflammatory response upon myocardial infarction via endothelial Arg1. *Circ Res.* (2015) 117:967–77. doi: 10.1161/CIRCRESAHA.115.306919
20. Kaur H, Takefuji M, Ngai CY, Carvalho J, Bayer J, Wietelmann A, et al. Targeted ablation of periostin-expressing activated fibroblasts prevents adverse cardiac remodeling in mice. *Circ Res.* (2016) 118:1906–17. doi: 10.1161/CIRCRESAHA.116.308643
21. Yan X, Anzai A, Katsumata Y, Matsuhashi T, Ito K, Endo J, et al. Temporal dynamics of cardiac immune cell accumulation following acute myocardial infarction. *J Mol Cell Cardiol.* (2013) 62:24–35. doi: 10.1016/j.yjmcc.2013.04.023

22. Zhang Y, Kanter EM, Yamada KA. Remodeling of cardiac fibroblasts following myocardial infarction results in increased gap junction intercellular communication. *Cardiovasc Pathol.* (2010) 19:e233–40. doi: 10.1016/j.carpath.2009.12.002
23. Ramilowski JA, Goldberg T, Harshbarger J, Kloppmann E, Lizio M, Satagopam VP, et al. A draft network of ligand-receptor-mediated multicellular signalling in human. *Nat Commun.* (2015) 6:7866. doi: 10.1038/ncomms8866
24. Bajpai G, Schneider C, Wong N, Bredemeyer A, Hulsmans M, Nahrendorf M, et al. The human heart contains distinct macrophage subsets with divergent origins and functions. *Nat Med.* (2018) 24:1234–1245. doi: 10.1038/s41591-018-0059-x
25. Martini E, Kunderfranco P, Peano C, Carullo P, Cremonesi M, Schorn T, et al. Single-cell sequencing of mouse heart immune infiltrate in pressure overload-driven heart failure reveals extent of immune activation. *Circulation.* (2019) 140:2089–107. doi: 10.1161/CIRCULATIONAHA.119.041694
26. Qiu X, Mao Q, Tang Y, Wang L, Chawla R, Pliner HA, et al. Reversed graph embedding resolves complex single-cell trajectories. *Nat Methods.* (2017) 14:979–82. doi: 10.1038/nmeth.4402
27. Haider N, Bosca L, Zandbergen HR, Kovacic JC, Narula N, Gonzalez-Ramos S, et al. Transition of macrophages to fibroblast-like cells in healing myocardial infarction. *J Am Coll Cardiol.* (2019) 74:3124–35. doi: 10.1016/j.jacc.2019.10.036
28. Laslo P, Spooner CJ, Warmflash A, Lancki DW, Lee HJ, Sciammas R, et al. Multilineage transcriptional priming and determination of alternate hematopoietic cell fates. *Cell.* (2006) 126:755–66. doi: 10.1016/j.cell.2006.06.052
29. Nguyen HQ, Hoffman-Liebermann B, Liebermann DA. The zinc finger transcription factor Egr-1 is essential for and restricts differentiation along the macrophage lineage. *Cell.* (1993) 72:197–209. doi: 10.1016/0092-8674(93)90660-I
30. Dick SA, Macklin JA, Nejat S, Momen A, Clemente-Casares X, Althagafi MG, et al. Self-renewing resident cardiac macrophages limit adverse remodeling following myocardial infarction. *Nat Immunol.* (2019) 20:29–39. doi: 10.1038/s41590-018-0272-2
31. Gladka MM, Molenaar B, de Ruiter H, van der Elst S, Tsui H, Versteeg D, et al. Single-cell sequencing of the healthy and diseased heart reveals cytoskeleton-associated protein 4 as a new modulator of fibroblasts activation. *Circulation.* (2018) 138:166–80. doi: 10.1161/CIRCULATIONAHA.117.030742
32. Ruiz-Villalba A, Romero JP, Hernandez SC, Vilas-Zornoza A, Fortelny N, Castro-Labrador L, et al. Single-cell RNA-seq analysis reveals a crucial role for collagen triple helix repeat containing 1 (CTHRC1) cardiac fibroblasts after myocardial infarction. *Circulation.* (2020) 142:1831–47. doi: 10.1161/CIRCULATIONAHA.119.044557
33. Leiper J, Nandi M, Torondel B, Murray-Rust J, Malaki M, O'Hara B, et al. Disruption of methylarginine metabolism impairs vascular homeostasis. *Nat Med.* (2007) 13:198–203. doi: 10.1038/nm1543
34. van Duijvenboden K, de Bakker DEM, Man JCK, Janssen R, Günthel M, Hill MC, et al. Conserved NPPB+ border zone switches from MEF2- to AP-1-driven gene program. *Circulation.* (2019) 140:864–79. doi: 10.1161/CIRCULATIONAHA.118.038944
35. Quaife-Ryan GA, Sim CB, Ziemann M, Kaspi A, Rafehi H, Ramialison M, et al. Multicellular transcriptional analysis of mammalian heart regeneration. *Circulation.* (2017) 136:1123–39. doi: 10.1161/CIRCULATIONAHA.117.028252
36. Hofmann U, Frantz S. Role of T-cells in myocardial infarction. *Eur Heart J.* (2016) 37:873–9. doi: 10.1093/eurheartj/ehv639
37. Zheng C, Zheng L, Yoo JK, Guo H, Zhang Y, Guo X, et al. Landscape of infiltrating T cells in liver cancer revealed by single-cell sequencing. *Cell.* (2017) 169:1342–56.e16. doi: 10.1016/j.cell.2017.05.035
38. Frangogiannis NG. Regulation of the inflammatory response in cardiac repair. *Circ Res.* (2012) 110:159–73. doi: 10.1161/CIRCRESAHA.111.243162
39. Bansal R, Nakagawa S, Yazdani S, van Baarlen J, Venkatesh A, Koh AP, et al. Integrin alpha 11 in the regulation of the myofibroblast phenotype: implications for fibrotic diseases. *Exp Mol Med.* (2017) 49:e396. doi: 10.1038/emm.2017.213
40. Henderson NC, Arnold TD, Katamura Y, Giacomini MM, Rodriguez JD, McCarty JH, et al. Targeting of αv integrin identifies a core molecular pathway that regulates fibrosis in several organs. *Nat Med.* (2013) 19:1617–24. doi: 10.1038/nm.3282
41. Munger JS, Huang X, Kawakatsu H, Griffiths MJ, Dalton SL, Wu J, et al. The integrin alpha v beta 6 binds and activates latent TGF beta 1: a mechanism for regulating pulmonary inflammation and fibrosis. *Cell.* (1999) 96:319–28. doi: 10.1016/S0092-8674(00)80545-0
42. Booz GW, Baker KM. Molecular signalling mechanisms controlling growth and function of cardiac fibroblasts. *Cardiovasc Res.* (1995) 30:537–43. doi: 10.1016/S0008-6363(96)88507-5
43. Abraham S, Kogata N, Fässler R, Adams RH. Integrin beta1 subunit controls mural cell adhesion, spreading, and blood vessel wall stability. *Circ Res.* (2008) 102:562–70. doi: 10.1161/CIRCRESAHA.107.167908
44. Befani C, Liakos P. Hypoxia upregulates integrin gene expression in microvascular endothelial cells and promotes their migration and capillary-like tube formation. *Cell Biol Int.* (2017) 41:769–78. doi: 10.1002/cbin.10777
45. Swirski FK, Nahrendorf M. Cardioimmunology: the immune system in cardiac homeostasis and disease. *Nat Rev Immunol.* (2018) 18:733–44. doi: 10.1038/s41577-018-0065-8
46. Gordon S, Pluddemann A. Tissue macrophages: heterogeneity and functions. *BMC Biol.* (2017) 15:53. doi: 10.1186/s12915-017-0392-4
47. Epelman S, Lavine KJ, Beaudin AE, Sojka DK, Carrero JA, Calderon B, et al. Embryonic and adult-derived resident cardiac macrophages are maintained through distinct mechanisms at steady state and during inflammation. *Immunity.* (2014) 40:91–104. doi: 10.1016/j.immuni.2013.11.019
48. Davies LC, Taylor PR. Tissue-resident macrophages: then and now. *Immunology.* (2015) 144:541–8. doi: 10.1111/imm.12451

6

Hypertrophic Cardiomyopathy: From Phenotype and Pathogenesis to Treatment

Zeyi Cheng [1†], *Tingting Fang* [2†], *Jinglei Huang* [3], *Yingqiang Guo* [1], *Mahboob Alam* [4] *and Hong Qian* [1*]

[1] *Department of Cardiovascular Surgery, West China Hospital, Sichuan University, Chengdu, China,* [2] *Department of Cardiology, West China Hospital, Sichuan University, Chengdu, China,* [3] *School of Medicine, Lanzhou University, Lanzhou, China,* [4] *Division of Cardiovascular Medicine, Department of Medicine, Baylor College of Medicine, Houston, TX, United States*

Correspondence:
Hong Qian
qianhong2222@126.com

† These authors have contributed equally to this work

Hypertrophic cardiomyopathy (HCM) is a very common inherited cardiovascular disease (CAD) and the incidence is about 1/500 of the common population. It is caused by more than 1,400 mutations in 11 or more genes encoding the proteins of the cardiac sarcomere. HCM presents a heterogeneous clinical profile and complex pathophysiology and HCM is the most important cause of sudden cardiac death (SCD) in young people. HCM also contributes to functional disability from heart failure and stroke (caused by atrial fibrillation). Current treatments for HCM (medication, myectomy, and alcohol septal ablation) are geared toward slowing down the disease progression and symptom relief and implanted cardiac defibrillator (ICD) to prevent SCD. HCM is, however, entering a period of tight translational research that holds promise for the major advances in disease-specific therapy. Main insights into the genetic landscape of HCM have improved our understanding of molecular pathogenesis and pointed the potential targets for the development of therapeutic agents. We reviewed the critical discoveries about the treatments, mechanism of HCM, and their implications for future research.

Keywords: hypertrophic cardiomyopathy, phenotype, pathogenesis, treatment, review

INTRODUCTION

Hypertrophic cardiomyopathy (HCM) is a heterogeneous myocardial disease characterized by left ventricular hypertrophy and in the cases of hypertrophic obstructive cardiomyopathy (HOCM), it is characterized by asymmetric septal hypertrophy. In the majority of the cases, the average interventricular septal thickness is 26 mm, which cannot be fully explained by the loading conditions of the left ventricle (1, 2). There are several types of HCM based on the distribution of hypertrophy: symmetric, asymmetric, apical, and focal (3). In addition to the hypertrophy, the abnormalities of the mitral valve and subvalvular apparatus lead to the systolic anterior motion (SAM) and left ventricular outflow tract (LVOT) obstruction in about two-thirds of the HCM cases, the characteristic features of HOCM, as well as the microvascular dysfunction and subendocardial ischemia (3). Due to a combination of these factors, patients with HCM frequently experience reduced exercise capacity, dyspnea, and/or chest pain. HCM is mainly inherited in an autosomal dominant pattern, linked with mutations (nucleotide sequence variants) in 11 or more

TABLE 1 | A list of the genes in which the pathogenic mutations are associated with hypertrophic cardiomyopathy (HCM).

Gene	HCM frequence	Protein or associated phenotypes
Sarcomeric proteins		
MYH7	40-44%	β-myosin heavy chain 7
MYBPC3	35-40%	Myosin-binding protein C3
TNNT2	5-15%	Troponin T
TNNI3	5%	Troponin I
TPM1	3%	Tropomyosin α-1 chian
MYL2	1-2%	Regulatory myosin light chain
MYL3	1%	Essential myosin light chain
ACTC1	1%	Actin
TNNC1	<1%	Troponin C
Z-disk proteins		
LBD3	1-5%	ZASP-LIM binding domain 3
ACTN2	<1%	Alpha-Actinin-2
ANKRD1	<1%	Ankyrin repeat domain-containing protein-1
CSRP3	<1%	Muscle LIM Protein
MYOZ2	<1%	Myozenin-2
TCAP	<1%	Telethonin
VCL	<1%	Vinculin
NEXT	<1%	Nexilin
FLNC	<1%	Filamin C
Sarcomere-associated proteins		
DES	<1%	Desmin

It also includes the proteins and related phenotypes that are involved in these specific gene mutations and their proportion in the overall HCM.

genes encoding the proteins of myocardial sarcomere structure (~60% of all the causes and >90% of the genetically defined patients), and with beta-myosin heavy chain and myosin-binding protein C genes most commonly involved (**Table 1**; **Figure 1**) (4–6). Patients with HCM suffer from the cardiovascular death rates of 1-2% per year including the sudden cardiac death (SCD) ~ 1%, heart failure (HF) ~ 0.5%, and thromboembolism ~ 0.1% (2, 3). In recent years, there has been tremendous development in this field with a translation of the basic science discoveries into the new therapeutic methods. In this study, we reviewed the recent development in pharmacological and gene-based therapies, which we believe will result in a comprehensive understanding of the treatment of HCM in the future.

PATHOGENESIS

Gene mutation is the initiating pathogenesis of HCM affecting the proteins by playing a critical role in the function of the cardiac muscle unit "sarcomeres." The function of the sarcomere may weaken due to an abnormality in or shortage of any one of these proteins, which, in turn, affects the normal myocardial contractility. It is still not exactly described how the mutations in the sarcomere-related genes cause hypertrophy of the heart muscle (7, 8). However, there are several hypotheses that are as follows (**Figure 2**):

(1) Mutations in the sarcomere-related genes are associated with an increased affinity for calcium in the myofilaments, activate the calmodulin kinase II (CaMKII) pathway, and delay the downstream targets of the CaMKII sodium channels, thus increase the intracellular calcium and, thus, forming a vicious cycle (9–12). This results in the impaired relaxation and diastolic dysfunction of the myocardium.
(2) Mutations in the sarcomere-related genes in HCM can lead to inefficient contractility with a resultant increase in the ATP demand. This impairs the structure and function of the mitochondria leading to energy supply disorders (13–16). Microvascular dysfunction further exacerbates the myocardial energy deficiency of HCM and restricts the transport of the oxidative metabolites. The imbalance between the energy supply and demand leads to the myocardial cells in a state of peroxidation and then produces various reactive oxygen species (ROS), resulting in the glutathione acylation of the muscle filaments [cardiac myosin-binding protein C (cMyBP-C)] (17, 18). Functionally, this modification increases the myofilament calcium sensitivity and inhibits the kinetics of cross-bridge cycling, leading to the diastolic dysfunction and ultimately aggravating the HCM phenotype (18–21).
(3) Due to the mutations in the sarcomere-related genes, the accumulation of the harmful proteins results in a toxic effect on the myocardial contractile devices and myocardial cells (22).
(4) Sarcomeric protein transcription and posttranslational modifications, as well as the other modified genes, also promote the development of HCM. Studies have shown that polymorphism of angiotensin I can contribute to the hypertrophic phenotype (23). These modified factors stimulate non-cardiac cell proliferation such as fibroblasts (23), thereby promoting the development of HCM. In conclusion, the functional changes at the cellular and molecular levels could be target of innovative therapies.

The structural abnormalities of HCM include the following:

(1) Abnormal myofibrils and abnormal arrangement of the cardiomyocytes (24).
(2) Coronary artery microvascular dysfunction. Thickening of the blood vessel wall leading to asymptomatic myocardial ischemia, further inducing myocardial injury and fibrosis (25, 26). Interstitial connective tissue increases significantly. Fibrosis is patchy or widely distributed around the cells and poor remodeling of the myocardial tissue ultimately leads to irreversible dysfunction such as severe HF and SCD (27, 28).

NOVEL THERAPIES

Calcium Desensitizer

Ca^{2+} overload, CaMKII, and increased I_{NaL} play a very important role that drive the myocardial remodeling from the earliest stage of the development of hypertrophy, diastolic dysfunction, and the

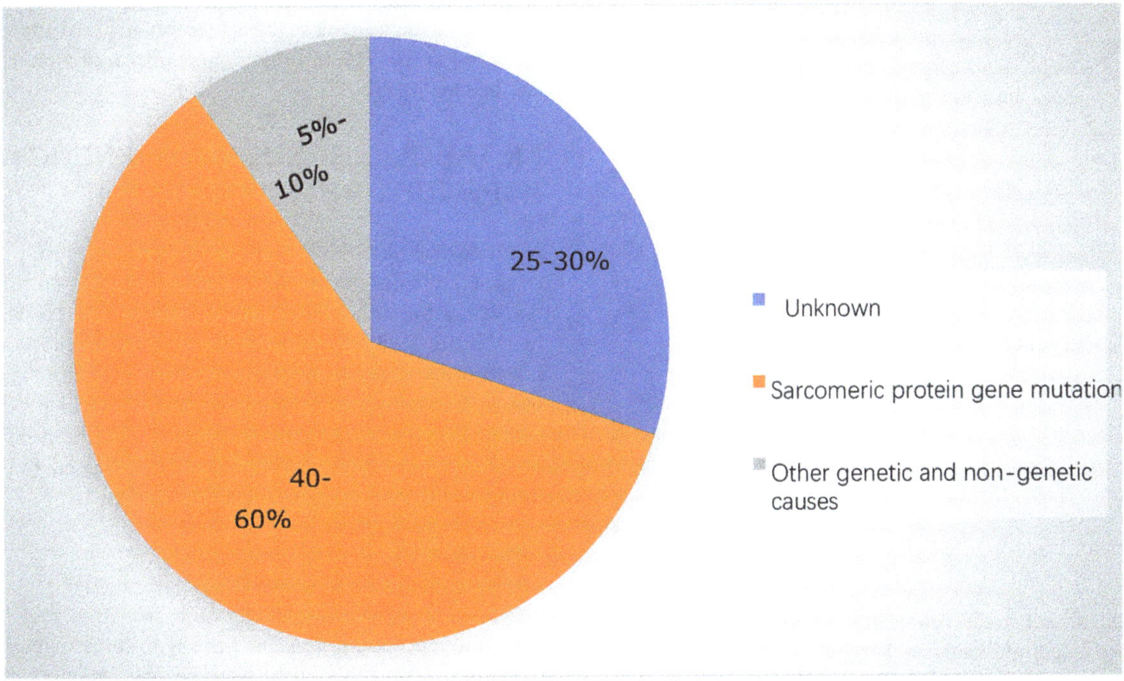

FIGURE 1 | The majority of the cases in adolescents and adults are caused by mutations in the sarcomere protein genes.

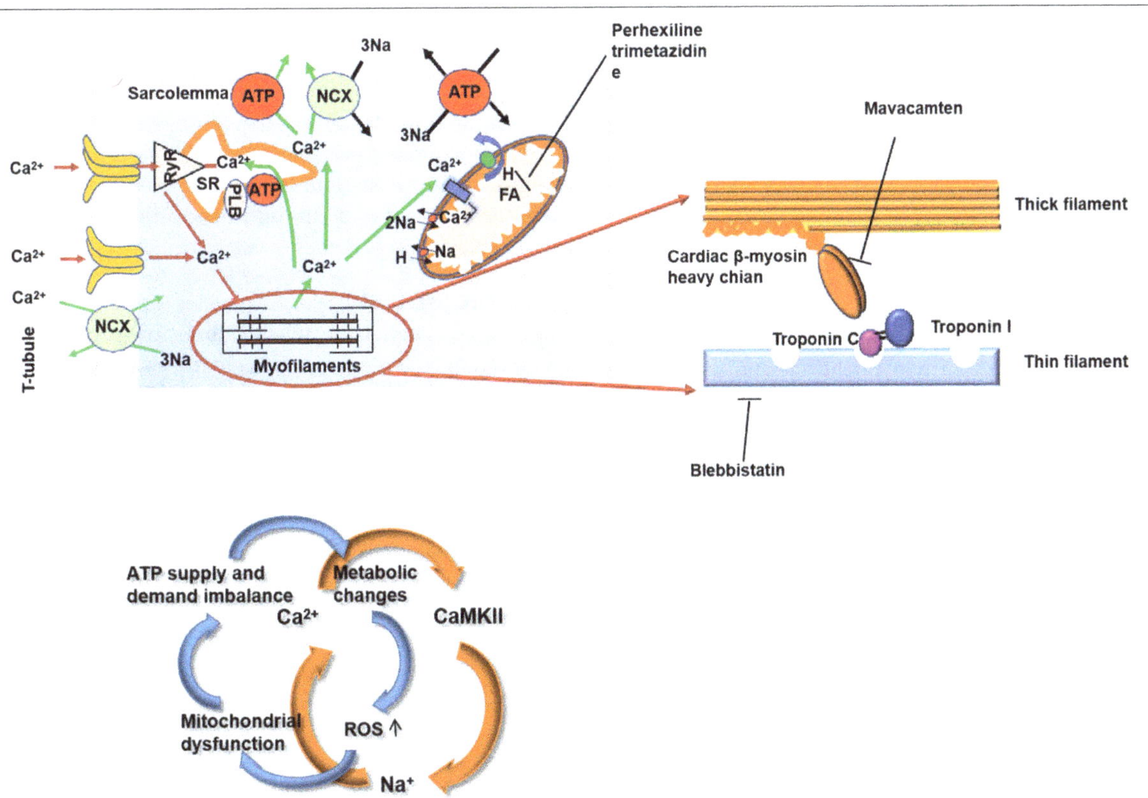

FIGURE 2 | The structure of the myocardium and the mechanism of myocardial contraction are the potential targets for HCM therapy. HCM, hypertrophic cardiomyopathy; RyR, ryanodine receptor; SR, sarcoplasmic reticulum; NCX, sodium/calcium exchange pump; PLB, phospholamban; ROS, reactive oxygen species; FA, fatty acid.

TABLE 2 | Table for the novel therapies.

Novel therapies	Targets	Mechanisms
Blebbistatin	Troponin T mutation	sensitivityofCa2+↓
Parvalbumin	Ca^{2+}	Decrease the concentration of Ca2+
SERCA2a	Ca^{2+}	SERCA2 a protein expression increased
Diltiazem	L-type calcium channels	Upregulation of the SR protein

TABLE 3 | Table for metabolic therapy.

Novel therapies	Targets	Mechanisms
Perhexiline	CPT1/2	shifting LCFA→ glucose
Mavacamten	β-myosin heavy chain	stabilizes the super relaxed state
Omecamtiv mecarbil	Ca^{2+}	accelerating ATP generation

arrhythmogenic substrate (5, 6). There are many studies aimed at an increased calcium sensitivity (**Figure 2**).

Blebbistatin

Blebbistatin is an inhibitor of actin-myosin interaction functioning independently of Ca^{2+} influx (29). Studies have shown that blebbistatin, in a mouse model of HCM caused by troponin T mutation, can reduce the sensitivity of Ca^{2+} to myofilaments and the incidence of arrhythmias; meanwhile, several studies Grillo et al. also reported that reducing the sensitivity of Ca^{2+} to myofilaments can be a target for the HCM treatment (29–32).

Parvalbumin

Parvalbumin is a Ca^{2+} buffering molecule not expressed in the cardiomyocytes; when the concentration of Ca^{2+} increases, parvalbumin will release Mg^{2+} and binds to Ca^{2+}. Piguet et al. and Coutu et al. found that parvalbumin can correct the myocardial diastolic dysfunction in the rat and mouse HCM models (33, 34).

SERCA2a

In a mouse model of HCM caused by a tropomyosin mutation, SERCA2a, an SR protein, was transported by the adenovirus to 1-day-old mice. After several weeks, The sarco/endoplasmic reticulum calcium ATPase 2a isoform (SERCA2a) protein expression increased in the heart of the mouse and significantly improved the morphology of the heart. In HCM mice knocked out with SERCA2a inhibitory protein, phosphoprotein gene [phospholamban (PLN)] can also increase the absorption of Ca^{2+} by the sarcoplasmic reticulum (SR) and improve the phenotype (35).

Diltiazem

Diltiazem can inhibit the L-type calcium channels (34). Early application of diltiazem caused the upregulation of the SR protein and eased the development of the HCM phenotype (36). In recent years, a study by Ho CY et al. found that diltiazem may relieve left ventricular remodeling in the asymptomatic sarcomere mutation carriers (NCT00319982) (37). The summarized novel therapies can be seen in **Table 2**.

METABOLIC REGULATION-ENERGY EXPENDITURE HYPOTHESIS

In HCM, the mutations in the sarcomere gene result in reduced contractile efficiency of the sarcomere and an increase in ATP consumption. The characteristic of the HCM substrate metabolism is the preferential use of fatty acid (FA) oxidation, but in order to adapt to the consumption of more ATP, energy metabolism transfers to glucose metabolism to produce more ATP. This increased glucose metabolism, however, results in the accumulation of pyruvate and lactate produced by glycolysis, which is harmful to the myocardium (**Figure 2**).

Perhexiline

Perhexiline improves the energy production efficiency by transferring the substrate utilization from the free fatty acids (FFAs) to glucose and improves the symptoms, exercise capacity (VO_2max), and function of heart in the patients with systolic heart failure caused by the ischemic and non-ischemic factors that are very effective (38). Perhexiline promotes the use of carbohydrates as the substrate for the myocardial energy by inhibiting carnitine palmitoyltransferase 1 (CPT1); meanwhile, CPT2 resulting in increased efficiency of the myocardial oxygen utilization (39). Perhexiline would be likely to induce an increase of at least 13% efficiency of the myocardial oxygen utilization (40). Perhexiline appears to exert the important anti-inflammatory (in part *via* nicotinamide adenine dinucleotide phosphate oxidase inhibition) and nitric oxide-potentiating effects that may occur independently of CPT inhibition (NCT00500552) (41).

Mavacamten

During the period of myosin force production, there is an autoinhibited state, also referred to as a super-relaxed state. With certain myosin mutations, the HCM sarcomere spends lesser time in this state, resulting in the hyperactivation and excess utilization of ATP. The small molecule mavacamten stabilizes this inhibited state, effectively extend the time that myosin is inhibited. Mavacamten is specific for β-myosin heavy chain. Many studies in the mouse HCM models have pointed out that the early treatment of phenotype-negative HCM mice can prevent HCM hypertrophy and other features (42). Administration to the HCM mice reduced the hypertrophic phenotype and reduced the expression of the fibrotic genes (43). The gradient of 8 out of 21 participating patients had significantly reduced LVOT to <30 mm Hg. It also resulted in the reduced serum N-terminal pro B-type natriuretic peptide (NT-proBNP) levels in patients with HCM. This is the biomarker associated with increased wall stress and myocardial injury (NCT03470545) (43). The trial was designed to evaluate the dose of mavacamten in the non-obstructive HCM. This study found that the mavacamten treatment group had no significant

TABLE 4 | Table for the gene therapy.

Method	Medicinal product	Targeted	Results	Research status
Genome editing	CRISPR/Cas9	mutated gene	repaired by homology-directed repair with a repair template	genetic correction in HCM hiPSC1-3 (55–57), and correct HCM caused by a GAGT-deletion in exon 16 of the MYBPC3 gene (58).
Exonskipping	antisense oligonucleotide	exonic splicing enhancer sequences of an inframe mutated exon	preventing binding of proteins involved in the splicing process	in newborn mice abolished cardiac dysfunction and prevented the development of leftventricularhypertrophy (59).
	CRISPR/Cas9	mutated DNA sequence	Permanently cut in-frame the mutated exon.	
Allele-specific silencing	specific RNA interferene molecule	mutant mRNA	knocked-down mutant mRNA	eliminate the mutant allele and delay the progression of cardiomyopathy in Myh6-targeted knock-in mice (63).
RNA trans-splicing	specific RNA interferene molecule	pre-mRNA	competes with cis-splicing	successful 5′trans-splicing in the context of HCM in cardiomyocytes and *in vivo* in Mybpc3-targeted knock-in mice and hiPSC (61, 62, 64).
Gene replacement	full-length cDNA	mutated DNA	functional full-length protein	in Mybpc3-targeted knock-in mice/hiPSCs, which were retrieved from an HCM patient carrying a truncating MYBPC3 muta -tion (49, 65, 66).

toxicity compared to the placebo group, proving that the drug was well-tolerated (NCT03442764) (44).

Omecamtiv Mecarbil

Omecamtiv mecarbil (OM) is being tested in treating hypercontractility by accelerating ATP generation, thus increasing myosin head binding to actin, resulting in an enhanced force-producing situation (45). The effects of OM are dependent on the intracellular Ca^{2+} levels (46). OM has shown promising clinical practical values, progressing to phase III trials (NCT02929329). The summarized metabolic therapy can be seen in **Table 3**.

CARDIAC GENE THERAPY

In the past decades, gene therapy got tremendous development in the field of HCM. From the current evidence, gene therapy seems a very promising treatment in HCM caused by the mutations in the genes that encode the sarcomeric proteins.

The key problem for gene therapy is the effective and safe delivery of the gene therapy drugs into the body of the patient. It has been shown that the adeno-associated virus serotype 9 (AAV9) is a very promising candidate for cardiac gene transfer after systemic delivery in mouse and large animal HCM models (47). The SERCA2a gene therapy phase II trial also showed a very exciting result of the safety and feasibility of AAV1-mediated gene transfer (48). However, this investigation has not shown significant positive outcomes in the treated patients (49, 50). The defect of AAV-mediated gene therapy is that the human body easily generates neutralizing antibodies against AAV. These neutralizing antibodies seriously impact the outcomes of gene therapy; another question is an increased readministration rate. This could be avoided by the pharmacological modulation of the immune response and/or use of another AAV serotype (51, 52).

Fortunately, the difficulty of delivering the gene therapy medicinal product into the body of the patient has been resolved to some extent. Various methods were developed to suppress the expression of the genetic defects on the DNA or RNA levels as well as genome editing (42, 53–58), exon skipping (59, 60), allele-specific silencing, (61–63) spliceosome-mediated RNA trans-splicing (61–64), and gene replacement therapy (49, 65, 66). Due to the advancement in genome modification technologies, antisense oligonucleotides, clustered regularly interspaced short palindromic repeats (CRISPR)/Cas9, wild-type complementary DNA (cDNA) (wild-type MYBPC3 cDNA) sequences, and RNA interference molecules are clustered regularly interspaced. Specific editing that promotes the genetic mutations of an individual may lead to the individual-based pharmacological approaches in HCM. The summarized gene therapy can be seen in **Table 4**.

FUTURE DIRECTIONS

Since there are many promising treatments for HCM, it is still a complex disease that requires further study based on pathophysiology and genetics. It is necessary to further study the mechanism of gene mutations and the secondary events caused by HCM. Thus, we need to develop new therapies based on gene editing or molecular regulatory pathways. Meanwhile, a large amount of basic medical research on the pathogenesis and treatment of HCM needs to be further transformed into clinical application. In conclusion, HCM is the main hereditary disease of the heart and the sarcomeric protein gene mutation is the most common cause of HCM. HCM is hereditary cardiomyopathy. Continued study and improved understanding of the genetic mediators of HCM will help to guide the development of effective targeted therapies, small molecules that can target the key molecular pathways or events in the heart to prevent the natural course of HCM. Increasing the treatment options for

HCM may block the progression of the HCM disease, but it is not possible to completely correct the mutant gene and there are still genetic risks. Finally, a better understanding of the structural and metabolic disorders caused by the gene mutations is very helpful for developing the new therapies of HCM.

AUTHOR CONTRIBUTIONS

YG: conception. MA and ZC: administrative support. HQ: study design. TF: collection and assembly of data. JH: data analysis and drawing. All authors: manuscript writing and final approval of manuscript.

ACKNOWLEDGMENTS

Thanks to Prof. Alam for his guidance and polishing of the English language in this article.

REFERENCES

1. Maron BJ, Maron MS. The 20 advances that have defined contemporary hypertrophic cardiomyopathy. *Trends Cardiovasc Med.* (2015) 25:54-64. doi: 10.1016/j.tcm.2014.09.004
2. Masarone D, Kaski JP, Pacileo G, Elliott PM, Bossone E, Day SM, et al. Epidemiology and clinical aspects of genetic cardiomyopathies. *Heart Fail Clin.* (2018) 14:119–28. doi: 10.1016/j.hfc.2017.12.007
3. Gersh BJ, Maron BJ, Bonow RO, Dearani JA, Fifer MA, Link MS, et al. 2011 ACCF/AHA guideline for the diagnosis and treatment of hypertrophic cardiomyopathy: a report of the American College of Cardiology Foundation/American Heart Association Task Force on Practice Guidelines. *Circulation.* (2011) 124:e783–831. doi: 10.1161/CIR.0b013e318223e2bd
4. Santos Mateo JJ, Sabater Molina M, Gimeno Blanes JR. Hypertrophic cardiomyopathy. *Med Clin.* (2018) 150:434-42. doi: 10.1016/j.medcle.2017.09.029
5. Hensley N, Dietrich J, Nyhan D, Mitter N, Yee MS, Brady M. Hypertrophic cardiomyopathy: a review. *Anesth Analg.* (2015) 120:554–69. doi: 10.1213/ANE.0000000000000538
6. Makavos G, Kappaairis C, Tselegkidi ME, Karamitsos T, Rigopoulos AG, Noutsias M, et al. Hypertrophic cardiomyopathy: an updated review on the diagnosis, prognosis, and treatment. *Heart Fail Rev.* (2019) 24:439-59. doi: 10.1007/s10741-019-09775-4
7. Wolf CM. Hypertrophic cardiomyopathy: genetics and clinical perspectives. *Cardiovasc Diagn Ther.* (2019) 9(Suppl 2):S388-415. doi: 10.21037/cdt.2019.02.01
8. Marian AJ, Braunwald E. Hypertrophic cardiomyopathy: genetics, pathogenesis, clinical manifestations, diagnosis, and therapy. *Circ Res.* (2017) 121:749–70. doi: 10.1161/CIRCRESAHA.117.311059
9. Coppini R, Ferrantini C, Del Lungo M, Stillitano F, Sartiani L, Tosi B, et al. Response to letter regarding article, late sodium current inhibition reverses electromechanical dysfunction in human hypertrophic cardiomyopathy. *Circulation.* (2013) 128:e157. doi: 10.1161/CIRCULATIONAHA.113.004016
10. Coppini R, Mazzoni L, Ferrantini C, Gentile F, Pioner JM, Laurino A, et al. Ranolazine prevents phenotype development in a mouse model of hypertrophic cardiomyopathy. *Circ Heart Fail.* (2017) 10:e003565. doi: 10.1161/CIRCHEARTFAILURE.116.003565
11. Ferrantini C, Coppini R, Pioner JM, Gentile F, Tosi B, Mazzoni L, et al. Pathogenesis of hypertrophic cardiomyopathy is mutation rather than disease specific: a comparison of the cardiac troponin T E163R and R92Q mouse models. *J Am Heart Assoc.* (2017) 6:e005407. doi: 10.1161/JAHA.116.005407
12. Ferrantini C, Pioner JM, Mazzoni L, Gentile F, Tosi B, Rossi A, et al. Late sodium current inhibitors to treat exercise-induced obstruction in hypertrophic cardiomyopathy: an *in vitro* study in human myocardium. *Br J Pharmacol.* (2018) 175:2635–52. doi: 10.1111/bph.14223
13. Witjas-Paalberends ER, Ferrara C, Scellini B, Piroddi N, Montag J, Tesi C, Stienen GJ, et al. Faster cross-bridge detachment and increased tension cost in human hypertrophic cardiomyopathy with the R403Q MYH7 mutation. *J Physiol.* (2014) 592:3257–72. doi: 10.1113/jphysiol.2014.274571
14. Belus A, Piroddi N, Scellini B, Tesi C, D'Amati G, Girolami F, et al. The familial hypertrophic cardiomyopathy- associated myosin mutation R403Q accelerates tension generation and relaxation of human cardiac myofibrils. *J Physiol.* (2008) 586:3639–44. doi: 10.1113/jphysiol.2008.155952
15. Nediani A, Borchi E, Giordano C, Baruzzo S, Ponziani V, Sebastiani M, et al. NADPH oxidase-dependent redox signaling in human heart failure: relationship between the left and right ventricle, *J Mol Cell Cardiol.* (2007) 42:826–34. doi: 10.1016/j.yjmcc.2007.01.009
16. Sebastiani M, Giordano C, Nediani C, Travaglini C, Borchi E, Zani M, et al. Induction of mitochondrial biogenesis is a maladaptive mechanism in mitochondrial cardiomyopathies. *J Am Coll Cardiol.* (2007) 50:1362-9. doi: 10.1016/j.jacc.2007.06.035
17. Becker RC, Owens AP, 3rd, Sadayappan S. Tissue-level inflammation and ventricular remodeling in hypertrophic cardiomyopathy. *J Thromb Thrombolysis.* (2020) 49:177–83. doi: 10.1007/s11239-019-02026-1
18. Miceli C, Santin Y, Manzella N, Coppini R, Berti A, Stefani M, et al. Oleuropein aglycone protects against MAO-A-Induced autophagy impairment and cardiomyocyte death through activation of TFEB. *Oxid Med Cell Longev.* (2018) 2018:8067592. doi: 10.1155/2018/8067592
19. Santin Y, Sicard P, Vigneron F, Guilbeau-Frugier C, Dutaur M, Lairez O, et al. Oxidative stress by monoamine Oxidase-A impairs transcription factor EB activation and autophagosome clearance, leading to cardiomyocyte necrosis and heart failure. *Antioxid Redox Signal.* (2016) 25:10–27. doi: 10.1089/ars.2015.6522
20. Singh SR, Zech ATL, Geertz B, Reischmann-Dusener S, Osinska H, Prondzynski M, et al. Carrier, activation of autophagy ameliorates cardiomyopathy in Mybpc3-targeted knockin mice. *Circ Heart Fail.* (2017) 10:e004140. doi: 10.1161/CIRCHEARTFAILURE.117.004140
21. Xu X, Roe ND, Weiser-Evans MC, Ren J. Inhibition of mammalian target of rapamycin with rapamycin reverses hypertrophic cardiomyopathy in mice with cardiomyocyte-specific knockout of PTEN. *Hypertension.* (2014) 63:729-39. doi: 10.1161/HYPERTENSIONAHA.113.02526
22. Marston S, Copeland O, Jacques A, Livesey K, Tsang V, McKenna WJ, et al. Evidence from human myectomy samples that MYBPC3 mutations cause hypertrophic cardiomyopathy through haploinsufficiency. *Circ Res.* (2009) 105:219–22. doi: 10.1161/CIRCRESAHA.109.202440
23. Geske JB, Ommen SR, Gersh BJ. Hypertrophic cardiomyopathy: clinical update. *JACC Heart Fail.* (2018) 6:364–75. doi: 10.1016/j.jchf.2018.02.010
24. Maron BJ. Clinical course and management of hypertrophic cardiomyopathy. *N Engl J Med.* (2018) 379:655–68. doi: 10.1056/NEJMra1710575
25. Veselka J, Anavekar NS, Charron P. Hypertrophic obstructive cardiomyopathy. *Lancet.* (2017) 389:1253-67. doi: 10.1016/S0140-6736(16)31321-6
26. Teekakirikul P, Zhu W, Huang HC, Fung E. Hypertrophic cardiomyopathy: an overview of genetics and management. *Biomolecules.* (2019) 9:878. doi: 10.3390/biom9120878
27. Daubert C, Gadler F, Mabo P, Linde C. Pacing for hypertrophic obstructive cardiomyopathy: an update and future directions. *Europace.* (2018) 20:908-20. doi: 10.1093/europace/eux131
28. Maron BJ, Rowin EJ, Maron MS, Braunwald E. Nonobstructive hypertrophic cardiomyopathy out of the shadows: known from the

beginning but largely ignored ... until now. *Am J Med.* (2017) 130:119–23. doi: 10.1016/j.amjmed.2016.09.015
29. Huke S, Venkataraman R, Faggioni M, Bennuri S, Hwang HS, Baudenbacher F, et al. Focal energy deprivation underlies arrhythmia susceptibility in mice with calcium-sensitized myofilaments. *Circ Res.* (2013) 112:1334–44. doi: 10.1161/CIRCRESAHA.113.301055
30. Baudenbacher F, Schober T, Pinto JR, Sidorov VY, Hilliard F, Solaro RJ, et al. Myofilament Ca2+ sensitization causes susceptibility to cardiac arrhythmia in mice. *J Clin Invest.* (2008) 118:3893–903. doi: 10.1172/JCI36642
31. Pohlmann L, Kröger I, Vignier N, Schlossarek S, Krämer E, Coirault C, et al. Cardiac myosin-binding protein C is required for complete relaxation in intact myocytes. *Circ Res.* (2007) 101:928–38. doi: 10.1161/CIRCRESAHA.107.158774
32. Fiset C, Giles WR. Cardiac troponin T mutations promote life-threatening arrhythmias. *J Clin Invest.* (2008) 118:3845–7. doi: 10.1172/JCI37787
33. Piguet F, de Montigny C, Vaucamps N, Reutenauer L, Eisenmann A, Puccio H. Rapid and complete reversal of sensory ataxia by gene therapy in a novel model of Friedreich Ataxia. *Mol Ther.* (2018) 26:1940–52. doi: 10.1016/j.ymthe.2018.05.006
34. Coutu P, Bennett CN, Favre EG, Day SM, Metzger JM. Parvalbumin corrects slowed relaxation in adult cardiac myocytes expressing hypertrophic cardiomyopathylinked alpha-tropomyosin mutations. *Circ Res.* (2004) 94:1235–41. doi: 10.1161/01.RES.0000126923.46786.FD
35. Peña JR, Szkudlarek AC, Warren CM, Heinrich LS, Gaffin RD, Jagatheesan G, et al. Neonatal gene transfer of Serca2a delays onset of hypertrophic remodeling and improves function in familial hypertrophic cardiomyopathy. *J Mol Cell Cardiol.* (2010) 49:993–1002. doi: 10.1016/j.yjmcc.2010.09.010
36. Flenner F, Geertz B, Reischmann-Düsener S, Weinberger F, Eschenhagen T, Carrier L, et al. Diltiazem prevents stress-induced contractile deficits in cardiomyocytes, but does not reverse the cardiomyopathy phenotype in Mybpc3knock-in mice. *J Physiol.* (2017) 595:3987–99. doi: 10.1113/JP273769
37. Ho CY, Lakdawala NK, Cirino AL, Lipshultz SE, Sparks E, Abbasi SA, et al. Diltiazem treatment for pre-clinical hypertrophic cardiomyopathy sarcomere mutation carriers: a pilot randomized trial to modify disease expression. *JACC Heart Fail.* (2015) 3:180–8. doi: 10.1016/j.jchf.2014.08.003
38. Abozguia K, Elliott P, McKenna W, Phan TT, Nallur-Shivu G, Ahmed I, et al. Metabolic modulator perhexiline corrects energy deficiency and improves exercise capacity in symptomatic hypertrophic cardiomyopathy. *Circulation.* (2010) 122:1562–9. doi: 10.1161/CIRCULATIONAHA.109.934059
39. Horowitz JD, Chirkov YY. Perhexiline and hypertrophic cardiomyopathy: a new horizon for metabolic modulation. *Circulation.* (2010) 122:1547–9. doi: 10.1161/CIRCULATIONAHA.110.981464
40. Gehmlich K, Dodd MS, Allwood JW, Kelly M, Bellahcene M, Lad HV, et al. Changes in the cardiac metabolome caused by perhexiline treatment in a mouse model of hypertrophic cardiomyopathy. *Mol Biosyst.* (2015) 11:564–73. doi: 10.1039/C4MB00594E
41. Drury NE, Licari G, Chong CR, Howell NJ, Frenneaux MP, Horowitz JD, et al. Relationship between plasma, atrial and ventricular perhexiline concentrations in humans: insights into factors affecting myocardial uptake. *Br J Clin Pharmacol.* (2014) 77:789–95. doi: 10.1111/bcp.12254
42. Carroll KJ, Makarewich CA, McAnally J, Anderson DM, Zentilin L, Liu N, et al. A mouse model for adult cardiac-specific gene deletion with CRISPR/Cas9. *Proc Natl Acad Sci USA.* (2016) 113:338–43. doi: 10.1073/pnas.1523918113
43. Olivotto I, Oreziak A, Barriales-Villa R, Abraham TP, Masri A, Garcia-Pavia P, et al. Mavacamten for treatment of symptomatic obstructive hypertrophic cardiomyopathy (EXPLORER-HCM): a randomised, double-blind, placebo-controlled, phase 3 trial. *Lancet.* (2020) 396:759–69. doi: 10.1016/S0140-6736(20)31792-X
44. Ho CY, Mealiffe ME, Bach RG, Bhattacharya M, Choudhury L, Edelberg JM, et al. evaluation of mavacamten in symptomatic patients with nonobstructive hypertrophic cardiomyopathy. *J Am Coll Cardiol.* (2020) 75:2649–60. doi: 10.1016/j.jacc.2020.03.064
45. Malik FI, Hartman JJ, Elias KA, Morgan BP, Rodriguez H, Brejc K, et al. Cardiac myosin activation: a potential therapeutic approach for systolic heart failure. *Science.* (2011) 331:1439–43. doi: 10.1126/science.1200113
46. Kampourakis T, Zhang X, Sun YB, Irving M. Omecamtiv mercabil and blebbistatin modulate cardiac contractility by perturbing the regulatory state of the myosin filament. *J Physiol.* (2018) 596:31–46. doi: 10.1113/JP275050
47. Ishikawa K, Fish KM, Tilemann L, Rapti K, Aguero J, SantosGallego CG, et al. Cardiac I1c overexpression with reengineered AAV improves cardiac function in swine ischemic heart failure. *Mol Ther.* (2014) 22:2038–45. doi: 10.1038/mt.2014.127
48. Jessup M, Greenberg B, Mancini D, Cappola T, Pauly DF, Jaski B, et al. Calcium upregulation by percutaneous administration of gene therapy in cardiac disease (CUPID): a phase 2 trial of intracoronary gene therapy of sarcoplasmic reticulum Ca2+-ATPase in patients with advanced heart failure. *Circulation.* (2011) 124:304–13. doi: 10.1161/CIRCULATIONAHA.111.022889
49. Mearini G, Stimpel D, Geertz B, Weinberger F, Krämer E, Schlossarek S, et al. Mybpc3 gene therapy for neonatal cardiomyopathy enables long term disease prevention in mice. *Nat Commun.* (2014) 5:5515. doi: 10.1038/ncomms6515
50. Murrey DA, Naughton BJ, Duncan FJ, Meadows AS, Ware TA, Campbell KJ, et al. Feasibility and safety of systemic rAAV9-hNAGLU delivery for treating mucopolysaccharidosis IIIB: toxicology, biodistribution, and immunological assessments in primates. *Hum Gene Ther Clin Dev.* (2014) 25:72–84. doi: 10.1089/humc.2013.208
51. Pleger ST, Shan C, Ksienzyk J, Bekeredjian R, Boekstegers P, Hinkel R, et al. Cardiac AAV9-S100A1 gene therapy rescues post-ischemic heart failure in a preclinical large animal model. *Sci Transl Med.* (2011) 3:92ra64. doi: 10.1126/scitranslmed.3002097
52. Ziegler T, Kraus M, Husada W, Gesenhues F, Jiang Q, Pinkenburg O, et al. Steerable induction of the Thymosin beta4/MRTF-A pathway *via* AAV-based over expression induces therapeutic neo-vascularization. *Hum Gene Ther.* (2018) 29:1407–15. doi: 10.1089/hum.2017.013
53. Guo Y, Van Dusen NJ, Zhang L, Gu W, Sethi I, Guatimosim S, et al. Analysis of cardiac myocyte maturation using CASAA V, a platform for rapid dissection of cardiac myocyte gene function *in vivo*. *Circ Res.* (2017) 120:1874–88. doi: 10.1161/CIRCRESAHA.116.310283
54. Johansen AK, Molenaar B, Versteeg D, Leitoguinho AR, Demkes C, Spanjaard B, et al. Postnatal cardiac gene editing using CRISPR/Cas9 with AA V9-mediated delivery of short guide RNAs results in mosaic gene disruption. *Circ Res.* (2017) 121:1168–81. doi: 10.1161/CIRCRESAHA.116.310370
55. Ben Jehuda R, Eisen B, Shemer Y, Mekies LN, Szantai A, Reiter I, et al. CRISPR correction of the PRKAG2 gene mutation in the patient's induced pluripotent stem cell-derived cardiomyocytes eliminates electrophysiological and structural abnormalities. *Heart Rhythm.* (2018) 15:267–76. doi: 10.1016/j.hrthm.2017.09.024
56. Mosqueira D, Mannhardt I, Bhagwan JR, Slimak KL, Katili P, Scott E, et al. CRISPR/Cas9 editing in human pluripotent stem cell-cardiomyocytes highlights arrhythmias, hypocontractility, and energy depletion as potential therapeutic targets for hypertrophic cardiomyopathy. *Eur Heart J.* (2018) 39:3879–92. doi: 10.1093/eurheartj/ehy249
57. Wang L, Kim K, Parikh S, Gabriel Cader A, Bersell KR, He H, et al. Hypertrophic cardiomyopathy-linked mutation in troponin T causes myofibrillar disarray and pro-arrhythmic action potential changes in human iPSC cardiomyocytes. *J Mol Cell Cardiol.* (2018) 114:320–7. doi: 10.1016/j.yjmcc.2017.12.002
58. Ma H, Marti-Gutierrez N, Park SW, Wu J, Lee Y, Suzuki K, et al. Correction of a pathogenic gene mutation in human embryos. *Nature.* (2017) 548:413–9. doi: 10.1038/nature23305
59. Gedicke-Hornung C, Behrens-Gawlik V, Reischmann S, Geertz B, Stimpel D, Weinberger F, et al. Rescue of cardiomyopathy through U7snRNA-mediated exon skipping in Mybpc3-targeted knock-in mice. *EMBO Mol Med.* (2013) 5:1128–45. doi: 10.1002/emmm.201202168
60. Vignier N, Schlossarek S, Fraysse B, Mearini G, Kramer E, Pointu H, et al. Nonsense-mediated mRNA decay and ubiquitin-proteasome system regulate cardiac myosin-binding protein C mutant levels in cardiomyopathic mice. *Circ Res.* (2009) 105:239–48. doi: 10.1161/CIRCRESAHA.109.201251
61. Mearini G, Stimpel D, Kramer E, Geertz B, Braren I, Gedicke-Hornung C, et al. Repair of Mybpc3 mRNA by 5′-trans-splicing in a mouse model of hypertrophic cardiomyopathy. *Mol Ther Nucleic Acids.* (2013) 2:e102. doi: 10.1038/mtna.2013.31

62. Prondzynski M, Kramer E, Laufer SD, Shibamiya A, Pless O, Flenner F, et al. Evaluation of MYBPC3 trans-splicing and gene replacement as therapeutic options in human iPSC-derived cardiomyocytes. *Mol Ther Nucleic Acids.* (2017) 7:475–86. doi: 10.1016/j.omtn.2017.05.008
63. Jiang J, Wakimoto H, Seidman JG, Seidman CE. Allele-specific silencing of mutant Myh6 transcripts in mice suppresses hypertrophic cardiomyopathy. *Science.* (2013) 342:111–4. doi: 10.1126/science.1236921
64. Azibani F, Brull A, Arandel L, Beuvin M, Nelson I, Jollet A, et al. Gene therapy *via* trans-splicing for LMNA-related congenital muscular dystrophy. *Mol Ther Nucleic Acids.* (2018) 10:376–86. doi: 10.1016/j.omtn.2017.12.012
65. Monteiro da Rocha A, Guerrero-Serna G, Helms A, Luzod C, Mironov S, Russell M, et al. Deficient cMyBP-C protein expression during cardiomyocyte differentiation underlies human hypertrophic cardiomyopathy cellular phenotypes in disease specific human ES cell derived cardiomyocytes. *J Mol Cell Cardiol.* (2016) 99:197–206. doi: 10.1016/j.yjmcc.2016.09.004
66. Wijnker PJ, Friedrich FW, Dutsch A, Reischmann S, Eder A, Mannhardt I, et al. Comparison of the effects of a truncating and a missense MYBPC3 mutation on contractile parameters of engineered heart tissue. *J Mol Cell Cardiol.* (2016) 97:82–92. doi: 10.1016/j.yjmcc.2016.03.003

7

Targeting the microRNA-34a as a Novel Therapeutic Strategy for Cardiovascular Diseases

Cun-Cun Hua [1‡], *Xin-Ming Liu* [1‡], *Li-Rong Liang* [2], *Le-Feng Wang* [1*†] *and Jiu-Chang Zhong* [1,2,3*†]

[1] Heart Center and Beijing Key Laboratory of Hypertension, Beijing Chaoyang Hospital, Capital Medical University, Beijing, China, [2] Department of Clinical Epidemiology and Tobacco Dependence Treatment Research, Beijing Institute of Respiratory Medicine, Beijing, China, [3] Beijing Institute of Respiratory Medicine, Capital Medical University, Beijing, China

***Correspondence:**
Jiu-Chang Zhong
jczhong@sina.com
Le-Feng Wang
drwlf311@sina.com

Cardiovascular diseases (CVDs) are still the main cause of morbidity and mortality worldwide and include a group of disorders varying from vasculature, myocardium, arrhythmias and cardiac development. MicroRNAs (miRs) are endogenous non-coding RNAs with 18–23 nucleotides that regulate gene expression. The miR-34 family, including miR-34a/b/c, plays a vital role in the regulation of myocardial physiology and pathophysiological processes. Recently, miR-34a has been implicated in cardiovascular fibrosis, dysfunction and related cardiovascular disorders as an essential regulator. Interestingly, there is a pivotal link among miR-34a, cardiovascular fibrosis, and Smad4/TGF-β1 signaling. Notably, both loss-of-function and gain-of-function approaches identified the critical roles of miR-34a in cardiovascular apoptosis, autophagy, inflammation, senescence and remodeling by modulating multifunctional signaling pathways. In this article, we focus on the current understanding of miR-34a in biogenesis, its biological effects and its implications for cardiac pathologies including myocardial infarction, heart failure, ischaemia reperfusion injury, cardiomyopathy, atherosclerosis, hypertension and atrial fibrillation. Thus, further understanding of the effects of miR-34a on cardiovascular diseases will aid the development of effective interventions. Targeting for miR-34a has emerged as a potential therapeutic target for cardiovascular dysfunction and related diseases.

Keywords: microRNA-34a, cardiovascular fibrosis, apoptosis, myocardial remodeling, heart dysfunction

INTRODUCTION

Cardiovascular diseases (CVDs) are regarded as the leading cause of human death worldwide (1). Extensive studies have focused on the pathogenesis of CVDs, but the underlying pathophysiological mechanism is still not clear. Therefore, investigations into the molecular basis of CVDs may elucidate a new pathway for treatment in clinical practice. MicroRNAs (miRs) are endogenous non-coding RNAs with 18–23 nucleotides that regulate gene expression by binding complementary sequences in the 3'UTR of mRNAs. MiRs are indispensable in various biological processes and are involved in cell differentiation and proliferation, cell death, and metabolism (2). In the cardiovascular system, miRs regulate cellular pathways in cardiac fibrosis, apoptosis, inflammation, autophagy and senescence. Recent studies have identified that miRs are involved in multiple CVDs. The role of miR-34 family in regulating cardiac function is notable.

The miR-34 precursor family was discovered computationally and identified experimentally later. Three mature miRs, miR-34a, miR-34b, and miR-34c, are processed by two different precursors. The miR-34 family is transcribed from two distinct sets of genes located on chromosomes 1 and 11 (3). MiR-34a expression is higher than miR34b/c expression in most human organs and tissues except in the lungs (4). Currently, miR-34a expression is mainly regulated by epigenetic modification, transcriptional regulation and other molecular mechanisms (5). Notably, miR-34a has been elucidated to play crucial roles in diverse cardiac biological pathways including apoptosis, inflammation, autophagy, aging and fibrosis, which ultimately contribute to cardiac dysfunction, suggesting the therapeutic potential of targeting miR-34a in CVDs. This review article will discuss the biological effects of miR-34a and summarize the current understanding of miR-34a in the development and prevention of CVDs, including myocardial infarction (MI), heart failure (HF), ischaemia reperfusion (I/R) injury, cardiomyopathy, atherosclerosis, hypertension and atrial fibrillation (AF).

BIOGENESIS AND BIOLOGICAL EFFECTS OF MIR-34A

MiRs are small non-coding RNAs which regulate gene expression by binding to complementary sequences in the 3'UTR of mRNAs. The miR-34 family was found to be increased in heart tissue from patients with cardiovascular diseases and encoded by two different genes (6). MiR-34a is encoded by its own transcript, while miR-34b and miR-34c are encoded by the same primary transcript (7). Similar to the biogenesis of all miRs, miR-34a is transcribed from the transcription start site in the nucleus by RNA polymerase II/III as a long hairpin molecule (pri-miR) and then cleaved by an RNase III Drosha to a ~70-nucleotide long stem-loop precursor (pre-miR). The pre-miR is transported from the nucleus to the cytoplasm and is further cleaved by an RNase III Dicer into 22-nucleotide long mature strands, which are consolidated into the RNA-induced silencing complex (**Figure 1**). This complex downregulates target transcripts by mRNA degradation or inhibition of translation (8, 9). The human miR-34a precursor is transcribed from chromosome 1 and maps to the distal region of chromosome 1p. It is encoded in the second exon of a gene located on chromosome 1p36.22 (10, 11). MiR-34a is involved in cellular diseases and is recognized as an essential regulator in cardiovascular diseases (12).

It has been reported that overexpression of miR-34a promotes apoptosis of MI by inhibiting the activity of silent information regulator 1 (SIRT1) (13). Phosphatase and tensin homolog (PTEN), a negative regulator of PI3K signaling, was downregulated, while miR-34a expression was increased and mRNA of SIRT1 was decreased in oxidative stress-induced epithelial cells (**Figure 2**) (14). In addition, Notch1, Smad4, and fork head box O3 (FOXO3) were verified as miR-34a target genes (**Figure 1**) (11, 15), all of which have actions relevant to cardiovascular diseases. In congenital heart disease (CHD), overexpression of miR-34a induced the deduction of embryonic endocardial cells (ECCs) and acceleration of cell apoptosis, further increasing the risk of CHD targeting Notch1 through the Notch signaling pathway (**Figure 2**) (16). Interestingly, hypoxia-induced HIF1α accelerated angiogenesis of trophoblast cells through the Notch1/ endothelial receptor type B (ETBR) signaling pathway (17). ETBR antagonist increases apoptosis and susceptibility to an apoptotic agent in human pulmonary arterial smooth muscle cells, further promoting vascular remodeling in pulmonary artery hypertension (**Figure 2**) (18). Additionally, miR-34a enhanced cardiac fibrosis after MI *via* targeting Smad4 related with TGF-β1 signaling pathway while miR-34a inhibition ameliorated the above changes (**Table 1**; **Figure 2**) (19). PNUTS, also known as PPP1R10, was identified as a target gene of miR-34a, a novel, SIRT1 independent of the miR-34a signaling pathway, plays a vital role in many cellular processes including cell cycle progression, DNA damage responses (DDR), and apoptosis. It has been reported that PNUTS plays a major role in the anti-senescence effect of doxorubicin (DOXO)-induced H9C2 cell aging. More importantly, inhibition of miR-34a improves cardiac function during aging and post MI by reducing cell death and fibrosis by targeting PNUTS, which is an essential regulator of endogenous cardiac regeneration (**Table 1**; **Figure 1**) (20, 29). MiR-34a accelerated the progression of atherosclerosis by regulating FOXO3 expression. It was reported that FOXO3 plays a critical role in restraining oxidative damage in ox-LDL-induced endothelial cell injury *via* the miR-34a/SIRT1/FOXO3 signaling pathway (**Table 1**; **Figure 2**) (21). FOXO3 inhibited the transcription of pro-apoptotic gene p53 upregulated modulator of apoptosis (PUMA) to promote cell apoptosis (**Figure 2**) (30). It was identified that inhibition of miR-34a-5p alleviated lipopolysaccharide-induced human umbilical vein endothelial cells (HUVECs) injury by targeting FOXM1 through activating the Nuclear factor-E2-related factor 2 (NRF2)/HO-1 pathway (**Figure 2**) (31).

Collectively, miR-34a plays a vital role in controlling cellular apoptosis, autophagy, inflammation, aging, fibrosis, and remodeling through Smad4/TGF-β1, FOXO3/PUMA, Notch1/ETBR, PTEN/PI3K/SIRT1 and FOXM1/NRF2/HO-1 signaling pathways.

MIR-34A AND APOPTOSIS IN THE CARDIOVASCULAR SYSTEM

Apoptosis as one of the cell death programs contributes significantly to multiple cardiovascular diseases such as MI, myocardial ischaemia/reperfusion injury (MIRI), and HF with reduced ejection fraction (32). MiR-34a is expressed abundantly in multiple cardiovascular disease induced apoptosis. A large number of studies have revealed that miR-34a regulates cellular apoptosis through p53-dependent or independent pathway. In p53-dependent pathway, miR-34a-induced apoptosis partly relies on the wild-type p53 genes at least, and p53 is induced by miR-34a, suggesting that miR-34a can also function in a feedback loop to p53 (11). The tumor suppressor p53 is critical for tumor prevention through regulating cell-cycle checkpoints, while loss of p53 function tends to result in human cancer (33). More importantly, ablation of p53 contributed to cardiomyocyte

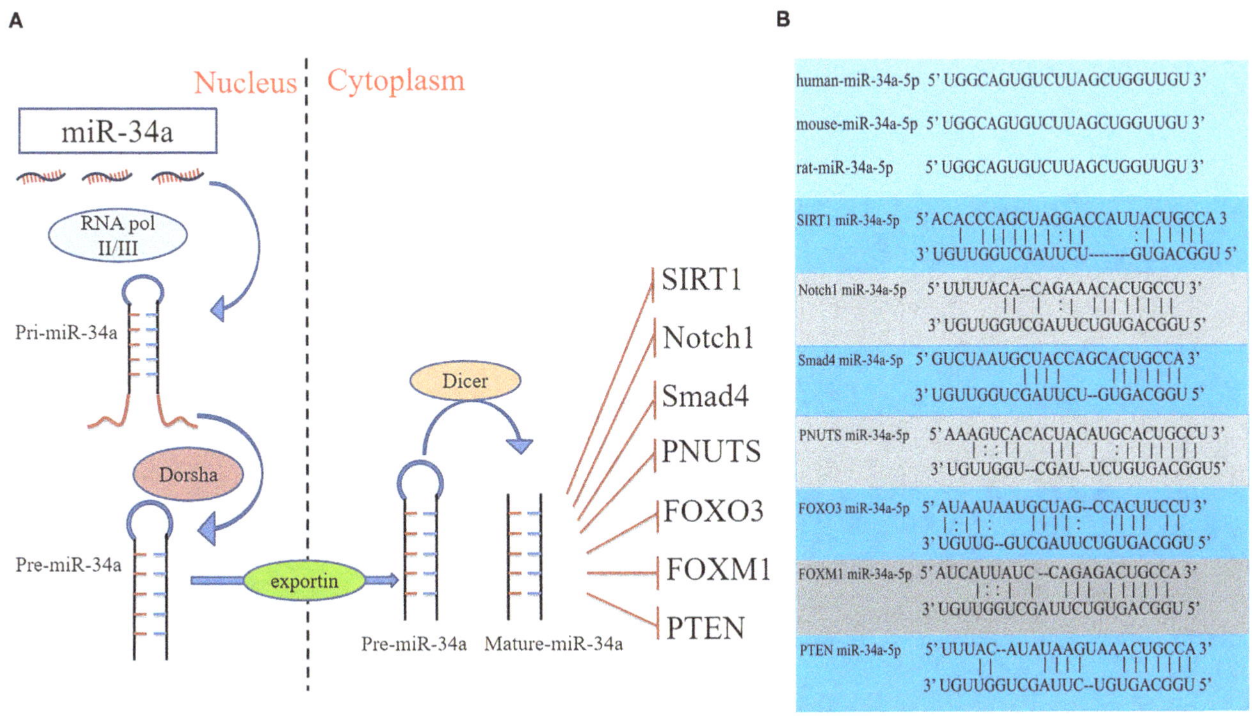

FIGURE 1 | Schematic diagram of the activities of miR-34a, and potential binding sites between miR-34a and the target genes. **(A)** Schematic diagram of the activities, and target genes of miR-34a. **(B)** The sequence of miR-34a-5p is conserved in humans, mice and rats. The potential miR-34a-5p-binding sites of target genes. FOXM1, Forkhead box M1; FOXO3, Fork head box O3; PTEN, Phosphatase and tensin homologue; SIRT1, Silent information regulator 1.

apoptosis and spontaneous hypertrophy in HF by regulating the cardiac transcriptome. This suggests that p53 plays a pleiotropic role in cardiac tissue homeostasis and function (34). As a target of p53, miR-34a targets Bcl2 and SIRT1 to aggravate myocardial injury by exacerbating apoptosis and infarct size, decreasing left ventricular function (35). Intriguingly, SIRT1, one of the main targets of miR-34a, mediates cellular responses involving apoptosis, autophagy and mitochondrial biogenesis, which suppress the activity of p53 by posttranscriptional deacetylation of the p53 protein (**Figure 1**) (9, 36, 37). Additionally, research have found that p53 and miR-34a interact in a positive feedback loop and target SIRT1 involved in cell cycle progression, cellular senescence and apoptosis. The above results indicated that miR-34a may regulate cardiac homeostasis and cellular apoptosis by modulating p53 function. Interestingly, the research has founded that the ratio of miR-34a to SIRT1 was increased in older patients' myocardial tissue rather than in young patients post MI, implying severe apoptosis in older patients and explained why older patients recovered more slowly than young patients.

It has been accepted that miR-34a modulates cellular apoptosis in cardiovascular system in a manner dependent on cell types. Recent study reported that miR-34a promotes apoptosis and angiogenesis of cardiac microvascular endothelial cells (CMECs), and upregulates inflammatory cytokines, thus worsening CMECs damage through the Notch signaling pathway (**Table 1**) (22). In hypoxia-induced cardiomyocytes, the expression of miR-34a-5p was increased while miR-34a-5p knockdown ameliorated cardiomyocyte apoptosis and cardiac dysfunction by upregulating ZEB1 and anti-apoptotic proteins such as aldehyde dehydrogenase 2 (38). In a diabetic cardiomyopathy rat model, granulocyte-colony stimulating factor ameliorated diastolic dysfunction and reduced cardiomyocyte apoptosis through downregulation of miR-34a and upregulation of Bcl2 (39). However, the effect of inhibition of miR-34a was not observed in cardiac progenitor cells, which showed reduced proliferation (39). Suppression of miR-34a activity may have diverse effects depending on cell types, thus it is necessary to eliminate off-target effects by introducing miR-based therapy.

The Notch signaling pathway is involved in processes related to cell differentiation, proliferation, apoptosis and survival. In a rat model of CHD, miR-34a targeted Notch1, improved the expression of Jagged1, Hes1, and Hey2, promoted the apoptosis rate and decreased the proliferation rate (**Figure 1**) (16). Similar to MIRI-induced microvascular injury, inhibition of miR-34a alleviates brain tissue damage and neuronal apoptosis by activating the Notch1/HIF-1α signaling pathway in a cerebral I/R-induced rat model (40). Additionally, adenosine deaminases acting on RNA 2 (ADAR2), an enzyme acting on double-stranded RNAs, promoted cardiomyocyte proliferation and inhibited DOXO-induced cell apoptosis *via* the ADAR2/miR-34a regulation axis, which involves the RNA editing activity of ADAR2 (41). These findings indicated that miR-34a promoted

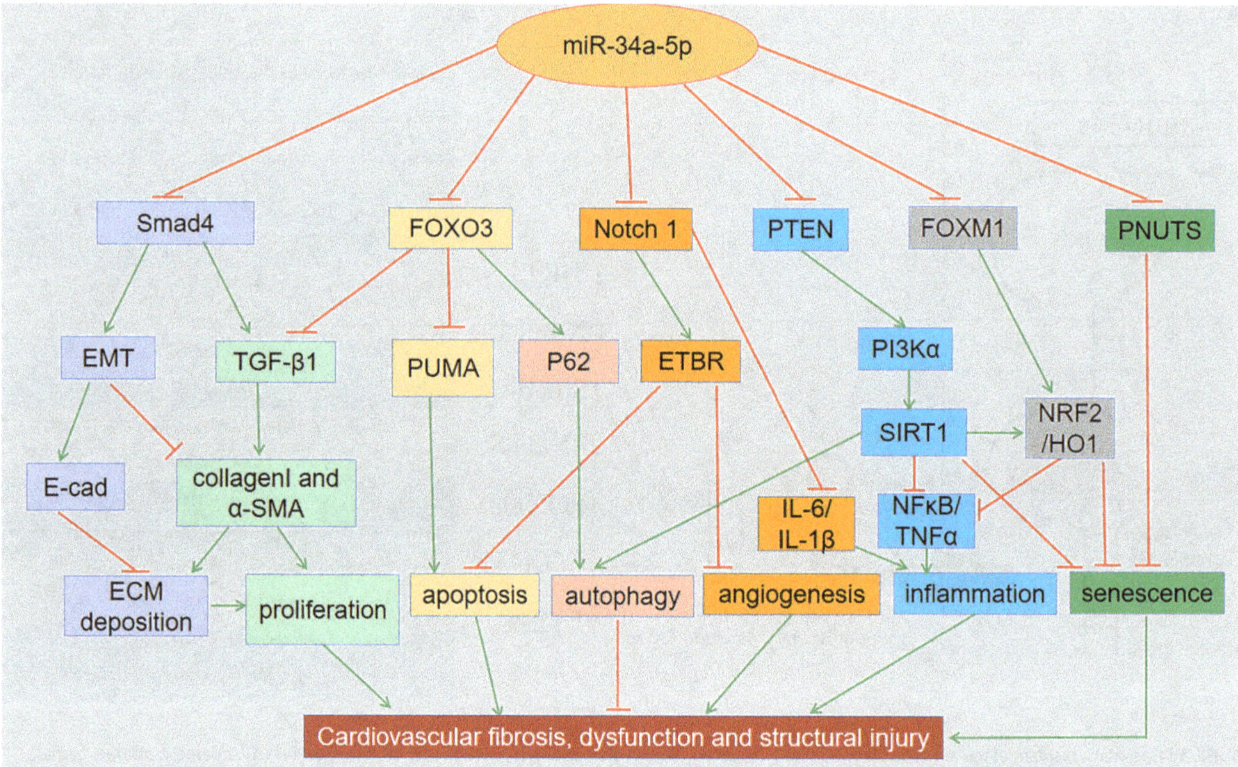

FIGURE 2 | The regulatory roles and underlying mechanisms of miR-34a in cardiovascular dysfunction and related disorders. MiR-34a has been shown to regulate cellular apoptosis, autophagy, inflammation, senescence and remodeling in various cardiac and vascular tissues and cells through Smad4/TGF-β1, FOXO3/PUMA, Notch1/ETBR, PTEN/PI3K/SIRT1, and FOXM1/NRF2/HO-1 signaling pathways, respectively. EMT, Epithelial-mesenchymal transition; ECM, Extracellular matrix; ETBR, endothelial receptor type B; FOXM1, Forkhead box M1; FOXO3, Forkhead box O3; NRF2, Nuclear factor-E2-related factor 2; PI3K, Phosphatidylinositol 3-kinase; PNUTS, Phosphatase-1 nuclear targeting subunit; PTEN, Phosphatase and tensin homologue; PUMA, p53-up-regulated modulator of apoptosis; SIRT1, Silent information regulator 1; TGF-β1, Transforming growth factor β1.

cardiomyocyte apoptosis and aggravated myocardial injury through different mechanisms.

MIR-34A AND AUTOPHAGY IN THE CARDIOVASCULAR SYSTEM

Autophagy plays a vital role in the development of various cardiovascular diseases (42). It has been reported that miR-34a suppresses autophagy in cancer cells (43). However, autophagy regulated by miR-34a has also been demonstrated in cardiovascular disease. The inhibition of miR-34a enhanced cardiomyocyte autophagy and further ameliorated cardiac function in diabetic cardiomyopathy (44). In addition, miR-34a has been shown to inhibit autophagy after cardiac I/R injury by regulating TNF-α expression, thereby ameliorating myocardial damage (45). Interestingly, miR-34a-5p was found to be elevated in human coronary artery endothelial cells (HCAECs) exposed to chronic intermittent hypoxia (CIH), further increasing autophagy-related proteins such as Beclin and LC3. These results indicated that miR-34a-5p contributed to CIH-induced HCAECs autophagy through Bcl2/Beclin signaling pathways. MiR-34a-5p has been recognized as a potential therapeutic target for autophagy induced by CIH which leads to CVDs (46). Accordingly, miR-34a inhibition improves cardiac function by regulating protective autophagy in CVDs.

MIR-34A AND CARDIOVASCULAR OXIDATIVE STRESS AND INFLAMMATION

MiR-34a is a driver of vascular and systemic inflammation, which promotes the progression of inflammation related disease (47). Overexpression of miR-34a enhanced radiation-induced oxidative stress in cardiomyocyte, while macrophage migration inhibition reduced cellular reactive oxygen species (ROS) through the miR-34a/SIRT1 signaling pathway (48). More importantly, inhibition of miR-34a mitigated oxidative stress induced by H_2O_2 to protect vascular endothelial cells by targeting SIRT1 (49). The role of inflammation in MIRI is still controversial. Enhancement of circulating monocyte levels and attenuated repair capacity after MI have been found in apolipoprotein E-null mice (50). In an additional study, anti-inflammatory therapy was shown to reduce the number of cardiac adverse events post MI (51). MI and MIRI have been shown to cause a burst of ROS accumulation. Down-regulation

TABLE 1 | The regulatory roles and underlying mechanisms of miR-34a in cardiovascular dysfunction and disorders.

Experimental model	Experimental intervention	Effects	References
MI mouse model	miR-34 family inhibitor	↑Vinculin, SIRT1, PNUTS, Notch1 ↑Bcl6, Sema4b ↓Left ventricular remodeling ↑Cardiac function	(6)
DOXO-induced myocardium	miR-34a inhibitor	↑Bcl2, SIRT1 ↓Apoptosis and senescence ↓Myocardial fibrosis and inflammation ↓Cardiac dysfunction	(12)
MI-induced rat myocardium	miR-34a mimic	↓Bcl2, SIRT1 ↑Bax ↑Apoptosis	(13)
MI rat model	miR-34a inhibitor	↓Apoptosis ↓TGF-β1 ↓CollagenI, α-SMA, ECM deposition	(19)
Cardiac fibroblast post MI	pre-miR-34a	↑Collagen I, α-SMA, fibronectin ↑TGF-β1, Smad4 ↑Proliferation, migration	(19)
Aged mouse	miR-34a inhibitor	↑PNUTS ↓Apoptosis, cell death ↓Cardiac hypertrophy ↑Cardiac contractile function	(20)
Mouse model of AMI	miR-34a inhibitor	↑PNUTS ↓Apoptosis ↓Fibrosis ↑Capillary density ↑Cardiac contractile function	(20)
ox-LDL-elicited HUVECs	miR-34a mimic	↑ROS, MDA ↓SOD, CAT, GSH,GPx, SIRT1, FOXO3a ↑Oxidative stress	(21)
Mouse CMECs	miR-34a mimic	↑IL-1β, IL-6 ↓Notch1, IL-10, VEGF, bFGF, HGF ↑Apoptosis ↓Cell viability and capillary-like structures of cells formation ability	(22)
ISO-induced rat myocardial fibrosis model	miR-34a inhibitor	↑c-Ski ↓Collagen I, α-SMA, TGF-β1 ↓Cardiac fibrosis ↓Cell proliferation	(23)
RBFox2 KO mice	miR-34a inhibitor	↑JPH2 ↓Anf ↑Cardiac function	(24)
H/R induced mouse cardiomyocytes	miR-34a inhibitor	↓Bax, caspase 3 ↑Bcl2 ↓ER stress and cell apoptosis	(25)
Apoe–/– mice fed with HFD	miR-34a inhibitor	↑Bcl2 ↓Bax, Caspase-3, and caspase-9 ↑Cell growth and viability ↓Atherosclerotic lesions	(26)
IS-induced HUVECs and HA VSMCs		↑miR-34a, p53 ↓Notch-1, SIRT1, Wnt-1, Jag1, ↓Proliferation, migration ↑Apoptosis	(27)
Wire injury CAVS mice	miR-34a inhibitor	↑Notch1 ↓Runx2, α-SMA, VCAM1, Cadherin ↓LVEDD ↓Intraventricular septum diameter ↓Aortic velocity, aortic valve tissue area ↓Calcium deposition	(28)

ALDH2, Aldehyde dehydrogenase 2; Anf, atrial natriuretic factor; ApoE–/–, Apolipoprotein E-defcient; α-SMA, α-smooth muscle actin; bFGF, Basic fibroblast growth factor; Bcl-2, B-cell lymphoma-2; Bax, Bcl-2 associated X protein; CAVS, Calcific aortic valve stenosis; CAT, catalase; CMECs, Cardiac microvascular endothelial cells; DOXO, doxorubicin; EF, ejection fraction; ER, Endoplasmic reticulum; FS, fractional shorting; GSH, glutathione; GPx, glutathione peroxidase; HCY, Homocystein; HGF, Human growth factor; HFD, high-fat diet; HUVECs, human umbilical vein endothelial cells; HAVSMCs, human aortic vascular smooth muscle cells; IL-1β, Interleukin 1 β; I/R, Ischemia/Reperfusion; IS, indoxyl sulfate; ISO, isoproterenol; LVEDD, left ventricular end-diastolic diameter; MI, Myocardial infarction; MDA, malondialdehyde; NF-kB, Nuclear factor kappa-B; ROS, reactive oxygen species; Runx2, Runt-related transcription factor 2; SIRT1, Silent information regulator 1; Sema4b, semaphorin 4B; SOD, superoxide dismutase; TGF-β, Transforming growth factor β; VCAM1, vascular cell adhesion molecule 1; VEGF, Vascular endothelial growth factor.

of miR-34a alleviates the inflammatory response induced by renal I/R by promoting Kruppel-like factor 4 (KLF4) levels in rats (52). Similarly, miR-34a is involved in cancer immunotherapy-mediated myocardial inflammation. Cancer immune therapy has become a well-known treatment for some cancers, but immune checkpoint inhibitors (ICIs) more often lead to cardiac injury. It has been reported that inhibition of miR-34a attenuates cardiomyocyte inflammation induced by ICIs targeting KLF4 which has a cardioprotective effect. This result indicated that targeting the miR-34a/KLF4 signaling pathway may be an effective approach for patients who experience ICISs therapy-induced cardiac injury (53). In general, treatment with the miR-34a inhibitor may alleviate cardiomyocyte inflammation and oxidative stress. However, further studies are needed to identify the role of miR-34 in the treatment of inflammation-mediated MI and MIRI.

MIR-34A AND CARDIOVASCULAR SENESCENCE

Age-related cardiac disease is driven by multiple molecular mechanisms such as telomere shortening, DDR, accumulation of somatic mutations, epigenetic changes, and alterations in non-coding RNAs regulating gene expression (54). Radiotherapy increases the survival of various cancer patients but leads to cardiac dysfunction, including cardiomyocyte senescence. A recent study demonstrated that the expression of miR-34a was obviously increased in the radiation-induced cardiac dysfunction to exert a pro-senescence effect on cardiomyocytes by regulating SIRT1 (**Figure 2**). Additionally, overexpression of miR-34a leads to a reduction in both the mRNA and protein levels of SIRT1/6, which are putative anti-aging enzymes, thereby promoting aging responses under oxidative stress (14). In the DOXO treated rat model, silencing of miR-34a ameliorated DOXO-induced myocardial senescence and protected cardiac function and integrity by targeting Bcl2 and SIRT1 (**Table 1**) (12). Suppression of miR-34a does not solely inhibit cardiomyocyte senescence but likewise plays a regulatory role in vascular senescence. A recent review generalized the role of miR-34a in vascular aging and senescence, demonstrating that miR-34a promoted vascular aging through targeting SIRT1 or regulating vascular cell adhesion protein1 and intercellular adhesion molecule 1 at least partially (55). More importantly, activation of FOXO3 promoted stress resistance in differentiated human vascular endothelial and smooth muscle cells which related to cellular aging (56). This may provide additional evidence that miR-34a promotes vascular aging and senescence by targeting FOXO3. The above results show that inhibition of miR-34a alleviated cellular senescence and further improved cardiac and vascular function, which may provide a new approach for protecting against radiotherapy-induced cardiac injury and HF.

MIR-34A AND CARDIOVASCULAR FIBROTIC REMODELING

Myocardial inflammation and oxidative stress play critical roles in cardiac fibrosis and remodeling (57). It has been well-documented that miR-34a contributes to cardiac fibrosis and aging (58). The important pathological reactions that affect ventricular remodeling post MI encompass myocardial apoptosis, myocardial pathological hypertrophy, cellular senescence, and extracellular matrix metabolism disorder (59). It was identified that miR-34a could modulate TGF-β1 induced myocardial proliferation and ECM deposition of rat cardiac fibroblasts by targeting c-ski. MiR-34a inhibitor alleviated rat cardiomyocyte proliferation and ECM deposition induced by TGF-β1 (**Table 1**; **Figure 2**) (23). A recent study indicated that sevoflurane preconditioning inhibited cardiomyocyte apoptosis and reduced cardiac injury in hypoxia/reoxygenation (H/R) stimulated H9C2 cells. MiR-34a-5p attenuated the protective effect of preconditioning with sevoflurane in H/R induced H9C2 cells *via* targeting syntaxin 1A (60). MiR-34a inhibition has been shown to alleviate ventricular remodeling and improve cardiac function after myocardial infarction in animal models (20). Inhibition of miR-34a-5p promoted adipose-derived stem cell proliferation and migration to protect the myocardium against MI damage by activating the expression of c1q/tumor necrosis factor related protein-9 (CTRP9) (61). Anti-miR-34 attenuates MI-induced ventricular remodeling and atrial enlargement and improves cardiac function by targeting Notch1 (**Table 1**) (6). Furthermore, miR-34a plays an important role in regulating vascular smooth muscle cell functions and neointima hyperplasia, indicating its potential treatment application for vascular diseases (62). The expression of miR-34a decreased in hypoxia-induced human pulmonary artery smooth muscle cells and the reduction in miR-34a increased proliferation, conversely, overexpression of miR-34a reversed the above effects by targeting platelet-derived growth factor receptor alpha (PDGFRA). PDGFRA is an important regulator in pulmonary artery hypertension mediates cell proliferation and vascular remolding (63). In this regard, in primary hypertension, miR-34a has not been reported to regulate vascular remolding *via* targeting PDGFRA. These miR-34a-mediated apoptosis, proliferation and necrosis ultimately contribute to cardiac remodeling (64). Contrary to most studies, a recent report shows that miR-34a ameliorates myocardial fibrosis by reducing type I collagen production, cell viability, and migration and improves cell function in diabetic cardiomyopathy (65). In general, miR-34a inhibition alleviated cardiac and vascular remodeling post ischaemic disease. Glucose metabolism-related cardiac fibrosis may result in differential targeting effects of miR-34a.

Taken together, these findings show that inhibition of miR-34a exerts a protective effect on the pathophysiology of cardiovascular diseases and is a potential therapeutic strategy for improving cardiac function.

ROLES OF MIR-34A IN MI AND HF

MI remains a leading cause of morbidity and mortality worldwide. The infarcted heart is characterized by a loss of cells from death and myocardial fibrotic scarring. Cardiac hypertrophy and fibrosis largely lead to thickening and stiffening of the ventricular wall, further contributing to cardiac remodeling that ultimately results in cardiac dysfunction and subsequent heart failure (66, 67). MiR-34a is involved in a variety of pathological process of AMI through regulating cardiomyocyte proliferation, migration, apoptosis and remodeling. The expression of miR-34a increased in an MI rat model, leading to myocardial apoptosis, fibrosis and cardiac dysfunction through the Wnt/β-catenin pathway, indicating that miR-34a may be a potential therapeutic target for MI (68). In this regard, a recent study demonstrated that miR-34a was highly expressed in the heart tissue of AMI, which promoted cell apoptosis and oxidative stress. The results indicated that inhibition of miR-34a attenuated myocardial injury by multiple gene regulation of cellular phenotypes (69). Recent studies have shown that some mature miRs are also modified by m6A/m5C methylation, and that these modified mature miRs are significantly differentially expressed among cancer tissues (70). Similarly in the cardiovascular system, methylation of miR-34a promoted by Bcl-6 has a cardioprotective effect on AMI *via* the EZH2/miR-34a/CTRP9 axis (69). In the early stage of AMI, prevention of heart failure and left ventricular remodeling are closely related to the prognosis of patients, and left ventricular remodeling after AMI is associated with poor prognosis (68). It is becoming increasingly clear that miRs are promising predictors for cardiovascular pathological processes, including MI, myocardial remodeling and progression to heart failure. Long-term remodeling is associated with increased risk of cardiovascular death. Thus, early identification of ventricular remodeling is essential for clinical medicine (71). MiR-34a is upregulated and associated with left ventricular diastolic dimension in the convalescent stage of AMI patients who survive AMI but ultimately experience HF within 1 year (72). In addition, miR-34a exacerbated cardiac fibrosis and left ventricular dysfunction in the early stage of HF post AMI. It was demonstrated that miR-34a serves as an available predictor for future progression of HF post AMI (73). The results implied that miR-34a is an important biomarker for predicting left ventricular (LV) remodeling after AMI. Elevated miR-34a levels impair myocardial excitation contraction coupling which further leads to cardiac dysfunction through targeting Jph2. Importantly, it was demonstrated that intervention of this pathway with miR-34a antagonist significantly alleviated the heart failure in RBFox2 KO mice (24). These results indicated that inhibition of miR-34a plays a key role in controlling cell viability and cardiomyocyte apoptosis further improving cardiac function in MI and HF.

ROLES OF MIR-34A IN I/R INJURY

Cardiovascular disease accounts for more than 40% of pathological occurrences, and the mortality and prevalence have increased in recent years (74). Ischaemic heart disease is a main cause of cardiovascular diseases, which mostly leads to MI and cardiac dysfunction (75, 76). The roles of miRs in I/R injury are mediated through the regulation of essential signaling pathways involved in necrosis, apoptosis, oxidative stress, inflammation, fibrosis and angiogenesis (77). It has been demonstrated that overexpression of miR-34a aggravates myocardial injury by increasing cell apoptosis and infarct size and decreasing LV function, while miR-34a suppression ameliorates myocardial I/R injury (35). Consistent with the above results, a recent study showed that miR-34a-5p inhibitor attenuated myocardial I/R injury by alleviating apoptosis rate and reducing infarct size and ROS accumulation through targeting Notch receptor 1 signaling (76). Crocin, one of the active components of saffron, has been identified to suppress I/R-induced endoplasmic reticulum stress and cardiomyocyte apoptosis through downregulation of miR-34a and activation of the SIRT1/NRF2 pathway (**Table 1**; **Figure 2**) (25). Accordingly, miR-34a inhibition protected cardiomyocytes against I/R injury, and future studies should be investigated the efficacy of treatment with miR-34a inhibitor in I/R patients and the underlying mechanisms.

ROLES OF MIR-34A IN CARDIOMYOPATHY

Cardiomyopathy is a disease that negatively affects cardiac function and can be classified into primary and secondary categories. Hypertrophic cardiomyopathy is the most common primary cardiomyopathy. More importantly, diabetes-induced cardiac dysfunction has been increasingly attracted worldwide; however, reports of mechanism of diabetic cardiomyopathy are limited (78–80). MiR-34a increased high glucose-induced inflammation, oxidative stress and cell death by targeting SIRT1 in H9C2 cells (81). MiR-34a was overexpressed to promote apoptosis in the diabetic heart and glucose control did not change the expression of miR-34a (82). In addition, transfection with miR-34a inhibitor significantly reduced cell apoptosis in diabetic cardiomyopathy. Treatment with dihydromyricetin decreased miR-34a expression further alleviating autophagy in high glucose-induced cardiomyocytes and in the heart tissue of diabetic mice to ameliorate cardiac dysfunction (44). Hypertension-induced hypertrophic cardiomyopathy increases the occurrence of cardiovascular events. MiR-34a has been shown to be a negative regulator in hypertrophic cardiomyopathy to aggravate myocardial cell inflammation and immune responses through TGF-β/Smad signaling pathway (83). In particular, silencing miR-34a alone serves a protective role in moderate cardiomyopathy while anti-miR-34a does not alter the severe hypertrophic cardiomyopathy phenotype (84).

ROLES OF MIR-34A IN ATHEROSCLEROSIS

The development of atherosclerosis is facilitated by the presence of concomitant risk factors, encompassing dyslipidaemial, leading to a chronic inflammatory reaction in the vessel wall. Endothelial cells (ECs) and vascular smooth muscle cells (VSMCs) are also involved in the development of atherosclerotic vascular disease (85). Macrophages play an important role in the pathogenesis of atherosclerosis by regulating inflammatory response and foam cell formation. MiR-34a regulated cholesterol effusion and inflammation in macrophages, reversed cholesterol transport, and promoted atherosclerosis by coordinating regulation of several genes related to the pathogenesis of atherosclerosis. Importantly, the inhibition of miR-34a significantly prevented the progression of atherosclerosis and reversed atherosclerosis *via* multiple signaling and different cell types (26, 85). In light of high level of miR-34a in vascular aging, it induces senescence and the acquisition of a senescence associated secretory phenotype in VSMCs and ECs. MiR-34a has been reported to trigger ECs aging through repression of SIRT1, whereas antagonism of miR-34a reduced ECs apoptosis and the development of atherosclerosis in $ApoE^{-/-}$ mice (26, 86, 87). Interestingly, a recent study indicated that miR-34a/SIRT1/FOXO3 may play a vital role in reversing ox-LDL-induced oxidative stress in HUVECs by genistein (**Figure 2**) (21). Indoxyl sulfate can promote the process of atherosclerosis through upregulating miR-34a expression and inhibiting the Notch signaling pathway (27). The miR-34a/HNF4α pathway may play a critical role in the pathogenesis of non-alcoholic fatty liver disease and regulate plasma lipid and lipoprotein metabolism. It was identified that miR-34a reduced the development of atherosclerosis in $ApoE^{-/-}$ mice by inhibiting HNF4α expression (**Table 1**) (26). Furthermore, a recent study suggested that miR-34a may be a promising target for the treatment of atherosclerosis as prevents cell growth and promotes apoptosis in atherosclerosis by regulating Bcl2, while deletion of miR-34a ameliorates atherosclerotic lesions in high-fat diet induced ApoE$^{-/-}$ mice (87). Interestingly, miRs in plasma are emerging as novel biomarkers for predicting multiple diseases. High level of miR-34a was related to coronary artery disease independently [OR [95% CI: 3.87 (1.56-9.56)]; $P = 0.003$] and the increased level was associated with expression of SIRT1, JAG1,CTNNB1, ATF1, and Notch2 inversely (88). Thus, miR-34a plays a central role by promoting inflammation, apoptosis and senescence in macrophages, ECs and VAMCs to exacerbated atherosclerosis progression.

ROLES OF MIR-34A IN HYPERTENSION

Primary hypertension is a common chronic disease that usually causes other health complications, such as coronary artery disease, stroke, renal failure and heart failure, and poses a great threat to human health (89, 90). Currently, the relationship between miR-34a and hypertension is relatively limited (91). Research has shown that miR-34a upregulated in the peripheral blood of patients with hypertension, and that upregulated miR-34a may promote vascular endothelial injury by targeting TIGF2 (89). The elevating miR-34a expression in hypertension increased the risk of vascular disease and related cardiovascular events. In hypertension-induced renal injury, urinary SIRT1 expression was decreased by miR-34a, indicating that SIRT1 is a potential method to evaluate renal injury in hypertensive patients (92). In contrary, a recent study showed that miR-34a reduces urinary microalbumin content in hypertensive mice and protects renal function targeting plasminogen activator inhibitor. The inhibition of miR-34a increased the levels of urinary microalbumin content and ACE protein, which contribute to renal damage in hypertensive mice (91). In general, miR-34a plays a critical role not only in hypertension but also in hypertension-related complications. The potential mechanisms between miR-34a and hypertension need further exploration.

ROLES OF MIR-34A IN AF

AF is the most common symptomatic cardiac arrhythmia in clinical medicine and shows an increasing prevalence with age. AF leads substantially to morbidity and mortality in the world (93). AF was divided into three groups at three durations (duration since diagnosis of AF). The 12-month and 24-month groups exhibited upregulated expression levels of miR-34a-5p (94). MiR-34a plays a critical role in promoting atrial electrical remodeling and the development of AF by inhibiting the expression of Ank-B (93). The present study revealed several novel persistent AF-associated miRs, including miR-34a-5p, which might target calcineurin1 and protein phosphatase three regulatory subunit B alpha to regulate persistent AF through the calcineurin-nuclear factor of activated T cells signaling pathway (95). These results provide valuable insights into the underlying mechanism of AF. The above results indicated that miR-34a may be a promising clinical diagnostic tool in the early stage of AF.

ANTI-MIR-34A THERAPY IN CVDS

It is well-known that miR-34a is a tumor suppressive miR in various tumor diseases. MiR-34a has been identified to have therapeutic potential for cancer. A recent study indicated that co-delivery 5-fluorouracil and miR-34a mimic improved the apoptotic effect and inhibited the metastasis of colorectal cancer cells (96). Further study demonstrated that pre-miR-34a transfection suppressed the expression of target genes, induced apoptosis and decreased the proliferation rate in gastric cancer (97). More importantly, this review showed that miR-34a plays a negative role in the progression of CVDs. Transfection with bone marrow-derived molecular cells promoted the release of IGF, which inhibited the expression of pre-miR-34a, thereby reducing cardiomyocyte apoptosis (98). Additionally, in calcific aortic valve stenosis model mice, locked nucleic acid-modified oligonucleotide (LNA)-miR-34a inhibitor attenuated the development of aortic valve stenosis and calcification (**Table 1**) (28). Inhibition of the miR-34 family attenuates pathological cardiac remodeling and atrial enlargement post AMI. Of interest, anti-miR-34a treatment ameliorated cardiac dysfunction by improving the cardiac molecular profile in females compared with males. More importantly, chronic administration of LNA-anti-miR-34 had no adverse effects on heart tissue morphology (99). The anti-miR-34 family, not anti-miR-34a only, shows a stronger therapeutic effect in cardiovascular disease, possibly due to regulating miRs and mRNA targets (100). Collectively, anti-miR-34a therapy is critical for CVDs and it is essential to explore the potential benefits of miR-34a inhibitor treatment in CVDs.

CONCLUSION AND PROSPECTION

MiR-34a plays a vital role in the process of cardiovascular diseases. Recently, clinical and experimental studies have demonstrated that miR-34a plays a crucial role in diverse cardiac biological pathways that induce cardiovascular injury and dysfunction. MiR-34a overexpression has been revealed to blunt autophagy and promote cardiovascular apoptosis, inflammation, fibrosis, remodeling, aging and heart dysfunction. More importantly, the inhibition of miR-34a has been shown to exert pro-autophagic, anti-apoptotic, anti-oxidant, and anti-fibrotic effects in the cardiovascular system. This review systematically outlined the regulatory roles of miR-34a in cardiovascular dysfunction and provided evidence to support miR-34a as a potential therapeutic target for the treatment of cardiovascular diseases. More preclinical and clinical trials are needed to identify the potential benefits and side effects of anti-miR-34a therapy in cardiovascular diseases.

AUTHOR CONTRIBUTIONS

C-CH and X-ML drafted the manuscript. L-RL revised the manuscript. L-FW and J-CZ designed and provided guidance for the manuscript. All authors have read and approved the final manuscript.

REFERENCES

1. Kalayinia S, Arjmand F, Maleki M, Malakootian M, Singh CP. MicroRNAs: Roles in cardiovascular development and disease. *Cardiovasc Pathol.* (2021) 50:107296. doi: 10.1016/j.carpath.2020.107296
2. Song R, Hu X, Zhang L. Mitochondrial MiRNA in cardiovascular function and disease. *Cells-Basel.* (2019) 8:1475. doi: 10.3390/cells8121475
3. Maroof H, Salajegheh A, Smith RA, Lam AK. Role of microRNA-34 family in cancer with particular reference to cancer angiogenesis. *Exp Mol Pathol.* (2014) 97:298–304. doi: 10.1016/j.yexmp.2014.08.002
4. Zhang L, Liao Y, Tang L. MicroRNA-34 family: A potential tumor suppressor and therapeutic candidate in cancer. *J Exp Clin Canc Res.* (2019) 38:1059. doi: 10.1186/s13046-019-1059-5
5. Li XJ, Ren ZJ, Tang JH. MicroRNA-34a: A potential therapeutic target in human cancer. *Cell Death Dis.* (2014) 5:e1327. doi: 10.1038/cddis.2014.270
6. Bernardo BC, Gao XM, Winbanks CE, Boey EJH, Tham YK, Kiriazis H, et al. Therapeutic inhibition of the miR-34 family attenuates pathological cardiac remodeling and improves heart function. *Proc Natl Acad Sci USA.* (2012) 109:17615–20. doi: 10.1073/pnas.1206432109
7. Zhang DG, Zheng JN, Pei DS. P53/microRNA-34-induced metabolic regulation: New opportunities in anticancer therapy. *Mol Cancer.* (2014) 13:115. doi: 10.1186/1476-4598-13-115
8. Misso G, Di Martino MT, De Rosa G, Farooqi AA, Lombardi A, Campani V, et al. Mir-34: A new weapon against cancer? *Mol Ther Nucleic Acids.* (2014) 3:e194. doi: 10.1038/mtna.2014.47
9. Rokavec M, Li H, Jiang L, Hermeking H. The p53/miR-34 axis in development and disease. *J Mol Cell Biol.* (2014) 6:214–30. doi: 10.1093/jmcb/mju003
10. Li WJ, Wang Y, Liu R, Kasinski AL, Shen H, Slack FJ, et al. MicroRNA-34a: Potent tumor suppressor, cancer stem cell inhibitor, and potential anticancer therapeutic. *Front Cell Dev Biol.* (2021) 9:640587. doi: 10.3389/fcell.2021.640587
11. He M, Gao L, Zhang S, Tao L, Wang J, Yang J, et al. Prognostic significance of miR-34a and its target proteins of FOXP1, p53, and BCL2 in gastric MALT lymphoma and DLBCL. *Gastric Cancer.* (2014) 17:431–41. doi: 10.1007/s10120-013-0313-3
12. Piegari E, Cozzolino A, Ciuffreda LP, Cappetta D, De Angelis A, Urbanek K, et al. Cardioprotective effects of miR-34a silencing in a rat model of doxorubicin toxicity. *Sci Rep-Uk.* (2020) 10:69038. doi: 10.1038/s41598-020-69038-3
13. Dong FF, Dong SH, Liang Y, Wang K, Qin YW, Zhao XX. MiR-34a promotes myocardial infarction in rats by inhibiting the activity of SIRT1. *Eur Rev Med Pharmacol Sci.* (2019) 23:7059–65. doi: 10.26355/eurrev_201908_18750
14. Baker JR, Vuppusetty C, Colley T, Papaioannou AI, Fenwick P, Donnelly L, et al. Oxidative stress dependent microRNA-34a activation *via* PI3Kα reduces the expression of sirtuin-1 and sirtuin-6 in epithelial cells. *Sci Rep-Uk.* (2016) 6:35871. doi: 10.1038/srep35871
15. Raddatz MA, Vander Roest MJ, Merryman WD. Notch1 suppression by microRNA-34a: A new mechanism of calcific aortic valve disease. *Cardiovasc Res.* (2020) 116:871–3. doi: 10.1093/cvr/cvz280
16. Wu K, Xiao Q, Yang Y, Xu J, Zhang F, Liu C, et al. MicroRNA-34a modulates the Notch signaling pathway in mice with congenital heart disease and its role in heart development. *J Mol Cell Cardiol.* (2018) 114:300–8. doi: 10.1016/j.yjmcc.2017.11.015
17. Yu N, Wu JL, Xiao J, Fan L, Chen SH, Li W. HIF-1alpha regulates angiogenesis *via* Notch1/STAT3/ETBR pathway in trophoblastic cells. *Cell Cycle.* (2019) 18:3502–12. doi: 10.1080/15384101.2019.1689481
18. Sakai S, Maruyama H, Kimura T, Tajiri K, Honda J, Homma S, et al. Antagonists to endothelin receptor type B promote apoptosis in human pulmonary arterial smooth muscle cells. *Life Sci.* (2016) 159:116–20. doi: 10.1016/j.lfs.2016.03.044
19. Huang Y, Qi Y, Du JQ, Zhang DF. MicroRNA-34a regulates cardiac fibrosis after myocardial infarction by targeting Smad4. *Expert Opin Ther Targets.* (2014) 18:1355–65. doi: 10.1517/14728222.2014.961424
20. Boon RA, Iekushi K, Lechner S, Seeger T, Fischer A, Heydt S, et al. MicroRNA-34a regulates cardiac ageing and function. *Nature.* (2013) 495:107–10. doi: 10.1038/nature11919
21. Zhang H, Zhao Z, Pang X, Yang J, Yu H, Zhang Y, et al. MiR-34a/sirtuin-1/foxo3a is involved in genistein protecting against ox-LDL-induced oxidative damage in HUVECs. *Toxicol Lett.* (2017) 277:115–22. doi: 10.1016/j.toxlet.2017.07.216
22. Li J, Gong J, Li X, Shen L, Xie Y, Zhang R. MicroRNA-34a promotes CMECs apoptosis and upregulate inflammatory cytokines, thus worsening CMECs damage and inhibiting angiogenesis by negatively targeting the Notch signaling pathway. *J Cell Biochem.* (2019) 120:1598–609. doi: 10.1002/jcb.27433
23. Zhang C, Zhang Y, Zhu H, Hu J, Xie Z. MiR-34a/miR-93 target c-Ski to modulate the proliferaton of rat cardiac fibroblasts and extracellular matrix deposition *in vivo* and *in vitro*. *Cell Signal.* (2018) 46:145–53. doi: 10.1016/j.cellsig.2018.03.005
24. Hu J, Gao C, Wei C, Xue Y, Shao C, Hao Y, et al. RBFox2-miR-34a-Jph2 axis contributes to cardiac decompensation during heart failure. *Proc Natl Acad Sci USA.* (2019) 116:6172–80. doi: 10.1073/pnas.1822176116
25. Wang X, Yuan B, Cheng B, Liu Y, Zhang B, Wang X, et al. Crocin alleviates myocardial Ischemia/Reperfusion-Induced endoplasmic reticulum stress *via* regulation of miR-34a/Sirt1/Nrf2 pathway. *Shock.* (2019) 51:123–30. doi: 10.1097/SHK.0000000000001116
26. Xu Y, Xu Y, Zhu Y, Sun H, Juguilon C, Li F, et al. Macrophage miR-34a is a key regulator of cholesterol efflux and atherosclerosis. *Mol Ther.* (2020) 28:202–16. doi: 10.1016/j.ymthe.2019.09.008
27. Li X, Lu Z, Zhou F, Jin W, Yang Y, Chen S, et al. Indoxyl sulfate promotes the atherosclerosis through up-regulating the miR-34a expression in endothelial cells and vascular smooth muscle cells in vitro. *Vasc Pharmacol.* (2020) 131:106763. doi: 10.1016/j.vph.2020.106763
28. Toshima T, Watanabe T, Narumi T, Otaki Y, Shishido T, Aono T, et al. Therapeutic inhibition of microRNA-34a ameliorates aortic valve calcification *via* modulation of Notch1-Runx2 signalling. *Cardiovasc Res.* (2020) 116:983–94. doi: 10.1093/cvr/cvz210
29. Dorn GN. MiR-34a and the cardiomyopathy of senescence: SALT PNUTS, SALT PNUTS! *Cell Metab.* (2013) 17:629–30. doi: 10.1016/j.cmet.2013.04.004
30. Natarajan SK, Stringham BA, Mohr AM, Wehrkamp CJ, Lu S, Phillippi MA, et al. FoxO3 increases miR-34a to cause palmitate-induced cholangiocyte lipoapoptosis. *J Lipid Res.* (2017) 58:866–75. doi: 10.1194/jlr.M071357
31. Zhang FM, Zheng WH, Wang HJ. MiR-34a-5p inhibition attenuates LPS-induced endothelial cell injury by targeting FOXM1. *Eur Rev Med Pharmacol Sci.* (2020) 24:10829–38. doi: 10.26355/eurrev_202010_23445
32. Del RD, Amgalan D, Linkermann A, Liu Q, Kitsis RN. Fundamental mechanisms of regulated cell death and implications for heart disease. *Physiol Rev.* (2019) 99:1765–817. doi: 10.1152/physrev.00022.2018
33. Ventura A, Kirsch DG, McLaughlin ME, Tuveson DA, Grimm J, Lintault L, et al. Restoration of p53 function leads to tumour regression *in vivo*. *Nature.* (2007) 445:661–5. doi: 10.1038/nature05541
34. Mak TW, Hauck L, Grothe D, Billia F. P53 regulates the cardiac transcriptome. *Proc Natl Acad Sci USA.* (2017) 114:2331–6. doi: 10.1073/pnas.1621436114
35. Fu BC, Lang JL, Zhang DY, Sun L, Chen W, Liu W, et al. Suppression of miR-34a expression in the myocardium protects against Ischemia-Reperfusion injury through SIRT1 protective pathway. *Stem Cells Dev.* (2017) 26:1270–82. doi: 10.1089/scd.2017.0062
36. Liang Y, Liu H, Zhu J, Song N, Lu Z, Fang Y, et al. Inhibition of p53/miR-34a/SIRT1 axis ameliorates podocyte injury in diabetic nephropathy. *Biochem Bioph Res Co.* (2021) 559:48–55. doi: 10.1016/j.bbrc.2021.04.025
37. Yacoub R, Lee K, He JC. The role of SIRT1 in diabetic kidney disease. *Front Endocrinol.* (2014) 5:166. doi: 10.3389/fendo.2014.00166
38. Shi K, Sun H, Zhang H, Xie D, Yu B. MiR-34a-5p aggravates hypoxia-induced apoptosis by targeting ZEB1 in cardiomyocytes. *Biol Chem.* (2019) 400:227–36. doi: 10.1515/hsz-2018-0195
39. Fomison-Nurse I, Saw E, Gandhi S, Munasinghe PE, Van Hout I, Williams M, et al. Diabetes induces the activation of pro-ageing miR-34a in the heart, but has differential effects on cardiomyocytes and cardiac progenitor cells. *Cell Death Differ.* (2018) 25:1336–49. doi: 10.1038/s41418-017-0047-6

40. Wang SP, Wang D, Li HX, Liu L, Duan XH. Influence of miR-34a on cerebral neuronal apoptosis in rats with cerebral ischemia reperfusion through the Notchl signaling pathway. *Eur Rev Med Pharmacol Sci.* (2019) 23:8049–57. doi: 10.26355/eurrev_201909_19021
41. Wu X, Wang L, Wang K, Li J, Chen R, Wu X, et al. ADAR2 increases in exercised heart and protects against myocardial infarction and doxorubicin-induced cardiotoxicity. *Mol Ther.* (2021) 30:1–15. doi: 10.1016/j.ymthe.2021.07.004
42. Bharath LP, Rockhold JD, Conway R. Selective autophagy in Hyperglycemia-Induced microvascular and macrovascular diseases. *Cells-Basel.* (2021) 10:2114. doi: 10.3390/cells10082114
43. Qiao P, Yao L, Zeng Z. Catalpol-mediated microRNA-34a suppresses autophagy and malignancy by regulating SIRT1 in colorectal cancer. *Oncol Rep.* (2020) 43:1053–66. doi: 10.3892/or.2020.7494
44. Ni T, Lin N, Lu W, Sun Z, Lin H, Chi J, et al. Dihydromyricetin prevents diabetic cardiomyopathy *via* miR-34a suppression by activating autophagy. *Cardiovasc Drugs Ther.* (2020) 34:291–301. doi: 10.1007/s10557-020-06968-0
45. Shao H, Yang L, Wang L, Tang B, Wang J, Li Q. MicroRNA-34a protects myocardial cells against ischemia-reperfusion injury through inhibiting autophagy *via* regulating TNFalpha expression. *Biochem Cell Biol.* (2018) 96:349–54. doi: 10.1139/bcb-2016-0158
46. Lv X, Wang K, Tang W, Yu L, Cao H, Chi W, et al. MiR-34a-5p was involved in chronic intermittent hypoxia-induced autophagy of human coronary artery endothelial cells *via* Bcl-2/beclin 1 signal transduction pathway. *J Cell Biochem.* (2019) 120:18871–82. doi: 10.1002/jcb.29207
47. Raucci A, Vinci MC. MiR-34a: A promising target for inflammaging and Age-Related diseases. *Int J Mol Sci.* (2020) 21:8293. doi: 10.3390/ijms21218293
48. Hu Y, Xia W, Hou M. Macrophage migration inhibitory factor serves a pivotal role in the regulation of radiation-induced cardiac senescencethrough rebalancing the microRNA-34a/sirtuin 1 signaling pathway. *Int J Mol Med.* (2018) 42:2849–58. doi: 10.3892/ijmm.2018.3838
49. Li T, Pang Q, Liu Y, Bai M, Peng Y, Zhang Z. Sulforaphane protects human umbilical vein endothelial cells from oxidative stress *via* the miR-34a/SIRT1 axis by upregulating nuclear factor erythroid-2-related factor 2. *Exp Ther Med.* (2021) 21:186. doi: 10.3892/etm.2021.9617
50. Panizzi P, Swirski FK, Figueiredo JL, Waterman P, Sosnovik DE, Aikawa E, et al. Impaired infarct healing in atherosclerotic mice with Ly-6C(hi) monocytosis. *J Am Coll Cardiol.* (2010) 55:1629–38. doi: 10.1016/j.jacc.2009.08.089
51. Ridker PM, Libby P, MacFadyen JG, Thuren T, Ballantyne C, Fonseca F, et al. Modulation of the interleukin-6 signalling pathway and incidence rates of atherosclerotic events and all-cause mortality: Analyses from the Canakinumab Anti-Inflammatory Thrombosis Outcomes Study (CANTOS). *Eur Heart J.* (2018) 39:3499–507. doi: 10.1093/eurheartj/ehy310
52. Shi YY, Ma YH, Zhang R, Li RS. Downregulation of miR-34a ameliorates inflammatory response and apoptosis induced by renal ischemia-reperfusion by promoting Kruppel-like factor 4 expression. *Eur Rev Med Pharmacol Sci.* (2020) 24:11683–9. doi: 10.26355/eurrev_202011_23813
53. Xia W, Zou C, Chen H, Xie C, Hou M. Immune checkpoint inhibitor induces cardiac injury through polarizing macrophages *via* modulating microRNA-34a/Kruppel-like factor 4 signaling. *Cell Death Dis.* (2020) 11:2778. doi: 10.1038/s41419-020-02778-2
54. Li H, Hastings MH, Rhee J, Trager LE, Roh JD, Rosenzweig A. Targeting Age-Related pathways in heart failure. *Circ Res.* (2020) 126:533–51. doi: 10.1161/CIRCRESAHA.119.315889
55. Raucci A, Macri F, Castiglione S, Badi I, Vinci MC, Zuccolo E. MicroRNA-34a: The bad guy in age-related vascular diseases. *Cell Mol Life Sci.* (2021) 78:7355–78. doi: 10.1007/s00018-021-03979-4
56. Yan P, Li Q, Wang L, Lu P, Suzuki K, Liu Z, et al. FOXO3-Engineered human ESC-Derived vascular cells promote vascular protection and regeneration. *Cell Stem Cell.* (2019) 24:447–61.e8. doi: 10.1016/j.stem.2018.12.002
57. Bacmeister L, Schwarzl M, Warnke S, Stoffers B, Blankenberg S, Westermann D, et al. Inflammation and fibrosis in murine models of heart failure. *Basic Res Cardiol.* (2019) 114:19. doi: 10.1007/s00395-019-0722-5
58. Verjans R, van Bilsen M, Schroen B. MiRNA deregulation in cardiac aging and associated disorders. *Int Rev Cell Mol Biol.* (2017) 334:207–63. doi: 10.1016/bs.ircmb.2017.03.004
59. Bian W, Tian F, Jiang L, Sun Y, Wu S, Gao B, et al. Influence of miR-34a on myocardial apoptosis in rats with acute myocardial infarction through the ERK1/2 pathway. *Eur Rev Med Pharmaco.* (2019) 23:3034–41. doi: 10.26355/eurrev_201904_17585
60. Wenlan L, Zhongyuan X, Shaoqing L, Liying Z, Bo Z, Min L. MiR-34a-5p mediates sevoflurane preconditioning induced inhibition of hypoxia/reoxygenation injury through STX1A in cardiomyocytes. *Biomed Pharmacother.* (2018) 102:153–9. doi: 10.1016/j.biopha.2018.03.002
61. Weng CF, Wu CF, Kao SH, Chen JC, Lin HH. Down-Regulation of miR-34a-5p potentiates protective effect of Adipose-Derived mesenchymal stem cells against ischemic myocardial infarction by stimulating the expression of C1q/Tumor necrosis Factor-Related protein-9. *Front Physiol.* (2019) 10:1445. doi: 10.3389/fphys.2019.01445
62. Chen Q, Yang F, Guo M, Wen G, Zhang C, Luong LA, et al. MiRNA-34a reduces neointima formation through inhibiting smooth muscle cell proliferation and migration. *J Mol Cell Cardiol.* (2015) 89:75–86. doi: 10.1016/j.yjmcc.2015.10.017
63. Wang P, Xu J, Hou Z, Wang F, Song Y, Wang J, et al. MiRNA-34a promotes proliferation of human pulmonary artery smooth muscle cells by targeting PDGFRA. *Cell Proliferat.* (2016) 49:484–93. doi: 10.1111/cpr.12265
64. Wang Q, Yu X, Dou L, Huang X, Zhu K, Guo J, et al. MiR-154-5p functions as an important regulator of angiotensin II-Mediated heart remodeling. *Oxid Med Cell Longev.* (2019) 2019:8768164. doi: 10.1155/2019/8768164
65. Zhang XL, Zhang G, Bai ZH. MiR-34a attenuates myocardial fibrosis in diabetic cardiomyopathy mice *via* targeting Pin-1. *Cell Biol Int.* (2021) 45:642–53. doi: 10.1002/cbin.11512
66. Reed GW, Rossi JE, Cannon CP. Acute myocardial infarction. *Lancet.* (2017) 389:197–210. doi: 10.1016/S0140-6736(16)30677-8
67. Xiao Y, Zhao J, Tuazon JP, Borlongan CV, Yu G. MicroRNA-133a and myocardial infarction. *Cell Transplant.* (2019) 28:831–8. doi: 10.1177/0963689719843806
68. Li JH, Dai J, Han B, Wu GH, Wang CH. MiR-34a regulates cell apoptosis after myocardial infarction in rats through the Wnt/beta-catenin signaling pathway. *Eur Rev Med Pharmacol Sci.* (2019) 23:2555–62. doi: 10.26355/eurrev_201903_17404
69. Lin JM, Hsu CH, Chen JC, Kao SH, Lin YC. BCL-6 promotes the methylation of miR-34a by recruiting EZH2 and upregulating CTRP9 to protect ischemic myocardial injury. *Biofactors.* (2021) 47:386–402. doi: 10.1002/biof.1704
70. Konno M, Koseki J, Asai A, Yamagata A, Shimamura T, Motooka D, et al. Distinct methylation levels of mature microRNAs in gastrointestinal cancers. *Nat Commun.* (2019) 10:3888. doi: 10.1038/s41467-019-11826-1
71. Lv P, Zhou M, He J, Meng W, Ma X, Dong S, et al. Circulating miR-208b and miR-34a are associated with left ventricular remodeling after acute myocardial infarction. *Int J Mol Sci.* (2014) 15:5774–88. doi: 10.3390/ijms15045774
72. Matsumoto S, Sakata Y, Suna S, Nakatani D, Usami M, Hara M, et al. Circulating p53-Responsive MicroRNAs are predictive indicators of heart failure after acute myocardial infarction. *Circ Res.* (2013) 113:322–6. doi: 10.1161/CIRCRESAHA.113.301209
73. Zhou R, Wang L, Zhao G, Chen D, Song X, Momtazi Borojeni AA, et al. Circulating exosomalmicroRNAs as emerging non-invasive clinical biomarkers in heart failure: Mega bio-roles of a nano bio-particle. *Iubmb Life.* (2020) 72:2546–62. doi: 10.1002/iub.2396
74. Xia YW, Wang SB. Microvesicles containing microRNA-21 induce myocardial fibrosis *via* AKT pathway. *Eur Rev Med Pharmacol Sci.* (2018) 22:4634–41. doi: 10.26355/eurrev_201807_15522
75. Vilahur G, Juan-Babot O, Pena E, Onate B, Casani L, Badimon L. Molecular and cellular mechanisms involved in cardiac remodeling after acute myocardial infarction. *J Mol Cell Cardiol.* (2011) 50:522–33. doi: 10.1016/j.yjmcc.2010.12.021
76. Wang Z, Wang Z, Wang T, Yuan J, Wang X, Zhang Z. Inhibition of miR-34a-5p protected myocardial ischemia reperfusion injury-induced apoptosis and reactive oxygen species accumulation through regulation of Notch Receptor 1 signaling. *Rev Cardiovasc Med.* (2019) 20:187–97. doi: 10.31083/j.rcm.2019.03.545

77. Ghafouri-Fard S, Shoorei H, Taheri M. Non-coding RNAs participate in the ischemia-reperfusion injury. *Biomed Pharmacother.* (2020) 129:110419. doi: 10.1016/j.biopha.2020.110419
78. Braunwald E. Cardiomyopathies: An overview. *Circ Res.* (2017) 121:711–21. doi: 10.1161/CIRCRESAHA.117.311812
79. Dadson K, Hauck L, Billia F. Molecular mechanisms in cardiomyopathy. *Clin Sci (Lond).* (2017) 131:1375–92. doi: 10.1042/CS20160170
80. Tan Y, Zhang Z, Zheng C, Wintergerst KA, Keller BB, Cai L. Mechanisms of diabetic cardiomyopathy and potential therapeutic strategies: Preclinical and clinical evidence. *Nat Rev Cardiol.* (2020) 17:585–607. doi: 10.1038/s41569-020-0339-2
81. Gao L, Wang X, Guo S, Xiao L, Liang C, Wang Z, et al. LncRNA HOTAIR functions as a competing endogenous RNA to upregulate SIRT1 by sponging miR-34a in diabetic cardiomyopathy. *J Cell Physiol.* (2019) 234:4944–58. doi: 10.1002/jcp.27296
82. Costantino S, Paneni F, Luscher TF, Cosentino F. MicroRNA profiling unveils hyperglycaemic memory in the diabetic heart. *Eur Heart J.* (2016) 37:572–6. doi: 10.1093/eurheartj/ehv599
83. Sun Y, Ren J, Wu WZ. Effect of MiR-34a on hypertension-induced hypertrophic cardiomyopathy in rats *via* the TGF-beta1/Smads signaling pathway. *Minerva Med.* (2021) 112:405–6. doi: 10.23736/S0026-4806.19.06192-5
84. Bernardo BC, Gao XM, Tham YK, Kiriazis H, Winbanks CE, Ooi JY, et al. Silencing of miR-34a attenuates cardiac dysfunction in a setting of moderate, but not severe, hypertrophic cardiomyopathy. *PLoS ONE.* (2014) 9:e90337. doi: 10.1371/journal.pone.0090337
85. Feinberg MW, Moore KJ. MicroRNA regulation of atherosclerosis. *Circ Res.* (2016) 118:703–20. doi: 10.1161/CIRCRESAHA.115.306300
86. Ito T, Yagi S, Yamakuchi M. MicroRNA-34a regulation of endothelial senescence. *Biochem Biophys Res Commun.* (2010) 398:735–40. doi: 10.1016/j.bbrc.2010.07.012
87. Su G, Sun G, Liu H, Shu L, Liang Z. Downregulation of miR-34a promotes endothelial cell growth and suppresses apoptosis in atherosclerosis by regulating Bcl-2. *Heart Vessels.* (2018) 33:1185–94. doi: 10.1007/s00380-018-1169-6
88. Gatsiou A, Georgiopoulos G, Vlachogiannis NI, Pfisterer L, Fischer A, Sachse M, et al. Additive contribution of microRNA-34a/b/c to human arterial ageing and atherosclerosis. *Atherosclerosis.* (2021) 327:49–58. doi: 10.1016/j.atherosclerosis.2021.05.005
89. Liu S, Yi F, Cheng W, Qu X, Wang C. Molecular mechanisms in vascular injury induced by hypertension: Expression and role of microRNA-34a. *Exp Ther Med.* (2017) 14:5497–502. doi: 10.3892/etm.2017.5216
90. Liu Y, Dong Y, Dong Z, Song J, Zhang Z, Liang L, et al. Expression profiles of circular RNA in aortic vascular tissues of spontaneously hypertensive rats. *Front Cardiovasc Med.* (2021) 8:814402. doi: 10.3389/fcvm.2021.814402
91. Liu R, Yang L, Wei Q. MiR-34a targets PAI-1 to regulate urinary microalbumin and renal function in hypertensive mice. *Eur J Med Res.* (2020) 25:7. doi: 10.1186/s40001-020-00404-7
92. Martinez-Arroyo O, Ortega A, Galera M, Solaz E, Martinez-Hervas S, Redon J, et al. Decreased urinary levels of SIRT1 as non-invasive biomarker of early renal damage in hypertension. *Int J Mol Sci.* (2020) 21:6390. doi: 10.3390/ijms21176390
93. Zhu Y, Feng Z, Cheng W, Xiao Y. MicroRNA34a mediates atrial fibrillation through regulation of AnkyrinB expression. *Mol Med Rep.* (2018) 17:8457–65. doi: 10.3892/mmr.2018.8873
94. Wang H, Chen Y, Tao T, Zhao X, Wang Y, Luo J, et al. Identification of microRNA biomarkers in serum of patients at different stages of atrial fibrillation. *Heart Lung.* (2020) 49:902–8. doi: 10.1016/j.hrtlng.2020.03.021
95. Xiao S, Zhou Y, Liu A, Wu Q, Hu Y, Liu J, et al. Uncovering potential novel biomarkers and immune infiltration characteristics in persistent atrial fibrillation using integrated bioinformatics analysis. *Math Biosci Eng.* (2021) 18:4696–712. doi: 10.3934/mbe.2021238
96. Xu J, Zhang G, Luo X, Wang D, Zhou W, Zhang Y, et al. Co-delivery of 5-fluorouracil and miRNA-34a mimics by host-guest self-assembly nanocarriers for efficacious targeted therapy in colorectal cancer patient-derived tumor xenografts. *Theranostics.* (2021) 11:2475–89. doi: 10.7150/thno.52076
97. Jafari N, Abediankenari S, Hossein-Nataj H. MiR-34a mimic or pre-mir-34a, which is the better option for cancer therapy? KatoIII as a model to study miRNA action in human gastric cancer cells. *Cancer Cell Int.* (2021) 21:178. doi: 10.1186/s12935-021-01872-5
98. Iekushi K, Seeger F, Assmus B, Zeiher AM, Dimmeler S. Regulation of cardiac microRNAs by bone marrow mononuclear cell therapy in myocardial infarction. *Circulation.* (2012) 125:1765–73. doi: 10.1161/CIRCULATIONAHA.111.079699
99. Bernardo BC, Ooi JY, Matsumoto A, Tham YK, Singla S, Kiriazis H, et al. Sex differences in response to miRNA-34a therapy in mouse models of cardiac disease: Identification of sex-, disease- and treatment-regulated miRNAs. *J Physiol.* (2016) 594:5959–74. doi: 10.1113/JP272512
100. Ooi JYY, Bernardo BC, Singla S, Patterson NL, Lin RCY, McMullen JR. Identification of miR-34 regulatory networks in settings of disease and antimiR-therapy: Implications for treating cardiac pathology and other diseases. *RNA Biol.* (2017) 14:500–13. doi: 10.1080/15476286.2016.1181251

8

Impaired Left Atrial Performance Resulting from Age-Related Arial Fibrillation is Associated with Increased Fibrosis Burden: Insights from a Clinical Study Combining with an *in vivo* Experiment

Kai-bin Lin [1†], Kan-kai Chen [1†], Shuai Li [1†], Ming-qi Cai [1], Min-jie Yuan [1], Yan-peng Wang [1], Xue Zhang [1], Meng Wei [1], Mei-Ling Yan [2], Xin-Xin Ma [3], Dong-Yan Zheng [3], Qi-han Wu [4], Jing-bo Li [1] and Dong Huang [1*]*

[1] Heart Center, Shanghai Jiaotong University Affiliated Sixth People's Hospital, School of Medicine, Shanghai Jiaotong University, Shanghai, China, [2] Department of Cardiology, Huadong Hospital, Fudan University, Shanghai, China, [3] Department of Ultrasound in Medicine, Shanghai Jiao Tong University Affiliated Sixth People's Hospital, Shanghai Institute of Ultrasound in Medicine, School of Medicine, Shanghai Jiaotong University, Shanghai, China, [4] NHC Key Lab of Reproduction Regulation (Shanghai Institute of Planned Parenthood Research), Fudan University, Shanghai, China

***Correspondence:**
Dong Huang
huangdong1004@126.com
Jing-bo Li
lijb@sjtu.edu.cn

† These authors have contributed equally to this work

Background: Atrial fibrillation (AF) is increasingly considered an age-related degenerative disease, whose process is associated with the development of impaired left atrial (LA) performance. However, the subtle dynamic changes of LA performance in AF during aging have yet to be fully elucidated. Atrial fibrosis is a key substrate for the development of AF, but the progression of fibrosis during aging and its relationship with LA dysfunction need to be further explored.

Methods: A total of 132 control individuals and 117 persistent AF patients were prospectively studied. Subjects were further stratified into three age groups (age group 1: younger than 65 years, age group 2: between 65 and 79 years old, and age group 3: older than 80 years). The two-dimensional speckle tracking imaging was carried out for analyzing the alterations in LA function underlying LA remodeling, whereas electroanatomic mapping was performed to investigate LA fibrosis burden. In animal study, aged mice and young mice served as research subjects. Echocardiography and histological staining were used to assess LA performance and fibrosis burden, respectively.

Results: Echocardiography showed progressive increases in LA dimension and LA stiffness index, and progressive decreases in LA global longitudinal strain and LA strain rates with advancing age in both AF and control cohorts, which was more prominent in AF cohort. Electroanatomic mapping showed progressive decrease in mean LA voltage and progressive increases in LA surface area, low-voltage area %, and LA volume with advancing age, whereas more significant alterations were observed in AF patients. Moreover, left atrial global longitudinal strain was positively correlated with mean LA voltage, whereas LA stiffness index was negatively related to mean LA voltage. In animal experiment, increased LA size and pulmonary artery dimension as well as longer P-wave duration and more prominent LA fibrosis were found in aged mice.

Conclusions: This study provides new evidence of subtle changes in structure and performance of left atrium and their association with atrial fibrosis in both AF and non-AF subjects during physiological aging. In addition, our study also provides normal values for LA structure and performance in both AF and non-AF conditions during aging. These measurements may provide an early marker for onset of AF and LA adverse remodeling.

Keywords: age, atrial fibrillation, fibrosis, left atrium performance, echocardiography

INTRODUCTION

Atrial fibrillation (AF) is a common arrhythmia associated with severe adverse clinical outcomes in practice. The incidence of AF ascends sharply with age, casting a heavy burden on health care systems (1). It was predicted that more than 8.3 million patients over the age of 60 will suffer from AF by the year 2030 in China (2). When AF is refractory and sustains with age, afflicted patients tend to develop severe left atrial (LA) dysfunction and heart failure with preserved ejection fraction (3).

Atrial fibrosis is the hallmark of structural remodeling in AF and is considered as the substrate for AF perpetuation (4). Aging contributes to the development of atrial fibrosis, which in turn impairs cardiac function (5). However, an early study illustrated that the degree of atrial fibrosis measured in magnetic resonance imaging was independent of AF duration (6). Furthermore, human autopsy studies indicated aging has a limited contribution to fibrosis development in AF patients (7, 8). When it comes to *in vitro* experiment, it was demonstrated that collagen incubation resulted in shortened action potential duration of pulmonary vein cardiomyocytes (9). However, aging independently prolonged atrial effective refractory period in human (10). Thus, there is a considerable controversy regarding the relationship between AF and fibrosis in the context of aging.

LA strain analysis allows us to quantify subtle cardiac alterations objectively under the background of physiological aging (11–13). Meanwhile, LA strain is applied to appraise the AF burden derived from atrial fibrosis (14). However, integrative analysis of the effect of aging and AF on LA function and their association with atrial fibrosis burden is still limited so far. The aim of the present clinical study was to demonstrate the impact of age-related AF on LA performance and characterize the relationship between LA dysfunction and atrial fibrosis burden. Additionally, animal experiments were also carried out in attempt to elucidating the overall mutual links in deep.

METHODS

Participants Enrollment

The clinical study was a prospective, single-center study designed to evaluate the alterations of LA function and fibrosis burden in age-related AF patients. It was registered at http://www.chictr.org.cn/index.aspx (ChiCTR-ROC-17011691). The individuals referred to Shanghai Jiaotong University affiliated Shanghai Sixth People's Hospital for catheter ablation between January 2017 and June 2020 were recruited for this study. The control candidates were defined as the patients who received ablation for supraventricular tachycardia with left accessory pathway, severe vasovagal syncope, or lone premature atrial contractions. Persistent AF was defined according to the 2014 American Heart Association/American College of Cardiology/Heart Rhythm Society and 2016 Focused Update of Canadian Cardiovascular Society guidelines for management of the patients with AF (15, 16). Patients with persistent AF undergoing initial catheter ablation were recruited to the AF group. The patients were excluded if diagnosed with or had a previous history of rheumatic heart diseases, cardiac surgery, ST-segment elevated myocardial infarction, and severe heart failure.

All patients were further stratified into three subgroups according to age: age group 1 (<65 years old), age group 2 (between 65 and 79 years old), and age group 3 (>80 years old).

Human Echocardiographic Assessment

In order to assess the LA performance with or without AF at different ages, all participants underwent echocardiography examination before ablation. The procedure was conducted as described in our previous study (17). The measurements of two-dimensional and tissue Doppler echocardiographic parameters, including LA dimension (LAD), left ventricular end-diastolic dimension (LVEDD), left ventricular end-diastolic posterior wall thickness, left ventricular septal wall thickness, left ventricular ejection fraction (LVEF), pulmonary artery dimension (PAD), E peak velocity and A peak velocity, were carried out using commercially available iE33 instruments (Philips Medical Systems, Koninklijke, the Netherlands) according to the guideline of the American Society of Echocardiography and the European Association of Cardiovascular Imaging (18–20). Left ventricular mass (LVM) index is calculated according to Devereux formula [LVM index = (LVM)/body surface area]. The measurement of LVM is according to the recommendations (18). Then two-dimensional speckle tracking echocardiography was performed offline by analysis of gray-scale images (four-chamber views) using commercially available software (TomTec Imaging Systems GmbH, Unterschleissheim, Germany). LA endocardial borders were manually traced in four-chamber and two-chamber views (**Figure 1A**), and LA was divided into six segments subsequently (**Figure 1B**). The software then generated longitudinal deformation curves and measured the mean values of strain and strain rates. Average of at least three beats was

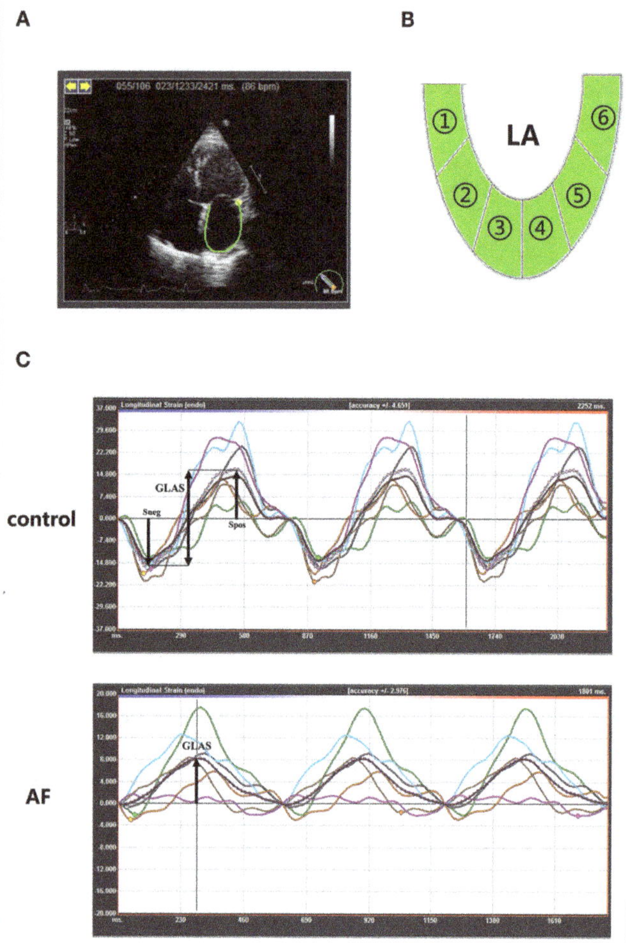

FIGURE 1 | Speckle-tracking echocardiography to quantify LA strain in control and AF patients at three age groups. **(A)** Representative apical four-chamber view echocardiogram of a control adult. Along the inner contour of the LA wall, we define the target region. **(B)** The six segments of the LA wall were into strain analysis. **(C)** The strain curves of six segments and average strain curve (dotted line). The GLAS of control patients were defined Spos minus Sneg. In AF patients, GLAS was identified as the value of Spos. GLAS, left atrial global longitudinal strain; Spos, longitudinal peak early-diastole strain; Sneg, longitudinal peak late-diastole strain.

taken in per measurement process. LA strain rates (SRa, SRe, and SRs) and LA global longitudinal strain were analyzed to evaluate LA performance. The LA global longitudinal strain (GLAS) was calculated as the value of longitudinal peak early-diastole strain (Spos, positive peak strain) minus longitudinal peak late-diastole strain (Sneg, negative peak strain). Because of impaired atrial contractility during AF rhythm, Sneg was close to 0. GLAS of AF patients was identified as the value of Spos (**Figure 1C**). On this basis, LA stiffness index based on strain imaging was defined as the ratio of E/e′ to GLAS [LA stiffness index = (E/e′ ratio)/GLAS] as demonstrated previously (21). All the procedures were performed by two fixed operators.

In this study, we also assessed all parameters' variability in a randomly selected subset of 10 patients referred to our previous study (17). The variability coefficients were all lower than 10% for all measurements in both interobserver and intraobserver analyses.

Electroanatomic Mapping

The mapping procedure of all enrolled adults was performed to appraise atrial fibrosis burden. Ensite NAVX system (Abbott, Chicago, IL, USA) was used for the reconstruction and voltage mapping. The mean voltage of LA was defined as the mean value of six-position voltage, including the roof and bottom of LA, anterior LA wall, posterior LA wall, lateral LA wall, and LA appendage. Abbott's 10-pole ring electrodes (81594, Abbott) were used in the measurement process. The fibrosis area was defined as the low-voltage area (LVA) whose endocardial bipolar voltage values were lower than 0.5 mV, observed in at least three adjacent voltage points as previously reported in our study (22). Electrogram quality was assessed by consensus of two experienced observers. A stable contact between the local atrial tissue and the parallel-aligned tip of the ablation catheter was required. The mapping points that displayed poor contact or an unstable electrogram signal were excluded. Quantitative evaluation of LA volume and mean LA voltage were assessed using three-dimensional mapping using standardized software (Abbott). The proportion of LVA in LA surface area (LVA%) was calculated as the formulate (LVA% $= \frac{sum\ of\ LVA}{LA\ surface\ area} * 100\%$). All individuals were graded based on the proportion of LVA (LVA%): non-LVA, mild (LVA% $\leq$10%), moderate (LVA% 10%–<20%), and severe (LVA% $\geq$20%) as the grading algorithm proposed by Wang et al. (23).

Animal Study Protocol

Young mice (3 months old) and senescent mice (27 months old) (C57BL/6, SIPPR-BK Laboratory Animal Co. Ltd., Shanghai, China) were used to evaluate the LA performance by high-frequency ultrasound following inhalation anesthesia of isoflurane (n = 15 for each group). Then, surface electrocardiogram (ECG) parameters were measured. Finally, they were sacrificed by cervical dislocation, and organs were immediately harvested.

Animal Echocardiographic Assessment

Echocardiography was performed using Vevo 770 imaging system (VisualSonics, Toronto, Ontario, Canada) equipped with a 30-MHz high-frequency scan head. During mild isoflurane anesthesia, the measurement procedure and ordinary echocardiographic parameters refer to a previous work (24). LA size was assessed under the apical four-chamber view. PAD was further measured under parasternal left ventricular long-axis view.

ECG Parameter Recording

All mice were anesthetized with 1% sodium pentobarbital at a dose of 0.1 mg/g. Surface limb leads were recorded continuously during the study through electrodes. ECG was shown and filtered (0.5–250 Hz) with a multiple electroconductive physiological recorder (Hongtong, Shanghai, China). ECG recordings at baseline were made at 100–400 mm/s paper speed. RR interval, P-wave duration, PR interval, and QT interval were calculated in lead II.

Fibrosis Area Measurement

Masson trichrome-stained sections were carried out to examine cardiac collagen accumulation. Collagen area fraction was determined as previously reported (25).

Statistical Analysis

Continuous variables were expressed as mean ± standard deviation for normally distributed data. Other continuous variables were presented as median (25th−75th percentile). Statistical significance of differences between groups was assessed using Student *t*-test for data or analysis of variance with normal distribution. Differences between quantitative non-normal variables were studied by non-parametric tests (Kruskal–Wallis *H*-test). All categorical variables were presented as frequencies and percentage, and the χ^2-test or Fisher exact test was used, as appropriate. Mantel-Haenszel χ^2-test was used to measure the correlation between two ordinal categorical variables. Pearson correlation was computed to evaluate the associations between two continuous variables. Stepwise multiple regression analysis was performed to evaluate the presence of collinearity for factors and determine the predictors for target continuous variables. Statistical analyses were performed using SPSS, version 17.0.2 (SPSS, Inc., Chicago, IL, USA). All P values were two-sided, and $P < 0.05$ was considered statistically significant.

RESULTS

Participants' Characteristics

A total of 303 candidates were enrolled. Fifty-four subjects were excluded because of poor image quality. The study cohort included 132 control individuals (supraventricular tachycardia with left accessory pathway for ablation: 42 cases; severe vasovagal syncope for catheter ablation of ganglionated plexi: 18 cases; premature atrial contractions for ablation: 72 cases) and 117 persistent AF patients, respectively. The clinical characteristics of the patients are presented in **Table 1**. In the AF group, AF duration prolonged with advanced age (age group 2 vs. age group 1, age group 3 vs. age group 2, all $P < 0.05$). There was no significant difference in the gender and BMI between control and AF patients across age-matched subgroups. There were more patients in age group 3 who also suffered from hypertension or diabetes mellitus, as compared with age group 1, with or without the presence of AF (all $P < 0.05$). In the AF group, the elderly patients (age group 2 and age group 3) had higher CHA_2DS_2-VASc scores than that in the young patients (age group 1, all $P < 0.05$). When it came to the HAS-BLED score, a graded increase was observed among different age groups (0.6 ± 0.1 vs. 1.8 ± 0.7 vs. 2.5 ± 1.0, all $P < 0.05$). The exposure to inhibitors of angiotensin-converting enzyme inhibitor/angiotensin receptor blocker, statins, and β-blocker therapy did not differ in the control and AF cohorts or among different age groups.

LA Dysfunction During Aging and the Effect of AF on LA Function

Table 2 summarizes echocardiographic characteristics of control individuals and AF patients in different subgroups. In three age-matched groups, similar LVEF was presented in the control individuals and AF patients. Meanwhile, in both control and AF cohorts, LVEDD, LV mass index, and E velocity remained stable along with age. In the control cohort, the elderly adults (age groups 2 and 3) showed higher A velocity in the comparison with young adults (age group 1), whereas the E/A ratio did not differ across different age groups ($P > 0.05$). PAD and E/e′

TABLE 1 | Baseline characteristics for all subgroups of patients.

	Control (*n* = 132)			AF patients (*n* = 117)		
	Age group 1 *n* = 67	Age group 2 *n* = 43	Age group 3 *n* = 22	Age group 1 *n* = 27	Age group 2 *n* = 48	Age group 3 *n* = 42
Age (year)	48.8 ± 7.5	72.8 ± 4.4	81.9 ± 2.1	54.8 ± 10.3	73.7 ± 5.3	82.1 ± 3.1
Male (%)	40 (59.3%)	24 (55.8%)	13 (59.1%)	17 (62.9%)	28 (58.3%)	24 (57.1%)
Time since diagnosis (month)	NA	NA	NA	8.5 (1–31)	13 (2–44)	18.5 (2–63)
BMI (kg/m^2)	21.7 ± 3.8	20.1 ± 4.9	18.3 ± 6.6	21.8 ± 4.2	20.4 ± 6.9	18.1+4.2
Hypertension, *n* (%)	20 (29.8%)	20 (46.5%)	12 (54.5%)	9 (33.3%)	29 (60.4%)	30 (71.4%)
DM, *n* (%)	8 (11.9%)	13 (30.2%)	7 (31.8%)	6 (22.2%)	10 (25.8%)	23 (54.8%)
CHA_2DS_2-VASc score	NA	NA	NA	1 (0-3)	2 (1–4)	3 (2–5)
HAS-BLED score	NA	NA	NA	0.6 ± 0.1	1.8 ± 0.7	2.5 ± 1.0
ACEI/ARB, *n* (%)	17 (25.4%)	18 (41.9%)	9 (40.9%)	8 (29.6%)	25 (52.1%)	26 (61.9%)
β-Blocker, *n* (%)	35 (52.2%)	26 (60.4%)	14 (63.6%)	12 (44.4%)	27 (56.3%)	26 (61.9%)
Statins, *n* (%)	27 (40.3%)	28 (65.1%)	15 (68.2%)	16 (59.2%)	34 (70.8%)	30 (71.4%)

AF, atrial fibrillation; BMI, body mass index; HF, heart failure; EF, ejection fraction; DM, diabetes mellitus; ACEI, angiotensin-converting enzyme inhibitor; ARB, angiotensin receptor blocker; NA, not applicable.

TABLE 2 | The echocardiographic characteristics for all age groups of patients.

		Control (n = 132)			AF patients (n = 117)			P-value in control individuals	P-value in AF patients
		Age group 1 n = 67	Age group 2 n = 43	Age group 3 n = 22	Age group 1 n = 27	Age group 2 n = 48	Age group 3 n = 42		
LVEF (%)		55.7 ± 6.8	55.9 ± 7.9	55.0 ± 11.8	54.8 ± 6.2	54.6 ± 8.7	53.9 ± 10.3	0.165	0.104
LVEDD (mm)		41.7 ± 2.6	42.4 ± 4.8	42.2 ± 3.5	42.3 ± 1.6	42.5 ± 2.9	42.7 ± 4.6	0.505	0.663
LVM index (g/m^2)		79.8 ± 14.8	80.4 ± 19.7	81.2 ± 18.4	80.9 ± 13.9	80.8 ± 20.7	81.0 ± 25.6	0.150	0.204
E velocity, m/s		0.80 ± 0.29	0.73 ± 0.25	0.73 ± 0.27	0.82 ± 0.22	0.79 ± 0.24†	0.75 ± 0.29†	0.247	0.115
A velocity, m/s		0.61 ± 0.14	0.67 ± 0.20	0.70 ± 0.21	NA	NA	NA	0.060	NA
E/A ratio		1.2 ± 0.4	1.1 ± 0.3	1.0 ± 0.4	NA	NA	NA	0.286	NA
E/e′ ratio		9.6 ± 1.6	9.5 ± 2.3	10.1 ± 2.6	9.8 ± 2.0	10.4 ± 3.9†	10.9 ± 4.0‡	0.074	0.051
PAD (mm)		22.4 ± 2.3	22.1 ± 2.7	23.9 ± 2.8	24.1 ± 3.6	24.2 ± 2.9†	24.9 ± 3.0	0.055	0.087
LAD (mm)		39.7 ± 3.6	41.3 ± 4.6	43.1 ± 5.2	41.7 ± 3.3*	43.1 ± 4.2†	46.4 ± 3.7‡	<0.001	<0.001
GLAS (%)		25.7 ± 7.2	23.2 ± 8.1	12.4 ± 3.6	18.4 ± 4.0***	12.7 ± 3.8†††	6.8 ± 2.1‡‡	<0.001	<0.001
LA stiffness index		0.4 ± 0.1	0.6 ± 0.3	0.9 ± 0.4	0.6 ± 0.2***	0.9 ± 0.4†††	1.6 ± 0.8‡‡‡	<0.001	<0.001
LA strain rate	SRa	−3.1 ± 0.8	−2.8 ± 0.8	−2.5 ± 0.7	−2.2 ± 0.6***	−2.1 ± 0.6†††	−1.4 ± 0.5‡‡‡	<0.001	<0.001
	SRs	2.6 ± 0.8	2.3 ± 0.7	1.9 ± 0.6	2.2 ± 0.6*	1.9 ± 0.6†	1.7 ± 0.4	<0.001	<0.001
	SRe	−2.0 ± 0.5	−1.4 ± 0.5	−1.0 ± 0.4	−1.5 ± 0.5*	−0.9 ± 0.3†††	−0.8 ± 0.3‡	<0.001	<0.001

AF, atrial fibrillation; LAD, left atrial dimension; LVEF, left ventricular ejection fraction; LVEDD, left ventricular end-diastolic dimension; GLAS, left atrial global longitudinal strain; SRs, global longitudinal left atrial stain rate; SRe, global longitudinal early–diastolic left atrial stain rate; SRa, global longitudinal late–diastolic left atrial stain rate; PAD, pulmonary artery dimension. $^*P < 0.05$ vs. control in age group 1; $^{***}P < 0.001$ vs. control in age group 1; $^†P < 0.05$ vs. control in age group 2; $^{†††}P < 0.001$ vs. control in age group 2; $^‡P < 0.05$ vs. control in age group 3; $^{‡‡}P < 0.01$ vs. control in age group 3; $^{‡‡‡}P < 0.001$ vs. control in age group 3. NA, not applicable.

ratio increased with age in both control and AF cohorts (age group 3 vs. age group 1, $P < 0.05$, respectively). Besides, AF patients had a significantly higher E/e′ ratio than control (all $P < 0.05$) in elderly patients (age groups 2 and 3), whereas the difference in PAD was observed only in age group 2. LAD, representing LA size, would help to identify abnormal atrial substrate and estimate the arrhythmia burden (26). A positive correlation between LAD and age was observed (control: r = 0.414; AF: r = 0.424, all $P < 0.001$; **Figure 2A**) Meanwhile, LAD was greater in AF patients compared to the control adults of corresponding age group (all $P < 0.05$; **Figure 2B**). GLAS was found to be negatively correlated with age in both control and AF cohorts (control: $r = -0.568$; AF: $r = -0.807$, all $P < 0.001$; **Figure 2C**), which was more significant in AF cohort (all $P < 0.001$; **Figure 2D**). Besides, stepwise multiple regression analysis showed that considering the covariates of gender, hypertension, and diabetes mellitus, age ($\beta = -0.37$, $P < 0.001$) and AF status ($\beta = -8.13$, $P < 0.001$) were both independently correlated with the GLAS. The LA stiffness index is a novel measure to estimate LA compliance and function (27). In the present study, LA stiffness exhibits a positive correlation with age in both cohorts (control: r = 0.616; AF: r = 0.638, all $P < 0.001$; **Figure 2E**), with the AF cohort showing a higher value than its age-matched control (all $P < 0.001$; **Figure 2F**). As for LA strain rates (SRa, SRs, and SRe), SRa and SRe were negatively correlated with age in both control individuals and AF subjects (SRa, control: $r = -0.381$, AF: $r = -0.335$, all $P < 0.001$; SRe, control: $r = -0.289$, AF: $r = -0.248$, all $P < 0.01$), whereas such correlation was not detected for SRs. It is worth noticing that in patients older than 80 years (age group 3), SRa, SRs, and SRe were all significantly lower in the AF cohort as compared with control cohort.

Evolution of Electrical Characteristics of LA in Patients With AF During Aging

LA electroanatomic mapping was performed to further confirm whether the marked alterations of LA performance were associated with atrial fibrosis in age-related AF patients (**Table 3**). **Figure 3** shows representative evolution patterns of LVA in control individuals and AF patients under the process of physiological aging. LA surface area and LA volume showed proportional increments, along with age, in both AF and control cohorts. Comparing with control subjects, AF patients showed greater LA volume and LA surface area than control subjects in corresponding age groups (**Figures 4A,B**). Mean LA voltage decreased with age in both cohorts, whereas it was lower in AF patients than in control subjects in corresponding age group (**Figure 4C**). In addition, stepwise multiple regression analysis illustrated that age ($\beta = -0.04$, $t = -16.33$, $P < 0.001$) and AF status ($\beta = -1.26$, $t = -19.61$, $P < 0.001$) were independently associated with mean LA voltage after adjustment for other factors (gender, hypertension, and diabetes mellitus). LVA% grades increased with age, irrespective of AF status (control: r = 0.369, AF: r = 0.392, all $P < 0.001$). Besides, in the comparison with age-matched control individuals, AF patients tended to have higher LVA% grades, although we only observed a significant difference in LVA% distribution in age groups 1 and 2 (all $P < 0.05$). Moreover, there was a significant positive linear relation between GLAS and mean LA voltage (control: r = 0.356, $P < 0.001$; AF: r = 0.787, $P < 0.001$; **Figure 4D**),

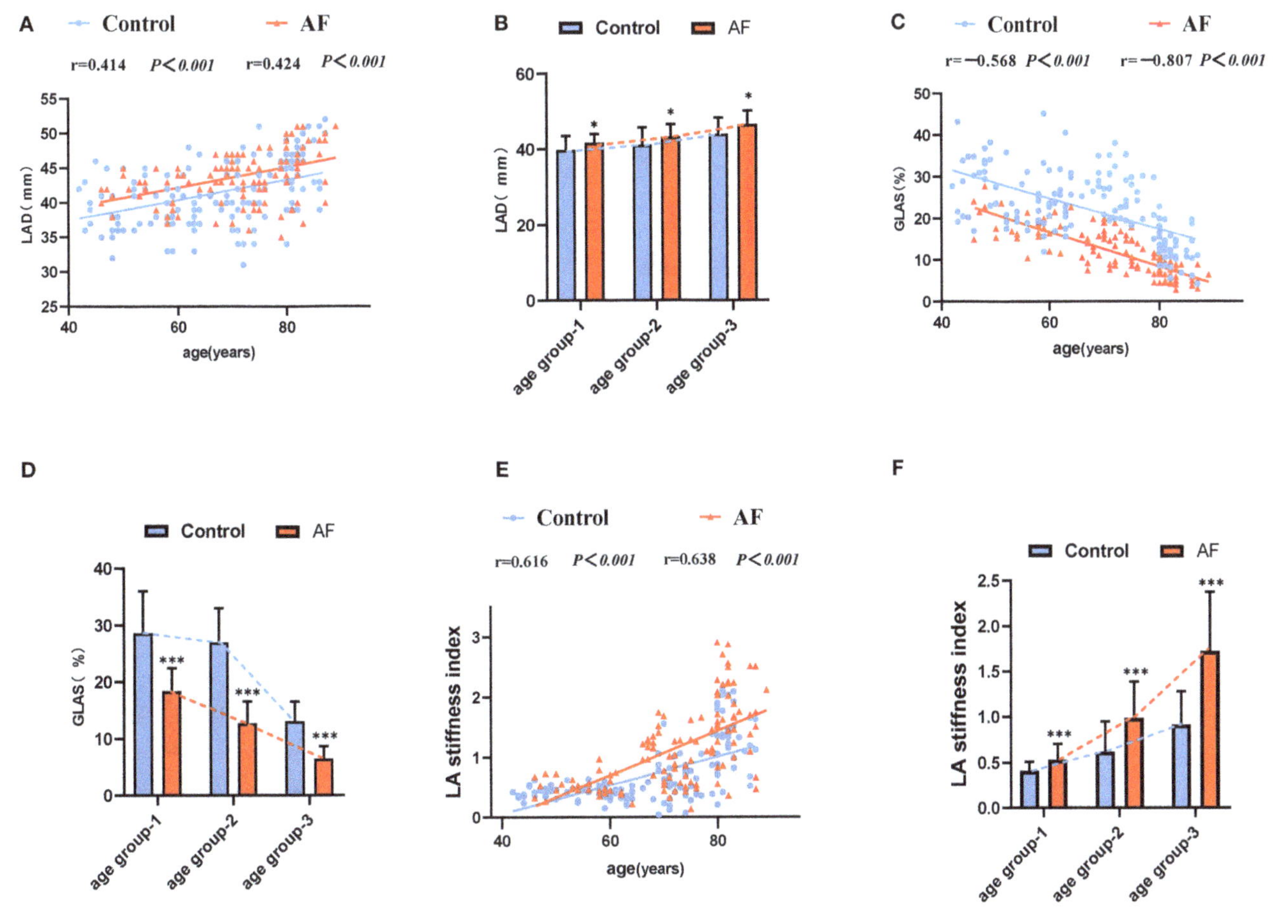

FIGURE 2 | The LA performance in the control individuals and AF patients during physiological aging. **(A)** Correlations of LAD and age in control adults and AF patients. **(B)** The effect of AF on LAD during aging. **(C)** Correlations of GLAS and age in control adults and AF patients. **(D)** The worse GLAS was shown in AF patients during aging. **(E)** A strong positive association between LA stiffness index and age. **(F)** Changes for LA stiffness index in the absence and presence of AF during aging. LAD, left atrial dimension; GLAS, left atrial global longitudinal strain. *$P < 0.05$ vs. control in age-match groups; **$P < 0.01$ vs. control in age-match groups; ***$P < 0.001$ vs. control in age-match groups.

TABLE 3 | The mapping results for all age groups of control and AF patient.

	Control (n = 132)			AF patients (n = 117)			P-value for control individuals	P-value for AF patients
	≤65y n = 67	66–80y n = 43	>80y n = 22	≤65y n = 27	66–80y n = 48	>80y n = 42		
LA surface area (cm^2)	107.1 ± 30.9	146.3 ± 30.9	152.4 ± 63.2	178.4 ± 50.2***	210.6 ± 47.5†††	240.6 ± 63.0‡‡‡	<0.001	<0.001
LA volume (cm^3)	88.6 ± 28.0	100.6 ± 36.0	118.1 ± 43.5	129.0±42.20***	148.7 ± 59.6†††	164.6 ± 63.0‡‡‡	<0.001	0.008
Mean LA voltage (mV)	3.4 ± 0.4	2.8 ± 0.3	1.6 ± 0.7	1.9 ± 0.4***	1.2 ± 0.4†††	1.0 ± 0.4‡‡‡	<0.001	<0.001
LVA% grouping, n (%)								
Non-LVA	63 (94.0%)	36 (83.7%)	13 (59.1%)	17 (62.9%)***	20 (41.6%)†††	8 (19.0%)	<0.001	0.005
Mild LVA	4 (6.0%)	5 (11.6%)	5 (22.7%)	6 (22.2%)	14 (29.17%)	11 (26.2%)		
Moderate LVA	0 (0%)	2 (4.6%)	2 (9.1%)	2 (3.7%)	10 (20.8%)	8 (19.0%)		
Severe LVA	0 (0%)	0 (0%)	2 (9.1%)	2 (3.7%)	4 (8.3%)	15 (35.7%)		

**P < 0.05 vs. control in age group 1; **P < 0.01 vs. control in age group 2; ***P < 0.001 vs. control in age group 1; †P < 0.05 vs. control in age group 2; ††P < 0.01 vs. control in age group 2; †††P < 0.001 vs. control in age group 2; ‡P < 0.05 vs. control in age group 3; ‡‡P < 0.01 vs. control in age group 3; ‡‡‡P < 0.001 vs. control in age group 3.*

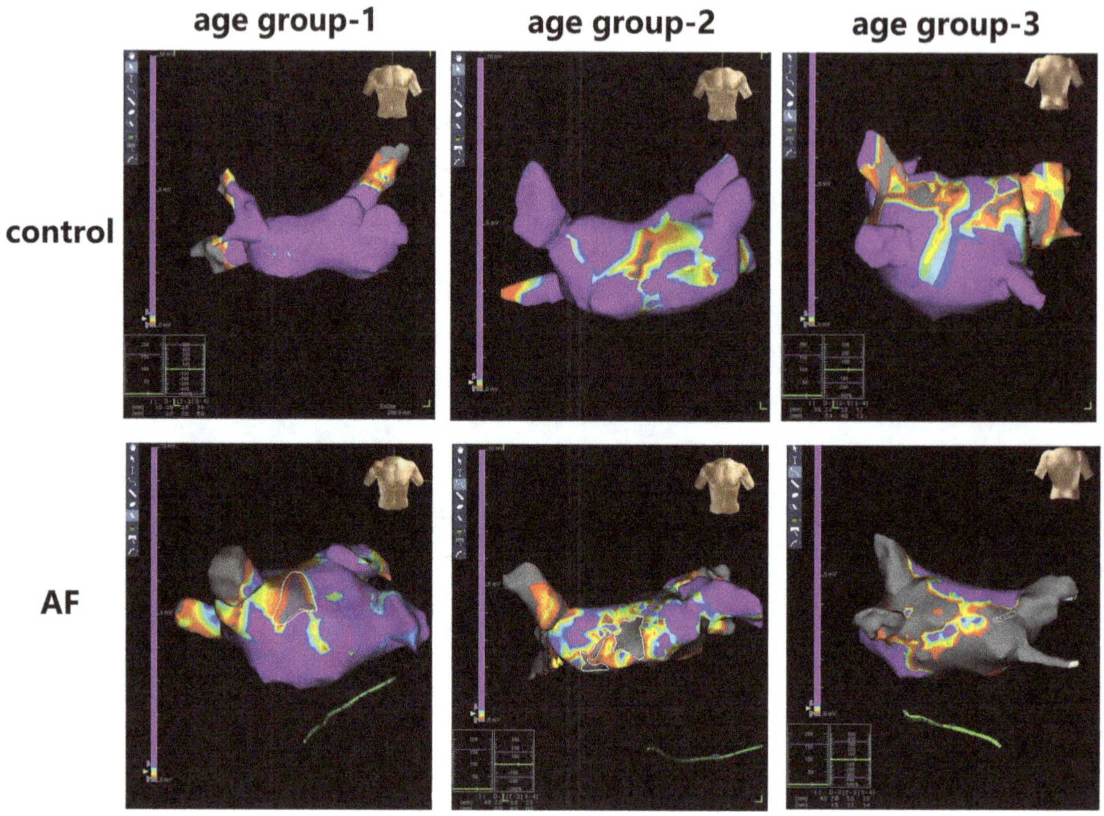

FIGURE 3 | Examples of LA fibrosis burden in control individuals and AF patients at three age groups. Different values of electrical voltage representing LA fibrosis are color-coded in purple to gray. Purple region, gray region and other color region represent completely healthy myocardial tissue with a voltage ≥0.5 mV, scar with a voltage ≤0.1 mV, and junction area at the voltage of 0.1- to 0.5-mV region, respectively.

whereas a negative correlation was found between LA stiffness index and mean LA voltage (control: $r = -0.605$, $P < 0.001$; AF: $r = -0.584$, $P < 0.001$; **Figure 4E**). Further adjustments for gender, hypertension, and diabetes mellitus did not materially alter these results.

An Evaluation for LA Remodeling Using High-Frequency Ultrasound and the Association With Atrial Fibrosis in Aged Mice

A preclinically experiment was also performed to investigate the relationship between age-related LA remodeling and atrial fibrosis burden. **Table 4** shows the echocardiographic and Doppler measurements of cardiac function in the young (3-month-old) and aged (27-month-old) male C57BL/6 mice. Interventricular septal thickness, left ventricular internal-diastolic dimension, and left ventricular end-diastolic volume were all significantly increased in aged mice as compared with young mice, indicating the presence of age-related cardiac remodeling. Despite the lack of statistical significance, a marginally increase in E/e′ ratio was observed in aged mice, suggesting a possible presence of age-related diastolic dysfunction.

In accordance with the clinical study, LVEF did not differ between young and old mice (59.16 ± 6.71 vs. 61.73 ± 4.16%, $P = 0.34$; **Figure 5A**), indicating the age-related cardiac alterations conformed to pathophysiologic progression of heart failure with preserved ejection fraction. Non-invasive LA volume and PA diameter were reported to be useful and state-independent measures of age-related cardiac diastolic dysfunction in mice (28). Representative B-mode images of LA and pulmonary artery in young and aged mice are shown in **Figure 5B**. LA area (4.57 ± 0.85 vs. 5.75 ± 0.75 mm^2, $P = 0.01$) and PAD (1.44 ± 0.07 vs. 1.71 ± 0.16 mm, $P = 0.02$) were both increased significantly in aged mice. PR interval did not differ between two groups (20.56 ± 2.16 vs 19.50 ± 2.89 ms, $P > 0.05$). Comparing with young mice, aged mice presented shorter RR interval (153.33 ± 9.01 vs 130.67 ± 8.00 ms, $P < 0.001$), along with longer P-wave duration (24.17 ± 2.27 vs. 32.60 ± 2.49 ms, $P < 0.01$; **Figure 5C**), indicating the increased inducibility of AF (29, 30). Moreover, in Masson trichrome stain, larger fibrosis areas were observed in aged mice (**Figure 5D**), suggesting aggravation of LA fibrosis during aging.

DISCUSSION

Impaired LA performance is increasingly considered as a predictor for aging and AF (31–33). Although a few circulating

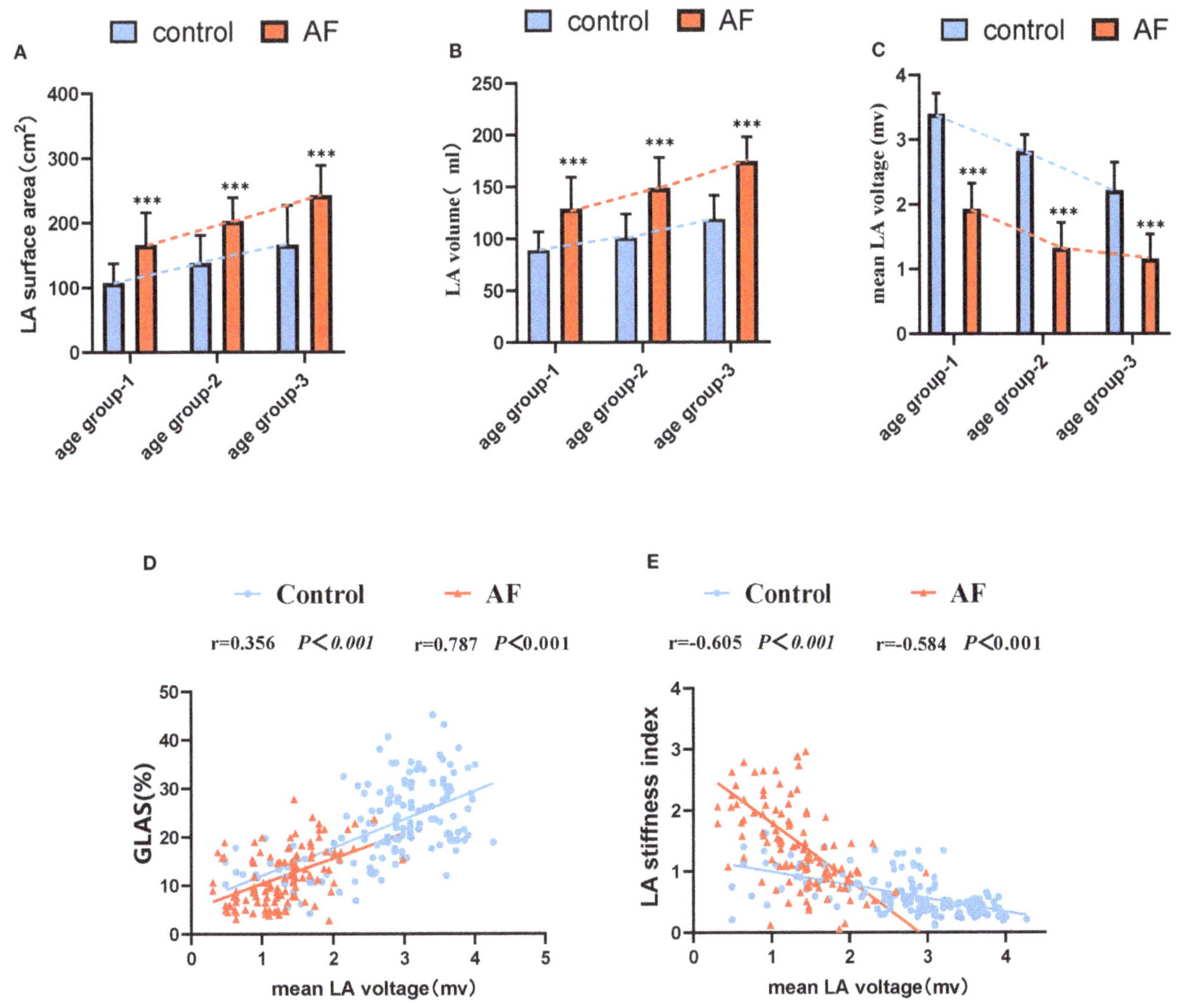

FIGURE 4 | The relationship between the LA dysfunction and fibrosis progression under the background of atrial aging. **(A,B)** In addition to increased LA surface area and LA volume significantly correlating with advanced age, alterations in two measurements were more apparent in AF patients in aging process. **(C)** Changes for mean LA voltage in the absence and presence of AF during aging. **(D,E)** Correlations of GLAS and LA stiffness index with mean LA voltage in control adults and AF patients. LA, left atrium; AF, atrial fibrillation; GLAS, left atrial global longitudinal strain. $^{*}P < 0.05$ vs. control in age-match groups; $^{**}P < 0.01$ vs. control in age-match groups; $^{***}P < 0.001$ vs. control in age-match groups.

molecules were reported to be correlated with age-related cardiovascular disease progress, none of them is capable of accurately manifesting cardiac performance in real time (34). Therefore, the present study aimed to evaluate subtle changes in LA performance due to AF during the process of aging. To our knowledge, this is the first report of evaluating subtle changes in mechanical and electrical characteristics of LA in AF patients and comparing them with non-AF control subjects during the process of aging. We found a negative correlation between LA performance and age, which was more prominent with the presence of AF. On that basis, we also illustrated through electroanatomic mapping that the alterations in LA performance were associated with development of LA fibrosis. Finally, in a murine model, we further validated the changes in LA performance and the relationship between impaired LA performance and fibrosis during aging.

In the present study, LAD tested by echocardiology, LA surface area, and LA volume tested by electroanatomic mapping all increased with age in both AF and control cohorts, with AF patients displaying a greater LA size evidenced by all three parameters compared with control individuals at corresponding age, indicating the LA remodeling progression in both AF and non-AF subjects during aging. However, a prior study reported aging does not significantly alter indexed LA size until the age of 80 years in normal healthy subjects (35). We suspected this discrepancy may have something to do with the control cohort

TABLE 4 | Non-invasive measurements of C57BL/6 male mice aged at 3 and 27 months under mild anesthesia.

	Young (n = 15)	Aged (n = 15)	P-value
HR (bpm)	411.8 ± 17.80	421.2 ± 29.30	0.100
IVS;d (mm)	0.88 ± 0.08	1.00 ± 0.09	0.056
IVS;s (mm)	1.28 ± 0.12	1.56 ± 0.25	0.060
LVID;d (mm)	4.03 ± 0.17	4.33 ± 0.18	0.030
LVID;s (mm)	2.78 ± 0.27	2.81 ± 0.11	0.790
LVPW;s (mm)	0.75 ± 0.13	0.70 ± 0.10	0.570
LVPW;d (mm)	1.03 ± 0.11	1.07 ± 0.09	0.680
E velocity (m/s)	0.70 ± 0.05	0.67 ± 0.11	0.392
A velocity (m/s)	0.48 ± 0.08	0.38 ± 0.08	0.035
E/A ratio	1.58 ± 0.37	1.50 ± 0.27	0.341
E/e′ ratio	18.66 ± 4.89	24.40 ± 7.00	0.054
FS (%)	31.17 ± 4.68	34.90 ± 2.69	0.054
LVEDV (uL)	71.72 ± 6.19	84.75 ± 8.87	0.030
LVESV (uL)	29.44 ± 7.10	30.07 ± 2.85	0.786

FS, fractional shortening; HR, heart rate; IVS;d, interventricular septal thickness at diastole; IVS;s, interventricular septal thickness at systole; LV, left ventricular; LVID;d, LV internal -diastolic dimension; LVID;s, LV internal-systolic dimension; LVPW;s, left ventricular posterior wall thickness at end systole; LVPW; d, left ventricular posterior wall thickness at end diastole; E/A, E–A peak velocity ratio; LVEDV, LV end-diastolic volume; LVESV, LV end-systolic volume; LVESD, LV end-systolic dimension; LVESV, LV end-systolic volume.

of the present study, which were patients who received ablation for other arrhythmia instead of healthy subjects. Previous studies showed that LA strain allows early detection of age-related LA dysfunction underlying LA remodeling (36). In current study, we demonstrated the age-related LA abnormalities in both control and AF patients *via* evaluating the dynamic changes in GLAS and LA strain rates, in accordance with work from other groups (37). Of note, in elderly patients with higher prevalence of hypertension and diabetes mellitus, LA remodeling and consequent LA dysfunction were more severe. Meanwhile, decreased GLAS and LA strain rates were observed in the AF patients comparing with the age-matched control individuals. LA stiffness index, measured in an invasive method, is considered as a novel index to assess LA dysfunction (15, 27, 38). The current study measured the LA stiffness index in a non-invasive manner based on strain imaging and systematically described its dynamic changes in AF and control patients in the context of aging. Similar to the results of invasive assessment (27), we observed that high LA stiffness index was associated with advanced age and the presence of AF. These findings illustrated the nature of consecutive progression of cardiac aging and the effect of AF on the longitudinal progression.

The relationship between fibrosis burden and LA performance in AF and non-AF subjects during aging was also evaluated in our study. The results of voltage mapping showed a graded decrease in mean LA voltage and a graded increase in LVA% grade alone with age, which is in accordance with an early observation in a large cross-sectional sample with AF (39). Of note, to our knowledge, this is the first study in which electroanatomic mapping results were acquired from non-AF subjects of different age groups. The results help to reveal the evolution pattern of LA electrical characteristics during aging. Moreover, in the current study, AF patients displayed lower LA voltage and higher LVA% grade as compared with non-AF subjects at corresponding age, except for subjects older than 80 years (age group 3), in which LVA% grades in AF cohort were not significantly different from those of control cohort. We deduce that the effect of aging might overrun the effect of AF in subjects older than 80 years. It is worth mentioning that we had excluded some measurements because of inadequate contact between the catheter and atrial wall, as was reported in a previous study (40). LA stiffness index has been proven to be related to LVA in AF patients (27, 40). LVA is affected by multiple factors, such as the size and shape of the heart. As a matter of fact, mean LA voltage appears to be a better way to describe overall LA interstitial fibrosis level (41, 42). In the present study, we discovered a significant positive link between the mean LA voltage and GLAS, and a significant negative link between the mean LA voltage and LA stiffness index. These findings provide further evidence to support the idea that aging enhances susceptibility of AF *via* promoting the progression of LA fibrosis.

Corresponding to our clinical findings, in the animal study, a prolonged P-wave duration was shown in aged mice, which provided further evidence for increased susceptibility of AF in aged subjects (43). A significant age-dependent increase of LAD was reported in a murine model with Acuson CV-70 (Siemens) (44). In the current study, aged mice showed expanded LA size (representing by LA area), in accordance with our clinical study. In the present study, increased PAD was observed in aged mice, which is consistent with the clinical findings. We also performed Masson trichrome stain to illustrate histological changes of LA during aging, the result showed a significant increase in LA fibrosis burden in aged mice, which was consistent with the electroanatomic mapping results in our clinical study.

There are also some limitations to the present study that could be addressed in the future. First, this is a single-center study with limited sample size, and the control cohort comprised patients who received ablation for other arrhythmias instead of healthy subjects, which may result in selection bias. Second, the accurate measurement of LA performance in a murine model can be challenging. The use of three-dimensional echocardiograph could potentially improve the sensitivity and accuracy of the tests. Lastly, in order to evaluate dynamic changes in LA performance during aging, a longitudinal study may be more convincing, especially when sample size is limited.

CONCLUSION

This study provides new evidences of subtle changes in mechanical and electrical characteristics of LA during process of aging in both AF and non-AF subjects. There was a negative correlation between LA performance and age, and the presence of AF further impairs LA performance in an additive manner, which is probably ascribed to increased atrial fibrosis burden, as evidenced by results from both electroanatomic mapping in human study and histological staining in animal experiment. In addition, our study also provides normal values for LA

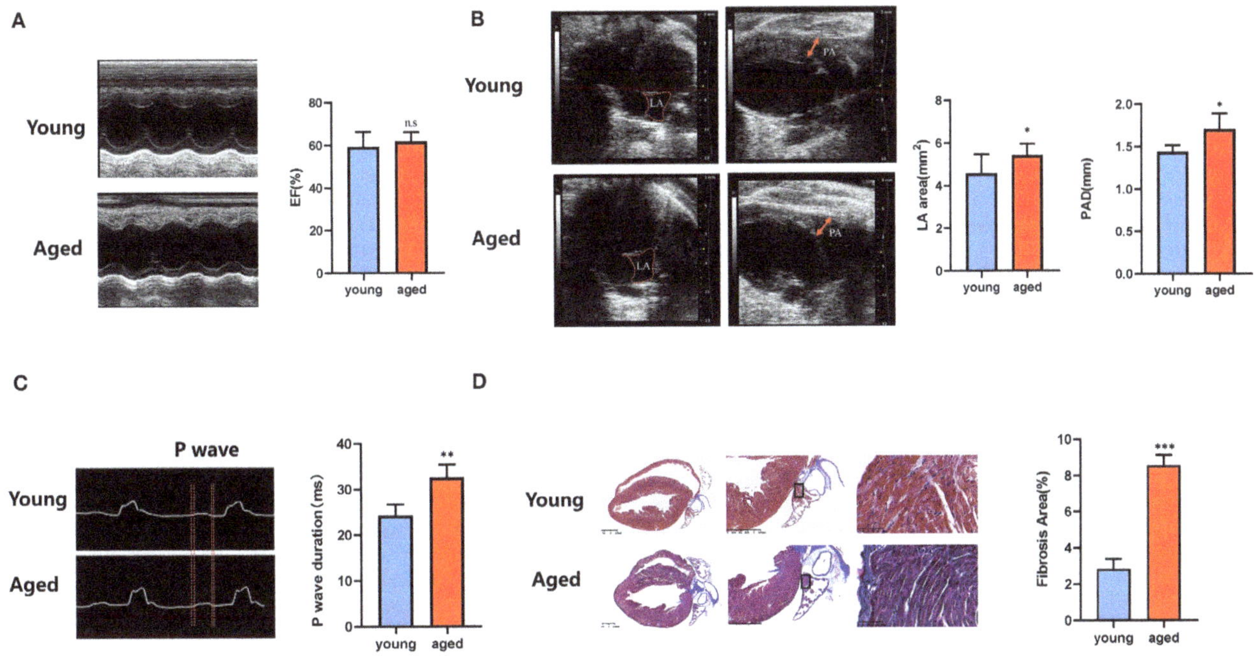

FIGURE 5 | Age-related LA remodeling is associated with atrial fibrosis in mice. **(A)** Representative echocardiographic images of ejection fraction analysis. **(B)** Representative B-mode echocardiographic recordings of LA area and PA diameter and quantification of LA area and PA diameter (right). **(C)** Representative electrocardiographic (ECG) recordings (left) in multiple electroconductive physiological recorder and quantification of P-wave duration. **(D)** Representative results of Masson staining of the left atrium sections obtained from young and old mice, and statistical results of fibrosis area in the left atrium. $n = 15$ in each group. n.s., no significant difference. $^{*}P < 0.05$, $^{**}P < 0.01$, $^{***}P < 0.001$.

mechanical and electrical characteristics in both AF and non-AF conditions during aging. These measurements may provide an early marker for the onset of AF.

AUTHOR CONTRIBUTIONS

K-bL, K-kC, and SL performed the clinical study, experiments, and drafted the original manuscript. M-jY, M-qC, M-LY, and XZ enrolled the patients and analysis part of clinical data. X-XM collected the ultrasound imaging and guided the cardiologists to analysis the data. D-YZ, MW, Y-pW, and Q-hW read critically and revised the manuscript. DH and J-bL reviewed and edited the manuscript. All authors contributed to the article and approved the submitted version.

REFERENCES

1. Schnabel RB, Yin X, Gona P, Larson MG, Beiser AS, McManus DD, et al. 50 year trends in atrial fibrillation prevalence, incidence, risk factors, and mortality in the Framingham Heart Study: a cohort study. *Lancet.* (2015) 386:154–62. doi: 10.1016/S0140-6736(14)61774-8
2. Tse HF, Wang YJ, Ahmed Ai-Abdullah M, Pizarro-Borromeo AB, Chiang CE, Krittayaphong R, et al. Stroke prevention in atrial fibrillation-an Asian stroke perspective. *Heart Rhythm.* (2013) 10:1082–8. doi: 10.1016/j.hrthm.2013.03.017
3. Reddy YNV, Obokata M, Verbrugge FH, Lin G, Borlaug BA. Atrial dysfunction in patients with heart failure with preserved ejection fraction and atrial fibrillation. *J Am Coll Cardiol.* (2020) 76:1051–64. doi: 10.1016/j.jacc.2020.07.009
4. Dzeshka MS, Lip GYH, Snezhitskiy V, Shantsila E. Cardiac fibrosis in patients with atrial fibrillation: mechanisms and clinical implications. *J Am Coll Cardiol.* (2015) 66:943–59. doi: 10.1016/j.jacc.2015.06.1313
5. Horn MA. Cardiac physiology of aging: extracellular considerations. *Comprehens Physiol.* (2015) 5:1069–121. doi: 10.1002/cphy.c140063
6. Mahnkopf C, Badger TJ, Burgon NS, Daccarett M, Haslam TS, Badger CT, et al. Evaluation of the left atrial substrate in patients with lone atrial fibrillation using delayed-enhanced MRI: implications for disease progression and response to catheter ablation. *Heart Rhythm.* (2010) 7:1475–81. doi: 10.1016/j.hrthm.2010.06.030
7. Corradi D, Callegari S, Manotti L, Ferrara D, Goldoni M, Alinovi R, et al. Persistent lone atrial fibrillation: clinicopathologic study of 19 cases. *Heart Rhythm.* (2014) 11:1250–8. doi: 10.1016/j.hrthm.2014.02.008
8. Platonov PG, Mitrofanova LB, Orshanskaya V, Ho SY. Structural abnormalities in atrial walls are associated with presence and persistency of atrial fibrillation but not with age. *J Am Coll Cardiol.* (2011) 58:2225–32. doi: 10.1016/j.jacc.2011.05.061
9. Lu Y-Y, Chen Y-C, Kao Y-H, Chen S-A, Chen Y-J. Extracellular matrix of collagen modulates arrhythmogenic activity of pulmonary veins through p38 MAPK activation. *J Mol Cell Cardiol.* (2013) 59:159–66. doi: 10.1016/j.yjmcc.2013.03.008
10. Taneja T, Mahnert BW, Passman R, Goldberger J, Kadish A. Effects of sex and age on electrocardiographic and cardiac electrophysiological properties in adults. *Pacing Clin Electrophysiol.* (2001) 24:16–21. doi: 10.1046/j.1460-9592.2001.00016.x
11. Okamatsu K, Takeuchi M, Nakai H, Nishikage T, Salgo IS, Husson S, et al. Effects of aging on left atrial function assessed by two-dimensional speckle tracking echocardiography. *J Am Soc Echocardiogr.* (2009) 22:70–5. doi: 10.1016/j.echo.2008.11.006

12. Miglioranza MH, Badano LP, Mihila S, Peluso D, Cucchini U, Soriani N, et al. Physiologic determinants of left atrial longitudinal strain: a two-dimensional speckle-tracking and three-dimensional echocardiographic study in healthy volunteers. *J Am Soc Echocardiogr.* (2016) 29:1023. doi: 10.1016/j.echo.2016.07.011
13. Abou R, Leung M, Tonsbeek AM, Podlesnikar T, Maan AC, Schalij MJ, et al. Effect of aging on left atrial compliance and electromechanical properties in subjects without structural heart disease. *Am Cardiol J.* (2017) 120:140–7. doi: 10.1016/j.amjcard.2017.03.243
14. Leung M, Abou R, van Rosendael PJ, van der Bijl P, van Wijngaarden SE, Regeer MV, et al. Relation of echocardiographic markers of left atrial fibrosis to atrial fibrillation burden. *Am J Cardiol.* (2018) 122:584–91. doi: 10.1016/j.amjcard.2018.04.047
15. January CT, Wann LS, Alpert JS, Calkins H, Cigarroa JE, Cleveland JC, et al. 2014 AHA/ACC/HRS guideline for the management of patients with atrial fibrillation: executive summary: a report of the American College of Cardiology/American Heart Association Task Force on practice guidelines and the Heart Rhythm Society. *Circulation.* (2014) 130:2071–104. doi: 10.1161/CIR.0000000000000040
16. Macle L, Cairns J, Leblanc K, Tsang T, Skanes A, Cox JL, et al. 2016 focused update of the canadian cardiovascular society guidelines for the management of atrial fibrillation. *Can J Cardiol.* (2016) 32:1170–85. doi: 10.1016/j.cjca.2016.07.591
17. Ma X-X, Zhang Y-L, Hu B, Zhu M-R, Jiang W-J, Wang M, et al. The usefulness of global left atrial strain for predicting atrial fibrillation recurrence after catheter ablation in patients with persistent and paroxysmal atrial fibrillation. *Arch Cardiovasc Dis.* (2017) 110:447–55. doi: 10.1016/j.acvd.2016.11.005
18. Lang RM, Bierig M, Devereux RB, Flachskampf FA, Foster E, Pellikka PA, et al. Recommendations for chamber quantification: a report from the American Society of Echocardiography's Guidelines and Standards Committee and the Chamber Quantification Writing Group, developed in conjunction with the European Association of Echocardiography, a branch of the European Society of Cardiology. *J Am Soc Echocardiogr.* (2005) 18:1440–63. doi: 10.1016/j.echo.2005.10.005
19. Nagueh SF, Smiseth OA, Appleton CP, Byrd BF 3rd, Dokainish H, Edvardsen T, et al. Recommendations for the evaluation of left ventricular diastolic function by echocardiography: an update from the American Society of Echocardiography and the European Association of Cardiovascular Imaging. *J Am Soc Echocardiogr.* (2016) 29:277–314. doi: 10.1016/j.echo.2016.01.011
20. Lang RM, Badano LP, Mor-Avi V, Afilalo J, Armstrong A, Ernande L, et al. Recommendations for cardiac chamber quantification by echocardiography in adults: an update from the American Society of Echocardiography and the European Association of Cardiovascular Imaging. *J Am Soc Echocardiogr.* (2015) 28:1–39. e14. doi: 10.1016/j.echo.2014.10.003
21. Kishima H, Mine T, Fukuhara E, Ashida K, Ishihara M. The association between left atrial stiffness and low-voltage areas of left atrium in patients with atrial fibrillation. *Heart Vessels.* (2019) 34:1830–8. doi: 10.1007/s00380-019-01423-z
22. Huang D, Li J-B, Zghaib T, Gucuk Ipek E, Balouch M, Spragg DD, et al. The extent of left atrial low-voltage areas included in pulmonary vein isolation is associated with freedom from recurrent atrial arrhythmia. *Can J Cardiol.* (2018) 34:73–9. doi: 10.1016/j.cjca.2017.10.012
23. Wang X-H, Li Z, Mao J-L, Zang M-H, Pu J. Low voltage areas in paroxysmal atrial fibrillation: The prevalence, risk factors and impact on the effectiveness of catheter ablation. *Int J Cardiol.* (2018) 269:139–44. doi: 10.1016/j.ijcard.2018.07.076
24. Wu J, Bu L, Gong H, Jiang G, Li L, Ma H, et al. Effects of heart rate and anesthetic timing on high-resolution echocardiographic assessment under isoflurane anesthesia in mice. *J Ultrasound Med.* (2010) 29:1771–8. doi: 10.7863/jum.2010.29.12.1771
25. Nakayama T, Sugano Y, Yokokawa T, Nagai T, Matsuyama T-A, Ohta-Ogo K, et al. Clinical impact of the presence of macrophages in endomyocardial biopsies of patients with dilated cardiomyopathy. *Eur J Heart Fail.* (2017) 19:490–8. doi: 10.1002/ejhf.767
26. Strisciuglio T, El Haddad M, Debonnaire P, De Pooter J, Demolder A, Wolf M, et al. Paroxysmal atrial fibrillation with high vs. low arrhythmia burden: atrial remodelling and ablation outcome. *Europace.* (2020) 22:1189–96. doi: 10.1093/europace/euaa071
27. Khurram IM, Maqbool F, Berger RD, Marine JE, Spragg DD, Ashikaga H, et al. Association between left atrial stiffness index and atrial fibrillation recurrence in patients undergoing left atrial ablation. *Circ Arrhythm Electrophysiol.* (2016) 9:e003163. doi: 10.1161/CIRCEP.115.003163
28. Medrano G, Hermosillo-Rodriguez J, Pham T, Granillo A, Hartley CJ, Reddy A, et al. Left atrial volume and pulmonary artery diameter are noninvasive measures of age-related diastolic dysfunction in mice. *J Gerontol A Biol Sci Med Sci.* (2016) 71:1141–50. doi: 10.1093/gerona/glv143
29. Hayashi H, Wang C, Miyauchi Y, Omichi C, Pak H-N, Zhou S, et al. Aging-related increase to inducible atrial fibrillation in the rat model. *J Cardiovasc Electrophysiol.* (2002) 13:801–8. doi: 10.1046/j.1540-8167.2002.00801.x
30. Chen LY, Soliman ZE. P wave indices-advancing our understanding of atrial fibrillation-related cardiovascular outcomes. *Front Cardiovasc Med.* (2019) 6:53. doi: 10.3389/fcvm.2019.00053
31. Vaziri SM, Larson MG, Benjamin EJ, Levy D. Echocardiographic predictors of nonrheumatic atrial fibrillation. The Framingham Heart Study. *Circulation.* (1994) 89:724–30. doi: 10.1161/01.CIR.89.2.724
32. Kizer JR, Bella JN, Palmieri V, Liu JE, Best LG, Lee ET, et al. Left atrial diameter as an independent predictor of first clinical cardiovascular events in middle-aged and elderly adults: the Strong Heart Study (SHS). *Am Heart J.* (2006) 151:412–8. doi: 10.1016/j.ahj.2005.04.031
33. Tsang TS, Abhayaratna WP, Barnes ME, Miyasaka Y, Gersh BJ, Bailey KR, et al. Prediction of cardiovascular outcomes with left atrial size: is volume superior to area or diameter? *J Am Coll Cardiol.* (2006) 47:1018–23. doi: 10.1016/j.jacc.2005.08.077
34. Angelini F, Pagano F, Bordin A, Picchio V, De Falco E, Chimenti I. Getting old through the blood: circulating molecules in aging and senescence of cardiovascular regenerative cells. *Front Cardiovasc Med.* (2017) 4:62. doi: 10.3389/fcvm.2017.00062
35. Boyd AC, Schiller NB, Leung D, Ross DL, Thomas L. Atrial dilation and altered function are mediated by age and diastolic function but not before the eighth decade. *JACC Cardiovasc Imaging.* (2011) 4:234–42. doi: 10.1016/j.jcmg.2010.11.018
36. Yoshida Y, Nakanishi K, Daimon M, Ishiwata J, Sawada N, Hirokawa M, et al. Alteration of cardiac performance and serum B-type natriuretic peptide level in healthy aging. *J Am Coll Cardiol.* (2019) 74:1789–800. doi: 10.1016/j.jacc.2019.07.080
37. van Grootel RWJ, Strachinaru M, Menting ME, McGhie J, Roos-Hesselink JW, van den Bosch EA. In-depth echocardiographic analysis of left atrial function in healthy adults using speckle tracking echocardiography and volumetric analysis. *Echocardiography.* (2018) 35:1956–65. doi: 10.1111/echo.14174
38. Nielsen JC, Lin YJ, de Oliveira Figueiredo MJ, Sepehri Shamloo A, Alfie A, Boveda S, et al. European Heart Rhythm Association (EHRA)/Heart Rhythm Society (HRS)/Asia Pacific Heart Rhythm Society (APHRS)/Latin American Heart Rhythm Society (LAHRS) expert consensus on risk assessment in cardiac arrhythmias: use the right tool for the right outcome, in the right population. *Heart Rhythm.* (2020) 17:e269–316. doi: 10.1016/j.hrthm.2020.05.004
39. Akoum N, Mahnkopf C, Kholmovski EG, Brachmann J, Marrouche FN. Age and sex differences in atrial fibrosis among patients with atrial fibrillation. *Europace.* (2018) 20:1086–92. doi: 10.1093/europace/eux260
40. Pilichowska-Paszkiet E, Baran J, Sygitowicz G, Sikorska A, Stec S, Kułakowski P, et al. Noninvasive assessment of left atrial fibrosis. Correlation between echocardiography, biomarkers, electroanatomical mapping. *Echocardiography.* (2018) 35:1326–34. doi: 10.1111/echo.14043
41. Kistler PM, Sanders P, Fynn SP, Stevenson IH, Spence SJ, Vohra JK, et al. Electrophysiologic and electroanatomic changes in the human atrium associated with age. *J Am Coll Cardiol.* (2004) 44:109–16. doi: 10.1016/j.jacc.2004.03.044
42. Jadidi AS, Cochet H, Shah AJ, Kim SJ, Duncan E, Miyazaki S, et al. Inverse relationship between fractionated electrograms and atrial fibrosis in persistent atrial fibrillation: combined magnetic resonance imaging and high-density mapping. *J Am Coll Cardiol.* (2013) 62:802–12. doi: 10.1016/j.jacc.2013.03.081
43. Luo T, Chang C-X, Zhou X, Gu S-K, Jiang T-M, Li Y-M. Characterization of atrial histopathological and electrophysiological changes in a mouse model of aging. *Int J Mol Med.* (2013) 31:138–46. doi: 10.3892/ijmm.2012.1174
44. Dai D-F, Santana LF, Vermulst M, Tomazela DM, Emond MJ, MacCoss MJ, et al. Overexpression of catalase targeted to mitochondria attenuates murine cardiac aging. *Circulation.* (2009) 119:2789–97. doi: 10.1161/CIRCULATIONAHA.108.822403

9

Novel Knowledge-Based Transcriptomic Profiling of Lipid Lysophosphatidylinositol-Induced Endothelial Cell Activation

Keman Xu[1], *Ying Shao*[1], *Fatma Saaoud*[1], *Aria Gillespie*[2], *Charles Drummer IV*[1], *Lu Liu*[3], *Yifan Lu*[1], *Yu Sun*[1], *Hang Xi*[3], *Çagla Tükel*[4], *Domenico Pratico*[5], *Xuebin Qin*[6], *Jianxin Sun*[7], *Eric T. Choi*[8], *Xiaohua Jiang*[1,3], *Hong Wang*[3] *and Xiaofeng Yang*[1,3]*

[1] Centers of Cardiovascular Research, Inflammation and Lung Research, Philadelphia, PA, United States, [2] Neural Sciences, Temple University Lewis Katz School of Medicine, Philadelphia, PA, United States, [3] Departments of Cardiovascular Sciences, Metabolic Disease Research, Thrombosis Research, Philadelphia, PA, United States, [4] Center for Microbiology & Immunology, Temple University Lewis Katz School of Medicine, Philadelphia, PA, United States, [5] Alzheimer's Center, Temple University Lewis Katz School of Medicine, Philadelphia, PA, United States, [6] National Primate Research Center, Tulane University, Covington, LA, United States, [7] Department of Medicine, Center for Translational Medicine, Thomas Jefferson University, Philadelphia, PA, United States, [8] Surgery (Division of Vascular and Endovascular Surgery), Temple University Lewis Katz School of Medicine, Philadelphia, PA, United States

***Correspondence:**
Xiaofeng Yang
xfyang@temple.edu

To determine whether pro-inflammatory lipid lysophosphatidylinositols (LPIs) upregulate the expressions of membrane proteins for adhesion/signaling and secretory proteins in human aortic endothelial cell (HAEC) activation, we developed an EC biology knowledge-based transcriptomic formula to profile RNA-Seq data panoramically. We made the following primary findings: first, G protein-coupled receptor 55 (GPR55), the LPI receptor, is expressed in the endothelium of both human and mouse aortas, and is significantly upregulated in hyperlipidemia; second, LPIs upregulate 43 clusters of differentiation (CD) in HAECs, promoting EC activation, innate immune trans-differentiation, and immune/inflammatory responses; 72.1% of LPI-upregulated CDs are not induced in influenza virus-, MERS-CoV virus- and herpes virus-infected human endothelial cells, which hinted the specificity of LPIs in HAEC activation; third, LPIs upregulate six types of 640 secretomic genes (SGs), namely, 216 canonical SGs, 60 caspase-1-gasdermin D (GSDMD) SGs, 117 caspase-4/11-GSDMD SGs, 40 exosome SGs, 179 Human Protein Atlas (HPA)-cytokines, and 28 HPA-chemokines, which make HAECs a large secretory organ for inflammation/immune responses and other functions; fourth, LPIs activate transcriptomic remodeling by upregulating 172 transcription factors (TFs), namely, pro-inflammatory factors NR4A3, FOS, KLF3, and HIF1A; fifth, LPIs upregulate 152 nuclear DNA-encoded mitochondrial (mitoCarta) genes, which alter mitochondrial mechanisms and functions, such as mitochondrial organization, respiration, translation, and transport; sixth, LPIs activate reactive oxygen species (ROS) mechanism by upregulating 18 ROS regulators; finally, utilizing the Cytoscape software, we found that three mechanisms, namely, LPI-upregulated TFs, mitoCarta genes, and ROS regulators, are integrated to promote HAEC activation. Our results provide novel insights into aortic EC activation, formulate an EC biology knowledge-based transcriptomic profile strategy, and identify new targets for the development of therapeutics for cardiovascular diseases, inflammatory conditions, immune diseases, organ transplantation, aging, and cancers.

Keywords: transcriptomic analysis, inflammation, secretomes, RNA-Seq analysis, aortic endothelial cell

INTRODUCTION

Atherosclerosis is a pathological process underlying the development of myocardial infarction, stroke, and peripheral arterial disease, which is a substantial cause of morbidity and mortality (1). Vascular inflammation contributes significantly to the atherosclerotic onset and the development of its complications (2–5). In addition to consistent findings across multiple mouse models (6), the Canakinumab Anti-inflammatory Thrombosis Outcomes Study (CANTOS) demonstrated that the inhibition of pro-inflammatory interleukin-1β (IL-1β) reduces the atherosclerotic burden in cardiovascular disease (7–9). The activation of endothelial cells (ECs) is the earliest event and a central pathological process associated with the onset of atherosclerosis. Based on our previous findings, we propose that:(1) ECs are innate immune cells (3–5), as they display innate immune functions similar to those of prototypical innate immune cells, such as macrophages (5, 10, 11) and monocytes (12–18). (2) In addition to increased secretion of cytokines and chemokines and upregulation of adhesion molecules, activated ECs also exhibit two new hallmarks of innate immune cells, namely, upregulation of both danger-associated molecular patterns (DAMPs) receptors and major histocompatibility complex (MHC) molecules for antigen presentation (19). (3) Endogenous metabolites that bind to their intrinsic receptors, rather than classical DAMP receptors, such as toll-like receptors (TLRs) and nod-like receptors/inflammasomes, can become conditional DAMPs, for example, lysophospholipids (19–23). (4) Similar to macrophages and monocytes, ECs have innate immune memory functions (trained immunity) (2, 3, 24–26). Although many transcriptomic data have been reported, there is no standard universal framework to analyze these data. To address this knowledge gap, we applied the ontology transcriptomic formula to characterize aortic endothelial cell activation.

There are four key features for conditional DAMPs as we proposed previously: (i) acting as endogenous metabolites; (ii) elevating in pathologically conditions; (iii) contributing to physiological signaling roles; (iv) binding to their intrinsic receptors and carrying out cytokine-like signal amplification functions (27). Conditional DAMPs include lysophospholipids, hyperhomocysteinemia (14–17, 28–30), and succinate (27) among others. Lysophospholipids are a group of bioactive lipids; some of which are pro-inflammatory molecules (31, 32), such as lysophosphatidylcholines (LPCs, lysoPC) (23, 33, 34), lysophosphatidic acid (LPA) (34–36), lysophosphatidylinositols (LPIs, lysoPIs) (19), and sphingosine-1-phosphate (37). LPA, LPCs, and LPIs are the characteristics of atherosclerotic aorta plaque in apolipoprotein E deficient (ApoE$^{-/-}$) and low-density lipoprotein receptor (LDLR$^{-/-}$) mice. One of the sub-species of LPIs, 18:0, has been reported and is mainly localized in the necrotic core of the plaque (38). In addition to pro-inflammatory molecules, we also proposed anti-inflammatory endogenous metabolites, such as lysophosphatidylethanolamine and lysophosphatidylserine, pro-resolving mediators (39), IL-35 (40), and itaconate (41, 42) as homeostasis-associated molecular patterns (20). As we have reported, most lysophospholipids (LPLs) contribute to aortic endothelial cell (EC) activation (23, 43, 44) and the progression of atherosclerosis (22). The molecular mechanisms underlying LPC-induced aortic EC activation included calcium influx-increased proton leaks *via* uncoupled mitochondrial electron transport chain, increased mitochondrial reactive oxygen species (mtROS), increased histone 3 lysine 14 acetylation (H3K14ac), and transcription factor AP-1 driven ICAM-1 upregulation (23, 43–46). In addition, we also reported that LPC induces caspase-1 activation and pyroptosis (inflammatory cell death) (33, 34, 47). Moreover, by RNA-Sequencing (RNA-Seq), we reported that LPC and LPIs induce prolonged EC activation by upregulating adhesion molecule ICAM-1, additional DAMP receptors such as CD36, and MHC molecules for antigen presentation (19). However, the transcriptomic formula of aortic EC activation in a panoramic view remained poorly characterized.

Low-throughput techniques used in current cardiovascular science research laboratories limit our understanding of aortic EC activation. Thus, high-throughput computational bioinformatics screening is often introduced to provide a whole picture at the beginning of an experimental project. As an initial step, RNA-Seq data can be profiled *via* various databases, for example, Gene Set Enrichment Analysis (GSEA) (19). To improve our panoramic understanding of the importance of aortic EC activation induced by conditional DAMP proinflammatory lipid LPIs, we hypothesized that transcriptomic profiling using high-throughput RNA-sequencing data can be formulated on an EC biology knowledge basis. We examined this new hypothesis by massive profiling. Aortic EC phenotypic research was studied from EC adhesion and secretory functions. LPIs induce aortic EC activation by upregulating EC biomarkers and membrane adhesion molecules (159 genes), clusters of differentiation (CDs) signaling (373 genes), six types of secretomic gene sets, namely, canonical secretome (2,640 genes with signal peptide) (13), caspase-1-gasdermin D (GSDMD) non-canonical secretome (964 genes), caspase-4-GSDMD non-canonical secretome (1,223 genes), exosome non-canonical secretome (6,560 genes) (48), Human Protein Atlas (HPA) database-classified cytokines (1,176 genes), and HPA-classified chemokines (200 genes) (49). Three mechanistic studies were included in this article to identify molecular mechanisms underlying the upregulation of these key features of EC activation, such as increased endothelial cell membrane adhesion functions and secretory functions. We focused on determining the expression changes in a complete list of 165 reactive oxygen species regulators (ROS regulatome) (50) and 1,158 nuclear DNA-encoded mitochondrial genes (mitoCarta genes), and a complete list of 1,496 human genome-encoded TFs (49) (**Figure 1**), as have we reported for CD4^{+}Foxp3^{+} regulatory T (Treg) cells (49). Our results have provided novel insights into aortic endothelial cell (EC) activation, formulated an EC biology knowledge-based transcriptomic profile strategy, and identify new targets for the future development of therapeutics for cardiovascular diseases, inflammations, immune diseases, transplantation, aging, and cancers (51).

MATERIALS AND METHODS

Gene List Generation

Eleven gene lists were generated in this manuscript for phenotypic and mechanistic studies of LPI-treated HAECs (**Figure 1**). One hundred fifty-nine EC biomarkers were modified from PMID: 29333215; 373 CD markers, 1,176 cytokines, 200 chemokines, and 1,496 TFs were generated from PMID: 33613572; 2,640 canonical secretomes were downloaded from the comprehensive protein database Human Protein Atlas (https://www.proteinatlas.org/); 964 non-canonical caspase-1-gasdermin D (GSDMD) secretomes were generated from PMID: 18329368;1,223 non-canonical caspase-4 (humans)/11 (mice) secretomes were extracted from PMID: 28196878; 6,560 exosome secretome downloaded from a comprehensive exosome database (http://www.exocarta.org/); 165 ROS regulators were downloaded from PMID: 33154757; 1,158 human nuclear genome DNA-encoded mitochondrion genes were downloaded from the Broad Institute at MIT (mitoCarta, https://www.broadinstitute.org/mitocarta/mitocarta30-inventory-mammalian-mitochondrial-proteins-and-pathways).

Microarray Datasets

Microarray datasets were collected from the National Institutes of Health (NIH)-National Center for Biotechnology Information (NCBI)-Gene Expression Omnibus (GEO) (https://www.ncbi.nlm.nih.gov/gds/) and ArrayExpress (https://www.ebi.ac.uk/arrayexpress/) databases and analyzed with online software GEO2R (https://www.ncbi.nlm.nih.gov/geo/geo2r/), as we have reported (3, 10, 52–54). Three GEO datasets were used in this manuscript, namely, GSE59226 (influenza virus infection), GSE 79218 (MERS-CoV infection for 0, 12, 24, 36, and 48 h), and GSE 1377 (Kaposi's sarcoma-associated herpes virus).

Metascape Analysis

Metascape (https://metascape.org/gp/index.html#/main/step1) was used for enrichment analysis. This website contains the core of most existing gene annotation portals. Our 11 gene lists mentioned in **Figure 1A** were compared with thousands of gene sets and ontology databases (KEGG, MSigDB, and GO) that were defined by their involvement in specific biological processes, pathway membership, enzymatic function, and protein localization. More details about Metascape can be found in cited references (55).

Cytoscape Analysis

The ClueGo v2.5.8 in Cytoscape (https://cytoscape.org/) v3.8.2 was applied to identify gene connections and interactions between functional terms/pathways, as we have reported (56). Eight ClueGO databases were used for our network analysis, namely, GO-Biological Process (17,776 terms/pathways with 18,058 available unique genes), GO-Cellular Component (1,975 terms/pathways with 18,983 available unique genes), GO-Immune System Process (1,195 terms/pathways with 3,625 available unique genes), GO-Molecular Function (5,468 terms/pathways with 18,336 available unique genes), KEGG (333 terms/pathways with 8,093 available unique genes), Reactome pathways (2,474 terms/pathways with 10,855 available unique genes), Reactome reactions (13,015 terms/pathways with 10,855 available unique genes), and Wiki Pathways (667 terms/pathways with 7,633 available unique genes).

RNA Sequencing (RNA-Seq) Data and Statistical Analysis

As we have reported previously, human aortic endothelial cells (HAECs) were treated with vehicle control or lysophosphatidylinositol (LPIs, 16:0) (10 μM) for 18 h. The RNA-Seq data are available in the Array Express database under accession number *E-MTAB-6605* (19).

The expression changes were listed in the results with $p < 0.05$ (statistical significance). Genes with expression changes more than log2 (1) in our RNA-Seq data were defined as upregulated, while those with expression decrease of more than log2 (1) were defined as downregulated (**Supplementary Tables**).

RESULTS

GPR55, a Specific Receptor for LPIs, Is Expressed on the Endothelium of Both Human and Mouse Aortas and Is Significantly Upregulated in Hyperlipidemia

To significantly improve our understanding of LPI-induced activation of HAECs with focus on EC activation key features, such as membrane protein adhesion and signaling and secretory function, an endothelial biology knowledge (3–5, 23, 24, 33, 34, 57–59)-based transcriptomic profile strategy was formulated, and 11 gene lists with 16,114 genes: (i) a comprehensive list of 373 cluster of differentiation (CD) markers (plasma membrane proteins) identified by specific monoclonal antibodies (https://en.wikipedia.org/wiki/List_of_human_clusters_of_differentiation); (ii) 159 updated EC-specific biomarkers (60); six types of secretomes namely, (iii) canonical

(A) Eleven gene lists were used for phenotypic and mechanistic studies of LPI-treated HAECs.

Group #	Classification (Total gene numbers)	Upregulated genes	Downregulated genes	Percentage of affected genes	Upregulated pathways
1	EC biomarkers (159)	10	3	8.2%	Response to wounding, regulation of nitric oxide biosynthetic process, regulation of cell adhesion, neutrophil degranulation
2	CD markers (373)	43	22	17.40%	Production of molecular mediator of immune response, regulation of cell adhesion, cell adhesion molecules, leukocyte migration, cytokine-cytokine receptor interaction
3	Canonical Secretome (2,640)	216	179	15%	Vasculature development, glycoprotein metabolic process, response to interleukin-1, myeloid leukocyte activation, regulation of cell adhesion
4	Caspase-1/Gasdermin D noncanonical secretome (964)	60	50	11.40%	Regulation of nuclease activity, myeloid cell differentiation, cellular response to oxidative stress
5	Caspase-4/11-Gasdermin D noncanonical secretome (1,223)	117	98	17.60%	Regulate exocytosis, autophagy, cytokine signaling in immune system
6	Exosome noncanonical secretome (6,560)	923	808	26%	Membrane trafficking, organelle localization, cytokine signaling in immune system, regulation of cell adhesion
7	Cytokines (1,176)	179	103	24%	Signaling by interleukins, regulation of cell adhesion, positive regulation of cytokine production
8	Chemokines (200)	28	14	21%	Chemokine production, signaling by interleukins, regulation of leukocyte migration, myeloid leukocyte activation, regulation of endothelial cell proliferation
9	ROS regulators (165)	18	17	21%	Reactive oxygen species metabolic process, Regulation of reactive oxygen species metabolic process, Superoxide metabolic process
10	Mitocarta (1,158)	152	164	27%	Mitochondrion organization Cellular respiration Mitochondrial gene expression Mitochondrial transport
11	Transcription factors (1,496)	172	104	18.40%	Kinase and transcription factor activation, myeloid cell differentiation, leukocyte differentiation

B Logic flow for transcriptomic ontology formula.

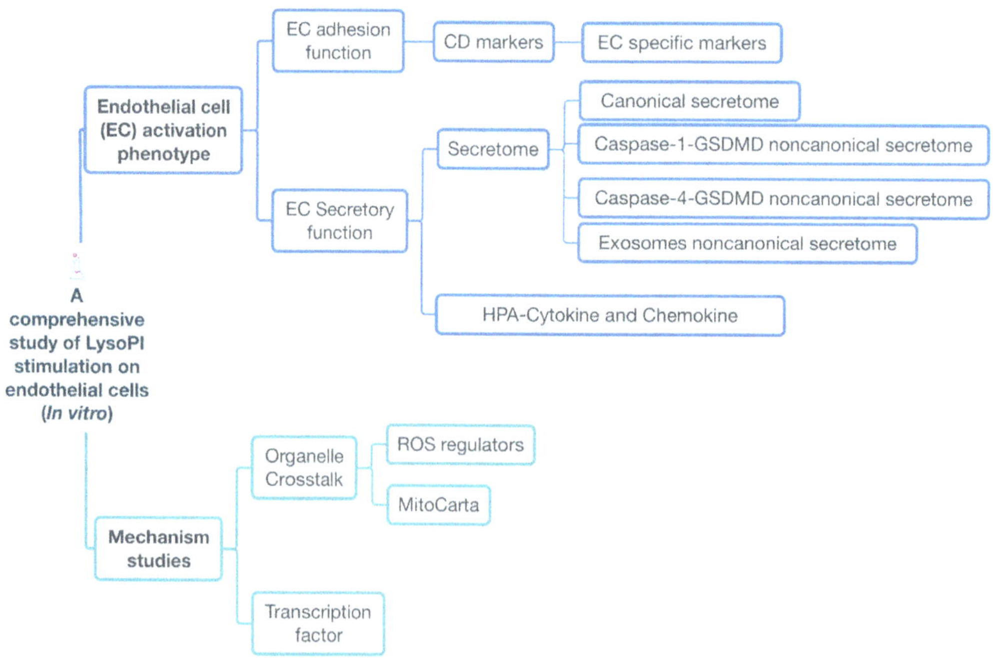

FIGURE 1 | Comprehensive analysis of lysophosphatidylinositol LPI)-treated human aorta endothelial cells (HAECs) at messenger RNA (mRNA) level from 11 different aspects. **(A)** Phenotypic and mechanistic studies. The table shows how a gene changes 18 h after HAECs were treated with 10 μM LPIs. The last column indicates that the pathways are promoted by LPI-upregulated genes. Pathways associated with endothelial cell activation are marked in red. **(B)** Logic flow for our knowledge-based transcriptomic profile strategy.

secretome with 2,640 genes (encoded by all human genome-encoded proteins with a signal peptide) as we have reported (13); (iv) DAMP-sensor caspase-1 (1, 26, 33, 34, 47, 61–65)-gasdermin D (GSDMD) (66) secretome (proteins secreted extracellularly *via* activated caspase-1 cleaved N-terminal GSDMD protein pore) with 961 genes (48, 67); (v) caspase-4-GSDMD secretome (proteins secreted extracellularly *via* activated caspase-4 cleaved N-terminal GSDMD protein pore) with 1,223 genes (48, 68), (vi) exosome secretome with 6,560 genes, as we have reported (48); (vii) a complete list of 1,176 Human Protein Atlas (HPA)-classified cytokines; viii) a complete list of 200 HPA-classified chemokines, as we have reported (49); (ix) a

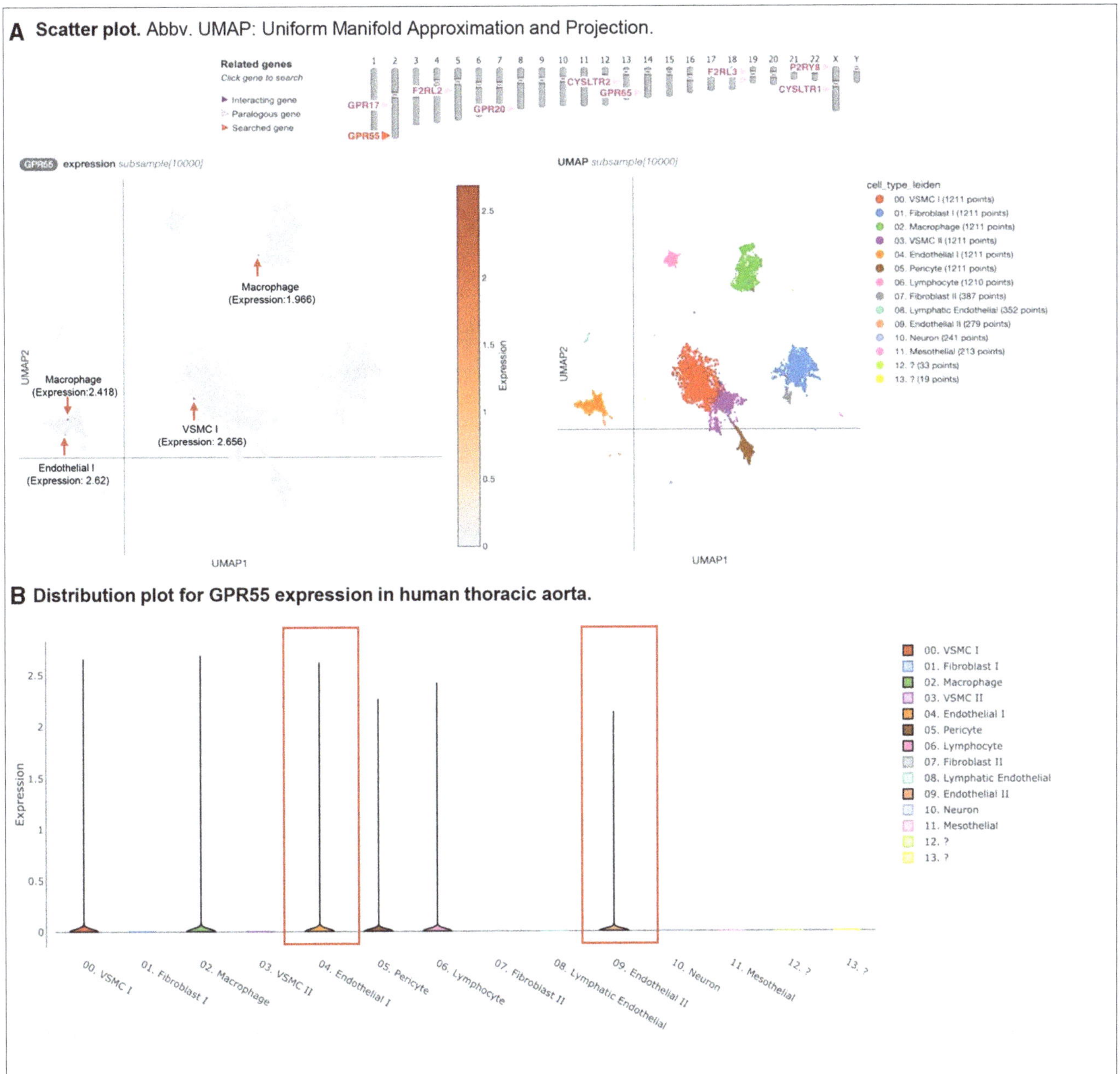

(C) Quantification of gene expression in human aortic cell types.

Cell Types	VSMCI	Macrophage	Endothelial I	Pericyte	Lymphocyte	Endothelial II
Maximum Expression [log 2 (TPM+1)]	2.656	2.69	2.62	2.261	2.417	2.131

FIGURE 2 | Continued

D **Distribution plot for GPR55 expression in mouse ascending aorta.**

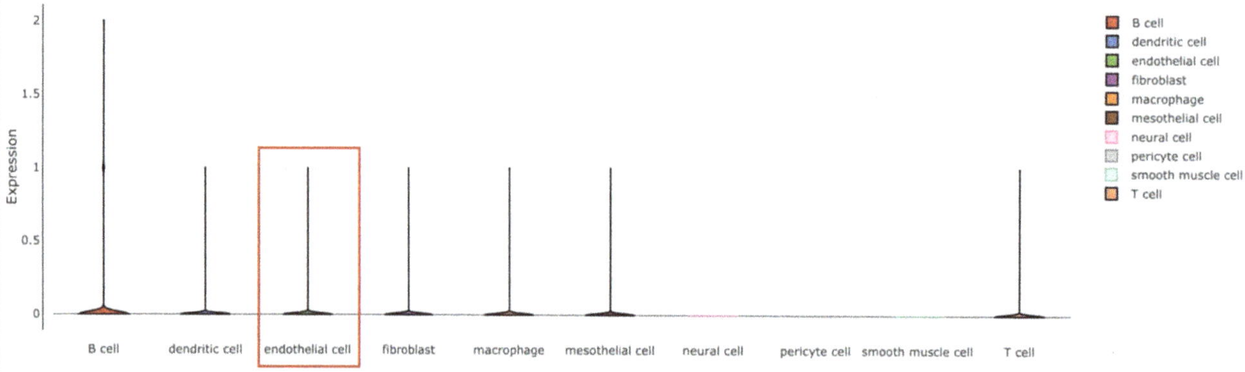

(E) Quantification of gene expression in mouse aortic cell types.

Cell Types	B cell	Dendritic cell	Endothelial cell	Fibroblast	Macrophage	Mesothelial cell	T cell
Maximum Expression	2	1	1	1	1	1	1

F **Distribution plot for GPR55 expression in ascending aorta of normal and high fat diet mice.**

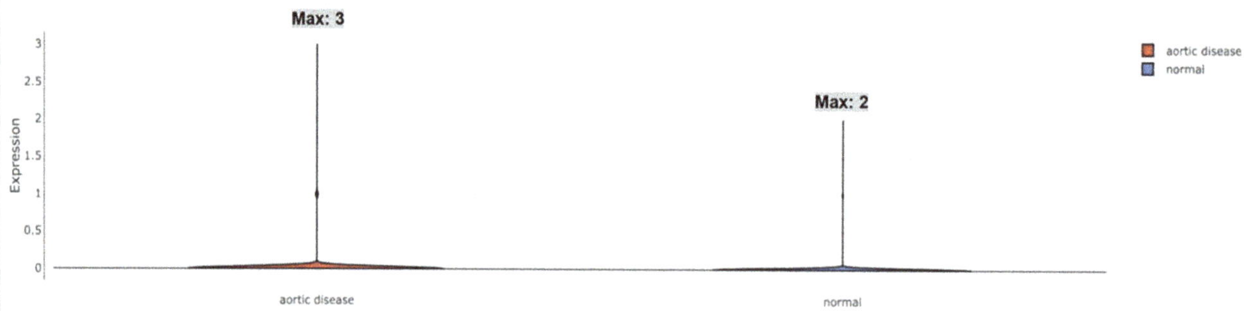

FIGURE 2 | G protein-coupled receptor 55 (GPR55) mRNA transcripts are found in endothelial cells in both human and mouse aortas. Moreover, the expression of GPR55 is upregulated in aortic disease. **(A)** Single-cell RNA-seq analyses were performed on the Single Cell RNA-Seq database of the Broad Institute of MIT and Harvard (Single-Cell RNA-Seq database portal for human thoracic aorta: https://singlecell.broadinstitute.org/single_cell/study/SCP1265/deep-learning-enables-genetic-analysis-of-the-human-thoracic-aorta?genes=GPR55#study-visualize (https://doi.org/10.1101/2020.05.12.091934); GPR55 expressions in macrophage, vascular smooth muscle cells, and endothelial cells of the human aorta are labeled with red arrows in the Scatter. **(B)** GPR55 expressions in endothelial cells of the human aorta were boxed in red in the Distribution. **(C)** The table shows the maximum expressions of GPR55 in each cell type. The expression unit should be the $\log_2$ (TPM+1). Note: **(A–C)** show the expression of GPR55 in humans. The single-cell transcriptional profiles in **(B,C)** from 54092 thoracic aortic cells singled out 14 clusters representing 13 cell types. **(D)** Single Cell RNA-Seq database portal for mouse study: https://singlecell.broadinstitute.org/single_cell/study/SCP1361/single-cell-transcriptome-analysis-reveals-cellular-heterogeneity-in-the-ascending-aorta-of-normal-and-high-fat-diet-mice?genes=Gpr55#study-visualize). GPR55 expressions in endothelial cells of mouse aorta were boxed in red in the Distribution. **(E)** The table shows the maximum expression of GPR55 in each cell type. **(F)** The expression of GPR55 increased in the high fat-fed aortic disease mouse model compared with the normal control mice. The expression unit should be the $\log_2$ (TPM+1). Note: The transcriptional profiles in **(D–F)** represent 24,001 aortic cells and 10 cell types.

complete list of 165 reactive oxygen species (ROS) regulators (regulatome), as we have reported (50); (x) a complete list of 1,496 human genome-encoded TFs from the Human Protein Atlas, as we have reported (3, 49); finally, (xi) a complete list of 1,158 human nuclear genome DNA-encoded mitochondria genes from the Broad Institute at MIT, were analyzed in this study (**Figure 1A**). As outlined in **Figure 1B**, all the examinations on EC membrane proteins, such as EC-specific biomarkers, CD markers, and the six types of secretomes were phenotypic studies. The three molecular mechanisms, namely TFs, mitoCarta genes, and ROS regulatome, were mechanistic studies.

As we mentioned in the introduction, G protein-coupled receptor 55 (GPR55, 319 amino acids, NIH-NCBI Protein database ID: NP_005674.2) is the specific receptor for LPIs (51, 69). The tissue RNA-Seq data from NIH-NCBI Gene database ID 9290 (https://www.ncbi.nlm.nih.gov/gene/9290) showed that significant GPR55 expressions (>0.5 reads per kilobase million, RPKM) were found in six tissues, such as the appendix, duodenum, lymph node, small intestine, spleen, and testis among 27 human tissues from 95 human individuals (**Supplementary Figure 1**). The expression of GPR55 was found in the human heart, although the GPR55 expression data from the vessel were not listed. However, the expressions of GPR55 in human and mouse aortic endothelial cells remained unknown. Hence, we hypothesized that GPR55 is expressed in human and mouse aortic endothelial cells. To examine this hypothesis, the human thoracic aorta single-cell RNA-Seq data were analyzed on the Single Cell^{Beta} Portal database of the Broad Institute at Massachusetts Institute of Technology (MIT) and Harvard (https://singlecell.broadinstitute.org/single_cell/study/SCP1265/deep-learning-enables-genetic-analysis-of-the-human-thoracic-aorta?genes=GPR55#study-summary). As shown in **Figures 2A,B**, the expressions of GPR55 were distributed in six aortic cell clusters identified in 54,092 cells, such as vascular smooth muscle cells, fibroblasts, macrophages, endothelial cells, pericytes, and lymphocytes. Of note, GPR55 expression in both subsets of EC made EC the only cell type with GPR55 expression among all subsets of the cell type (**Figure 2B**). The maximum GPR55 expression in EC reached 2.62 $\log_2$ (transcripts per million, TPM+1), ranking third among all the six cell types (**Figure 2C**). In addition, GPR55 was also expressed in ECs of the mouse aorta. Transcriptions of 24,001 aortic cells were profiled, and ten aortic cell types were identified (https://singlecell.broadinstitute.org/single_cell/study/SCP1361/single-cell-transcriptome-analysis-reveals-cellular-heterogeneity-in-the-ascending-aorta-of-normal-and-high-fat-diet-mice?genes=Gpr55#study-summary). GPR55 mRNA transcripts were found in B cells, dendritic cells, endothelial cells, fibroblasts, macrophages, mesothelial cells, and T cells of mouse aortas (**Figures 2D,E**). However, no significant expression of GPR55 was found in aortic neural cells, pericyte cells, and smooth muscle cells (**Figure 2D**). Moreover, GPR55 mRNA transcripts in aortic cells were expressed at much higher levels in the aortas of high-fat-fed mice than in the aortas of normal chow diet-fed healthy control mice (**Figure 2F**).

Taken together, these findings have demonstrated that first, LPI receptor GPR55 is expressed in human and mouse aortic endothelial cells; second, GPR55 is also expressed in human aortic vascular smooth muscle cells, fibroblasts, macrophages, pericytes, and lymphocytes, and mouse aortic B cells, dendritic cells, fibroblasts, macrophages, mesothelial cells, and T cells. Of note, the expression patterns of GPR55 in aortic endothelial cells, fibroblasts, macrophages, and lymphocytes are shared between human aortas and mouse aortas; *third*, high fat diet-induced hyperlipidemia upregulates aortic GPR55 expression, suggesting critical roles of GPR55 in hyperlipidemia-accelerated atherosclerosis (11, 14, 15, 33, 44, 47, 57, 70, 71). The results were well correlated with our report on LPI-induced activation of EC (19).

LPIs Upregulate 43 Out of 373 Clusters of Differentiation (CD) Markers in HAECs, Promoting EC Activation, Innate Immune Trans-Differentiation, and Immune and Inflammatory Responses; 72.1% of LPI-Upregulated CD Markers Are Not Induced in Three Types of Virus-Infected Human Endothelial Cells

Our recent report showed that LPIs upregulate the expressions of membrane proteins, such as E selectin (SELE), intercellular adhesion molecule 1 (ICAM1), CD74, human leukocyte antigen (HLA) allele-DRB1, and HLA-DMA in HAECs (19). EC expresses specific clusters of differentiation (CDs), such as CD31, which includes various membrane-bound or cytoplasmic molecules on its surface, helps in easier identification of ECs from other cell types, such as $CD4^+$ T cells (72–77), and can be defined by specific monoclonal antibodies (78). However, the overall LPI-modulated membrane protein expressions remained unknown. An excellent review summarized that 11 CDs expressed in ECs, namely, CD54 (ICAM1), CD102 (ICAM2), CD146 (MCAM), CD322 (JAM-B), CD106 (VCAM1), CD31 (PECAM1), CD155 (poliovirus receptor), CD99 (MIC2), CD62E (E-selectin), CD62P (P-selectin), and CD144 (VE-Cadherin), are involved in monocyte trafficking across the vessel wall (79). However, an important question remained whether the expression of all the other CDs is modulated in EC activation. We hypothesize that LPIs play a vital role in modulating the expressions of CDs and other EC adhesion molecules. To examine this hypothesis and study how LPIs change immunophenotyping and alter the behavior of ECs, we collected a complete list of 373 CD markers from a human protein database (https://www.proteinatlas.org/search/protein_class:CD$+$markers) and screened these CD markers in our LPI-treated HAEC RNA-Seq dataset (19). By comparing the RNA-Seq data of the LPI-treated HAECs with that of untreated HAEC controls, 21,252 genes were found to be significantly modulated ($p < 0.05$, $|\log 2FC| \geq 1$). As shown in **Supplementary Table S1**, 65 out of 373 (17.4%) CDs showed significant expression changes in LPI-treated HAECs. Among them, 43 CDs out of 373 (11.5%) were dramatically upregulated (**Figure 3A**). Of the 43 upregulated CD markers, we found that nine were involved in the regulation of cell adhesion, namely, selectin E (SELE, CD62E), intercellular adhesion molecule-1 (ICAM1, CD54, which are ligands for the leukocyte adhesion protein LFA-1), integrin a6 (ITGA6, CD49f, and beta4, which promote tumorigenesis where beta1 inhibits erbB2/HER2 signaling), ITGA1 (CD49a, which is involved in cell adhesion, inflammation, and fibrosis), ITGB1 (CD29, which is involved in cell adhesion and recognition in various processes such as embryogenesis, hemostasis, tissue repair, immune response, and cancer metastasis), lysosome-associated membrane protein 2 (LAMP2 and CD107b, which play an important role in chaperone-mediated autophagy),

(A) LPIs upregulated 43 CD markers in HAECs.

Gene symbol	Fold change	Gene symbol	Fold change
Upregulated genes: 43 (LPIs treated HAECs vs Control HAECs)			
CD36	6.231	HMMR	1.238
SELE	4.072	ITGA2	1.229
CD27	3.772	TNFSF4	1.222
IFITM1	2.631	ENTPD1	1.21
IL13RA2	2.523	ITGA6	1.205
GGT1	2.468	CD55	1.197
MME	2.352	CD46	1.194
CD74	1.986	LAMP2	1.191
IL7R	1.743	ADAM10	1.184
KIT	1.683	ABCG2	1.183
ICAM1	1.478	PRNP	1.18
SEMA7A	1.463	TFRC	1.163
TLR3	1.435	FAS	1.162
CD34	1.37	CD109	1.16
EVI2B	1.37	NECTIN3	1.148
DPP4	1.341	ITGA1	1.143
TNFSF10	1.339	ITGB1	1.135
PDCD1LG2	1.311	SLC44A1	1.115
CD274	1.307	LIFR	1.114
CD302	1.296	CD82	1.081
IFNGR1	1.289	IL3RA	1.054
CD164	1.266		

(B) LPIs-induced CDs mediate EC adhesion, immune cell responses, and inflammatory cell signaling.

	CD markers	Where to present	Interact with	Function	Sources/PMID
Regulation of cell adhesion	SELE	activated endothelium	PSGL-1, ESL-1, L-Selectin, Podocalyxin	Leukocyte recruitment, slow rolling	28680883, 10925300
	ICAM1	leukocyte, EC, plasma membrane	LFA-1, VLA-4	Leukocyte adhesion	19307690
	ITGA6	macrophage	TSPAN4, GIPC1	Cell adhesion	25973901, 27624978
	ITGA1	Ecs, SMCs	ITGB1, ITGB3, Ptpn2	Angiogenesis, cell-cell adhesion	18647959
	ITGB1	Ecs	ITGA3, ITGAV, ITGA1	Angiogenesis, cell-cell adhesion	18647959
	LAMP2	lysosomal membrane	E-selectin	Autophagy, adhesion	8660832
	IFITM1	Plasma membrane, early endosomes	CD81, CD19,CR2	Proliferation, adhesion,formation of functional blood vessels, stabilizes EC-EC interaction during endothelial lumen formation, Angiogenesis	24603679
	CD164	primitive hematopoietic progenitor cells	CD34	Cell adhesion molecules,hematopoiesis	10721766, 17892536
	Nectin3	T-lymphocytes	Nectin-2	Cell-cell adherens junction formation, transendothelial migration of monocytes	24116228
Immune cell responses	CD27	Lymphoid cells (naïve CD4+, NK cells, activated B cells, CD8+)	CD70	Play a decisive role in establishing T cell response and memory; CD 27 co-stimulation increases Treg responses	29045618

FIGURE 3 | Continued

(B) LPIs-induced CDs mediate EC adhesion, immune cell responses, and inflammatory cell signaling.

	CD markers	Where to present	Interact with	Function	Sources/PMID
	CD274/PD-L1	T cells, macrophage, vascular EC	PD-1	Regulation of T cell activity	17853943
	SEMA7A	EC, monocyte, T cell, Platelets, DC	Integrin beta-1	Endothelial dysfunction, leukocyte infiltration	17853943
	TNFSF4	Macrophage, CD4+,CD8+	ox40l	Co-activation of T cells and facilitates B-T cell interaction, cytokine production	17068285
Inflammatory responses	GGT1	Macrophage		influence plaque progression, trigger the production of reactive oxygen species, promote pro-oxidant reaction, up-regulated on memory T lymphocytes	18486136, 10545483
	CD74	Macrophage and VSMC		AKT and NFkB activation, monocyte infiltration, inflammation during atherogenesis	19423618
	IL7R	B cells and T cells	IL7	promote inflammation	12742982
	CD36	macrophage	oxLDL, oxPL	induce signaling cascade for inflammatory responses, macrophage trapping mechanism	24903227
	TLR3	EC, cell surface, and endosomes in macrophages	dsRNA	Endothelial dysfunction, endothelial activation, inflammatory vascular development	21493895

(C) The other cell signaling mediated by LPIs-induced CDs.

CD markers	Function	Sources/PMID
IFITM1	Restricting early events in viral infection; against both RNA and DNA virus; related to cytokine signaling in immune system; IFNgamma pathway	30567988
IL13RA2	Receptor for IL13 and overexpression in many cancers	25896327
MME	A common lymphocytic leukemia antigen; a glycoprotein expresses on normal tissues, such as kidney; neutral endopeptidase.	MME / CD10 - LSBio
CD34	Hematopoietic cells; a promising therapy for end-stage atherosclerosis	24646491
EVI2B	Required for granulocyte differentiation; control of cell cycle progression and survival of hematopoietic progenitor cells.	https://www.genecards.org/cgi-bin/carddisp.pl?gene$=$EVI2B
DPP4	A novel adipokine impairs insulin sensitivity; Obesity association; metabolic syndrome	21593202
TNFSF10	tumor necrosis factor (TNF) related apoptosis inducing ligand; p53-transcriptional target gene; protects against diabetes and atherosclerosis	19106633, 21965021
PDCD1LG2	Immune checkpoint receptor (PD-1) ligand downregulates proatherogenic T-cell responses	21393583
CD302	C type lectin receptor, functioning dendritic cell migration	27316686
IFNGR1	IFNgamma receptor, promote foam cell formation	29874587
HMMR	Cell locomotion, cell motility, macrophage chemotaxis	34335086
ITGA2	Single-nucleotide polymorphism is associated with coronary atherosclerosis	20485444
ENTPD1	Regulator of atherogenesis that is driven by shear stress	26121751
CD55	Restrict complement pathway activity at the level of C3 and protect arterial wall from atherosclerosis	19729477
CD46	Transmembrane protein inactivate C3b and C4b; Induce Autophagy	Cell Surface Pathogen Receptor CD46 Induces Autophagy - ScienceDirect
ADAM10	Binding partner of VEGFR2, Angiogenesis, Cleavage of VE-cadherin; Increase vascular permeability and EC migration	20814017
ABCG2	A member of ATP-binding cassette transporter superfamily, contributing to multidrug resistance	22509477
PRNP	Affect the prion disease susceptibility	26022925
TFRC	Transferrin receptor can import iron by binding transferrin; progression of cancers	30034931
FAS	Pro-apoptotic cell surface receptor; pro-inflammatory molecule	33488632
CD109	Internalization and degradation of TGFbeta receptor	21295082
SLC44A1	Mediator of choline transport across both plasma and mitochondrial membrane	19357133
LIFR	Polyfunctional cytokine affects the differentiation, survival, and proliferation	OMIM Entry - * 151443 - LEUKEMIA INHIBITORY FACTOR RECEPTOR; LIFR
CD82	Restrain pathological angiogensis by inhibiting EC movement	25149363
IL3RA	Cytokine receptor activity	IL3RA Gene - GeneCards | IL3RA Protein | IL3RA Antibody

FIGURE 3 | Continued

(D) Majority of LPIs-induced CD markers were not shared with the reported EC specific markers, suggesting that LPIs induce ECs innate immune trans-differentiation.

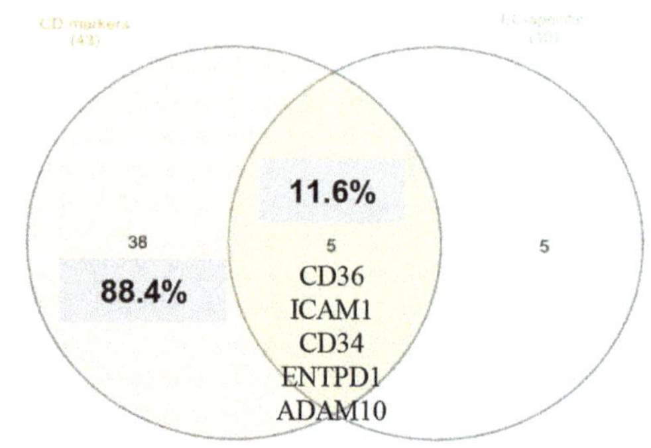

(E) The expressions of 16 out of 43 upregulated CDs also showed gene changes upon viral stimulation of ECs. Four of 16 CDs decreased upon virus stimulation but increased in LPIs treatments. The other 27 CDs are LPIs upregulated but virus infection no changed, which indicates the specificity for LPIs stimulation. *↑ Expression is consistent with LPI stimulated CDs. ↓ Expression is opposite of LPI stimulated CDs (LPI-specific group 1).

Expression	ID	Influenza virus infection (GSE59226)	MERS-CoV(icMERS) infection for 0 hr (GSE79218)	MERS-CoV(icMERS) infection for 12 hr (GSE79218)	MERS-CoV(icMERS) infection for 24 hr (GSE79218)	MERS-CoV(icMERS) infection for 36 hr (GSE79218)	MERS-CoV(icMERS) infection for 48 hr (GSE79218)
↑	IL7R	1.03	0.000001	0.000001	1.957338	1.647394	1.16601
↑	IL3RA	1.06	0.000001	−0.25735444	1.012712	0.247313	−0.34509
↑	ICAM1	−2.34	0.000001	2.59000745	3.093472	2.166789	0.000001
↑	FAS	−3.79	0.17608313	0.90609741	−0.55859	−0.50903	0.570957
↑	Ifitm1	−2.38	0.32868482	0.15805397	0.601549	0.920599	0.000001
↑	TNFSF10	−0.939	0.35543934	−1.50791028	−4.22693	−3.06942	−1.38672
↑	CD274	2.63	0.000001	0.65846262	0.866781	0.892408	0.828139
↑	CD74	0.806	0.000001	0.09087779	−0.14353	−0.17697	0.000001
↑	CD36	0.591	0.000001	−0.543872	−1.27092	−1.49171	−1.76812
↑	SELE	2.22	1.38410641	0.88052142	1.922168	0.947346	0.000001
↓	IFNGR1	−2.26	0.000001	0.000001	−1.07137	−1.40498	−0.72044
↑	ITGA6	−3.44	0.000001	−1.26917399	0.000001	0.510317	1.285312
↑	HMMR	−2.52	0.000001	0.000001	−0.68537	0.186594	1.946059
↓	ITGB1	−2.24	0.000001	−0.73254498	−1.02011	0.000001	0.000001
↓	TLR3	−2.05	0.000001	−0.55344746	−0.92855	−0.86757	0.000001
↓	ITGA2	−3.45	0.30550044	−0.75442646	−0.79849	0.000001	1.128331
LPI-induced specific CDs (LPI-specific group 2)	CD27, IL13RA2, GGT1, MME, KIT, SEMA7A, CD34, EVI2B, DPP4, PDCD1LG2, CD302, CD164, TNFSF4, ENTPD1, CD55, CD46, LAMP2, ADAM10, ABCG2, PRNP, TFRC, CD109, NECTIN3, ITGA1, SLC44A1, LIFR, CD82						

FIGURE 3 | Continued

F **Metascape pathway analysis for 43 up-regulated CD markers.** The pathways that are related to EC activation were boxed in red.

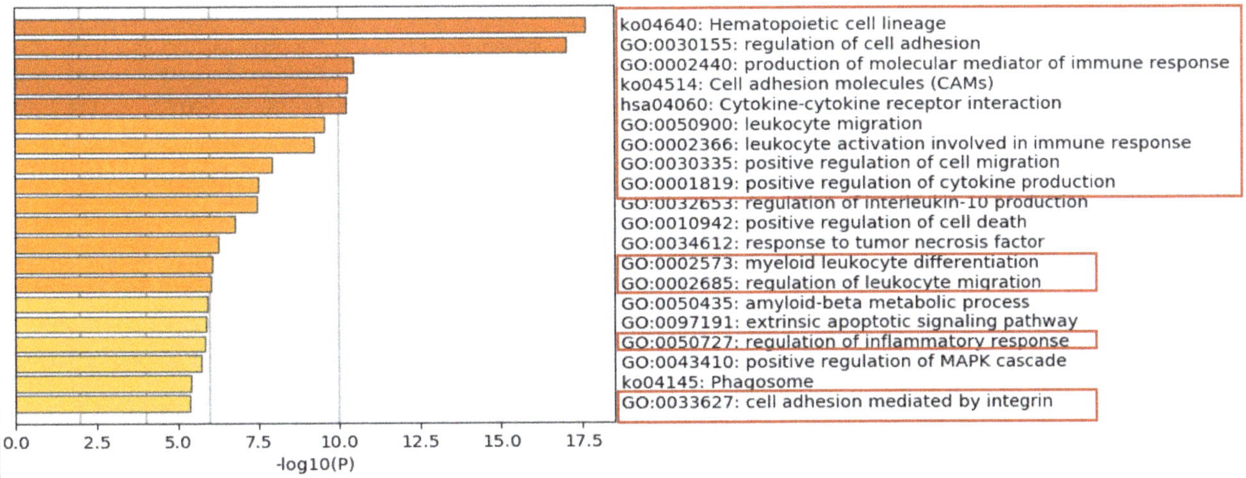

G **Schematic presentation for LPI-induced CD markers in HAECs.**

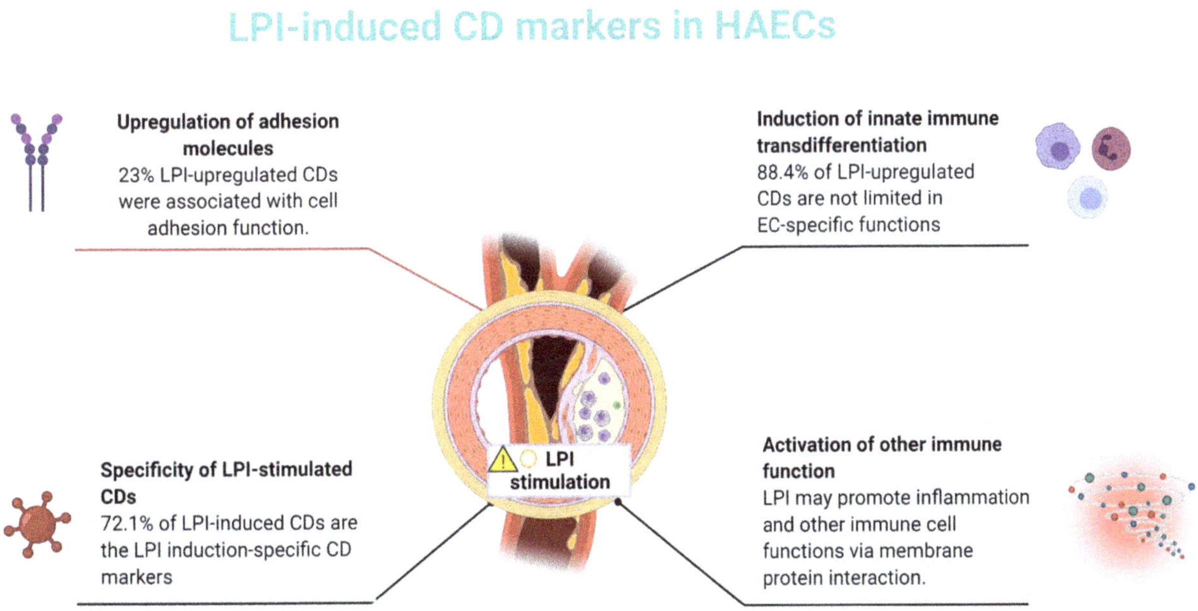

FIGURE 3 | LPIs upregulated EC adhesion molecules and cluster of differentiation (CD) marker-mediated signaling pathways. **(A)** 373 CD markers were used for database mining. Genes with $p < 0.05$ and $\log_2$ FC > |1| were selected as significantly changed genes. The total number of significantly changed CD markers is 65; upregulated genes account for 66.2% (43/65) and downregulated genes occupied 33.8% (22/65). Downregulated CDs can be found in **Supplementary Table S1**. **(B)** Eighteen out of 43 LPI-induced CDs mediate EC adhesion, immune cell responses, and inflammatory cell signaling. **(C)** Twenty-five out of 43 LPI-induced CDs mediates the other cell signaling. **(D)** One hundred fifty-nine endothelial cell-specific markers were generated (modified from PMID: 29333215). The LPI-upregulated EC-specific genes were compared with the upregulated CD markers. The Venn diagram indicated that five adhesion molecules showed in the overlapped area between endothelial cell-specific cell markers and LPI-stimulated CD markers. The functions of five overlapped CD markers and most of them participate in the cell adhesion process. **(E)** About 43 upregulated CDs were screened in seven virus-stimulated EC datasets (PMID:34248940). Sixteen out of 43 showed different changes in these seven datasets. **(F)** Upregulated genes of LPI-treated HAECs were analyzed by Metascape (https://metascape.org/gp/index.html#/main/step1). Pathways with high expression are related to the cell adhesion process, leukocyte migration, and inflammation. **(G)** A schematic presentation shows how LPIs regulate endothelial cells by mediating membrane protein interactions. ***(G)** was created with Biorender.com.

(A) Secretomes (canonical): LPI treated HAECs vs Control HAECs [upregulated genes: 216 (216/2640~8.2%)].

GENE	P value	Fold change	GENE	P value	Fold change	GENE	P value	Fold change	GENE	P value	Fold change
ACVR1C	0.0201	∞	TGFBR1	0.00297	1.319	ERO1A	0.00276	1.192	ENOX2	0.0353	1.104
CA9	0.0242	∞	CLEC2B	0.00117	1.314	MATR3	0.0154	1.19	TOGARAM1	0.0225	1.101
ISM1	0.00327	∞	RASA2	0.00315	1.314	FKBP14	0.0154	1.189	MMRN1	0.0173	1.099
NPNT	0.0126	∞	PDCD1LG2	0.0284	1.311	ADAMTS9	0.015	1.188	CXorf36	0.000143	1.098
RLN2	0.0242	∞	KRT10	0.0257	1.307	CFI	0.0095	1.187	HEXB	0.00676	1.098
WIF1	0.016	12.511	MSH3	0.000133	1.305	ITFG1	0.0000025	1.185	INHBA	0.0056	1.094
GNRH2	0.0317	8.996	CXCL1	0.000572	1.302	ADAM10	0.00193	1.184	ZNF449	0.0392	1.092
IL1RN	0.0479	7.785	IGFBP5	0.0186	1.301	FKBP7	0.00862	1.184	CDC23	0.0396	1.089
LYZ	0.0488	6.815	LOX	0.00109	1.301	MCEE	0.0249	1.184	BMP2	0.0134	1.083
CGB7	0.039	6.098	TFPI	0.000708	1.292	C2orf69	0.0162	1.183	GFOD1	0.0242	1.08
LYG2	0.01	5.997	CTSS	0.012	1.28	MFAP3	0.0169	1.182	HBEGF	0.045	1.077
CCL20	0.0155	4.781	SDHD	0.000547	1.279	PRNP	0.00662	1.18	SNCA	0.0353	1.073
CX3CL1	0.00443	4.511	TGFB3	0.0158	1.278	GLCE	0.0172	1.179	PRSS23	0.0423	1.069
CXCL11	0.0171	3.582	ASAH1	0.0227	1.276	GGH	0.0282	1.178	FSTL1	0.00538	1.055
CXCL6	0.000187	2.693	BCKDHB	0.00648	1.276	EMCN	0.00176	1.177	LRCH3	0.00486	1.046
MAMDC2	0.00233	2.682	TGFBR3	0.000782	1.274	DHX29	0.004	1.174			
CCL26	0.0496	2.635	DNAJB9	0.0165	1.271	PLAU	0.0494	1.171			
IL1A	0.0116	2.569	SPATA6	0.00587	1.268	ERP44	0.0434	1.169			
FGL2	0.0147	2.481	HMGB2	0.00233	1.267	GOLM1	0.00112	1.167			
FAM3D	0.0364	2.47	CD164	0.0027	1.266	B4GALT6	0.0000025	1.163			
GGT1	0.0277	2.468	GLIPR1	0.0251	1.26	IDE	0.0167	1.163			
TMEM108	0.0399	2.263	MTX2	0.00379	1.259	TFRC	0.00778	1.163			
TNFSF15	0.0314	2.143	GHR	0.0474	1.256	FAS	0.0271	1.162			
IL1B	0.00209	2.115	MINPP1	0.00891	1.252	MET	0.00986	1.162			
CXCL3	0.035	2.046	ADAMTS6	0.00481	1.248	EPS15	0.00127	1.161			
STC1	0.00191	1.994	ANTXR1	0.00843	1.24	ITM2B	0.00553	1.16			
CPXM1	0.0208	1.907	PON2	0.000283	1.239	PDZD2	0.038	1.16			
CXCL8	0.000266	1.849	NID2	0.00218	1.238	MSRB3	0.0209	1.159			
CSF3	0.00679	1.832	TRIM24	0.00814	1.236	METTL9	0.0136	1.157			
NLGN4Y	0.000245	1.821	CDC40	0.00142	1.235	EDEM3	0.0114	1.155			
LIPH	0.0282	1.802	DSE	0.0059	1.231	B2M	0.0378	1.153			
APOB	0.0203	1.788	HMGB1	0.00593	1.231	AK4	0.00392	1.152			
FLRT3	0.0143	1.786	AIMP1	0.00314	1.23	CLPX	0.0374	1.152			
IL7R	0.0261	1.743	TFAM	0.00563	1.23	CCBE1	0.0118	1.151			
IL33	0.000272	1.678	MGAT4A	0.0178	1.227	ERLEC1	0.0113	1.149			
RAPGEF5	0.000207	1.66	SDCBP	0.000634	1.227	CCNL1	0.0158	1.148			
CPA3	0.00101	1.642	TFPI2	0.000177	1.227	NUP155	0.0264	1.147			
CCL2	0.00112	1.639	ANXA1	0.00125	1.226	NTN4	0.000166	1.144			
SERPINE3	0.038	1.636	CTSO	0.0114	1.225	PDGFD	0.045	1.144			
ERP27	0.0075	1.584	FAM3C	0.0251	1.224	NFE2L3	0.000631	1.143			
NRG4	0.0211	1.557	HS2ST1	0.00624	1.222	ABHD10	0.0449	1.142			
NOG	0.0109	1.556	ADAMTS18	0.000145	1.221	FAM177A1	0.00292	1.141			
GNRH1	0.00293	1.532	GALNT1	0.000176	1.219	PDZD8	0.0159	1.14			
LRRC17	0.0017	1.514	SECISBP2	0.0225	1.216	SYAP1	0.00322	1.14			
MASP2	0.00387	1.504	EOGT	0.000538	1.214	PDCD6IP	0.00231	1.139			
UBXN8	0.00404	1.497	DNAJC3	0.000746	1.213	AGK	0.0208	1.137			
PAPLN	0.0454	1.47	CLN5	0.0012	1.211	ARSJ	0.00339	1.136			
ANGPT2	0.00182	1.452	PTGS2	0.0413	1.211	HSPA13	0.00495	1.134			
TLR3	0.0138	1.435	CEP57	0.00509	1.21	ATMIN	0.0213	1.131			

FIGURE 4 | Continued

(A) Secretomes (canonical): LPI treated HAECs vs Control HAECs [upregulated genes: 216 (216/2640~8.2%)].

GENE	P value	Fold change	GENE	P value	Fold change	GENE	P value	Fold change	GENE	P value	Fold change
ID1	0.00047	1.434	MRPS22	0.0103	1.207	GPD2	0.0269	1.13			
NAMPT	0.0000158	1.427	OCLN	0.0124	1.207	PCDH12	0.00786	1.13			
CXADR	0.00475	1.426	FGF2	0.00616	1.206	RSF1	0.00817	1.13			
INHBB	0.0212	1.42	FGF5	0.0078	1.203	PTEN	0.00361	1.127			
SEMA3A	0.00123	1.414	COL12A1	0.0403	1.202	SEL1L	0.00652	1.127			
EBAG9	0.00437	1.407	MIER1	0.0017	1.202	PTX3	0.0494	1.125			
CSGALNACT1	0.00134	1.393	POGLUT1	0.00192	1.201	ARSK	0.000526	1.124			
NT5C3A	0.0012	1.376	COG3	0.00734	1.2	MIA3	0.00907	1.124			
PROS1	0.0426	1.372	MRPL32	0.00321	1.2	RSPRY1	0.00247	1.123			
FABP5	0.0156	1.366	PIGK	0.0135	1.2	ADAMTS1	0.00243	1.121			
EXTL2	0.0000815	1.365	ERAP1	0.00111	1.199	AGA	0.0334	1.119			
DPP4	0.0109	1.341	CD55	0.00103	1.197	PLA2G12A	0.0152	1.119			
TNFSF10	0.00413	1.339	OXCT1	0.0173	1.196	SIAE	0.022	1.119			
C6orf120	0.000917	1.338	PLOD2	0.00644	1.196	QPCT	0.0374	1.118			
KDM6A	0.00304	1.327	KDELC2	0.0429	1.195	CHST1	0.00564	1.117			
DCN	0.0142	1.323	KITLG	0.00299	1.194	LAMA4	0.00265	1.117			
ERAP2	0.000668	1.323	MDFIC	0.00224	1.194	NUDT9	0.0333	1.117			
GBP1	0.0000777	1.322	C3orf58	0.00398	1.192	LIFR	0.0292	1.114			

(B) Secretomes (CASP1-dependent): LPI treated HAECs vs Control HAECs.

Upregulated genes: 60 (60/964~6.2%)

GENE	P value	Fold change	GENE	P value	Fold change	GENE	P value	Fold change	GENE	P value	Fold change
IDI1	0.00885	1.157	UBE2N	0.000591	1.172	OSTF1	0.00201	1.104	BZW1	0.0137	1.211
FLI1	0.00183	1.114	SSB	0.0036	1.236	EIF2A	0.000561	1.314	RAP1B	0.0183	1.199
VPS35	0.00354	1.148	CBX3	0.0277	1.23	SBDS	0.000145	1.262	PCNA	0.0472	1.118
PRDX3	0.000182	1.278	SUMO2	0.004	1.195	VPS29	0.0266	1.244	TMOD3	0.00269	1.2
ANXA3	0.000171	1.309	CDC42	0.0203	1.103	HMGB2	0.00233	1.267	CNN3	0.00813	1.123
PDCD5	0.0119	1.217	RAB10	0.0358	1.127	HMGB1	0.00593	1.231	ERH	0.025	1.355
EHBP1	0.00333	1.208	BTF3	0.00053	1.276	MTPN	0.000675	1.211			
ERO1A	0.00276	1.192	ELOC	0.0445	1.168	NACA	0.000108	1.287			
INHBA	0.0056	1.094	UAP1	0.000546	1.307	FUBP3	0.0000824	1.196			
API5	0.000681	1.214	FKBP3	0.00875	1.336	CDCA2	0.00343	1.134			
ANXA1	0.00125	1.226	CUL1	0.00166	1.152	GGH	0.0282	1.178			
UBE2A	0.0231	1.094	ATP5J	0.0339	1.497	FSTL1	0.00538	1.055			
NUDT5	0.0155	1.192	SF3B1	0.000758	1.213	FAM3C	0.0251	1.224			
TCEA1	0.00372	1.208	STX7	0.0001	1.185	CALD1	0.000488	1.184			
TWF1	0.00181	1.199	SRP72	0.000579	1.251	LPP	0.0145	1.143			
ETFA	0.00372	1.093	FAS	0.0271	1.162	CAB39	0.00937	1.202			
SFPQ	0.0369	1.065	CLIC4	0.00753	1.231	SRP19	0.0384	1.368			
MET	0.00986	1.162	ADK	0.022	1.153	SMC4	0.0265	1.083			

FIGURE 4 | Continued

(C) Secretomes (Caspase 4 dependent): LPI treated HAECs vs Control HAECs.
Upregulated genes: 117 (117/1223~9.6%)

Gene	P value	Fold change	Gene	P value	Fold change	Gene	P value	Fold change
FGL2	0.0147	2.481	RAP1B	0.0183	1.199	CDC42	0.0203	1.103
MX1	0.0118	1.71	ERAP1	0.00111	1.199	SYNC	0.0127	1.102
LXN	0.00194	1.502	EIF3J	0.0012	1.197	GBP2	0.0248	1.102
ICAM1	0.000258	1.478	TIGAR	0.00911	1.197	NAA15	0.0324	1.1
FABP4	0.00521	1.455	SNX6	0.0189	1.197	HEXB	0.00676	1.098
CASP1	0.00193	1.455	DNM1L	0.0000683	1.195	RBMX	0.00182	1.096
NAMPT	0.0000158	1.427	SUMO2	0.004	1.195	INHBA	0.0056	1.094
SRP19	0.0384	1.368	ERO1A	0.00276	1.192	ETFA	0.00372	1.093
PPIL3	0.0103	1.367	NUDT5	0.0155	1.192	CDV3	0.0294	1.093
FABP5	0.0156	1.366	LAMP2	0.00435	1.191	KIF2A	0.0139	1.082
ERH	0.025	1.355	ABCE1	0.0168	1.19	RBBP7	0.0115	1.077
FKBP3	0.00875	1.336	SGTB	0.00116	1.188	FKBP5	0.0188	1.067
VTA1	0.000652	1.329	STX7	0.0001	1.185	SFPQ	0.0369	1.065
GBP1	0.0000777	1.322	TNPO1	0.00114	1.181			
SUMO1	0.00481	1.321	GGCT	0.00908	1.179			
EIF2A	0.000561	1.314	HMGN1	0.00347	1.178			
NACA	0.000108	1.287	GGH	0.0282	1.178			
PRDX3	0.000182	1.278	GMFB	0.0499	1.175			
ASAH1	0.0227	1.276	VAPA	0.0075	1.174			
CLIC2	0.0418	1.274	NAA50	0.026	1.173			
HMGB2	0.00233	1.267	UBE2N	0.000591	1.172			
OLA1	0.000505	1.266	ERP44	0.0434	1.169			
SBDS	0.000145	1.262	ELOC	0.0445	1.168			
SCRN3	0.0136	1.25	GOLM1	0.00112	1.167			
PTPRE	0.00932	1.249	PSD3	0.0291	1.167			
PIN4	0.032	1.249	MOB1A	0.00557	1.166			
CUL2	0.00248	1.246	RAB1A	0.00162	1.165			
PGM2	0.00042	1.244	CAND1	0.0259	1.165			
VPS29	0.0266	1.244	IDE	0.0167	1.163			
CASP3	0.00581	1.238	FAS	0.0271	1.162			
HMGB1	0.00593	1.231	CD109	0.0355	1.16			
CLIC4	0.00753	1.231	BROX	0.0112	1.158			
AIMP1	0.00314	1.23	IDI1	0.00885	1.157			
CBX3	0.0277	1.23	XPO1	0.00563	1.155			
SNX2	0.00608	1.229	LIMS1	0.00203	1.155			
DCK	0.00437	1.229	BUB3	0.00612	1.153			
ARMT1	0.00629	1.229	ADK	0.022	1.153			
ANXA1	0.00125	1.226	DDI2	0.0211	1.153			
BDH2	0.0414	1.221	MTAP	0.00373	1.152			
IPO7	0.000408	1.219	BLM	0.00833	1.151			
PDCD5	0.0119	1.217	VPS35	0.00354	1.148			
FNTA	0.0000756	1.216	DEK	0.0313	1.139			
IMPA1	0.037	1.212	ZMYM4	0.0451	1.126			
MTPN	0.000675	1.211	UFC1	0.048	1.126			
EHBP1	0.00333	1.208	PTX3	0.0494	1.125			
UBA3	0.0449	1.208	CRK	0.000865	1.119			
UBE2K	0.00188	1.207	PCNA	0.0472	1.118			
VPS4B	0.0187	1.203	QPCT	0.0374	1.118			
OPTN	0.00296	1.203	NUDT9	0.0333	1.117			
CAB39	0.00937	1.202	SNX5	0.000777	1.114			
XPOT	0.00201	1.201	IPO5	0.0346	1.107			
TMOD3	0.00269	1.2	OSTF1	0.00201	1.104			

FIGURE 4 | Continued

(D) Secretomes (Exosome): LPI treated HAECs vs Control HAECs.
Upregulated genes (FC>|1.5|): 40 (40/6561~0.6%)

Exosome	P value	Fold change	Exosome	P value	Fold change
IL1RN	0.0479	7.785	IFIT1	0.0265	2.093
LYZ	0.0488	6.815	Ndufa13	0.0497	2.082
Cd36	0.000939	6.231	Nme2	0.0388	2.027
CCL20	0.0155	4.781	STC1	0.00191	1.994
Cx3cl1	0.00443	4.511	CD74	0.0201	1.986
PYGM	0.0284	4.385	IFIT3	0.00791	1.907
CRYAB	0.0147	3.484	CXCL8	0.000266	1.849
Pdzk1	0.0324	3.164	CSF3	0.00679	1.832
SLC6A15	0.0478	3.153	MYO1B	0.000466	1.792
RPL29P11	0.00246	2.757	Apob	0.0203	1.788
MAMDC2	0.00233	2.682	Sod2	0.000254	1.778
IFITM1	0.0183	2.631	MX1	0.0118	1.71
LYPD3	0.0234	2.624	DCLK1	0.00424	1.707
FOXF1	0.0255	2.574	KIT	0.000128	1.683
IL13RA2	0.0389	2.523	Cpa3	0.00101	1.642
FGL2	0.0147	2.481	CCL2	0.00112	1.639
GGT1	0.0277	2.468	STK26	0.00157	1.615
LST1	0.0378	2.41	MASP2	0.00387	1.504
MME	0.00022	2.352			
PKHD1L1	0.0075	2.318			
NEK10	0.00569	2.233			
SYCP3	0.0346	2.157			

FIGURE 4 | LPIs significantly upregulate secretomic genes of canonical secretomes, non-canonical caspase-1-Gasdermin D (GSDMD), caspase-4-GSDMD, and exosome secretomes in HAECs. **(A)** Among 2,640 canonical secretomes, 216 were significantly upregulated in LPI-treated HAECs. The upregulated genes accounted for 8.2% of the total canonical secretomes. **(B)** Sixty non-canonical caspase 1 dependent secretomes were significantly elevated in LPI-treated HAECs. **(C)** One hundred seventeen non-canonical caspase 4 dependent secretomes were dramatically increased in LPI-treated HAECs. **(D)** Forty exosomes were dramatically increased in LPI-stimulated HAECs. *Genes in **(A–C)** were selected with $p < 0.05$ and $\log_2$ FC > |1| as significantly changed genes, while genes in exosome listed $p < 0.05$ and $\log_2$ FC > |1.5| as significantly changed genes. The full list of 923 LPI-upregulated exosomes can be found in **Supplementary Table S3**. *Created with Biorender.com.

interferon-induced transmembrane protein 1 (IFITM1, which inhibits the entry of viruses, viral fusion, and release to the cytoplasm), CD164 (multi-glycosylated core protein 24, which regulates the proliferation, adhesion, and migration of hematopoietic progenitor cells), and nectin cell adhesion molecule 3 (nectin3 and CD113, which function as adhesion molecules at adherens junctions). These CDs were also functional in leukocyte recruitment, cell-cell interaction, and slow rolling (80–90). The second group of five upregulated CDs, namely CD27 (a tumor necrosis factor receptor (TNFR), a superfamily member and co-stimulation receptor), semaphoring 7A (SEMA7A), CD108, (which promotes axonal growth and T cell development), TNFSF4 (CD134, OX40 ligand, a co-stimulation receptor), and GGT1[CD224, which promotes clear cell renal cell carcinoma initiation and progression (91)], played roles in co-stimulating T cell immune responses, promoting cancer growth (92), and establishing immune memory (93–97). In addition, the third group of four inflammation-related CDs, such as MHC HLA-DR gamma chain (CD74) for MHC class II antigen presentation, interleukin-7 receptor (IL7R, which plays a critical role in the development of lymphocytes in a process called VDJ recombination), scavenger receptor class B, member 3 (CD36) for oxidized low-density lipoprotein (oxLDL) cell internalization (98), and toll-like receptor 3 (TLR3) for binding to double-stranded RNA/unmethylated CpG DNA and cooperating with scavenger receptor SREC-I to trigger inflammatory innate immune response (99), were dramatically upregulated in LPI-treated HAECs (**Figure 3B**) (100–103). Moreover, the fourth group included 25 CDs involved in many cellular functions, such as viral infection (IFITM1), interferon-gamma receptor signaling (IFITM1, IFNGR1), growth factor/cytokine receptors (TNFSF10, ADAM10, TFRC, FAS, CD109, IL13RA2, IL3RA, LIFR, DPP4), immune checkpoint receptors (PDCD1LG2), complement signaling (CD55, CD46), and hematopoiesis and stem cells [CD34, EVI2B, and KIT (104)] (**Figure 3C**).

To better understand the alteration of endothelial cell surface markers induced by LPIs, we further gathered a list of 159 endothelial cell-specific biomarkers (60)

(**Supplementary Table S2**). **Figure 3D** shows that five CD markers (11.6%) out of 43 LPI-upregulated CDs were shared with 5 out of 10 LPI-upregulated EC-specific cell biomarkers: CD36, ICAM1, CD34, ectonucleoside triphosphate diphosphohydrolase 1 (ENTPD1), and ADAM metallopeptidase domain 10 (ADAM10). Among these five CD markers, ICAM1, CD34, and ADAM10 directly mediate cell-cell adhesion. For example, the classic adhesion molecule ICAM1 on the surface of EC could interact with the molecule LFA-1 on lymphocytes, leading to a pro-inflammatory signaling cascade (82). CD34, a marker for human hematopoietic progenitor cells, exhibits E-selectin binding activity, facilitating leukocyte rolling and adhesion (105). ADAM10 showed a significantly high expression in atherosclerotic plaque, and its activity was necessary for chemotaxis/migration of monocytes and ECs (106). Of note, the LPIs upregulating 38 out of 43 CDs (88.4%) that did not overlap with EC-specific markers suggested that as high as 88.4% of the CDs upregulated by LPIs are functional in various aspects and not limited to EC-specific functions. These results have demonstrated that the LPI stimulation of aortic ECs may induce innate immune trans-differentiation of ECs, as we have reported (19), and non-EC-specific functions.

In order to identify CD markers specifically induced by LPIs, we examined the expressions of 43 LPI-induced CD markers in the microarray datasets of seven virus-infected human endothelial cells, such as influenza virus-infected human umbilical vein endothelial cells (HUVEC), middle east respiratory syndrome coronavirus (MERS-CoV, homologous to severe acute respiratory syndrome coronavirus 2, SARS-CoV2, or COVID-19)-infected human microvascular endothelial cells, and Kaposi's sarcoma-associated herpes virus(KSHV)-infected human dermal endothelial cells, as we have reported (3). As shown in **Figure 3E**, the 43 LPI-induced CD markers can be classified into three groups: (1) 12 LPIs were upregulated, and pathogen-associated molecular pattern (PAMP)-triggered (virus-infection) was upregulated (activated endothelial cell shared), namely, IL7R, IL3RA, ICAM1, FAS, Ifitm1, TNFSF10, CD274, CD74, CD36, SELE, ITGA6, and HMMR; (2) 4 LPIs were upregulated, but virus infection was downregulated (LPI-specific group 1), such as IFNGR1, ITGB1, TLR3, and ITGA2; 3) 27 LPIs were upregulated but virus infection was not changed (LPI-specific group 2) namely, CD27, IL13RA2, GGT1, MME, KIT (CD117, stem cell growth factor receptor), SEMA7A (CD108), CD34 (107), EVI2B, DPP4 (CD26, its inhibitors approved for treating type 2 diabetes), PDCD1LG2, CD302, CD164, TNFSF4 (OX40 ligand, CD252), ENTPD1, CD55, CD46, LAMP2, ADAM10, ABCG2 (CDw338, breast cancer resistant protein), PRNP, TFRC, CD109, NECTIN3, ITGA1, SLC44A1, LIFR, and CD82. Of note, future work is needed to determine whether LPIs upregulated CDs share with the CDs upregulated in responses to the stimulation of PAMPs/DAMPs and conditional DAMPs (20, 21).

In addition to analyzing the functions of upregulated CD markers, Metascape was used for pathway analysis (https://metascape.org/gp/index.html#/main/step1) for small gene sets in comparison with that analyzed by IPA. Twenty pathways, using upregulated CD markers from LPI-treated HAECs (**Figure 3F**), were identified, such as the top 10 functions of hematopoietic cell lineage, regulation of cell adhesion, production of molecular mediator of the immune response, cell adhesion molecules (CAMs), cytokine-cytokine receptor interaction, leukocyte migration, leukocyte activation involved in immune response, positive regulation of cell migration, positive regulation of cytokine production, and regulation of IL-10 production. Among these 20 pathways, 11 were related to EC activation (boxed), namely, the top 2–9 functions mentioned above, and myeloid leukocyte differentiation, regulation of inflammatory response, and cell adhesion mediated by integrin. Of note, the "regulation of cell adhesion" showed extraordinarily high enrichment up to around log10 (16).

Our results on LPI-induced CD markers in HAECs demonstrated that, first, of the total 65 LPI-changed CD markers, 66.2% were significantly upregulated by LPI stimulation, and that only 33.8% were downregulated by LPIs. Among the LPI-upregulated CD markers, 23% were associated with cell adhesion; 9.3 and 9.3% were related to immune response and inflammation, respectively. These results suggest that LPIs induce aortic EC activation through the upregulation of various adhesion molecules, *via* which LPIs may initiate inflammation by recruiting immune cell accumulation; second, by comparing LPI-upregulated CD markers with EC-specific markers, we found that LPI stimulation upregulates CDs that are significantly different from EC-specific markers, suggesting that LPIs may induce the innate immune trans-differentiation of ECs, as we have reported (19), LPI-activated HAECs may carry out many non-EC-specific functions; third, 31 out of the 43 LPI-induced CD markers (72.1%) are LPI induction-specific CD markers that are not induced in three types of virus-infected endothelial cells, which significantly enhance our understanding of CD markers upregulated in activated ECs; fourth, in addition to inducing EC activation, LPI-induced CD markers may promote other immune cell functions and inflammatory responses *via* membrane protein interactions (**Figure 3G**).

LPI-Activated Aortic ECs Upregulate Six Types of Secretomic Genes, Canonical Secretome, Caspase-1-Gasdermin D (GSDMD) Non-Canonical Secretome, Caspase-4/11-GSDMD Non-Canonical Secretome, Exosome Non-Canonical Secretome, HPA-Classified Cytokines, and HPA-Classified Chemokines, Which Makes HAECs a Large Secretory Organ for Inflammation, Immune Responses, and Other Functions

Secretome refers to a collection of actively secreted proteins for a destination outside the nucleus and cytoplasm of the cells. Those proteins are actively transported within the secretory pathways and participate in various signaling functions, such as cytokines, chemokines, adhesion molecules (108), angiogenesis, and wound healing (109). ECs are secretory cells, and protein secretion plays a pivotal role in EC functions, as we and others have reported/reviewed (1, 3, 4, 40, 44, 50, 110, 111). Especially during EC activation, secreted proteins are responsible for cell-cell interaction, affecting vascular tone, cell adhesion, and inflammation (112). The 18 cytokines secreted from EC (110) included pro-inflammatory cytokines, such as tumor necrosis factor-α (TNF-α), interleukin-1 (IL-1), IL-3, IL-5, IL-6, IL-8, IL-11, IL-15, monocyte chemoattractant protein-1 (MCP-1), granulocyte-macrophage colony-stimulating factor (GM-CSF) (3, 57), CD40/CD40L, endothelin-1, regulated upon activation, normal T cell expressed and presumably secreted (RANTES, C-C motif ligand 5, CCL5) and anti-inflammatory cytokine IL1 receptor antagonist (IL1ra), IL10 (59), IL13, transforming growth factor-β (TGF-β), and IL-35 (40, 44, 58, 59, 111). We hypothesize that LPI treatment drives HAEC activation *via* the upregulation of inflammatory and adhesion-related secreted proteins. To gain a comprehensive understanding of how the LPI stimulation of HAECs regulates the secretory functions of ECs, we collected six secretomic gene lists:(1) 2,640 conventional secretomes (with signal peptide) were downloaded from the comprehensive protein database Human Protein Atlas (https://www.proteinatlas.org/), as we have reported (13); (2) 964 non-canonical caspase-1-gasdermin D (GSDMD) secretomes (67); (3) 1,223 non-canonical caspase-4 (humans)/11 (mice) secretomes (68), and 4) 6,560 exosome secretomes downloaded from a comprehensive exosome database (http://www.exocarta.org/) (113), as we have reported (48). As shown in **Figure 4A**, 216 (8.2%) out of the 2,640 canonical secretomic genes were dramatically increased in LPI-treated HAECs. Similarly, 60 (6.2%) out of the 964 caspase-1-GSDMD non-canonical secretomic genes and 117 (9.6%) out of the 1,223 caspase-4-GSDMD non-canonical secretomic genes were significantly upregulated in the LPI-activated HAECs, respectively (**Figures 4B,C**). In addition, 40 out of the 6,560 total exosome secretomic genes showed dramatic elevation, with >log2FC 1.5 (fold change) (**Figure 4D**).

Of note, secretomes secrete a variety of biologically active molecules, such as (1) growth factors, (2) hormones, (3) cytokines [myokines/exerkines from muscle (113), adipokines from adipose tissues (114), cardiokines from the heart (115), hepatokines from the liver (116), osteokines from bones (116), nephrokines from kidney (113), and neurokines from the brain (113)]; (4) chemokines (117), and (5) many other secretory molecules with poorly characterized functions (13, 48, 49). Cytokines and chemokines released from endothelium have long been documented to be essential in promoting leukocyte recruitment, and inflammation during atherosclerosis, as we and others have reported/reviewed (1, 3, 4, 40, 44, 50, 110, 111). However, the vital question remained whether ECs secrete large pools of cytokines and chemokines during LPI-induced EC activation. Thus, we collected two lists of 1,176 cytokines and 200 chemokines (49) classified by the Human Protein Atlas (HPA, https://www.proteinatlas.org/) and examined the expression changes in the HPA-classified cytokines and chemokines, and their interactors in the LPI-treated HAEC RNA-Seq dataset. Of note, some cytokines and chemokines were overlapped with secretory proteins classified in other secretomes. As shown in **Figure 5A**, the expressions of 179 (15.2%) out of 1,176 HPA-classified cytokines showed a significant increase, and the expressions of 28 (14%) out of 200 HPA-classified chemokines were significantly upregulated (**Figure 5B**).

The Metascape (https://metascape.org/gp/index.html#/main/step1) database analysis with six types of upregulated secretomes, cytokines, and chemokines in LPI-activated HAECs in **Figure 6** demonstrated that the LPI-upregulated canonical secretome had top 10 functional pathways, namely, NABA matrisome associated, extracellular structure organization, glycoprotein metabolic process, vasculature development, myeloid leukocyte activation, regulation of cell adhesion, positive regulation of cell migration, IL-10 signaling, cellular response to growth factor stimulus, and VEGFA-VEGFR2 signaling (**Figure 6A**). The LPI-upregulated caspase-1-GSDMD non-canonical secretome had top 10 functional pathways, namely, regulation of nuclease activity, homeostasis of the number of cells, renal cell carcinoma, negative regulation of protein complex assembly, myeloid cell differentiation, CDC5L complex, cellular response to oxidative stress, 7q11.23 copy number variation syndrome, neutrophil degranulation, and nucleotide excision repair (**Figure 6B**). The LPI-upregulated caspase-4-GSDMD non-canonical secretome had top 10 functional pathways, namely, regulated exocytosis, autophagy, cytokine signaling in the immune system, cellular component disassembly, viral life cycle, response to an inorganic substance, response to tumor necrosis factor, apoptotic signaling pathway, cellular protein catabolic process, and regulation of nuclease activity (**Figure 6C**). The LPI-upregulated exosome non-canonical secretome had top 10 functional pathways, namely, membrane trafficking, endomembrane system organization, organelle localization, vesicle organization, actin filament-based process, regulated exocytosis, protein localization to the membrane, cellular protein catabolic process, endocytosis, and autophagy (**Figure 6D**). The LPI-upregulated cytokines had top 10 functions, namely, signaling by interleukins, regulation of cell adhesion, cytokinesis, cytokine-cytokine receptor interaction, response to molecule of bacterial origin, transmembrane receptor protein tyrosine kinase signaling, positive regulation of locomotion, Kaposi sarcoma-associated herpesvirus infection, positive regulation of cytokine production, and regulation of MAPK cascade (**Figure 6E**). The LPI-upregulated chemokines had top 10 functions, namely, chemokine production, response to chemokine, cellular response to interleukin-1, signaling by interleukins, positive regulation of response to external stimulus, regulation of leukocyte migration, positive regulation of vasculature development, regulation of the multi-organism process, positive regulation of cytokine biosynthetic process, and influenza A-related process (**Figure 6F**).

To find potential connections among the LPI-treated HAEC secretory protein molecules, we created a Venn diagram for the pathways of canonical secretome, caspase-1 secretome, caspase-4 secretome, exosome secretome, HPA cytokines, and HPA chemokines. As shown in **Figure 7A**, among the 118 secretomic gene pathways identified by the Metascape analysis, the majority of the pathways were secretome-specific; and 12 pathways were shared among the six types of secretomic genes. The caspase-1-GSDMD secretome shared homeostasis of numbers of cells with HPA-cytokines; the caspase-1-GSDMD secretome shared endocytosis with the exosome secretome; the exosome secretome shared positive regulation of hydrolase activity with the HPA cytokines, and three types of secretomes, canonical, exosome, HPA cytokines, shared regulation of cell adhesion; the canonical secretome and HPA chemokines shared myeloid leukocyte activation; the canonical secretome and HPA cytokines shared response to wounding and response to interleukin-1; the caspase-4-GSDMD and exosome secretomes shared three pathways, regulated exocytosis, autophagy, and cytokine signaling in the immune system; three types of secretomes, namely, caspase-4-GSDMD, exosome, and HPA chemokines, shared viral life cycle; caspase-4-GSDMD and HPA cytokines shared response to tumor necrosis factor.

The results have demonstrated for the first time that first, in contrast to the 20 cytokines reported to be secreted from ECs as mentioned above (110), activated aortic ECs are a large secretory organ that can upregulate the transcripts of large numbers (640 genes) of secretory proteins, potentially secrete six long lists of cytokines (179 genes), chemokines (28 genes), and 433 secretomic genes (216 + 60 + 117 + 40 = 433) and modulate the functions of innate and adaptive immune cells, inflammatory cells, other vascular cells, and non-vascular cells *via* three manners, such as autocrine, paracrine, and endocrine (**Figure 7B**); second, around 10% of secretomes in each category (canonical, caspase-1-GSDMD, caspase-4-GSDMD, exosome, HPA-cytokines, HPA-chemokines) showed significant upregulation after LPI stimulation. The

(A) Cytokines: LPI treated HAECS vs Control HAECS.
Upregulated genes: 179 (179/1176~15.2%)

Gene symbol	Fold change	Gene symbol	Fold change	Gene symbol	Fold change	Gene symbol	Fold change	Gene symbol	Fold change	Gene symbol	Fold change
IL1RN	7.785	MAP10	1.478	GHR	1.256	PTGS2	1.211	MOB1A	1.166	CDC42	1.103
CD36	6.231	SEMA7A	1.463	DOCK4	1.254	IFNAR1	1.209	PKN2	1.165	SETD2	1.1
CCL20	4.781	IFIH1	1.462	PTPRE	1.249	KRAS	1.208	ELF1	1.164	ZNF654	1.1
BCL2A1	4.685	CASP1	1.455	ADAMTS6	1.248	OCLN	1.207	PRPF40A	1.156	USP8	1.096
CX3CL1	4.511	FABP4	1.455	CHMP5	1.248	FGF2	1.206	IQCB1	1.154	INHBA	1.094
SELE	4.072	TLR3	1.435	OPN1SW	1.247	CKAP2	1.206	B2M	1.153	RASA1	1.093
NR4A3	3.948	NAMPT	1.427	PIK3CG	1.246	CUL3	1.205	ZNF302	1.153	NPTN	1.092
CXCL11	3.582	INHBB	1.42	FMNL2	1.244	E2F8	1.203	PIK3CB	1.152	DOCK1	1.086
CXCL6	2.693	NUSAP1	1.402	PTPN12	1.243	VPS4B	1.203	DOCK10	1.15	BMP2	1.083
CCL26	2.635	DLG1	1.377	C12orf66	1.241	PRKCI	1.203	ACTR3	1.148	SOS1	1.083
FOXF1	2.574	CEP55	1.364	CASP3	1.238	ECT2	1.202	RIPK2	1.145	SETX	1.083
IL1A	2.569	DENND1B	1.352	NMI	1.237	CAB39	1.202	NFAT5	1.141	PIK3CA	1.076
IL13RA2	2.523	GAN	1.346	SH3GL2	1.236	HSP90AA1	1.199	DOCK9	1.139	VIM	1.073
FAM3D	2.47	TNFSF10	1.339	TNFSF18	1.232	KRR1	1.199	PDCD6IP	1.139	PRKACB	1.068
MME	2.352	PTPN2	1.335	SEH1L	1.232	PELI1	1.198	IK	1.138	MKKS	1.06
TNFSF15	2.143	DCN	1.323	HMGB1	1.231	SASH1	1.198	ITGB1	1.135	YWHAZ	1.055
IL1B	2.115	GBP1	1.322	KIAA1143	1.231	AIDA	1.198	RPS6KA5	1.129	IL3RA	1.054
LTB	2.075	HIF1A	1.322	AIMP1	1.23	CD55	1.197	PTX3	1.125	FRYL	1.053
CXCL3	2.046	CELF2	1.317	MITD1	1.228	KITLG	1.194	GPAM	1.124	JAK1	1.05
CD74	1.986	CD274	1.307	RORA	1.228	CBFB	1.191	JAK2	1.123		
CXCL8	1.849	CAV1	1.306	MERTK	1.226	SH3GLB1	1.19	SIRT1	1.123		
CSF3	1.832	CXCL1	1.302	ANXA1	1.226	ACTR2	1.185	SNX18	1.12		
FLRT3	1.786	CDC7	1.3	CHMP2B	1.225	KLHL9	1.184	CRK	1.119		
IL7R	1.743	ANLN	1.292	FAM3C	1.224	RPL6	1.183	IGF2BP3	1.117		
KIT	1.683	IFNGR1	1.289	ZC3H15	1.224	IQGAP1	1.178	LIFR	1.114		
SH2D3A	1.681	DDX58	1.288	CMTM6	1.223	TIA1	1.178	COPS2	1.112		
IL33	1.678	PIK3R1	1.287	TNFSF4	1.222	FAM76A	1.178	SOCS6	1.111		
CCL2	1.639	FASTKD2	1.281	STAM2	1.218	MAPK8	1.176	PTPN4	1.11		
FOS	1.586	TGFB3	1.278	POU2F1	1.217	SOCS5	1.175	POU4F1	1.108		
NOG	1.556	IFI16	1.277	VLDLR	1.217	TBK1	1.172	FOXN3	1.108		
LRRC17	1.514	RAB11A	1.272	LGR4	1.216	SNX9	1.171	DOCK5	1.107		
ICAM1	1.478	TAB3	1.263	EIF2AK2	1.213	PIK3C3	1.168	FOXO3	1.106		

FIGURE 5 | Continued

(B) Chemokines: LPI treated HAECS vs Control HAECS.
Upregulated genes: 28 (28/200~14%)

Gene symbol	Fold change	Gene symbol	Fold change
CCL20	4.781	LRCH1	1.371
CX3CL1	4.511	HIF1A	1.322
CXCL11	3.582	CXCL1	1.302
MCOLN2	2.764	CD164	1.266
CXCL6	2.693	DDX3X	1.235
CCL26	2.635	HMGB1	1.231
EGR1	2.156	CMTM6	1.223
IL1B	2.115	TNFSF4	1.222
CXCL3	2.046	ITCH	1.221
CD74	1.986	EIF2AK2	1.213
CXCL8	1.849	RIPK2	1.145
IL33	1.678	ACKR4	1.138
CCL2	1.639	ITGB1	1.135
TLR3	1.435	JAK1	1.05

FIGURE 5 | Cytokines and chemokines showed significant upregulation in LPI-treated HAECs compared with the control HAECs. **(A)** One hundred seventy-nine cytokines were significantly upregulated in LPI-treated HAECs. **(B)** Twenty-eight chemokines were significantly upregulated in LPI-treated HAECs.

percentages of LPI-upregulated cytokines and chemokines are higher than that of the four types of secretomes, around 15% in each. A similar percentage also occurred in the LPI-stimulated exosome secretomic genes, 923 (923/6,560 in total, ~14.1%) with $p < 0.05$ and $\log_2 FC > 1$; third, based on the comparison of top 10 functional pathways related to the LPI-upregulated secretomic genes, canonical secretome, caspase-1-GSDMD non-canonical secretome, caspase-4-GSDMD non-canonical secretome, and exosome non-canonical secretome in LPI-activated aortic EC may carry out different functions in EC adhesion, immune and inflammatory cell activation, regulation of leukocyte migration, regulation of cellular response to stress, and many other functions; fourth, a previous report has suggested that pools of human coronary artery ECs and human umbilical vein ECs have polarized secretomes, such as apical secretome and basolateral secretome. The majority of EC secretomes with 840 proteins and extracellular vesicles (EVs), such as exosome (53)) secretome, are polarized to the apical surface (112). A future proteomic study is needed to determine the polarized secretomes of LPI-activated aortic ECs (**Figure 7B**).

LPIs Activate a Transcription Mechanism by Upregulating 172 Transcription Factors, Some of Which, NR4A3, FOS, KLF3, and HIF1A, Play Significant Roles in Promoting Inflammation and Atherosclerosis

To identify molecular mechanisms underlying LPI-induced transcriptomic changes in CDs and EC-specific biomarkers, and six types of secretomic genes, we first examined the LPI-induced transcriptomic remodeling of the master gene transcription factors. We previously reported that three transcription factors (TFs), GATA-binding protein 3 (GATA3), B cell lymphoma 6 (Bcl-6), and histone deacetylase 6 (HDAC6), regulate $CD4^+Foxp3^+$ regulatory T cell (Treg) plasticity and determine Treg conversion into either novel antigen-presenting cell-like Treg or Th1-Treg (118). This result suggests that other T helper cell subsets, such as type 2 CD4+ T helper cell (Th2), and TFs such as GATA3, follicular T helper cell (Tfh) TF Bcl-6, and HDAC6, cooperate with Foxp3 to determine Treg transcriptomes and functions. Moreover, three upregulated TFs, Jun (AP-1 transcription factor subunit), hypoxia-inducible factor-1α (HIF1A), and endothelial PAS domain protein 1 (EPAS1, HIF-2α), collaborate with other pathways and membrane receptors to potentially trans-differentiate $CD14^+$ thrombus leukocytes into angiogenic endothelial cells (12). The expressions of 232 transcription regulators are differentially regulated in 28 sets of endothelial cell microarrays in response to the stimulation of a broad spectrum of pathophysiologically relevant pathogen-associated molecular patterns (PAMPs)/danger-associated molecular patterns (DAMPs) (3). We hypothesized that LPIs activate HAECs by upregulating a set of specific TFs. To test this hypothesis, we collected 1,496 TFs from the comprehensive protein database Human Protein Atlas (HPA, https://www.proteinatlas.org/search/cytokine), as we reported recently (13). As shown in **Figure 8A**, 172 out of the total 1,496 TFs (11.5%, $\log_2 FC > 1$, $p < 0.05$) were significantly upregulated in LPI-activated HAECs. In addition, the numbers of LPI-induced upregulation for more than $\log_2 FC$ 2 folds, more than $\log_2 FC$ 1.5-fold, more than $\log_2 FC$ 1.4-fold, more than $\log_2 FC$ 1.3-fold, and more than $\log_2 FC$ 1.2-fold were 5, 3, 8, 15, and 49 TFs,

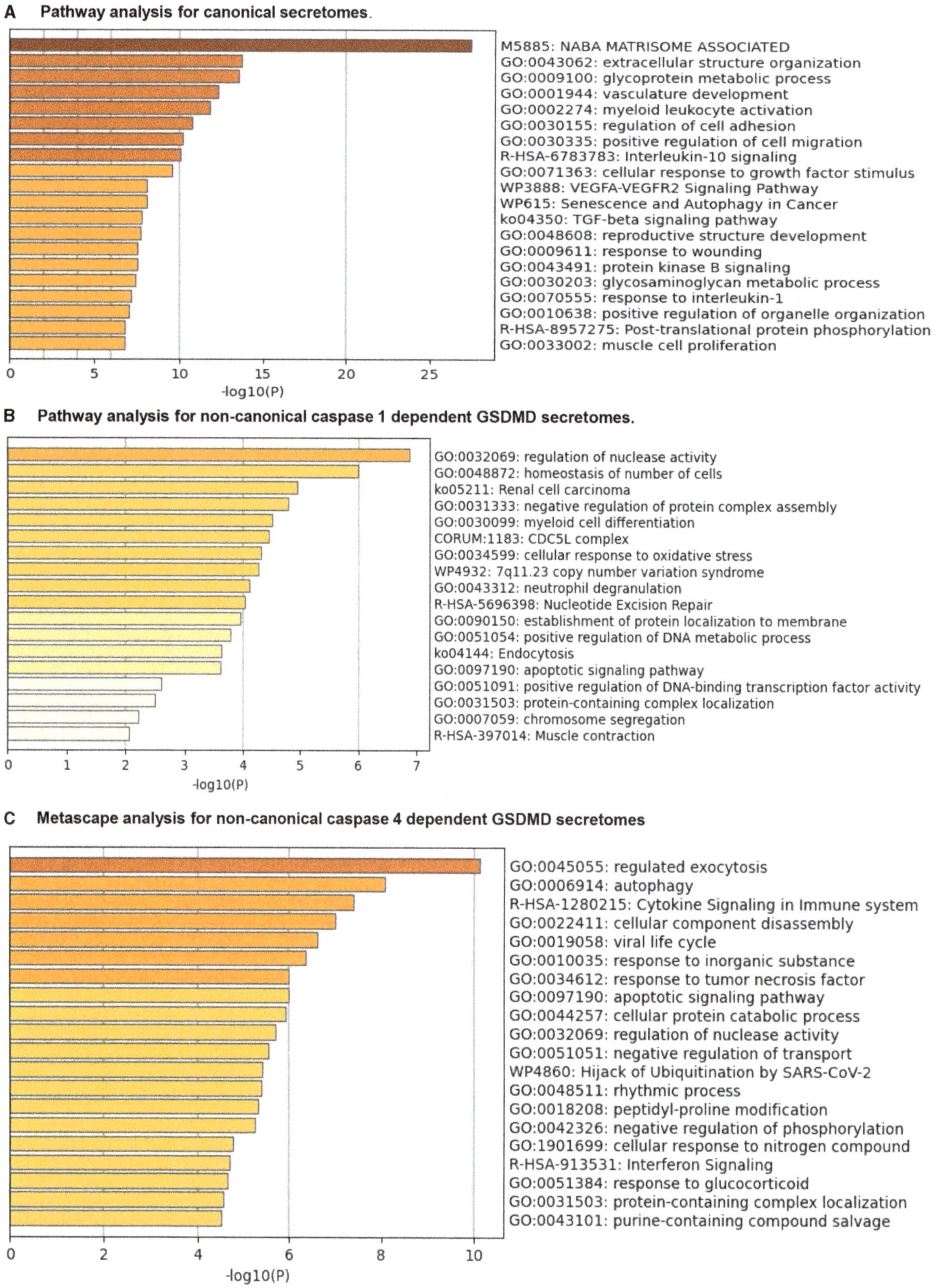

FIGURE 6 | Continued

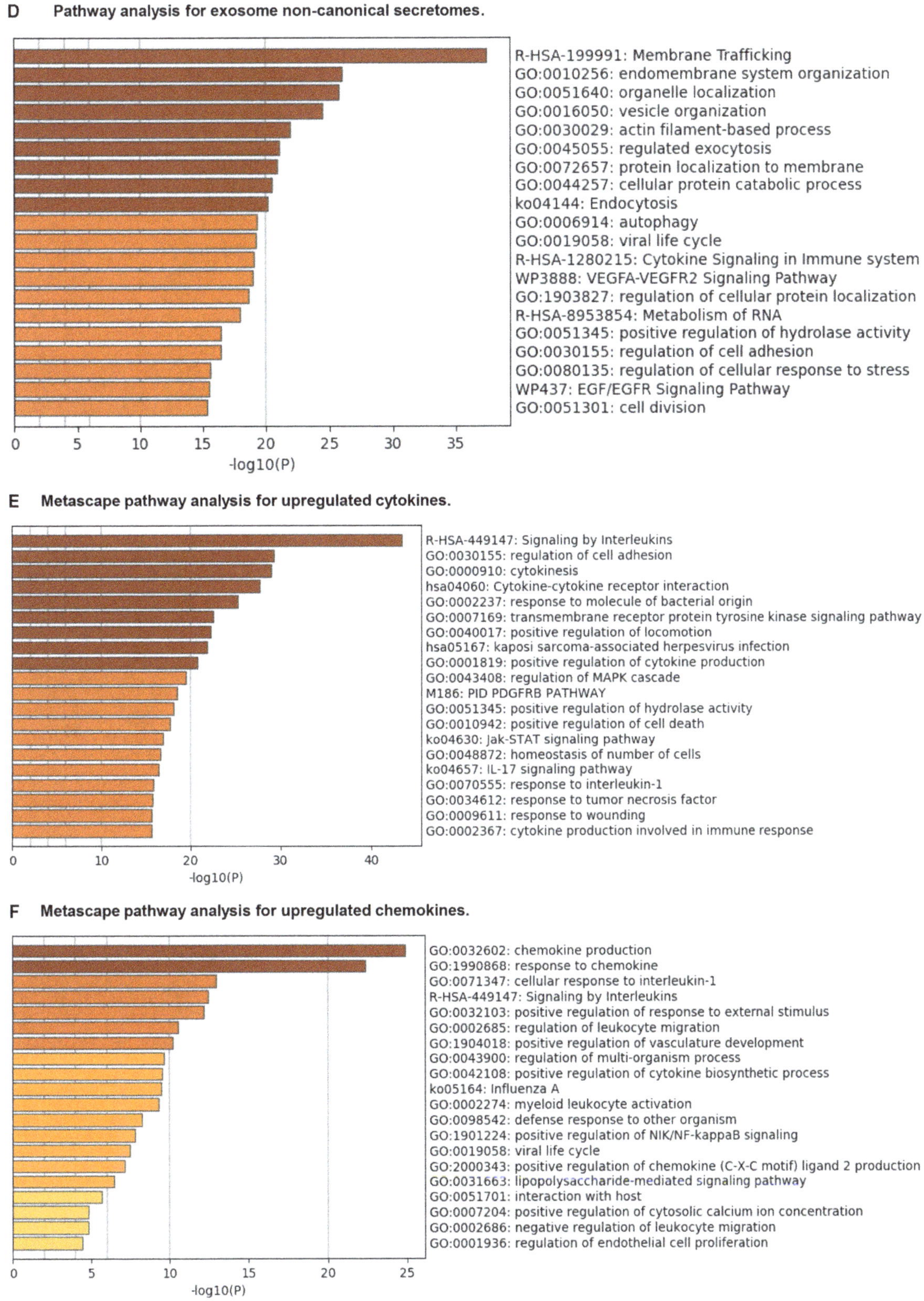

FIGURE 6 | Metascape pathway analysis for upregulated six secretomes and cytokine and chemokines in LPI-treated HAECs. **(A)** Pathway analysis for canonical secretomes. **(B)** Pathway analysis for caspase-1-dependent non-canonical GSDMD secretomes. **(C)** Pathway analysis for caspase-4-dependent non-canonical GSDMD secretomes. **(D)** Pathway analysis for exosomes non-canonical secretomes. **(E)** Metascape pathway analysis for upregulated cytokines. **(F)** Metascape pathway analysis for upregulated chemokines.

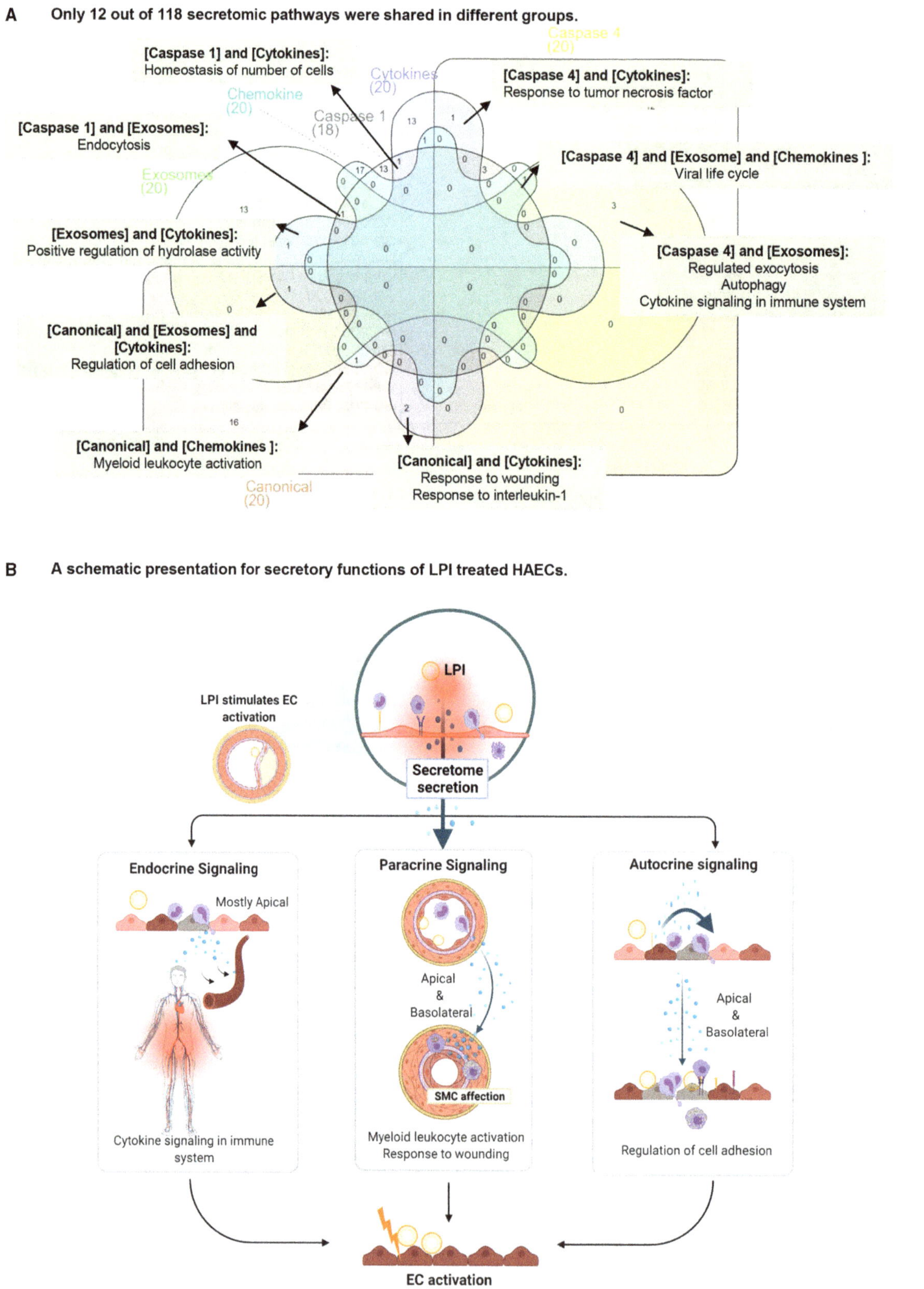

FIGURE 7 | The majority of secretory pathways are mutually exclusive in LPI-stimulated HAECs. **(A)** Venn diagram was used to check the overlapped pathways among six secretomic groups. *(**B**) was created with Biorender.com.

respectively. Among the highly LPI-upregulated TFs, nuclear receptor subfamily 4 group A member 3 (NR4A3) was a novel target of p53 contributing to apoptosis (119); FoxF1 was a therapy target of Hedgehog-related cancers (120); FOS (AP-1 TF subunit) was one of the TFs linked to ERK/MAPK activation (121), inflammation, and atherosclerosis (122); Kruppel-Like Factor 3 (KLF3) was one of the key mechanosensitive master switches in gene expression in promoting atherosclerosis (123); hypoxia-inducible factor-1α (HIF1A) was a master regulator of EC biology for diabetic atherosclerosis (124).

The Metascape analysis in **Figure 8B** shows that LPI-upregulated TFs had 20 significant pathways, namely, herpes simplex virus 1 infection, nuclear events (kinase and transcription factor activation), pri-miRNA transcription by RNA polymerase II, myeloid cell differentiation, SMAD2-3 nuclear pathway [main signal transducers for transforming growth factor-β (TGF-β)], cardiac chamber morphogenesis, muscle structure development, rhythmic process, cell fate commitment, blood vessel development, positive regulation of transcription in response to chemical stimulus, DNA-template transcription-initiation, transcription misregulation in cancer, gland development, cellular response to organic cyclic compound, leukocyte differentiation, brain development, circadian regulation of gene expression, neuronal stem cell regulation maintenance, and homeostasis of the number of cells.

Taken together, the results have demonstrated that first, LPIs upregulate 172 (11.5%) out of 1,496 TFs and 80 (5.3%) TFs ($log_2FC > 1.2$, $p < 0.05$), suggesting that LPIs have a broad effect on aortic EC transcriptome; second, some LPI-upregulated TFs, such as NR4A3, FOS, KLF3, and HIF1A, play significant roles in promoting inflammation and atherosclerosis; third, other Metascape analysis-identified inflammatory pathways include myeloid cell differentiation, positive regulation of transcription in response to chemical stimulus, cellular response to organic cyclic compound, and leukocyte differentiation.

LPIs Activate a Mitochondrial Mechanism in Aortic ECs by Upregulating152 Nuclear DNA-Encoded Mitochondrial Genes (MitoCarta) and Promote the Mitochondrial Organization, Respiration, Translation, and Transport

Our previous reports showed that LPC induces aortic EC activation by increasing mitochondrial reactive oxygen species (mtROS) and proton leaks uncoupled from ATP synthesis (23, 44–46, 125) and that similar to LPC, LPIs also induces the upregulation of ICAM1 and aortic EC activation (19). We hypothesized that LPIs activate aortic ECs *via* a mitochondrion-dependent mechanism and modulate the transcription of genomic (nuclear) DNA-encoded mitochondrial genes (mitoCarta genes). To test this hypothesis, we collected the mitoCarta gene list from the Broad Institute at MIT (https://www.broadinstitute.org/mitocarta/mitocarta30-inventory-mammalian-mitochondrial-proteins-and-pathways). **Figure 9A** shows that LPIs upregulated 152 (13.1%) out of 1,158 mitoCarta genes. In addition, the Metascape analysis showed that the LPI-upregulated mitoCarta genes had functions of mitochondrion organization, cellular respiration, mitochondrial translation, mitochondrial gene expression, mitochondrial transport, propanoate metabolism, small-molecule catabolic process, ribose phosphate metabolic process, mitochondrial membrane organization, regulation of cellular respiration, mitochondrial biogenesis, metabolism of lipids, tRNA aminoacylation for protein translation, citric acid cycle (TCA cycle), ribosome disassembly, glycerol-3-phosphate metabolic process, protein depalmitoylation, mitochondrial iron-sulfur cluster biogenesis, protein complex oligomerization, and regulation of mitochondrial membrane potential (**Figure 9B**). Taken together, the results have demonstrated that LPI-activated aortic ECs activate a mitochondrial mechanism by upregulating 152 nuclear DNA-encoded mitochondrial genes (MitoCarta) and promote the mitochondrial organization, cellular respiration, translation, transport, and membrane organization.

LPIs Activate the Reactive Oxygen Species (ROS) Mechanism in Activated HAECs by Upregulating 18 Out of 165 ROS Regulators

It has been reported that ROS plays a key role in regulating pathophysiological signaling in endothelial cell activation (126) and cardiovascular diseases (127). We also reported that mitochondrial ROS plays a significant role in mediating EC activation (23, 44, 59). In addition, we recently proposed a new working model in which ROS is an integrated cellular network for sensing homeostasis and alarming DAMPs (128). We hypothesized that LPIs modulate the expressions of ROS regulators in HAECs. We collected 165 ROS regulators classified in the Gene Set Enrichment Analysis (GSEA) (https://www.gsea-msigdb.org/gsea/index.jsp) database, as we have reported (50). **Figure 9C** shows that LPIs upregulated 18 (10.9%) out of 165 ROS regulators in activated HAECs. In addition, the Metascape analysis showed that LPIs upregulated ROS regulators and promoted the functions of ROS metabolic process, regulation of ROS metabolic process, superoxide metabolic process, regulation of intrinsic apoptotic signaling, generation of precursor metabolites and energy, positive regulation of oxidoreductase activity, mitochondrion organization, positive regulation of cell death, cellular response to hypoxia, response to gamma radiation, regulation of cysteine-type endopeptidase activity involved in apoptosis, response to monosaccharide, folate metabolism, regulation of response to endoplasmic reticulum stress, response to cyclic adenosine 3', 5'-monophosphate (cAMP), regulation of smooth muscle cell proliferation, and cellular response to biotic stimulus (**Figure 9D**). Taken together, the results have demonstrated that first, LPIs upregulate 18 (10.9%) out of 165 ROS regulators in activated HAECs, suggesting that LPIs activate human aortic endothelial cells potentially *via* ROS-mediated mechanisms; second, LPIs upregulate many pathways in regulating ROS metabolic process, mitochondrial metabolism, and cell death.

(A)

Transcription factors: LPI treated HAECS vs Control HAECS.
Upregulated genes: 172/1496~ 11.5%

Gene symbol	Fold change	Gene symbol	Fold change	Gene symbol	Fold change	Gene symbol	Fold change	Gene symbol	Fold change
ZNF705G	5.477	ZNF22	1.28	MIER1	1.202	BNC1	1.153	NR3C1	1.113
NR4A3	3.948	HIVEP2	1.276	NCOA2	1.202	ZNF302	1.153	FOXN3	1.108
FOXF1	2.574	FOXN2	1.273	CDC5L	1.2	ZNF79	1.152	POU4F1	1.108
ID2	2.259	CREM	1.267	CREB1	1.2	MEF2A	1.151	FOXO3	1.106
EGR1	2.156	SMARCE1	1.267	LRRFIP1	1.199	MXD1	1.149	NFE2L2	1.105
ZNF19	1.915	HEY1	1.26	ZNF350	1.199	PLAG1	1.147	ZNF430	1.102
FOS	1.586	ID3	1.259	ZNF281	1.198	BNC2	1.146	ZNF654	1.1
ZNF860	1.584	ETS1	1.255	ARNTL2	1.195	ZHX1	1.146	RC3H2	1.097
ZNF280C	1.488	MITF	1.25	ETV1	1.195	HBP1	1.145	CREBL2	1.095
MEF2C	1.475	ZNF484	1.249	TCF12	1.192	ELK4	1.144	MAX	1.093
ID1	1.434	BBX	1.247	ZFY	1.192	KLF6	1.143	ZNF776	1.093
ZBTB2	1.432	PLAGL1	1.245	ZNF800	1.19	LYAR	1.143	ZNF449	1.092
ZNF551	1.431	THAP1	1.245	ZFX	1.187	NFE2L3	1.143	ZNF175	1.088
NFKBIZ	1.428	ZNF664	1.245	ZBTB33	1.181	PBRM1	1.143	JARID2	1.086
ZNF585B	1.418	ZNF547	1.241	ZNF277	1.18	SMAD4	1.143	NFYB	1.085
ZNF614	1.41	ATF1	1.239	AEBP2	1.179	ZNF268	1.143	HMG20A	1.075
ZNF502	1.397	IKZF5	1.239	MEIS2	1.179	FOXJ3	1.141	ZKSCAN1	1.075
ZNF813	1.389	ZNF25	1.237	ZKSCAN2	1.179	NFAT5	1.141	SFPQ	1.065
ZNF891	1.375	ELK3	1.232	PROX1	1.178	E2F3	1.139	NR2F1	1.051
ZNF674	1.373	ZNF180	1.231	REST	1.175	GABPA	1.139	NR2F2	1.035
BACH1	1.371	TFAM	1.23	SMAD5	1.175	ZNF697	1.137		
ZNF124	1.361	RORA	1.228	ZNF100	1.171	NFIA	1.135		
ZNF613	1.355	ZBTB6	1.227	PURB	1.17	HMGXB4	1.133		
SMAD1	1.351	ELF2	1.226	SMARCA5	1.17	MTF1	1.132		
ZNF433	1.342	ZFP1	1.226	ZNF440	1.17	SOX4	1.13		
CREB3L1	1.34	ZNF507	1.226	TEAD1	1.169	KLF10	1.129		
ZNF597	1.337	TRERF1	1.222	ZNF652	1.168	TFEC	1.127		
HIF1A	1.322	ZEB2	1.221	ZNF880	1.165	NFIB	1.124		
SP4	1.32	ZNF160	1.221	ELF1	1.164	ZNF468	1.123		
ZNF143	1.305	MECOM	1.219	CEBPG	1.163	DMTF1	1.122		
KLF3	1.3	RBPJ	1.219	SP3	1.162	ZNF644	1.121		
ZNF701	1.295	POU2F1	1.217	MIER3	1.161	SMAD2	1.12		
ZC3H8	1.293	VEZF1	1.215	KLF11	1.16	RARB	1.119		
PRRX1	1.29	ATF2	1.213	ZBED5	1.159	SP100	1.118		
ZNF121	1.289	HES1	1.213	ZNF451	1.159	ZNF148	1.116		
ZNF347	1.287	ZNF195	1.211	ZNF24	1.158	FLI1	1.114		
ZNF766	1.282	ZNF700	1.211	ZBTB38	1.157	ZNF426	1.114		
TCF4	1.281	E2F8	1.203	CLOCK	1.154	ETV3	1.113		

B Metascape analysis for 172 LPI upregulated pathways.

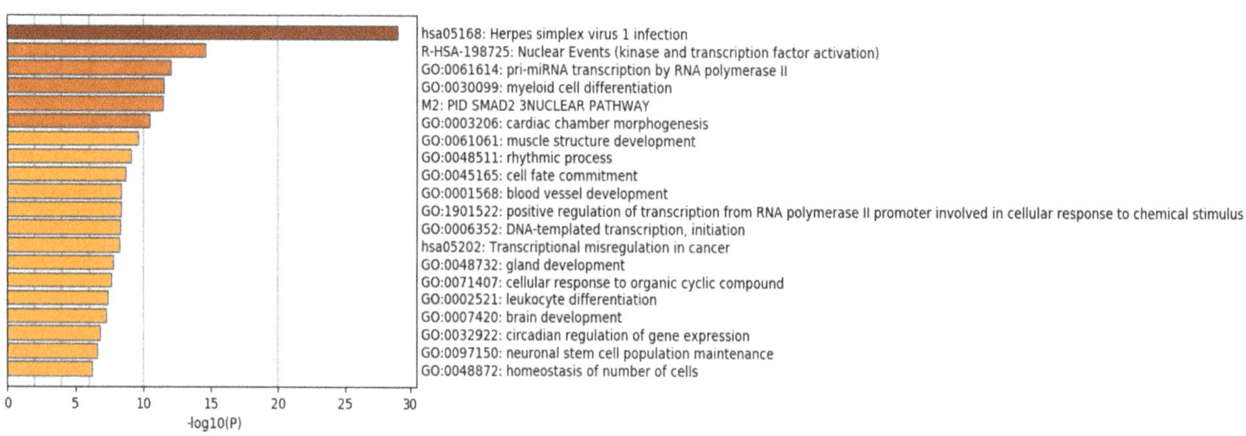

FIGURE 8 | One hundred seventy-two LPI-upregulated transcription factors (TFs) were identified, which mediates 20 pathways after screening for a total of 1,496 TFs. **(A)** Around 11.5% of the genes (172/1496) showed significant upregulation among total TFs. **(B)** Metascape pathways and biological process enrichment analysis for upregulated genes in the LPI group.

(A) MitoCarta: LPI treated HAECS vs Control HAECS.

Upregulated genes: 152 (152/1,158~13.1%)					
Gene symbol	**Fold change**	**Gene symbol**	**Fold change**	**Gene symbol**	**Fold change**
PMPCB	1.174	CCDC58	1.489	OXR1	1.144
SDHD	1.279	MCEE	1.184	LYPLAL1	1.241
LRPPRC	1.196	MUT	1.137	MGST1	1.097
GFM1	1.201	PNPLA8	1.217	MTPAP	1.261
ISCA1	1.189	MRPL32	1.2	DNM1L	1.195
COX11	1.278	ME2	1.133	TMEM126B	1.338
ETFA	1.093	SLC30A9	1.197	NIPSNAP3A	1.203
BCKDHB	1.276	RMND1	1.146	HSDL1	1.1
ATP5J	1.497	ABCB10	1.131	IDI1	1.157
DLD	1.238	GK	1.153	MTFR1	1.132
TIMM9	1.13	NARS2	1.157	DDAH1	1.179
MTIF2	1.182	ZADH2	1.12	TRMT10C	1.308
PRDX3	1.278	SLC25A24	1.207	MMADHC	1.198
MRPL40	1.156	IDE	1.163	OSBPL1A	1.183
MRPL1	1.233	TMEM70	1.107	GDAP1	1.372
SOD2	1.778	XPNPEP3	1.129	MTIF3	1.277
CLPX	1.152	PDP1	1.145	PTS	1.162
NDUFS4	1.342	ECHDC1	1.21	TARS	1.175
HSDL2	1.194	NDUFA13	2.082	PSMA6	1.244
ISCU	1.072	HSD17B4	1.107	AGPAT5	1.168
GFM2	1.143	MRPL50	1.26	NUDT5	1.192
NDUFAF4	1.27	RARS2	1.068	BOLA3	1.24
MFN1	1.155	NDUFA11	1.369	NCEH1	1.181
PPTC7	1.215	TEFM	1.261	FASTKD2	1.281
OXCT1	1.196	MRPS22	1.207	PNPT1	1.191
MTO1	1.069	LAP3	1.135	TMBIM4	1.268
NDUFA5	1.216	MRPS33	1.154	SCP2	1.256
MTX2	1.259	LYRM2	1.147	PTPN4	1.11
SUCLG2	1.204	TFAM	1.23	NUDT9	1.117
YARS2	1.111	TMEM65	1.173	MSRB3	1.159
AK3	1.256	NLN	1.143	GPAM	1.124
CYCS	1.226	GRPEL2	1.492	CRYZ	1.203
LYRM7	1.251	MRPL39	1.274	TOMM20	1.163
MRPL3	1.089	LYPLA1	1.298	COA7	1.099
PCCA	1.134	MTRF1L	1.297	BNIP3L	1.32
TMEM126A	1.14	YME1L1	1.24	RARS	1.125
ECHDC2	1.205	TCAIM	1.16	PDE12	1.132
HIBADH	1.086	SDR39U1	1.414	ANGEL2	1.226
TIMM17A	1.234	MRPS31	1.215	PAICS	1.178
ATP5F1	1.23	SLC25A32	1.266	PMAIP1	1.389
COQ10B	1.3	SLC25A40	1.184	SLC30A6	1.242
CBR4	1.122	SLC25A36	1.183	EMC2	1.221
NDUFA12	1.208	STOM	1.084	SPTLC2	1.076
GPD2	1.13	LIPT1	1.129	AGK	1.137
CCDC90B	1.148	UQCR11	1.77	PREPL	1.088
SSBP1	1.12	MRPL42	1.287	FASTKD3	1.199
HSCB	1.21	ABHD10	1.142	SERAC1	1.176
MRPS10	1.139	RFK	1.35	PLGRKT	1.215
AK4	1.152	RHOT1	1.169	SECISBP2	1.216
CISD1	1.19	PTRH2	1.316	C2orf69	1.183
				CLIC4	1.231
				TRMT11	1.494

FIGURE 9 | Continued

B Metascape pathway analysis for the upregulated genes of mitocarta.

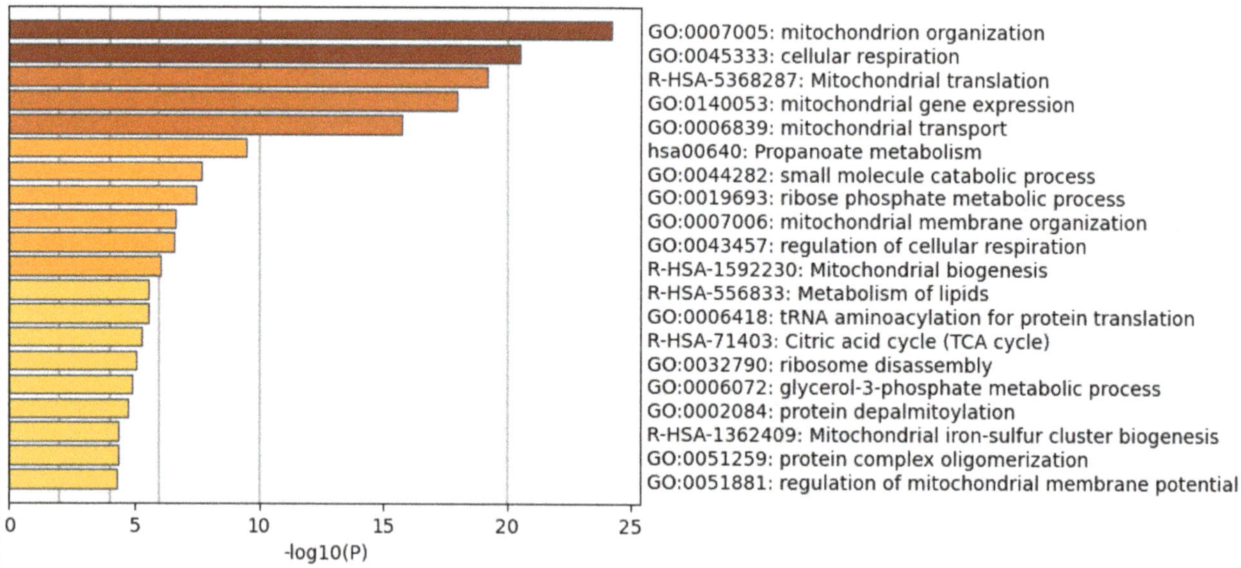

(C) LPIs upregulate 18 out of 165 ROS regulators in HAECs.

ROS regulators: LPI treated HAECS vs Control HAECS.
Upregulated genes: 18 (18/165~10.9%).

Symbol	Log2FC	Symbol	Log2FC
CRYAB	3.484	CYB5R4	1.26
DHFR	1.102	PMAIP1	1.389
GNAI3	1.272	RFK	1.35
HIF1A	1.322	SELENOS	1.056
BIRC2	1.197	TIGAR	1.197
NDUFS4	1.342	SOD2	1.778
NFE2L2	1.105	TGFBR2	1.164
NOX4	1.25	STK17A	1.12
NDUFA13	2.082	CD36	6.231

D Metascape pathway analysis for the upregulated genes of mitochondrial ROS.

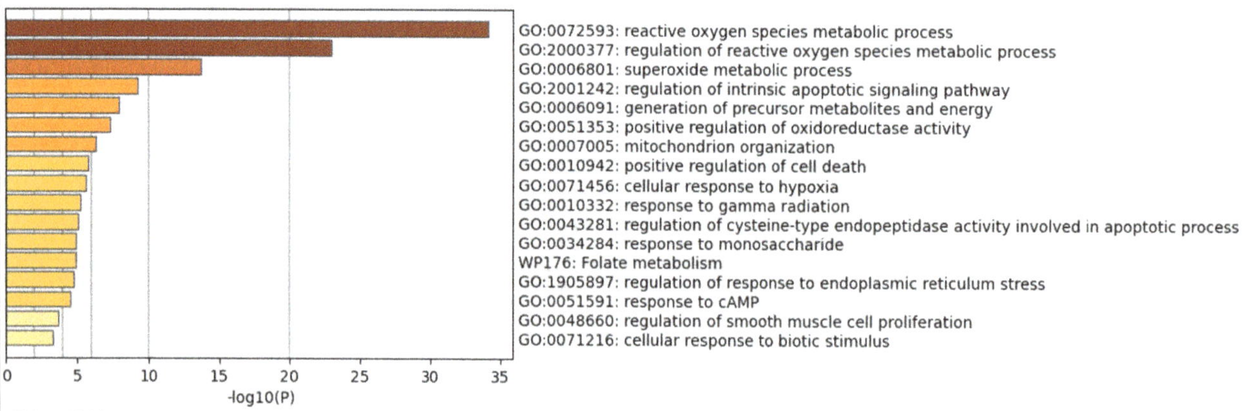

FIGURE 9 | Mitochondrion-related genes showed significant upregulation in LPI-treated HAECs compared with the control HAECs. **(A)** One hundred fifty-two out of 1,158 mitocarta genes were significantly upregulated in LPI-treated HAECs. **(B)** Metascape pathway analysis for the upregulated genes of mitocarta. **(C)** Eighteen mitochondrial reactive oxygen species (ROS) regulators were significantly upregulated in LPI-treated HAECs. **(D)** Metascape pathway analysis for the upregulated genes of mitochondrial ROS.

Cytoscape Results Have Demonstrated That Three Molecular Mechanisms, Such as 172 LPI-Upregulated TFs, 152 LPI-Upregulated MitoCarta Genes, and 18 LPI-Upregulated ROS Regulators, Are Integrated to Regulate HAEC Activation

We further hypothesized that three molecular mechanisms underlying the LPI activation of human aortic endothelial cells can be connected. To examine this hypothesis, we used the Cytoscape (https://cytoscape.org/) database to visualize and integrate the complex network among 172 LPI-upregulated TFs, 152 LPI-upregulated mitoCarta genes, and 18 LPI-upregulated ROS regulators. As shown in **Figure 10A**, three groups of genes are loaded in the function ClueGO of the Cytoscape database, and the visual style is set as the clusters with assigned colors. The three groups of genes included 172 LPI-upregulated TFs (shown in cluster 1, red), 152 LPI-elevated Mitocarta genes (shown in cluster 2, blue), and 18 LPI-increased ROS regulators (shown in cluster 3, purple). In the search for potential connections between three color clusters, two selection criteria were used. First, the GO tree interval was set between GO levels 4–10 to identify the representative and specific pathways, meaning mapped genes represent 4 to 50% of the total associated genes. When the pathways were selected to be only presented when the *p*-value of the pathway was less than .05, 185 terms/pathways were identified. The second criteria/step were to find potential connections among the lists of LPIs stimulated TF (Red Cluster), MitoCarta genes (Blue Cluster), and ROS regulators (Purple Cluster). Thus, the genes in all three clusters (Red, Blue, Purple colors) were selected for further analysis. After the first and second screening, five terms/pathways were chosen that genes associated with the term/pathways were from different, overlapping clusters (all clusters < 60%). The representative genes are shown in **Figure 10B**, and include: (i) mitochondrial biogenesis (13% associated genes to the term, 41% for cluster 1, 50% for cluster 2, and 9% for cluster3); (ii) regulation of cellular response to oxidative stress (13% associated genes to the term, 38% for cluster 1, 20% for cluster 2, and 42% for cluster3); (iii) regulation of oxidative stress-induced cell death (11% associated genes to the term, 50% for cluster 1, 17% for cluster 2, and 33% for cluster3); (iv) transcriptional activation of mitochondrial biogenesis (16% associated genes to the term, 52% for cluster 1, 36% for cluster 2, and 11% for cluster3); and (v) mitochondrion localization (12% associated genes to the term, 27% for cluster 1, 56% for cluster 2, and 17% for cluster 3). **Figure 10C** shows the overlapped genes between each term. Taken together, the Cytoscape results have demonstrated that three molecular mechanisms, such as 172 LPI-upregulated TFs, 152 LPI-upregulated mitoCarta genes, and 18 LPI-upregulated ROS regulators, are integrated to promote HAEC activation.

DISCUSSION

We proposed a novel concept that ECs are innate immune cells. Inflammatory mechanisms and endothelial cell activation play essential roles in promoting the progression of cardiovascular diseases, inflammatory diseases, autoimmune diseases, transplantation immune responses, cancer metastasis, and aging diseases (1, 3–6, 23, 33, 34, 44, 47, 57, 58, 61, 70, 92, 129). Significant progress has been made in elucidating molecular mechanisms underlying endothelial cell activation. However, several important issues remain to be addressed: (1) whether aortic endothelial cell activation induces conditional DAMP (20, 21). LPIs upregulate additional membrane proteins for signaling in addition to mediating inflammatory cell adhesion to EC and trans-EC migration; (2) how many secretory proteins can be upregulated during aortic EC activation, and whether aortic ECs are equipped to upregulate various secretomes during EC activation induced by LPIs; (3) whether LPIs activate aortic ECs *via* remodeling ROS regulatome, mitochondrial reprogramming, and TF machinery reshaping. To address these questions, we developed an EC biology knowledge-based transcriptomic formula to analyze RNA-Seq data in a panoramic manner. We made the following important findings: first, GPR55, a specific receptor for LPIs, is expressed in the endothelium of both human and mouse aortas, and is significantly upregulated in hyperlipidemia; second, LPIs upregulate 43 out of 373 clusters of differentiation (CDs) markers in HAECs, promoting EC activation, innate immune trans-differentiation, and immune and inflammatory responses; and 72.1% of LPI-upregulated CD markers are not induced in three types of virus-infected human endothelial cells; third, LPI-activated aortic ECs upregulate six types of secretomic genes, canonical secretome, caspase-1-gasdermin D (GSDMD) non-canonical secretome, caspase-4/11-GSDMD non-canonical secretome, exosome non-canonical secretome, HPA-classified cytokines, and HPA-classified chemokines, which makes HAECs a large secretory organ for inflammation, immune responses, and other functions; fourth, LPIs activate a transcription mechanism by upregulating 172 TFs, some of which, namely, NR4A3, FOS, KLF3, and HIF1A, play significant roles in promoting inflammation and atherosclerosis; fifth, LPIs activate a mitochondrial mechanism in aortic ECs by upregulating 152 nuclear DNA-encoded mitochondrial genes (MitoCarta) and promote mitochondrial organization, cellular respiration, translation, and transport, and membrane organization; sixth, LPIs activate reactive oxygen species (ROS) mechanism in activated HAECs by upregulating 18 out of 165 ROS regulators; seventh, the Cytoscape analysis results have demonstrated that three novel molecular mechanisms, namely, 172 LPI-upregulated TFs, 152 LPI-upregulated mitoCarta genes, and 18 LPI-upregulated ROS regulators, are integrated to regulate HAEC activation.

Our findings on hyperlipidemia-increased GPR55 expression in mouse aortas were correlated with several reports: (1) patients with Crohn's disease (a type of inflammatory bowel disease) manifest higher (12.5-fold) GPR55 mRNA expression in inflamed compared with non-inflamed colonic tissues ($p < 0.0001$) (130); (2) circulating LPIs and the liver expression of GPR55 are upregulated in patients with nonalcoholic steatohepatitis (NASH); the *in vivo* knockdown of GPR55 is sufficient to improve liver damage in mice fed with a high-fat diet and in mice fed with a methionine-choline-deficient diet (131); and

3) O-1602, the most potent agonist of GPR55, induces lipid accumulation in hepatocytes, which is reversed by treatment with CID16020046, an antagonist of GPR55 (132). Our findings on the LPI upregulation of 640 secretomic genes in activating HAECs and promoting inflammation were well correlated with several reviews (69) and reports: GPR55 antagonist CID16020046 protects oxLDL-induced inflammation in HAECs (133); LPIs, especially the albumin-bound form, induce pro-inflammatory cytokines TNF-a and IL-6 in macrophages *via* the GPR55/MAPKP38 pathway (134); GPR55 antagonist has anti-inflammatory effects in LPS-activated primary microglial cells (135); GPR55 knockout mice show reduced inflammation scores as compared with wild-type mice in an intestinal inflammation model (2.5% dextran sulfate sodium model) (136). Our findings

A Ontology network among LPI-upregulated TFs, mitoCarta genes, and ROS regulators.

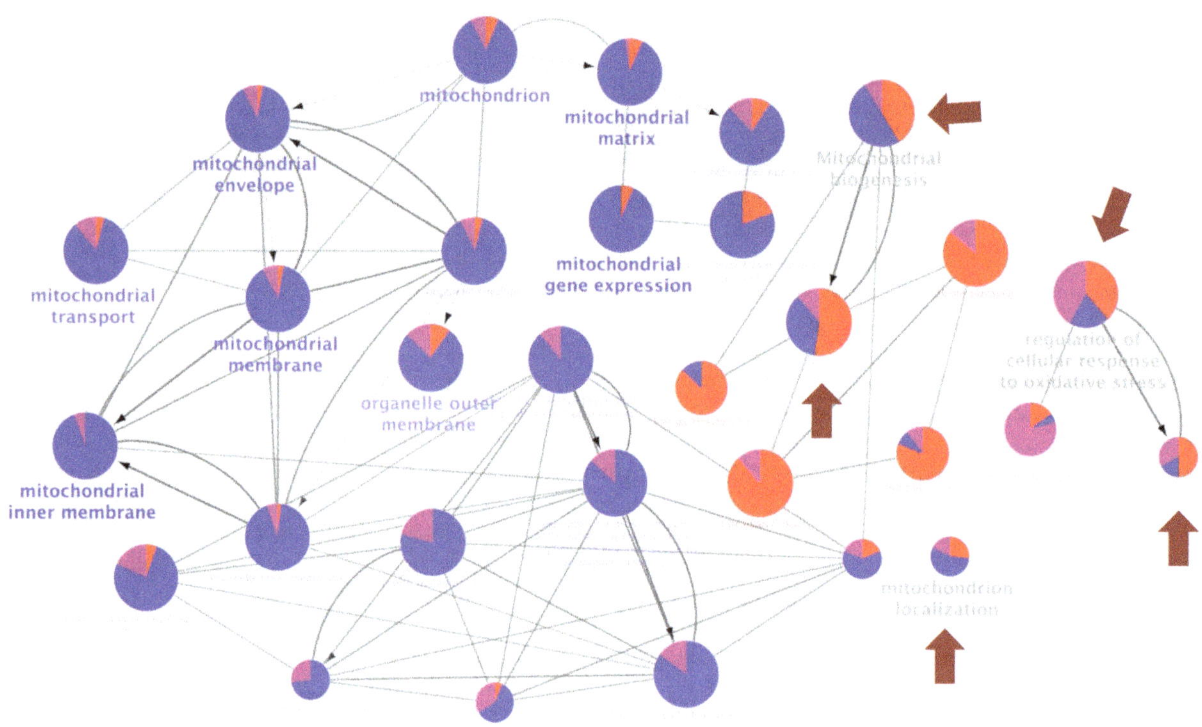

(B) detailed data distribution for five terms/pathways.

Term	Term *P* Value	% Associated genes	%Genes Cluster #1	%Genes Cluster #2	%Genes Cluster #3	TF-Cluster #1 (Red)	Mitocarta genes-Cluster #2 (Blue)	ROS regulator-Cluster #3 (Purple)
Mitochondrion localization	1.81E-04	11.8	26.8	55.7	17.4	[HIF1A, MEF2A]	[DNM1L, LRPPRC, MFN1, RHOT1]	[HIF1A]
Regulation of cellular response to oxidative stress	1.62E-07	12.8	38.4	20	41.6	[FOXO3, HIF1A, NFE2L2, NR4A3, REST, SFPQ]	[OXR1, PNPLA8, SOD2]	[CD36, DHFR, HIF1A, NFE2L2, SOD2]
Regulation of oxidative stress-induced cell death	3.15E-05	10.7	50.1	17.3	32.6	[FOXO3, HIF1A, NFE2L2, NR4A3, REST, SFPQ]	[OXR1, SOD2]	[HIF1A, NFE2L2, SOD2]
Mitochondrial biogenesis	5.08E-08	12.6	41.2	49.9	8.9	[ATF2, CREB1, GABPA, MEF2C, NCOA2, TFAM]	[ATP5PB, ATP5PF, CYCS, MTX2, SOD2, SSBP1, TFAM]	[SOD2]
Transcriptional activation of mitochondrial biogenesis	2.99E-07	16.1	52.4	36.3	11.4	[ATF2, CREB1, GABPA, MEF2C, NCOA2, TFAM]	[CYCS, SOD2, SSBP1, TFAM]	[SOD2]

FIGURE 10 | Continued

C Venn diagram showed the overlapped genes between the 'parent terms' and the 'child terms'.

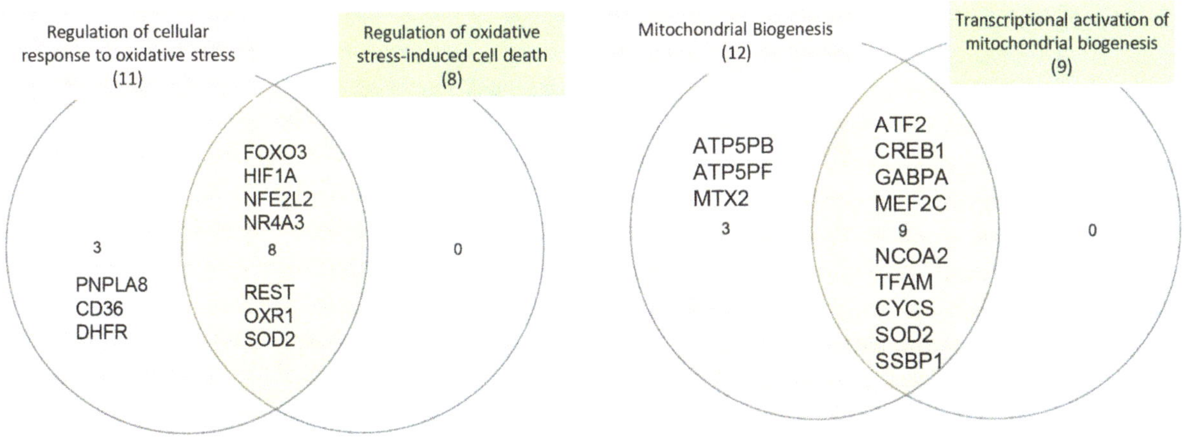

FIGURE 10 | Network data integration database Cytoscape analysis (https://cytoscape.org/) was performed to analyze the network connection among 172 upregulated LPI TFs, LPI-increased mitocarta genes, and LPI-upregulated ROS regulators. **(A)** Ontology network among LPI-upregulated TFs, mitoCarta genes, and ROS regulators. The cluster of 172 LPI-increased TFs is shown in red, the cluster of 152 LPI-upregulated mitoCarta genes is shown in blue, and the cluster of 18 LPI-elevated ROS regulators is shown in purple. One node represents a term/pathway, and the node size stands for significance. The bigger the node size, the higher the significance. (the smallest node in this figure is $p < 0.05$). The proportion of the colors in each node indicates the percentage of genes that contribute to this term/pathway from each cluster. The red arrow highlights five terms/pathways, indicating that the three clusters of genes equally contribute to a term/pathway. We focus on these five pathways, and the other 25 shown in this figure are closely related to the five. The gray lines indicate the connection between each term. The thicker the line, the stronger the correlation. The gray arrow starts from "parent term" to "child term." The child term is more specialized than its parent term. **(B)** Detailed data distribution for five terms/pathways. The associated genes% represent how many genes from our three clusters matched to the genes of terms in the database. The gene clusters #1, #2, #3 indicate how many percentages of each cluster of genes contribute to the term/pathway. **(C)** Venn diagram shows the overlapped genes between the "parent terms" and the "child terms."

on the LPI upregulation of 172 transcription factors in activated HAECs were well-correlated with the previous report that LPIs induce the activation of several TFs, such as nuclear factor of activated T-cells (NFAT), nuclear factor κ of activated B cells (NF-κB), and serum response element, translocation of NFAT and NF-κB, and GPR55 internalization (137). Of note, GPR55 is a non-cannabinoid receptor 1 or 2 (CB1/CB2) receptor that exhibits affinity for endogenous plant and synthetic cannabinoids. It was reported that LPI-mediated calcium release and mitogen-activated protein kinase (MAPK)-extracellular signal-regulated kinase (ERK) activation depend on the stable expression of GPR55 and that LPIs cannot have the above-mentioned calcium release and MAPK/ERK activation when CB_1 or CB_2 is expressed in the cells (137), suggesting the contexture (cannabinoid receptor 1 or 2 expression levels) dependence of LPI pro-inflammatory functions.

As shown in **Figure 11**, we proposed a novel working model to integrate all the findings. First, LPI receptor GPR55 is expressed in human and mouse aortic endothelial cells as well as other aortic cell types and is upregulated in hyperlipidemic conditions, suggesting that LPIs/GPR55 signaling is increased in aortic endothelial cells in cardiovascular diseases such as hyperlipidemia. In addition, LPI pro-inflammatory functions may depend on the contexture (cannabinoid receptor 1 or 2 expression levels). Second, by screening 12,763 secretory protein genes in six types of secretomes, we have demonstrated for the first time that human aortic endothelial cells are a large secretory organ. Under stimulation by LPIs, a prototypic conditional DAMP, pro-inflammatory lipid, and human aortic endothelial cells can upregulate as many as 640 secretomic genes *via* six types of secretomic mechanisms, namely, canonical secretome with all human proteins having a signal peptide *via* exocytic direction along the endoplasmic reticulum-Golgi-plasma membrane route, caspase-1-GSDMD non-canonical secretome without a signal peptide but secreted *via* the N-terminal Gasdermin D protein pore/channel, caspase-4(humans)/11 (mice)-GSDMD non-canonical secretome without a signal peptide but secreted *via* the N-terminal Gasdermin D protein pore/channel, exosome non-canonical secretome without a signal peptide but secreted *via* exosomes and docking on target cells with exosome docking mechanism but not cytokine/chemokine receptors, and HPA-classified cytokines and chemokines. In contrast to 18 traditional EC-secreted cytokines and chemokines (110), such as TNF-α, IL-1, IL-3, IL-5, IL-6, IL-8, IL-11, IL-15, MCP-1, GM-CSF (3, 57), CD40/CD40L, endothelin-1, RANTES, IL1ra, IL10 (59), IL13 and TGF-β, and IL-35 (40, 44, 58, 59, 111), these large numbers of secretomic proteins play significant roles in promoting EC activation, inflammatory cell and immune cell recruitment, cancer cell metastasis, immune cell development and regulation, vascular smooth muscle cell function regulation, and many other functions *via* autocrine, paracrine, and endocrine manners, either by apical secretion and/or basolateral secretion. Third,

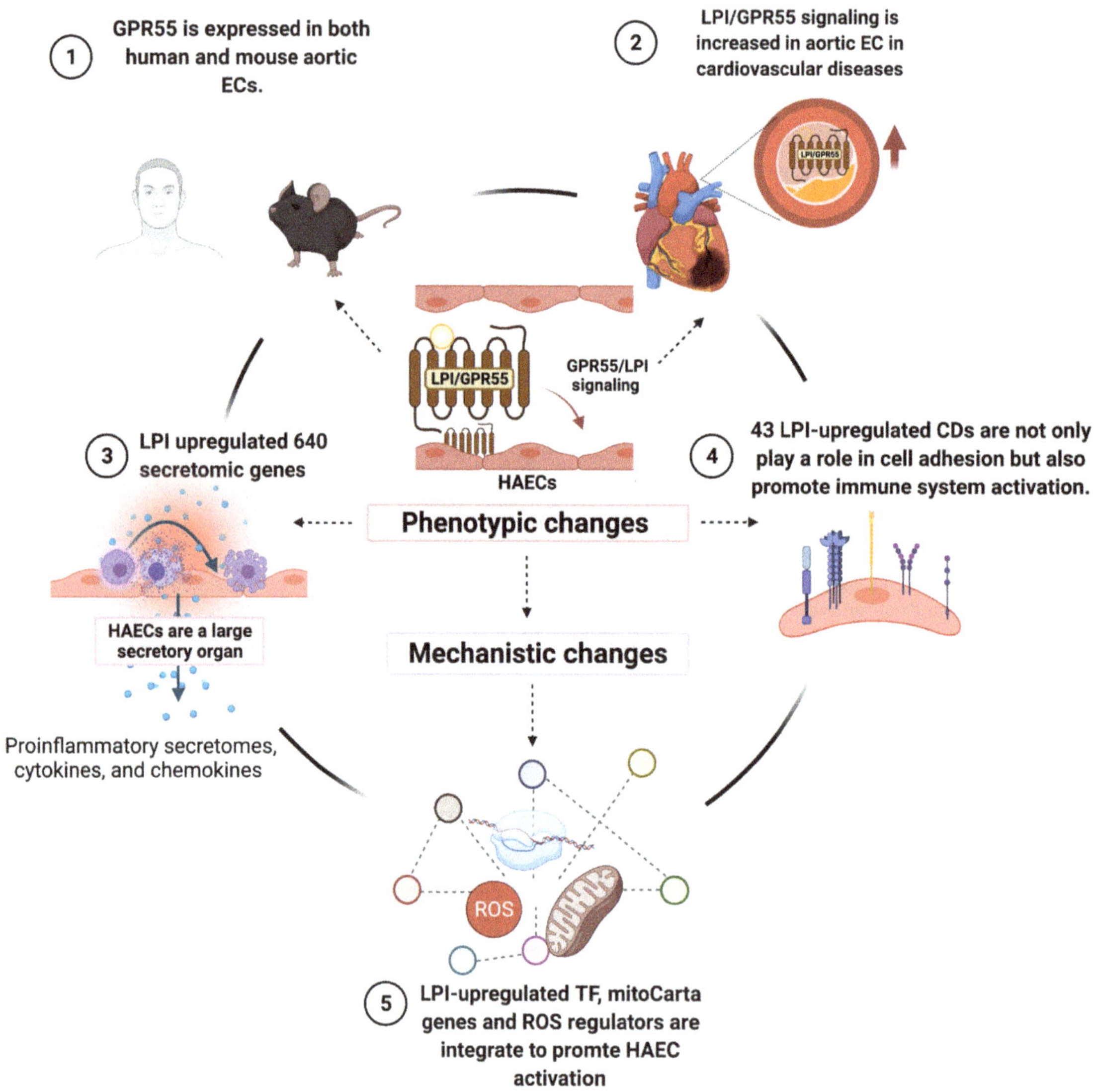

FIGURE 11 | Working model. LPI receptor GPR55 is expressed in both human and mouse aortic endothelial cells. LPIs/GPR55 signaling is upregulated in aortic endothelial cells in hyperlipidemia. We first proposed human aortic endothelial cells as a large secretory organ, which can mediate up to 640 secretomic genes upon LPI stimulation. A large number of secretory proteins contribute a significant role in mediating EC activation and inflammation. LPI-stimulated specific CD markers not only participate in cell adhesion but also play an essential role in immune cell activation, proliferation, and differentiation. All these phenotypic changes may be caused by the mechanisms of synergy among LPI-increased TFs, mitoCarta genes, and ROS regulators. *This figure was created with Biorender.com.

by screening 373 clusters of differentiation markers and 159 EC-specific biomarkers, we have demonstrated for the first time that LPIs upregulate 43 CD markers, five of which are shared with 159 EC-specific biomarkers, and 12 of which are shared with other human endothelial cell activation induced by an influenza virus infection, MERS-CoV infection, and KSHV infection, respectively. In contrast to traditional EC adhesion molecules, such as ICAM1, VCAM1, and SELE, as we and others have reported (33, 58), the 43 LPI-upregulated CD markers not only play significant roles in endothelial cell adhesion and inflammatory and immune cell recruitment but also promote inflammatory cell and immune cell activation, proliferation, differentiation, and immune tolerance. Fourth, three novel molecular mechanisms, namely, 172 LPI-upregulated transcription factors, 152 LPI-upregulated mitoCarta genes, and 18 LPI-upregulated ROS regulators, are integrated to promote HAEC activation.

Our results have provided novel insights into aortic endothelial cell (EC) activation, formulated an EC biology knowledge-based transcriptomic profile strategy, and identified new targets for the future development of therapeutics for cardiovascular diseases, inflammations, immune diseases, transplantation, aging, and cancers. One limitation of all the RNA-Seq data analyses is that due to the low-throughput nature of verification techniques in every laboratory, including ours, we could not verify every result we found with the analyses of high-throughput data, which are similar to all the studies with RNA-Seq (19, 59), single-cell RNA-Seq, metabolomics (23), chromatin immunoprecipitation (CHIP)-Seq (24, 44), and other-omics data (11, 138, 139). We acknowledge that carefully designed *in vitro* and *in vivo* experimental models will be needed in the future to verify the LPI-upregulated genes further and the underlying mechanisms we report here (9, 140).

AUTHOR CONTRIBUTIONS

KX carried out data gathering and data analysis and prepared the tables and figures. YSh, FS, AG, CD, LL, YL, YSu, HX, DP, XQ, JS, EC, XJ, and HW aided in the analysis of data. XY supervised the experimental design, data analysis, and manuscript writing. All the authors read and approved the final manuscript.

REFERENCES

1. Yang XF, Yin Y, Wang H. Vascular inflammation and atherogenesis are activated via receptors for pamps and suppressed by regulatory T cells. *Drug Discov Today Ther Strateg.* (2008) 5:125–42. doi: 10.1016/j.ddstr.2008.11.003
2. Drummer C. 4th, Saaoud F, Shao (邵颖) Y, Sun (孙宇) Y, Xu (徐克曼) K, Lu (路一凡) Y, et al. Trained immunity and reactivity of macrophages and endothelial cells. *Arteriosclerosis, Thrombosis, Vascular Biology.* (2021) 41:1032–46. doi: 10.1161/ATVBAHA.120.315452
3. Shao Y, Saredy J, Xu K, Sun Y, Saaoud F, Drummer C, et al. Endothelial immunity trained by coronavirus infections, DAMP stimulations and regulated by anti-oxidant NRF2 may contribute to inflammations, myelopoiesis, covid-19 cytokine storms and thromboembolism. *Front Immunol.* (2021) 12:653110. doi: 10.3389/fimmu.2021.653110
4. Shao Y, Saredy J, Yang WY, Sun Y, Lu Y, Saaoud F, et al. Vascular endothelial cells and innate immunity. *Arteriosclerosis, Thrombosis, Vascular Biology.* (2020) 40:e138–52. doi: 10.1161/ATVBAHA.120.314330
5. Mai J, Virtue A, Shen J, Wang H, Yang XF. An evolving new paradigm: endothelial cells–conditional innate immune cells. *J Hematol Oncol.* (2013) 6:61. doi: 10.1186/1756-8722-6-61
6. Shao Y, Cheng Z, Li X, Chernaya V, Wang H, Yang XF. Immunosuppressive/anti-inflammatory cytokines directly and indirectly inhibit endothelial dysfunction–a novel mechanism for maintaining vascular function. *J Hematol Oncol.* (2014) 7:80. doi: 10.1186/s13045-014-0080-6
7. Fidler TP, Xue C, Yalcinkaya M, Hardaway B, Abramowicz S, Xiao T, et al. The AIM2 inflammasome exacerbates atherosclerosis in clonal haematopoiesis. *Nature.* (2021) 592:296–301. doi: 10.1038/s41586-021-03341-5
8. Ridker PM, Everett BM, Thuren T, MacFadyen JG, Chang WH, Ballantyne C, et al. CANTOS trial group. Antiinflammatory therapy with canakinumab for atherosclerotic disease. *The New England journal of medicine.* (2017) 377:1119–31. doi: 10.1056/NEJMoa1707914
9. Liu M, Saredy J, Zhang R, Shao Y, Sun Y, Yang WY, et al. Approaching inflammation paradoxes-proinflammatory cytokine blockages induce inflammatory regulators. *Front Immunol.* (2020) 11:554301. doi: 10.3389/fimmu.2020.554301
10. Lai B, Wang J, Fagenson A, Sun Y, Saredy J, Lu Y, et al. Twenty novel disease group-specific and 12 new shared macrophage pathways in eight groups of 34 diseases including 24 inflammatory organ diseases and 10 types of tumors. *Front Immunology.* (2019) *10*:2612. doi: 10.3389/fimmu.2019.02612
11. Johnson C, Drummer Iv C, Shan H, Shao Y, Sun Y, Lu Y, et al. A novel subset of $CD95^+$ pro-inflammatory macrophages overcome miR155 deficiency and may serve as a switch from metabolically healthy obesity to metabolically unhealthy obesity. *Front Immunol.* (2021) 11:619951. doi: 10.3389/fimmu.2020.619951
12. Fu H, Vadalia N, Xue ER, Johnson C, Wang L, Yang WY, et al. Thrombus leukocytes exhibit more endothelial cell-specific angiogenic markers than peripheral blood leukocytes do in acute coronary syndrome patients, suggesting a possibility of trans-differentiation: a comprehensive database mining study. *J Hematol Oncol.* (2017) 10:74. doi: 10.1186/s13045-017-0440-0
13. Zhang R, Saredy J, Shao Y, Yao T, Liu L, Saaoud F, et al. End-stage renal disease is different from chronic kidney disease in upregulating ROS-modulated proinflammatory secretome in PBMCs - A novel multiple-hit model for disease progression. *Redox Biol.* (2020) 34:101460. doi: 10.1016/j.redox.2020.101460
14. Zhang D, Fang P, Jiang X, Nelson J, Moore JK, Kruger WD, et al. Severe hyperhomocysteinemia promotes bone marrow-derived and resident inflammatory monocyte differentiation and atherosclerosis in LDLr/CBS-deficient mice. *Circ Res.* (2012) 111:37–49. doi: 10.1161/CIRCRESAHA.112.269472
15. Zhang D, Jiang X, Fang P, Yan Y, Song J, Gupta S, et al. Hyperhomocysteinemia promotes inflammatory monocyte generation and accelerates atherosclerosis in transgenic cystathionine beta-synthase-deficient mice. *Circulation.* (2009) 120:1893–902. doi: 10.1161/CIRCULATIONAHA.109.866889
16. Fang P, Li X, Shan H, Saredy JJ, Cueto R, Xia J, et al. $Ly6C^+$ inflammatory monocyte differentiation partially mediates hyperhomocysteinemia-induced vascular dysfunction in type 2 diabetic db/db Mice. *Arteriosclerosis, Thrombosis, Vascular Biology.* (2019) 39:2097–119. doi: 10.1161/ATVBAHA.119.313138
17. Fang P, Zhang D, Cheng Z, Yan C, Jiang X, Kruger WD, et al. Hyperhomocysteinemia potentiates hyperglycemia-induced inflammatory monocyte differentiation and atherosclerosis. *Diabetes.* (2014) 63:4275–90. doi: 10.2337/db14-0809
18. Yang J, Fang P, Yu D, Zhang L, Zhang D, Jiang X, et al. Chronic kidney disease induces inflammatory CD40+ monocyte differentiation via homocysteine elevation and DNA hypomethylation. *Circ Res.* (2016) 119:1226–41. doi: 10.1161/CIRCRESAHA.116.308750
19. Li X, Wang L, Fang P, Sun Y, Jiang X, Wang H, et al. Lysophospholipids induce innate immune transdifferentiation of endothelial cells, resulting in prolonged endothelial activation. *J Biol Chem.* (2018) 293:11033–45. doi: 10.1074/jbc.RA118.002752
20. Wang X, Li YF, Nanayakkara G, Shao Y, Liang B, Cole L, et al. Lysophospholipid receptors, as novel conditional danger receptors and homeostatic receptors modulate inflammation-novel paradigm and therapeutic potential. *J Cardiovasc Transl Res.* (2016) 9:343–59. doi: 10.1007/s12265-016-9700-6
21. Shao Y, Nanayakkara G, Cheng J, Cueto R, Yang WY, Park JY, et al. Lysophospholipids and their receptors serve as conditional DAMPs and DAMP receptors in tissue oxidative and inflammatory injury. *Antioxid Redox Signal.* (2018) 28:973–86. doi: 10.1089/ars.2017.7069
22. Li YF Li RS, Samuel SB, Cueto R, Li XY, Wang H, et al. Lysophospholipids and their G protein-coupled receptors in atherosclerosis. *Frontiers in Bioscience (Landmark edition).* (2016) 21:70–88. doi: 10.2741/4377
23. Li X, Fang P, Li Y, Kuo YM, Andrews AJ, Nanayakkara G, et al. Mitochondrial reactive oxygen species mediate lysophosphatidylcholine-induced endothelial cell activation. *Arteriosclerosis, Thrombosis, Vascular Biology.* (2016) 36:1090–100. doi: 10.1161/ATVBAHA.115.306964
24. Lu Y, Sun Y, Drummer C. 4th, Nanayakkara GK, Shao Y, Saaoud F, et al. jabb Increased acetylation of H3K14 in the genomic regions that encode trained immunity enzymes in lysophosphatidylcholine-activated human aortic endothelial cells - Novel qualification markers for chronic disease risk factors and conditional DAMPs redox. *Biology.* (2019) 24:101221. doi: 10.1016/j.redox.2019.101221
25. Zhong C, Yang X, Feng Y, Yu J. Trained immunity: an underlying driver of inflammatory atherosclerosis. *Front Immunol.* (2020) 11:284. doi: 10.3389/fimmu.2020.00284
26. Fagenson AM, Xu K, Saaoud F, Nanayakkara G, Jhala NC, Liu L, et al. Liver ischemia reperfusion injury, enhanced by trained immunity, is attenuated in caspase 1/caspase 11 double gene knockout mice. *Pathogens (Basel, Switzerland).* (2020) 9:879. doi: 10.3390/pathogens9110879

27. Zasłona Z, O'Neill L. Cytokine-like roles for metabolites in immunity. *Mol Cell.* (2020) 78:814–23. doi: 10.1016/j.molcel.2020.04.002
28. Wang H, Jiang X, Yang F, Gaubatz JW, Ma L, Magera MJ, et al. Hyperhomocysteinemia accelerates atherosclerosis in cystathionine beta-synthase and apolipoprotein E double knock-out mice with and without dietary perturbation. *Blood.* (2003) 101:3901–7. doi: 10.1182/blood-2002-08-2606
29. Jiang X, Yang F, Tan H, Liao D, Bryan RM. Jr, et al. Hyperhomocystinemia impairs endothelial function and eNOS activity via PKC activation. *Arteriosclerosis, Thrombosis, Vascular Biology.* (2005) 25:2515–21. doi: 10.1161/01.ATV.0000189559.87328.e4
30. Jamaluddin MD, Chen I, Yang F, Jiang X, Jan M, Liu X, et al. Homocysteine inhibits endothelial cell growth via DNA hypomethylation of the cyclin A gene. *Blood.* (2007) 110:3648–55. doi: 10.1182/blood-2007-06-096701
31. Chiurchiù V, Leuti A, Maccarrone M. Bioactive lipids and chronic inflammation: managing the fire within. *Front Immunol.* (2018) 9:38. doi: 10.3389/fimmu.2018.00038
32. Chapman MJ, Orsoni A, Tan R, Mellett NA, Nguyen A, Robillard P, et al. LDL subclass lipidomics in atherogenic dyslipidemia: effect of statin therapy on bioactive lipids and dense LDL. *J Lipid Res.* (2020) 61:911–32. doi: 10.1194/jlr.P119000543
33. Yin Y, Li X, Sha X, Xi H, Li YF, Shao Y, et al. Early hyperlipidemia promotes endothelial activation via a caspase-1-sirtuin 1 pathway. *Arteriosclerosis, Thrombosis, Vascular Biology.* (2015) 35:804–16. doi: 10.1161/ATVBAHA.115.305282
34. Lopez-Pastrana J, Ferrer LM Li YF, Xiong X, Xi H, Cueto R, et al. Inhibition of caspase-1 activation in endothelial cells improves angiogenesis: a novel therapeutic potential for ischemia. *J Biol Chem.* (2015) 290:17485–94. doi: 10.1074/jbc.M115.641191
35. An D, Hao F, Zhang F, Kong W, Chun J, Xu X, et al. CD14 is a key mediator of both lysophosphatidic acid and lipopolysaccharide induction of foam cell formation. *J Biol Chem.* (2017) 292:14391–400. doi: 10.1074/jbc.M117.781807
36. Smyth SS, Kraemer M, Yang L, Van Hoose P, Morris AJ. Roles for lysophosphatidic acid signaling in vascular development and disease. *Biochimica et biophysica acta Molecular and cell biology of lipids.* (2020) 1865:158734. doi: 10.1016/j.bbalip.2020.158734
37. Green CD, Maceyka M, Cowart LA, Spiegel S. Sphingolipids in metabolic disease: The good, the bad, the unknown. *Cell Metab.* (2021) 33:1293–306. doi: 10.1016/j.cmet.2021.06.006
38. Cao J, Goossens P, Martin-Lorenzo M, Dewez F, Claes B, Biessen E, et al. Atheroma-specific lipids in ldlr$^{-/-}$ and apoe$^{-/-}$ mice using 2D and 3D Matrix-assisted laser desorption/ionization mass spectrometry imaging. *J Am Soc Mass Spectrom.* (2020) 31:1825–32. doi: 10.1021/jasms.0c00070
39. Serhan CN, Levy BD. Resolvins in inflammation: emergence of the pro-resolving superfamily of mediators. *J Clin Invest.* (2018) 128:2657–69. doi: 10.1172/JCI97943
40. Li X, Fang P, Yang WY, Wang H, Yang X. IL-35, as a newly proposed homeostasis-associated molecular pattern, plays three major functions including anti-inflammatory initiator, effector, and blocker in cardiovascular diseases. *Cytokine.* (2019) 122:154076. doi: 10.1016/j.cyto.2017.06.003
41. Mills EL, Ryan DG, Prag HA, Dikovskaya D, Menon D, Zaslona Z, et al. Itaconate is an anti-inflammatory metabolite that activates Nrf2 via alkylation of KEAP1. *Nature.* (2018) 556:113–7. doi: 10.1038/nature25986
42. Hooftman A, O'Neill L. The Immunomodulatory Potential of the Metabolite Itaconate. *Trends Immunol.* (2019) 40:687–98. doi: 10.1016/j.it.2019.05.007
43. Li X, Fang P, Yang WY, Chan K, Lavallee M, Xu K, et al. Mitochondrial ROS, uncoupled from ATP synthesis, determine endothelial activation for both physiological recruitment of patrolling cells and pathological recruitment of inflammatory cells. *Can J Physiol Pharmacol.* (2017) 95:247–52. doi: 10.1139/cjpp-2016-0515
44. Li X, Shao Y, Sha X, Fang P, Kuo YM, Andrews AJ, et al. IL-35 (Interleukin-35) suppresses endothelial cell activation by inhibiting mitochondrial reactive oxygen species-mediated site-specific acetylation of H3K14 (Histone 3 Lysine 14). *Arteriosclerosis, Thrombosis, Vascular Biology.* (2018) 38:599–609. doi: 10.1161/ATVBAHA.117.310626
45. Cheng J, Nanayakkara G, Shao Y, Cueto R, Wang L, Yang WY, et al. Mitochondrial proton leak plays a critical role in pathogenesis of cardiovascular diseases. *Adv Exp Med Biol.* (2017) 982:359–70. doi: 10.1007/978-3-319-55330-6_20
46. Nanayakkara GK, Wang H, Yang X. Proton leak regulates mitochondrial reactive oxygen species generation in endothelial cell activation and inflammation - A novel concept. *Arch Biochem Biophys.* (2019) 662:68–74. doi: 10.1016/j.abb.2018.12.002
47. Yin Y, Pastrana JL Li X, Huang X, Mallilankaraman K, Choi ET, et al. Inflammasomes: sensors of metabolic stresses for vascular inflammation. *Frontiers in Bioscience (Landmark edition).* (2013) 18:638–49. doi: 10.2741/4127
48. Ni D, Tang T, Lu Y, Xu K, Shao Y, Saaoud F, et al. Canonical secretomes, innate immune caspase-1-, 4/11-gasdermin D non-canonical secretomes and exosomes may contribute to maintain treg-ness for treg immunosuppression, tissue repair and modulate anti-tumor immunity via ROS pathways. *Front Immunol.* (2021) 12:678201. doi: 10.3389/fimmu.2021.678201
49. Zhang R, Xu K, Shao Y, Sun Y, Saredy J, Cutler E, et al. Tissue treg secretomes and transcription factors shared with stem cells contribute to a treg niche to maintain treg-ness with 80% innate immune pathways, and functions of immunosuppression and tissue repair. *Front Immunol.* (2021) 11:632239. doi: 10.3389/fimmu.2020.632239
50. Fu H, Sun Y, Shao Y, Saredy J, Cueto R, Liu L, et al. Interleukin 35 delays hindlimb ischemia-induced angiogenesis through regulating ros-extracellular matrix but spares later regenerative angiogenesis. *Front Immunol.* (2020) 11:595813. doi: 10.3389/fimmu.2020.595813
51. Falasca M, Ferro R. Role of the lysophosphatidylinositol/GPR55 axis in cancer. *Adv Biol Regul.* (2016) 60:88–93. doi: 10.1016/j.jbior.2015.10.003
52. Yang Q, Nanayakkara GK, Drummer C, Sun Y, Johnson C, Cueto R, et al. Low-intensity ultrasound-induced anti-inflammatory effects are mediated by several new mechanisms including gene induction, immunosuppressor cell promotion, and enhancement of exosome biogenesis and docking. *Front Physiol.* (2017) 8:818. doi: 10.3389/fphys.2017.00818
53. Yang Q, Zhang R, Tang P, Sun Y, Johnson C, Saredy J, et al. Ultrasound may suppress tumor growth, inhibit inflammation, and establish tolerogenesis by remodeling innatome via pathways of ROS. immune checkpoints, cytokines, trained immunity/tolerance. *Journal Of Immunology Research.* (2021)2021:6664453. doi: 10.1155/2021/6664453
54. Wang J, Lai B, Nanayakkara G, Yang Q, Sun Y, Lu Y, et al. Experimental data-mining analyses reveal new roles of low-intensity ultrasound in differentiating cell death regulatome in cancer and non-cancer cells via potential modulation of chromatin long-range interactions. *Front Oncol.* (2019) 9:600. doi: 10.3389/fonc.2019.00600
55. Zhou Y, Zhou B, Pache L, Chang M, Khodabakhshi AH, Tanaseichuk O, et al. Metascape provides a biologist-oriented resource for the analysis of systems-level datasets. *Nature Communications.* (2019) *10:*1523. doi: 10.1038/s41467-019-09234-6
56. Jan M, Cueto R, Jiang X, Lu L, Sardy J, Xiong X, et al. Molecular processes mediating hyperhomocysteinemia-induced metabolic reprogramming, redox regulation and growth inhibition in endothelial cells. *Redox Biol.* (2021) 45:102018. doi: 10.1016/j.redox.2021.102018
57. Mai J, Nanayakkara G, Lopez-Pastrana J, Li X, Li YF, Wang X, et al. Interleukin-17A promotes aortic endothelial cell activation via transcriptionally and post-translationally activating p38 mitogen-activated protein kinase (MAPK) pathway. *J Biol Chem.* (2016) 291:4939–54. doi: 10.1074/jbc.M115.690081
58. Sha X, Meng S, Li X, Xi H, Maddaloni M, Pascual DW, et al. Interleukin-35 inhibits endothelial cell activation by suppressing MAPK-AP-1 pathway. *J Biol Chem.* (2015) 290:19307–18. doi: 10.1074/jbc.M115.663286
59. Li X, Fang P, Sun Y, Shao Y, Yang WY, Jiang X, et al. Anti-inflammatory cytokines IL-35 and IL-10 block atherogenic lysophosphatidylcholine-induced, mitochondrial ROS-mediated innate immune activation, but spare innate immune memory signature in endothelial cells. *Redox Biol.* (2020) 28:101373. doi: 10.1016/j.redox.2019.101373
60. Goncharov NV, Nadeev AD, Jenkins RO, & Avdonin PV. (2017). Markers and Biomarkers of Endothelium: When Something Is Rotten in the State. *Oxidative Medicine And Cellular Longevity.* (2017). 9759735. doi: 10.1155/2017/9759735
61. Yin Y, Yan Y, Jiang X, Mai J, Chen NC, Wang H, et al. Inflammasomes are differentially expressed in cardiovascular and other tissues.

Int J Immunopathol Pharmacol. (2009) 22:311–22. doi: 10.1177/039463200902200208

62. Li YF, Huang X, Li X, Gong R, Yin Y, Nelson J, et al. Caspase-1 mediates hyperlipidemia-weakened progenitor cell vessel repair. *Frontiers in Bioscience (Landmark edition).* (2016) 21:178–91. doi: 10.2741/4383
63. Ferrer LM, Monroy AM, Lopez-Pastrana J, Nanayakkara G, Cueto R, Li YF, et al. Caspase-1 plays a critical role in accelerating chronic kidney disease-promoted neointimal hyperplasia in the carotid artery. *J Cardiovasc Transl Res.* (2016) 9:135–44. doi: 10.1007/s12265-016-9683-3
64. Li YF, Nanayakkara G, Sun Y, Li X, Wang L, Cueto R, et al. Analyses of caspase-1-regulated transcriptomes in various tissues lead to identification of novel IL-1β-, IL-18- and sirtuin-1-independent pathways. *J Hematol Oncol.* (2017) 10:40. doi: 10.1186/s13045-017-0406-2
65. Wang L, Fu H, Nanayakkara G, Li Y, Shao Y, Johnson C, et al. Novel extracellular and nuclear caspase-1 and inflammasomes propagate inflammation and regulate gene expression: a comprehensive database mining study. *J Hematol Oncol.* (2016) 9:122. doi: 10.1186/s13045-016-0351-5
66. Broz P, Pelegrín P, Shao F. The gasdermins, a protein family executing cell death and inflammation. *Nature Reviews Immunology.* (2020) 20:143–57. doi: 10.1038/s41577-019-0228-2
67. Keller M, Rüegg A, Werner S, Beer HD. Active caspase-1 is a regulator of unconventional protein secretion. *Cell.* (2008) 132:818–31. doi: 10.1016/j.cell.2007.12.040
68. Lorey MB, Rossi K, Eklund KK, Nyman TA, Matikainen S. Global characterization of protein secretion from human macrophages following non-canonical caspase-4/5 inflammasome activation. *Molecular & Cellular Proteomics: MCP.* (2017) 16:S187–S199. doi: 10.1074/mcp.M116.064840
69. Alhouayek M, Masquelier J, Muccioli GG. Lysophosphatidylinositols, from cell membrane constituents to GPR55 ligands. *Trends Pharmacol Sci.* (2018) 39:586–604. doi: 10.1016/j.tips.2018.02.011
70. Virtue A, Johnson C, Lopez-Pastraña J, Shao Y, Fu H, Li X, et al. MicroRNA-155 deficiency leads to decreased atherosclerosis, increased white adipose tissue obesity, and non-alcoholic fatty liver disease: a novel mouse model of obesity paradox. *J Biol Chem.* (2017) 292:1267–87. doi: 10.1074/jbc.M116.739839
71. Saaoud F, Wang J, Iwanowycz S, Wang Y, Altomare D, Shao Y, et al. Bone marrow deficiency of mRNA decaying protein Tristetraprolin increases inflammation and mitochondrial ROS but reduces hepatic lipoprotein production in LDLR knockout mice. *Redox Biol.* (2020) 37:101609. doi: 10.1016/j.redox.2020.101609
72. Yang XF, Weber GF, Cantor H, A. novel Bcl-x isoform connected to the T cell receptor regulates apoptosis in T cells. *Immunity.* (1997) 7:629–39. doi: 10.1016/S1074-7613(00)80384-2
73. Yang Y, Yang F, Xiong Z, Yan Y, Wang X, Nishino M, et al. An N-terminal region of translationally controlled tumor protein is required for its antiapoptotic activity. *Oncogene.* (2005) 24:4778–88. doi: 10.1038/sj.onc.1208666
74. Yang Y, Xiong Z, Zhang S, Yan Y, Nguyen J, Ng B, et al. Bcl-xL inhibits T-cell apoptosis induced by expression of SARS coronavirus E protein in the absence of growth factors. *The Biochemical Journal. (2005)* 392:135–143. doi: 10.1042/BJ20050698
75. Yan Y, Xiong Z, Zhang S, Song J, Huang Y, Thornton AM, et al. CD25high T cells with a prolonged survival inhibit development of diabetes. *Int J Immunopathol Pharmacol.* (2008) 21:767–80. doi: 10.1177/039463200802100401
76. Xiong Z, Song J, Yan Y, Huang Y, Cowan A, Wang H, et al. Higher expression of Bax in regulatory T cells increases vascular inflammation. *Frontiers in bioscience: a journal and virtual library.* (2008) 13:7143–55. doi: 10.2741/3217
77. Xiong Z, Yan Y, Song J, Fang P, Yin Y, Yang Y, et al. Expression of TCTP antisense in CD25(high) regulatory T cells aggravates cuff-injured vascular inflammation. *Atherosclerosis.* (2009) 203:401–8. doi: 10.1016/j.atherosclerosis.2008.07.041
78. Rakocevic J, Orlic D, Mitrovic-Ajtic O, Tomasevic M, Dobric M, Zlatic N, et al. Endothelial cell markers from clinician's perspective. *Exp Mol Pathol.* (2017) 102:303–13. doi: 10.1016/j.yexmp.2017.02.005
79. Gerhardt T, Ley K. Monocyte trafficking across the vessel wall. *Cardiovasc Res.* (2015) 107:321–30. doi: 10.1093/cvr/cvv147
80. Kappelmayer J, & Nagy B, Jr (2017). The Interaction of Selectins and PSGL-1 as a Key Component in Thrombus Formation and Cancer Progression. BioMed research international, (2017). 6138145. doi: 10.1155/2017/6138145
81. Hu Y, Kiely JM, Szente BE, Rosenzweig A, & Gimbrone MA, Jr (2000). E-selectin-dependent signaling via the mitogen-activated protein kinase pathway in vascular endothelial cells. Journal of immunology (Baltimore, Md.: 1950), 165: 2142–2148. doi: 10.4049/jimmunol.165.4.2142
82. Lawson C, Wolf S. ICAM-1 signaling in endothelial cells. *Pharmacological reports: PR.* (2009) 61:22–32. doi: 10.1016/S1734-1140(09)70004-0
83. Chistiakov DA, Bobryshev YV, Orekhov AN. Changes in transcriptome of macrophages in atherosclerosis. *J Cell Mol Med.* (2015) 19:1163–73. doi: 10.1111/jcmm.12591
84. Hu T, Zhou R, Zhao Y, Wu G. Integrin α6/Akt/Erk signaling is essential for human breast cancer resistance to radiotherapy. *Sci Rep.* (2016) 6:33376. doi: 10.1038/srep33376
85. Abair TD, Bulus N, Borza C, Sundaramoorthy M, Zent R, Pozzi A. Functional analysis of the cytoplasmic domain of the integrin {alpha}1 subunit in endothelial cells. *Blood.* (2008) 112:3242–54. doi: 10.1182/blood-2007-12-126433
86. Kannan K, Stewart RM, Bounds W, Carlsson SR, Fukuda M, Betzing KW, et al. Lysosome-associated membrane proteins h-LAMP1 (CD107a) and h-LAMP2 (CD107b) are activation-dependent cell surface glycoproteins in human peripheral blood mononuclear cells which mediate cell adhesion to vascular endothelium. *Cell Immunol.* (1996) 171:10–9. doi: 10.1006/cimm.1996.0167
87. Popson SA, Ziegler ME, Chen X, Holderfield MT, Shaaban CI, Fong AH, et al. Interferon-induced transmembrane protein 1 regulates endothelial lumen formation during angiogenesis. *Arteriosclerosis, Thrombosis, Vascular Biology.* (2014) 34:1011–9. doi: 10.1161/ATVBAHA.114.303352
88. Watt SM, Chan JY. CD164–a novel sialomucin on CD34+ cells. *Leuk Lymphoma.* (2000) 37:1–25. doi: 10.3109/10428190009057625
89. Kleemann R, Verschuren L, van Erk MJ, Nikolsky Y, Cnubben NH, Verheij ER, et al. Atherosclerosis and liver inflammation induced by increased dietary cholesterol intake: a combined transcriptomics and metabolomics analysis. *Genome Biol.* (2007) 8:R200. doi: 10.1186/gb-2007-8-9-r200
90. Devilard E, Xerri L, Dubreuil P, Lopez M, Reymond N. Nectin-3 (CD113) interacts with Nectin-2 (CD112) to promote lymphocyte transendothelial migration. *PLoS ONE.* (2013) 8:e77424. doi: 10.1371/journal.pone.0077424
91. Bansal A, Sanchez DJ, Nimgaonkar V, Sanchez D, Riscal R, Skuli N, et al. Gamma-Glutamyltransferase 1 Promotes Clear Cell Renal Cell Carcinoma Initiation and Progression. *Molecular Cancer Research: MCR.* (2019) 17:1881–92. doi: 10.1158/1541-7786.MCR-18-1204
92. Shen H, Wu N, Nanayakkara G, Fu H, Yang Q, Yang WY, et al. Co-signaling receptors regulate T-cell plasticity and immune tolerance. *Frontiers in bioscience (Landmark edition).* (2019) 24:96–132. doi: 10.2741/4710
93. Winkels H, Meiler S, Lievens D, Engel D, Spitz C, Bürger C, et al. CD27 co-stimulation increases the abundance of regulatory T cells and reduces atherosclerosis in hyperlipidaemic mice. *Eur Heart J.* (2017) 38:3590–9. doi: 10.1093/eurheartj/ehx517
94. Gotsman I, Grabie N, Dacosta R, Sukhova G, Sharpe A, Lichtman AH. Proatherogenic immune responses are regulated by the PD-1/PD-L pathway in mice. *J Clin Invest.* (2007) 117:2974–82. doi: 10.1172/JCI31344
95. van Wanrooij EJ, van Puijvelde GH, de Vos P, Yagita H, van Berkel TJ, Kuiper J. Interruption of the Tnfrsf4/Tnfsf4 (OX40/OX40L) pathway attenuates atherogenesis in low-density lipoprotein receptor-deficient mice. *Arteriosclerosis, thrombosis, vascular biology.* (2007) 27:204–10. doi: 10.1161/01.ATV.0000251007.07648.81
96. Franzini M, Corti A, Martinelli B, Del Corso A, Emdin M, Parenti GF, et al. Gamma-glutamyltransferase activity in human atherosclerotic plaques–biochemical similarities with the circulating enzyme. *Atherosclerosis.* (2009) 202:119–27. doi: 10.1016/j.atherosclerosis.2008.03.023
97. Karp DR, Carlisle ML, Mobley AB, Nichols TC, Oppenheimer-Marks N, Brezinschek RI, et al. Gamma-glutamyl transpeptidase is up-regulated on memory T lymphocytes. *Int Immunol.* (1999) 11:1791–800. doi: 10.1093/intimm/11.11.1791

98. Sommariva E, Stadiotti I, Casella M, Catto V, Dello Russo A, Carbucicchio C, et al. Oxidized LDL-dependent pathway as new pathogenic trigger in arrhythmogenic cardiomyopathy. *EMBO Mol Med.* (2021) 13:e14365. doi: 10.15252/emmm.202114365
99. Murshid A, Borges TJ, Lang BJ, Calderwood SK. The Scavenger Receptor SREC-I Cooperates with Toll-Like Receptors to Trigger Inflammatory Innate Immune Responses. *Front Immunol.* (2016) 7:226. doi: 10.3389/fimmu.2016.00226
100. Martín-Ventura JL, Madrigal-Matute J, Muñoz-Garcia B, Blanco-Colio LM, Van Oostrom M, Zalba G, et al. Increased CD74 expression in human atherosclerotic plaques: contribution to inflammatory responses in vascular cells. *Cardiovasc Res.* (2009) 83:586–94. doi: 10.1093/cvr/cvp141
101. Damås JK, Waehre T, Yndestad A, Otterdal K, Hognestad A, Solum NO, et al. Interleukin-7-mediated inflammation in unstable angina: possible role of chemokines and platelets. *Circulation.* (2003) 107:2670–6. doi: 10.1161/01.CIR.0000070542.18001.87
102. Park YM. CD36, a scavenger receptor implicated in atherosclerosis. *Exp Mol Med.* (2014) 46:e99. doi: 10.1038/emm.2014.38
103. Zimmer S, Steinmetz M, Asdonk T, Motz I, Coch C, Hartmann E, et al. Activation of endothelial toll-like receptor 3 impairs endothelial function. *Circ Res.* (2011) 108:1358–66. doi: 10.1161/CIRCRESAHA.111.243246
104. Yang XF. Immunology of stem cells and cancer stem cells. *Cell Mol Immunol.* (2007) 4:161–71.
105. AbuSamra DB, Aleisa FA, Al-Amoodi AS, Jalal Ahmed HM, Chin CJ, Abuelela AF, et al. Not just a marker: CD34 on human hematopoietic stem/progenitor cells dominates vascular selectin binding along with CD44. *Blood advances.* (2017) 1:2799–816. doi: 10.1182/bloodadvances.2017004317
106. Donners MM, Wolfs IM, Olieslagers S, Mohammadi-Motahhari Z, Tchaikovski V, Heeneman S, et al. A disintegrin and metalloprotease 10 is a novel mediator of vascular endothelial growth factor-induced endothelial cell function in angiogenesis and is associated with atherosclerosis. *Arteriosclerosis, Thrombosis, Vascular Biology.* (2010) 30:2188–95. doi: 10.1161/ATVBAHA.110.213124
107. Nelson J, Wu Y, Jiang X, Berretta R, Houser S, Choi E, et al. Hyperhomocysteinemia suppresses bone marrow CD34+/VEGF receptor 2+ cells and inhibits progenitor cell mobilization and homing to injured vasculature-a role of β1-integrin in progenitor cell migration and adhesion. *FASEB Journal.* (2015) 29:3085–99. doi: 10.1096/fj.14-267989
108. Uhlén M, Karlsson MJ, Hober A, Svensson AS, Scheffel J, Kotol D, et al. The human secretome. *Science Signaling.* (2019) *12:* eaaz0274. doi: 10.1126/scisignal.aaz0274
109. Fromer MW, Chang S, Hagaman A, Koko KR, Nolan RS, Zhang P, et al. The endothelial cell secretome as a novel treatment to prime adipose-derived stem cells for improved wound healing in diabetes. *J Vasc Surg.* (2018) 68:234–44. doi: 10.1016/j.jvs.2017.05.094
110. Kofler S, Nickel T, & Weis M. Role of cytokines in cardiovascular diseases: a focus on endothelial responses to inflammation. *Clinical Science (London, England: 1979).* (2005) 108:205–213. doi: 10.1042/CS20040174
111. Li X, Mai J, Virtue A, Yin Y, Gong R, Sha X, et al. IL-35 is a novel responsive anti-inflammatory cytokine–a new system of categorizing anti-inflammatory cytokines. *PLoS One.* (2012) 7:e33628. doi: 10.1371/journal.pone.0033628
112. Wei H, Sundararaman A, Dickson E, Rennie-Campbell L, Cross E, Heesom KJ, et al. Characterization of the polarized endothelial secretome. *FASEB Journal.* (2019) 33:12277–87. doi: 10.1096/fj.201900262R
113. Safdar A, Tarnopolsky MA. Exosomes as Mediators of the Systemic Adaptations to Endurance Exercise. *Cold Spring Harb Perspect Med.* (2018) 8:a029827. doi: 10.1101/cshperspect.a029827
114. Scheja L, Heeren J. The endocrine function of adipose tissues in health and cardiometabolic disease. *Nature Reviews Endocrinology.* (2019) 15:507–24. doi: 10.1038/s41574-019-0230-6
115. Planavila A, Fernández-Solà J, Villarroya F. Cardiokines as modulators of stress-induced cardiac disorders. *Adv Protein Chem Struct Biol.* (2017) 108:227–56. doi: 10.1016/bs.apcsb.2017.01.002
116. Gonzalez-Gil AM, Elizondo-Montemayor L. The Role of Exercise in the Interplay between Myokines, Hepatokines, Osteokines, Adipokines, and Modulation of Inflammation for Energy Substrate Redistribution and Fat Mass Loss: A Review. *Nutrients.* (2020) *12:*1899. doi: 10.3390/nu12061899
117. L PK, Kandoi S, Misra R, S V, K R, Verma RS. The mesenchymal stem cell secretome: A new paradigm towards cell-free therapeutic mode in regenerative medicine. *Cytokine & Growth Factor Reviews.* (2019) 46:1–9. doi: 10.1016/j.cytogfr.2019.04.002
118. Xu K, Yang WY, Nanayakkara GK, Shao Y, Yang F, Hu W, et al. GATA3, HDAC6, and BCL6 regulate FOXP3+ treg plasticity and determine treg conversion into either novel antigen-presenting cell-like treg or Th1-treg. *Front Immunol.* (2018) 9:45. doi: 10.3389/fimmu.2018.00045
119. Fedorova O, Petukhov A, Daks A, Shuvalov O, Leonova T, Vasileva E, et al. Orphan receptor NR4A3 is a novel target of p53 that contributes to apoptosis. *Oncogene.* (2019) 38:2108–22. doi: 10.1038/s41388-018-0566-8
120. Katoh M. Genomic testing, tumor microenvironment and targeted therapy of Hedgehog-related human cancers. *Clinical Science (London, England: 1979).* (2019) 133:953–970. doi: 10.1042/CS20180845
121. Lu N, Malemud CJ. Extracellular Signal-Regulated Kinase: A Regulator of Cell Growth, Inflammation, Chondrocyte and Bone Cell Receptor-Mediated Gene Expression. *Int J Mol Sci.* (2019) 20:3792. doi: 10.3390/ijms20153792
122. Nailwal NP, Doshi GM. Role of intracellular signaling pathways and their inhibitors in the treatment of inflammation. *Inflammopharmacology.* (2021) 29:617–40. doi: 10.1007/s10787-021-00813-y
123. Dunn J, Simmons R, Thabet S, Jo H. The role of epigenetics in the endothelial cell shear stress response and atherosclerosis. *Int J Biochem Cell Biol.* (2015) 67:167–76. doi: 10.1016/j.biocel.2015.05.001
124. Pirri D, Fragiadaki M, & Evans PC. Diabetic atherosclerosis: is there a role for the hypoxia-inducible factors? *Bioscience Reports.* (2020) *40:* BSR20200026. doi: 10.1042/BSR20200026
125. Li X, Fang P, Mai J, Choi ET, Wang H, Yang XF. Targeting mitochondrial reactive oxygen species as novel therapy for inflammatory diseases and cancers. *J Hematol Oncol.* (2013) 6:19. doi: 10.1186/1756-8722-6-19
126. Pattillo CB, Pardue S, Shen X, Fang K, Langston W. Jourd'heuil D, et al. ICAM-1 cytoplasmic tail regulates endothelial glutathione synthesis through a NOX4/PI3-kinase-dependent pathway. *Free Radical Biology & Medicine.* (2010) 49:1119–28. doi: 10.1016/j.freeradbiomed.2010.06.030
127. Ray PD, Huang BW, Tsuji Y. Reactive oxygen species (ROS) homeostasis and redox regulation in cellular signaling. *Cell Signal.* (2012) 24:981–90. doi: 10.1016/j.cellsig.2012.01.008
128. Sun Y, Lu Y, Saredy J, Wang X, Drummer Iv C, Shao Y, et al. ROS systems are a new integrated network for sensing homeostasis and alarming stresses in organelle metabolic processes. *Redox Biol.* (2020) 37:101696. doi: 10.1016/j.redox.2020.101696
129. Shao Y, Chernaya V, Johnson C, Yang WY, Cueto R, Sha X, et al. Metabolic Diseases Downregulate the Majority of Histone Modification Enzymes, Making a Few Upregulated Enzymes Novel Therapeutic Targets—"Sand Out and Gold Stays." *J Cardiovasc Transl Res.* (2016) 9:49–66. doi: 10.1007/s12265-015-9664-y
130. Włodarczyk M, Sobolewska-Włodarczyk A, Cygankiewicz AI, Jacenik D, Krajewska WM, Stec-Michalska K, et al. G protein-coupled receptor 55 (GPR55) expresses differently in patients with Crohn's disease and ulcerative colitis. *Scand J Gastroenterol.* (2017) 52:711–5. doi: 10.1080/00365521.2017.1298834
131. Fondevila MF, Fernandez U, Gonzalez-Rellan MJ, Da Silva Lima N, Buque X, Gonzalez-Rodriguez A, et al. The L-α-Lysophosphatidylinositol/G Protein-Coupled Receptor 55 System Induces the Development of Nonalcoholic Steatosis and Steatohepatitis. *Hepatology (Baltimore, Md).* (2021) 73:606–24. doi: 10.1002/hep.31290
132. Kang S, Lee AY, Park SY, Liu KH, Im DS. O-1602 Promotes Hepatic Steatosis through GPR55 and PI3 Kinase/Akt/SREBP-1c Signaling in Mice. *Int J Mol Sci.* (2021) 22:3091. doi: 10.3390/ijms22063091
133. Wang Y, Pan W, Wang Y, Yin Y. The GPR55 antagonist CID16020046 protects against ox-LDL-induced inflammation in human aortic endothelial cells (HAECs). *Archives of biochemistry and biophysics.* (2020) 681:108254. doi: 10.1016/j.abb.2020.108254
134. Kurano M, Kobayashi T, Sakai E, Tsukamoto K, Yatomi Y. Lysophosphatidylinositol, especially albumin-bound form, induces inflammatory cytokines in macrophages. *FASEB Journal.* (2021) 35:e21673. doi: 10.1096/fj.202100245R

135. Saliba SW, Jauch H, Gargouri B, Keil A, Hurrle T, Volz N, et al. Anti-neuroinflammatory effects of GPR55 antagonists in LPS-activated primary microglial cells. *J Neuroinflammation.* (2018) 15:322. doi: 10.1186/s12974-018-1362-7
136. Stančić A, Jandl K, Hasenöhrl C, Reichmann F, Marsche G, Schuligoi R, et al. The GPR55 antagonist CID16020046 protects against intestinal inflammation. *Neurogastroenterology Motility.* (2015) 27:1432–45. doi: 10.1111/nmo.12639
137. Kargl J, Brown AJ, Andersen L, Dorn G, Schicho R, Waldhoer M, et al. A selective antagonist reveals a potential role of G protein-coupled receptor 55 in platelet and endothelial cell function. *J Pharmacol Exp Ther.* (2013) 346:54–66. doi: 10.1124/jpet.113.204180
138. Li A, Sun Y, Drummer C. 4th, Lu Y, Yu D, Zhou Y, et al. Increasing upstream chromatin long-range interactions may favor induction of circular RNAs in LysoPC-activated human aortic endothelial cells. *Front physiology.* (2019) 10:433. doi: 10.3389/fphys.2019.00433
139. Johnson C, Drummer C, 4th, Virtue A, Gao T, Wu S, Hernandez M, et al. increased expression of resistin in microrna-155-deficient white adipose tissues may be a possible driver of metabolically healthy obesity transition to classical obesity. *Frontiers in physiology.* (2018) 9:1297. doi: 10.3389/fphys.2018.01297
140. Liu M, Wu N, Xu K, Saaoud F, Vasilopoulos E, Shao Y, et al. Organelle crosstalk regulators are regulated in diseases, tumors, and regulatory t cells: novel classification of organelle crosstalk regulators. *Frontiers in Cardiovascular Medicine.* (2021) 8:713170. doi: 10.3389/fcvm.2021.713170

10

Cardiac Fibroblast-Specific Knockout of PGC-1α Accelerates AngII-Induced Cardiac Remodeling

Hong-jin Chen [1], *Xiao-xi Pan* [1*], *Li-li-qiang Ding* [1], *Cheng-chao Ruan* [2] *and Ping-jin Gao* [1]

[1] *Department of Cardiovascular Medicine, State Key Laboratory of Medical Genomics, Shanghai Key Laboratory of Hypertension, Department of Hypertension, Shanghai Institute of Hypertension, Ruijin Hospital, Shanghai Jiao Tong University School of Medicine, Shanghai, China,* [2] *Shanghai Key Laboratory of Bioactive Small Molecules, Department of Physiology and Pathophysiology, School of Basic Medical Sciences, Fudan University, Shanghai, China*

Correspondence:
Xiao-xi Pan
pxx313@sjtu.edu.cn

Cardiac remodeling consisted of ventricular hypertrophy and interstitial fibrosis is the pathological process of many heart diseases. Fibroblasts as one of the major cells in the myocardium regulate the balance of the generation and degeneration of collagen, and these cells transform toward myofibroblasts in pathological state, contributing to the remodeling of the heart. Peroxisome proliferator-activated receptor-γ (PPAR-γ) coactivator-1α (PGC-1α) is vital to the function of mitochondria, which contributes to the energy production and reactive oxidative species (ROS)-scavenging activity in the heart. In this study, we found that fibroblast-specific PGC-1α KO induced cardiac remodeling especially fibrosis, and Angiotensin II (AngII) aggravated cardiac fibrosis, accompanied with a high level of oxidative stress response and inflammation.

Keywords: cardiac fibroblast, fibrosis, PGC-1α, cardiac remodeling, AngII

INTRODUCTION

Cardiac remodeling is the main pathological mechanism of heart failure which is characterized by left ventricular hypertrophy and interstitial fibrosis (1, 2). Hypertension is the most common cause of cardiac remodeling, in which the renin–angiotensin system (RAS) plays an important role. AngII is a key trigger of heart remodeling, which stimulates the expression of TGF-β through the angiotensin type 1 receptor, contributing to cardiac hypertrophy and fibrosis (3). The myocardium is composed of several cell types and vascular and neuronal networks. The types of cells include cardiomyocytes, cardiac fibroblasts (CFs), and endothelial cells. Also, there is abundant and complex extracellular matrix (ECM) in the interstitium, including several types of collagen proteins. Among these, type I collagen proteins account for more than 70% (4), which is critical to maintaining the structural integrity of the heart and generates a stress-tolerant network. CFs are a key source of ECM and are responsible for the homeostasis of the ECM, contributing to tissue repair and fibrosis (5). Acute stimulation or progressive damage induces necrosis or apoptosis of cardiomyocytes, followed by phagocytosis of neighboring cells. Myofibroblasts surround the injury area and produce interstitial collagen, resulting in cardiac remodeling (6, 7), but extensive ECM accumulation will lead to the dysfunction of the myocardium and finally result in heart failure. In fact, there are no activated myofibroblasts in the healthy myocardium, and CFs transfer to myofibroblasts and migrate to the injured area upon cardiac damage (8). In addition, myofibroblasts are also derived from epithelial and endothelial cells through the process of epithelial–mesenchymal transition (EMT) and endothelial–mesenchymal transition (EndMT), respectively (9, 10). Moreover, myofibroblasts are characterized by the expression of alpha-smooth muscle actin (α-SMA), Cofilin, Palladin 4lg, and other markers (11–13). As mentioned above, in physiological conditions, the synthesis and degeneration of collagen are in dynamic equilibrium. CF has been reported to secrete the collagenase and stromelysin, which have the ability to degrade surrounding interstitial collagens (14). In an injured heart, increased synthesis of collagen that exceeds the rate of degradation can lead to cardiac fibrosis. CFs are crucial in regulating the process of cardiac remodeling, but the exact mechanism remains unclear.

Peroxisome proliferator-activated receptor gamma (PPARγ) coactivator-1 alpha (PGC-1α) is an important coactivator of several nuclear receptors and regulates mitochondrial function in various organs and tissues, including the heart, brain, and liver (15). Initially, PGC-1α was found in the brown adipose tissue and skeletal muscle of the mice exposed to cold conditions, and it plays a key role in thermogenesis (16). As the research of PGC-1α moves along, researchers found that activated PGC-1α stimulates mitochondrial oxidative metabolism. Thus, PGC-1α is highly expressed in the heart, brain, and kidney (17–19). The decreased expression of PGC-1α has been found in many diseases, which is often accompanied by a change of metabolic substrate from fatty acid to glucose (20, 21). Previous study has reported that the reduction of PGC-1α exacerbated non-alcohol fatty liver disease which eventually evolved into liver fibrosis. Moreover, this pathological process was accompanied by increased inflammation and oxidative damage (22). In terms of the heart, PGC-1α knockout mice exhibit lower treadmill running times and cardiac function decline after exercise compared to wild-type (WT) mice (23, 24). The synthesis and degeneration of collagen are energy-consuming and enzyme-dependent processes. The myocardium is mainly composed of cardiomyocytes and CFs, and both of them express PGC-1α. Although whole-body PGC-1α knockout mice have been reported to have heart dysfunction, the role of CF-specific PGC-1α in the heart is still unclear.

In the present study, we investigated the role of PGC-1α in CF. The activated fibroblasts have been considered the primary cause of cardiac fibrosis, and PGC-1α is essential to maintaining the function of CFs. Thus, we suppose that PGC-1α in CFs takes part in regulating the process of heart remodeling. Herein, we utilized the Cre-Loxp system to construct CF-specific PGC-1α knockout mouse and further examined its effects on the heart. In addition, we cultured CFs *in vitro* to study the function of PGC-1α.

MATERIALS AND METHODS

Animal Study

PGC-1α^{flox} (C57BL/6J background), SM22$\alpha^{Cre/ER}$ (C57BL/6J background) mice were obtained from the Jackson Laboratory (Bar Harbor, ME, USA). PGC-1$\alpha^{flox/flox}$ mice were bred with SM22$\alpha^{Cre/ER}$ mice to produce SM22$\alpha^{Cre/ER}$;PGC-1$\alpha^{flox/-}$ heterozygote mice. Then, heterozygote mice were bred with PGC-1$\alpha^{flox/flox}$ mice to produce SM22$\alpha^{Cre/ER}$;PGC-1$\alpha^{flox/flox}$ (SP) homozygote mice. The WT mice and SP mice we used in the study are all 2- to 3-month-old male mice. The animal study was approved in accordance with institutional guidelines established by the Committee of Ethics on Animal Experiments at Shanghai Jiao Tong University School of Medicine.

Identification of Transgenic Mice

SP mice were identified by tail DNA PCR using primers for SM22α and PGC-1α (**Supplementary Table 2**). Mouse tail DNA was extracted by Mouse Tail Genomic DNA Kit (CWBIO). PCR was performed for 34 cycles with each cycle at 95°C for 30 s, 62°C for 30 s, and 72°C for 30 s. Finally, DNA agarose gel electrophoresis was used to identify mouse genotype (**Supplementary Figure 1**).

AngII-Induced Cardiac Remodeling

WT mice and SP mice were assigned to sham group and AngII group, respectively. AngII group mice were implanted subcutaneously with osmotic mini-pumps (Alzet, model: 2004, ALZET® Osmotic Pumps, Cupertino, CA, USA) to deliver AngII (1.44 mg/kg/day) for 28 days. The sham group received the same amount of saline.

Cell Culture

Primary CFs were isolated from 3 to 4-day-old male mice, as described previously (25). Cells were cultured in DMEM with 20% FBS and 1% penicillin and streptomycin. Then, CFs in the AngII group were stimulated by AngII (10^{-7} M) for 12 h.

Recombinant Lentiviruses

Lentiviruses carrying small hairpin RNA (shRNA) were produced and purified by GeneChem. The PGC-1α shRNA sequence was ACTATTGAGCGAACCTTAA, and the no-target control shRNA sequence was TTCTGCGAACGTGTCACGT. The viruses were used to infect CFs for 72 h (MOI = 10).

Histology and Immunostaining

Aortas fixed in formalin and embedded in paraffin were sectioned at 5 μm. Masson or wheat germ agglutinin (WGA) staining was performed using standard procedures. For immunofluorescence staining, the paraffin-embedded and frozen sections of the heart were incubated with primary antibodies for α-SMA (1:100) (19245S, CST, Danvers, MA, USA), Col1a1 (1:100) (GB11022, Servicebio, Wuhan, China), and F4/80 (1:100) (ab6640, Abcam, Cambridge, UK). Antigen retrieval of the paraffin section was obtained by heating the tissue slides in 0.01 M citrate buffer, pH 6.0, at 100°C for 5 min.

Quantitative Real-Time PCR

Total RNA was extracted from tissues and cultured cells using TRIzol (Invitrogen, Carlsbad, CA, USA) followed by chloroform extraction according to the manufacturer's protocol. Total RNA was reverse transcribed into single-stranded cDNA by incubation with reverse transcriptase (EZBioscience, Roseville, MN, USA). Real-time qRT-PCR was performed with SYBR Premix Ex Taq kits with ROX (TaKaRa) according to the manufacturer's instructions. Signals were detected on an ABI PRISM 7900 machine (Applied Biosystems, Foster City, CA, USA). β-Actin was used as a standard reference. Reactions were done at 95°C for 30 s followed by 40 cycles of 95°C for 5 s and 60°C for

30 s. Sequences of primers used in this study are provided in **Supplementary Table 1**.

Western Blotting

Frozen tissues were powdered and then homogenized in ice-cold RIPA buffer (50 mM Tris–HCl (pH 7.4); 10% Nonidet P-40; 0.25% sodium deoxycholate; 150 mM NaCl; 1 mM EDTA; 0.5 M NaF; 10 mM sodium pyrophosphate) supplemented with Protease Inhibitor Cocktail (BioTool Swiss, Kirchberg, Switzerland) and a phosphatase inhibitor (BioTool). Cultured cells were directly lysed in RIPA buffer. Proteins were applied into 10% SDS-PAGE gel and blotted onto a PVDF membrane (Merck Millipore, Burlington, MA, USA). Furthermore, blots were incubated with α-SMA (1:1,000) (19245S, CST), TGF-β (1:1,000) (3711S, CST), Col1a1 (1:1,000) (GB11022, Servicebio), iNOS (1:1,000) (ab178945, Abcam), and GAPDH (1:1,000) (5174S, CST) antibodies overnight at 4°C and then incubated with an HRP-conjugated antibody for 2 h at room temperature. The signal was detected by chemiluminescence.

Statistics

Differences between two independent groups were determined using Student's t-test (two-tailed). To compare more than two groups, one-way analysis of variance (ANOVA) was conducted followed by *post-hoc* Dunnett's testing for multiple-group comparison by GraphPad Prism (GraphPad Software, San Diego, CA, USA). Data represent mean ± SEM. The significant level was set at $p < 0.05$.

RESULTS

CF-Specific PGC-1αKO Aggravates Cardiac Fibrosis

To determine whether the absence of PGC-1α in CFs could impact on heart health, WT and CF-specific PGC-1α KO mice were treated with AngII for 28 days. SM22α$^{Cre/ERT}$;PGC-1α$^{flox/flox}$ (SP) mice were utilized to study the role of CF-specific PGC-1α KO in cardiac remodeling, including interstitial fibrosis and cardiac hypertrophy. Masson's trichrome (Masson) staining was performed to analyze interstitial fibrosis. Histology analysis showed that WT mice developed significant heart fibrosis under administration of AngII for 28 days. More importantly, dramatic cardiac fibrosis was observed in both SP mice with and without the stimulation of AngII, and the SP-AngII group exhibited a higher level of fibrosis. Furthermore, SP mice developed more severe fibrosis than WT mice after AngII infusion (**Figure 1A**). In immunofluorescent staining of Col1a1 and α-SMA, increased expressions of Col1a1 and α-SMA were detected in WT mice after the stimulation of AngII. CF-specific PGC-1α KO induced collagen deposition in the heart, and AngII infusion aggravated it (**Figure 1B**). Then, qPCR was performed to explore the level of gene expression. The mRNA levels of fibrosis markers including collagen type I alpha 1 chain (*Col1a1*), collagen type III alpha 1 chain (*Col3a1*), *TGF-β*, and *α-SMA* were increased in specific PGC-1αKO mice compared to WT mice. Under the stimulation of AngII, the heart of SP-AngII mice presented upregulation of fibrosis-associated genes compared with that of control-AngII mice (**Figure 1C**). PGC-1αKO promoted the expressions of Col1a1, TGF-β, and α-SMA in heart (**Figure 1D**). These results indicated that PGC-1α plays an important role in maintaining the normal function of CFs, which can further influence heart health.

CF-Specific PGC-1αKO Aggravates Cardiac Hypertrophy

To study the possible influence of fibroblast-specific knockout of PGC-1α in cardiac hypertrophy, the following experiments were carried out. Both AngII treatment and CF-PGC1a KO induced the increase in the heart weight to body weight ratio, but there was no significant difference between the SP-sham and SP-AngII groups (**Figure 2A**). Masson and WGA staining results showed that ventricular wall thickness and cardiomyocyte size were increased in both WT mice and SP mice after the stimulation of AngII. Without the infusion of AngII, there were elevated ventricular wall thickness and cardiomyocyte size in SP mice compared with WT mice (**Figure 2B**). Besides, CF-specific PGC-1α KO resulted in elevated mRNA expression of hypertrophic relative factors, including atrial natriuretic peptide (*ANP*), atrial natriuretic peptide (*ANP*), brain natriuretic peptide (*BNP*), *Gata4*, and myosin heavy chain β (β*MHC*) compared with WT mice (**Figure 2C**). These findings suggested that CF-specific PGC-1α KO aggravated cardiac hypertrophy, which was independent of the stimulation of AngII.

CF-Specific PGC-1αKO Activates the Oxidative Stress Response in the Heart

PGC-1α is considered as a suppressor in oxidative stress response (26). To explore whether the knockdown of PGC-1α in CFs could aggravate the oxidative stress in heart, the following experiments were carried out. Dihydroethidium (DHE) staining was utilized to examine the level of ROS. The results showed that the intensity and the proportion of DHE-positive cells were elevated in both WT mice and CF-PGC-1αKO mice after the stimulation of AngII. The heart of SP mice exhibited a higher level of ROS production than that of WT mice in both sham and AngII infusion (**Figures 3A,B**). The protein expression of inducible nitric oxide synthase (iNOS) was increased in both WT mice and SP mice after the stimulation of AngII. Moreover, the content of iNOS was at a higher level in SP mice compared to WT mice without the treatment of AngII (**Figure 3C**). In addition, the mRNA level of iNOS in the heart was measured. The results of analysis were identical to the expression of protein (**Figure 3D**). These data showed that PGC-1α knockdown in CFs aggravated the oxidative stress response in the heart.

CF-Specific PGC-1αKO Aggravates the Inflammatory Response in the Heart

Inflammation is an important process in cardiac remodeling. The accumulation of inflammatory cells in the heart is closely associated with development of cardiac fibrosis. Furthermore, the activation of fibroblasts is responsive for elevated pro-inflammatory cytokines, which promotes the proliferation and migration of myofibroblasts and accelerates the synthesis of

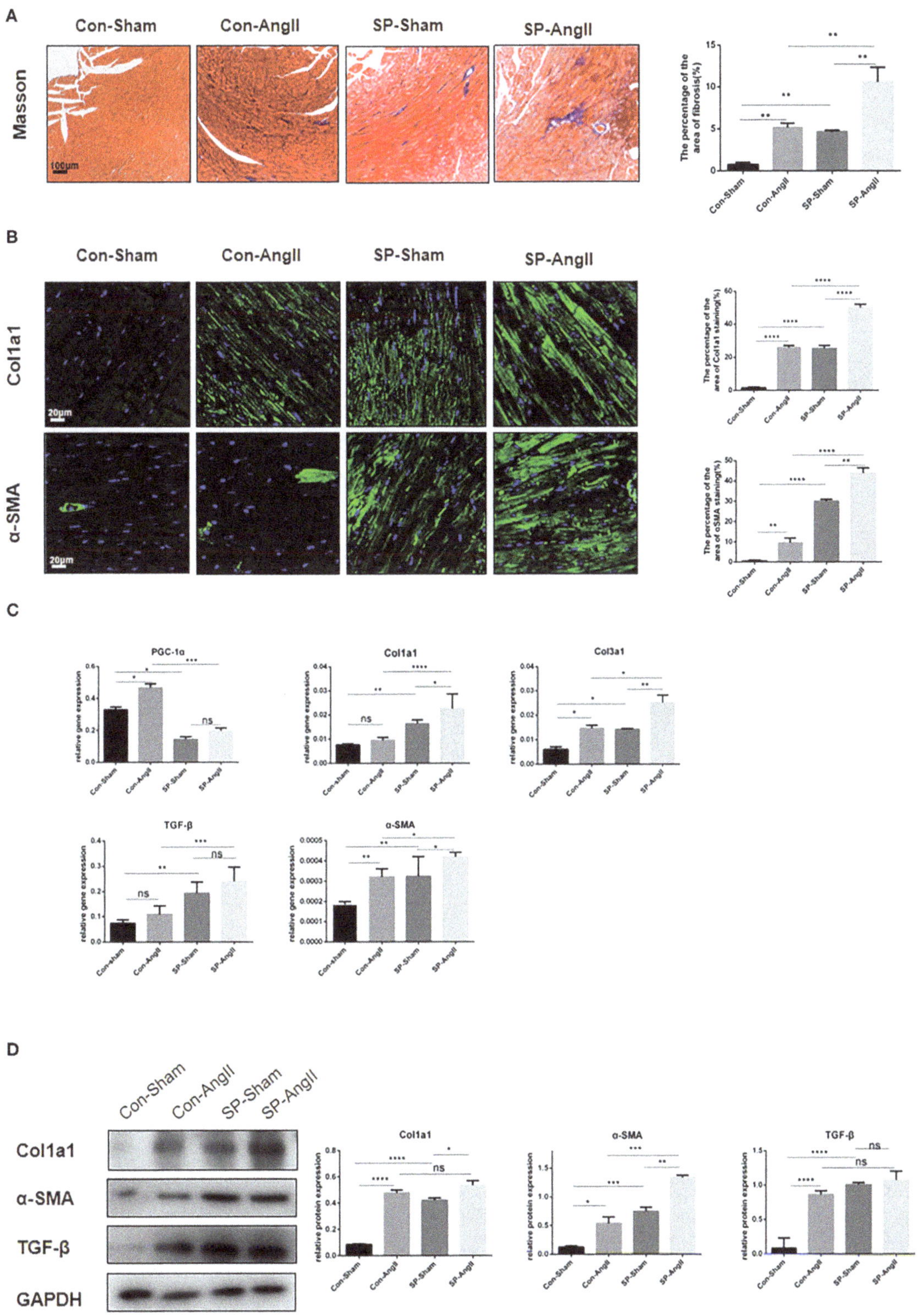

FIGURE 1 | Cardiac fibroblast-specific PGC-1αKO aggravates cardiac remodeling. **(A)** Representative cross sections of the heart stained for Masson and quantitative analysis of the area of fibrosis (Masson staining). **(B)** Representative immunofluorescent staining of Col1a1 and α-SMA and quantitative analysis of immunofluorescent staining of Col1a1 and α-SMA. **(C)** qPCR analysis of mRNA expression levels of *PGC-1α* and fibrotic genes (*Col1a1*, *Col3a1*, *α-SMA*, *TGF-β*). **(D)** Representative Western blot and analysis of the expression of fibrotic proteins (Col1a1, α-SMA, TGF-β). N.S. indicates no significant difference. $^{*}p < 0.05$, $^{**}p < 0.01$, $^{***}p < 0.001$, $^{****}p < 0.0001$. Data represent mean ± SEM ($n = 5$ per group).

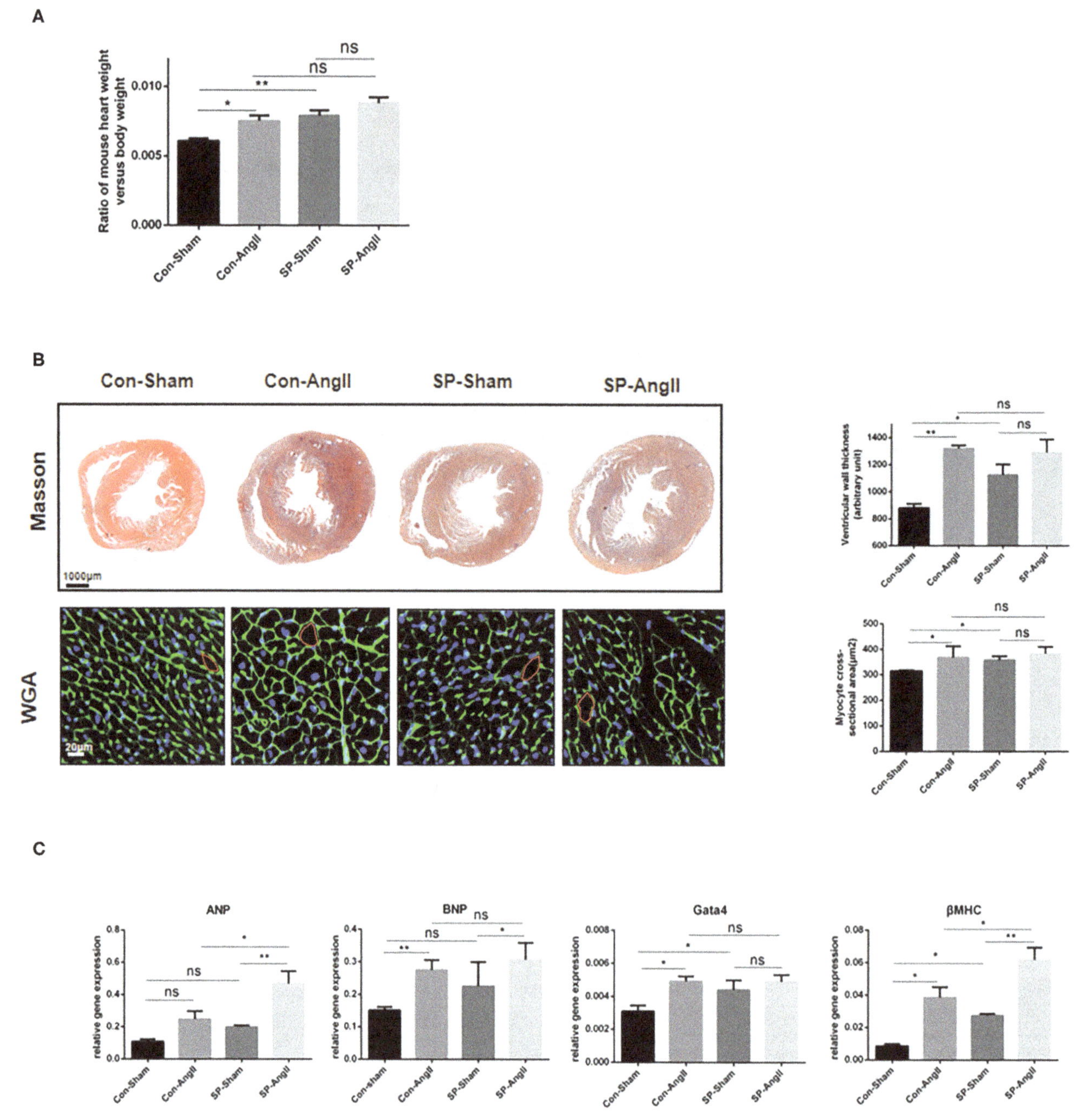

FIGURE 2 | Cardiac fibroblast-specific PGC-1αKO aggravates cardiac hypertrophy. **(A)** Quantitative analysis of the ratio of the weight of mouse heart to body weight. **(B)** Representative cross sections of the heart stained for Masson and WGA. Quantitative analysis of the thickness of ventricular wall (Masson staining) and cardiomyocyte size (WGA staining). **(C)** qPCR analysis of mRNA expression levels of hypertrophic markers (ANP, BNP, Gata4, βMHC). N.S. indicates no significant difference. $^{*}p < 0.05$, $^{**}p < 0.01$. Data represent mean ± SEM ($n = 5$ per group).

collagen (12, 27). To confirm the effect of PGC-1αKO in CFs on inflammation, qPCR was carried out to examine the mRNA levels of genes coding pro-inflammatory cytokines, including tumor necrosis factor-α (*TNF-α*), interleukin 6 (*IL-6*), macrophage inflammatory protein (*MIP-1α*), and monocyte chemotactic protein 1 (*MCP-1*). After the treatment of AngII, the levels of the above genes were elevated dramatically in WT mice. CF-PGC1a KO mice showed upregulation of *TNF-α*, *IL-6*, *MIP-1α*, and *MCP-1* compared to WT mice, and AngII enhanced the MCP-1 expression in SP-AngII mice (**Figure 4A**). Consistent

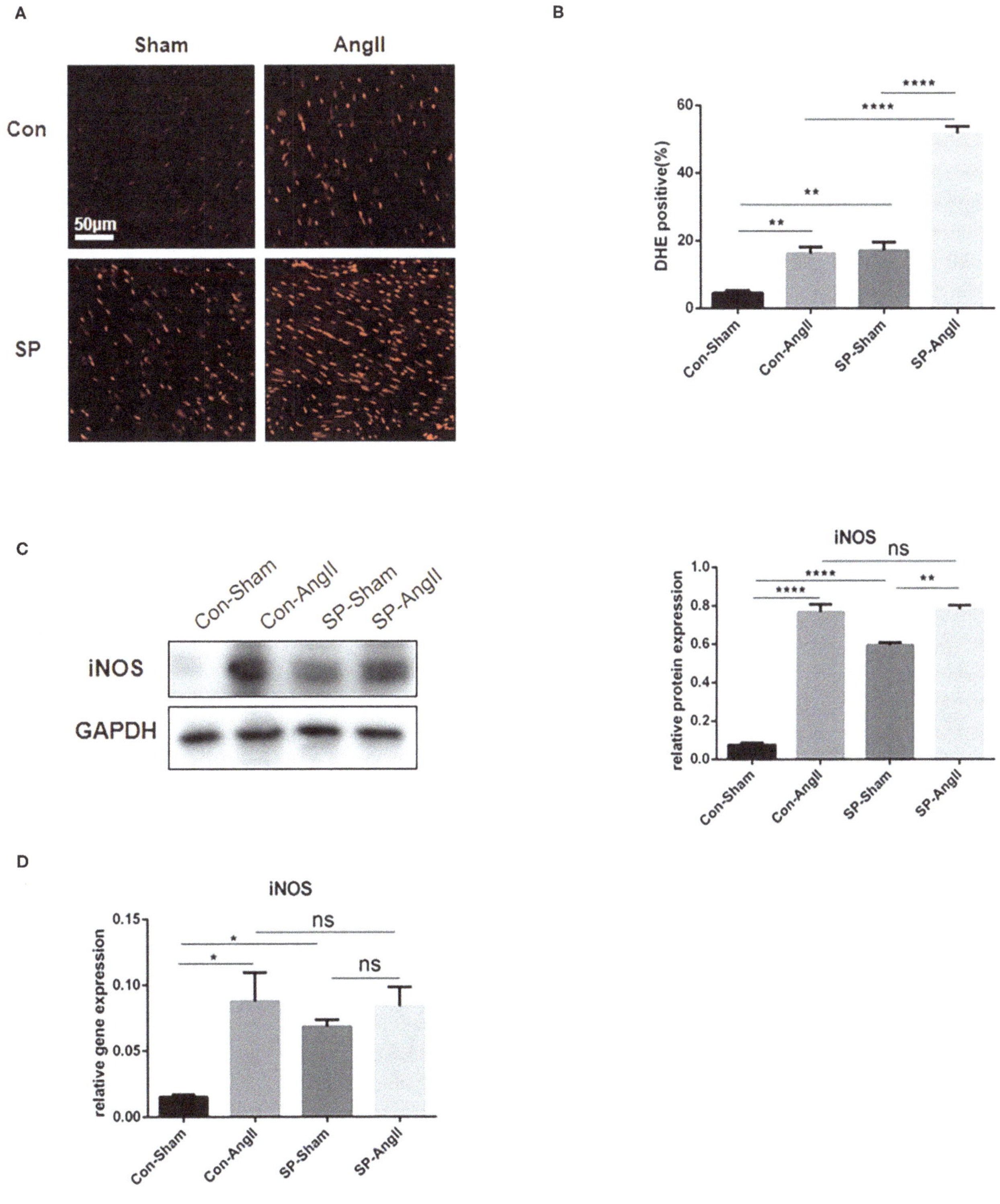

FIGURE 3 | Cardiac fibroblast-specific PGC-1αKO activates the oxidative stress response in the heart. **(A)** Representative cross sections of the heart stained for DHE. **(B)** Quantitative analysis of reactive oxidative stress as assessed by DHE staining. **(C)** Representative Western blot and analysis of the expression of iNOS. **(D)** qPCR analysis of the mRNA expression levels of *iNOS*. N.S. indicates no significant difference. $^{*}p < 0.05$, $^{**}p < 0.01$. Data represent mean ± SEM ($n = 3$–5 per group).

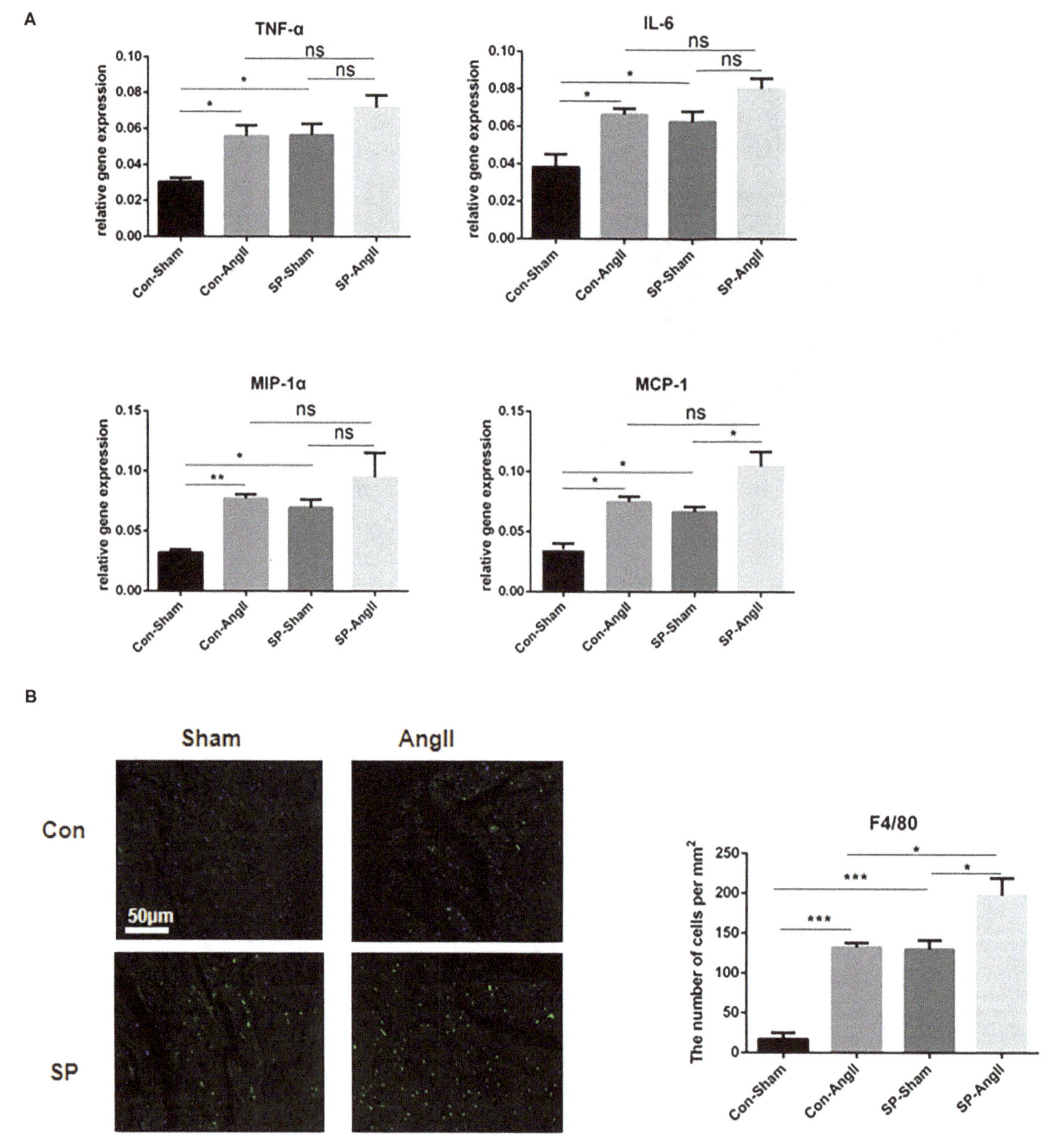

FIGURE 4 | Cardiac fibroblast-specific PGC-1αKO aggravates the inflammatory response in the heart. **(A)** qPCR analysis of the mRNA expression levels of inflammatory genes (*TNF-α*, *IL-6*, *MCP-1*, *MIP-1α*). N.S. indicates no significant difference. **(B)** Representative cross sections of the heart stained for F4/80 and quantitative analysis of the number of positive cells. $^{*}p < 0.05$, $^{**}p < 0.01$, $^{***}p < 0.001$. Data represent mean ± SEM ($n = 5$ per group).

with this, there was more amount of macrophage infiltration in the heart of SP mice than WT mice. Moreover, AngII induced inflammation response (**Figure 4B**). Based on the results, we concluded that PGC-1α in CFs might take part in the regulation of inflammation.

PGC-1α KO in CF Promotes the Expression of Fibrosis-Related Genes

To rule out the effect of cardiomyocytes, CFs were cultured *in vitro* to find direct evidence that PGC-1α plays a vital role in maintaining the function of CFs. Lentivirus PGC-1α RNA

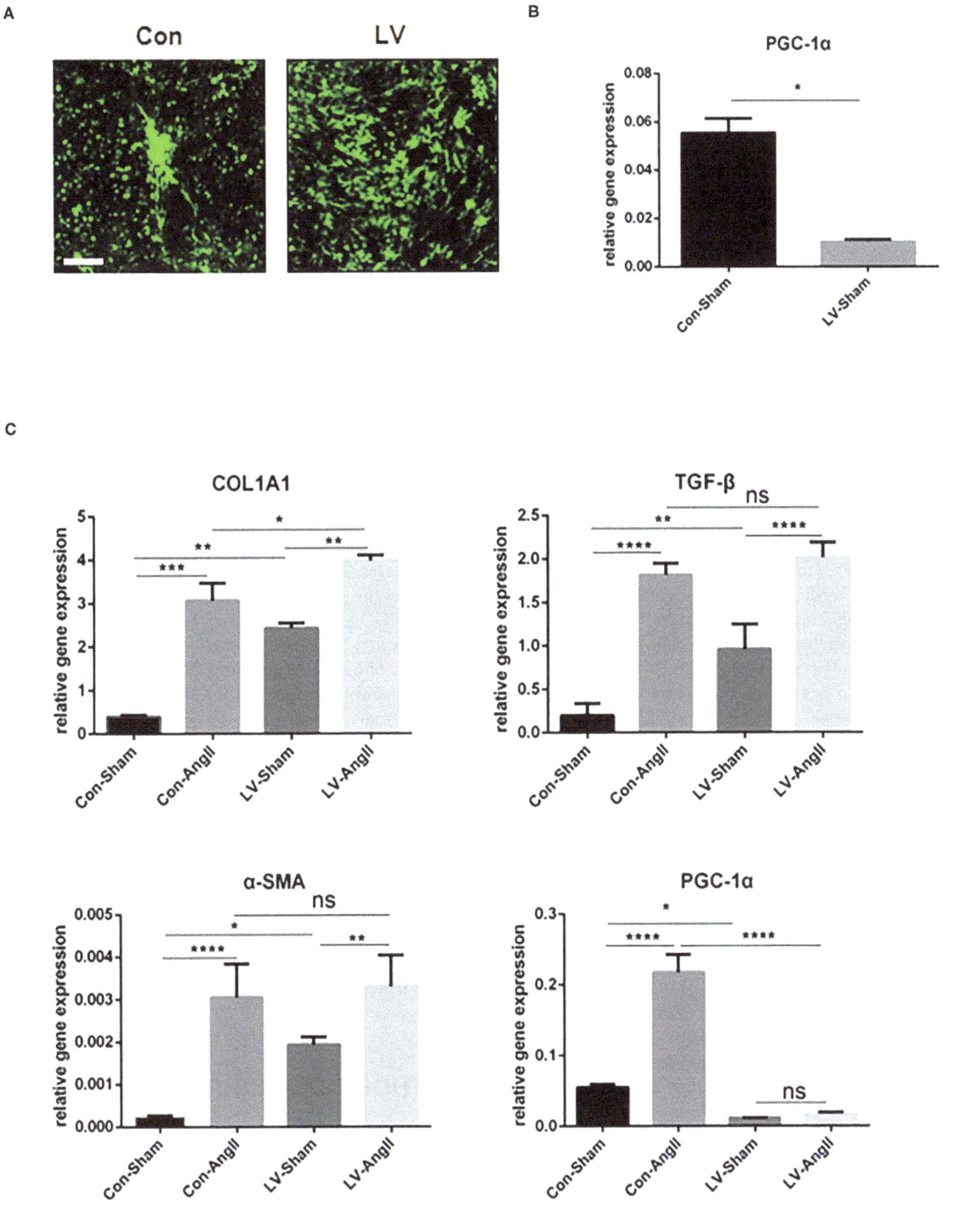

FIGURE 5 | PGC-1α KO in cardiac fibroblast promotes the expression of fibrosis-related genes. **(A)** Representative CF treated with PGC-1α-knockdown lentivirus (LV) and control virus (Con). **(B)** qPCR analysis of the mRNA expression levels of PGC-1α in the LV and Con CF groups. **(C)** qPCR analysis of mRNA expression levels of fibrotic genes (*Col1a1*, *α-SMA*, *TGF-β*). N.S. indicates no significant difference. $^{*}p < 0.05$, $^{**}p < 0.01$, $^{***}p < 0.001$. Data represent mean ± SEM ($n = 3$ independent experiments).

interference (RNAi) was used to knock down PGC-1α expression in CFs (**Figures 5A,B**). Without the stimulation, cells knocked down of PGC-1α were detected to have higher mRNA levels of *Col1a1*, *TGF-β*, and *α-SMA* at baseline. AngII stimulation resulted in an increased expression of fibrosis markers, including *Col1a1*, *TGF-β*, and α-SMA in both experimental group and control group. Also, there is no significant difference in the expression of TGF-β and α-SMA between Con-AngII and LV-AngII cells (**Figure 5C**). These results indicated that PGC-1α may be involved in mediating the activation of CFs.

DISCUSSION

An increasing number of studies have emphasized the relationship between heart remodeling and metabolism. PGC-1α is an important regulator of mitochondrial biology and energy metabolism, and the repression of PGC-1α accelerates cardiac dysfunction and the clinical signs of heart failure (24). Some mechanistic studies have shown that the protective role of PGC-1α in heart requires the activation of Sirtuin 1 (SIRT1), which is a redox-sensitive enzyme. Furthermore, the SIRT1-PGC-1α axis is vital to the performance of cardiac protection through decreasing inflammation, oxidative stress, fibrosis, and so on (28, 29). However, the underlying mechanism of PGC-1α-mediated cardiac remodeling is still unclear. Herein, we unveil the specific role of PGC-1α in regulating the function of CFs, which accelerates cardiac remodeling including cardiac fibrosis and cardiomyocytes hypertrophy.

Reduced PGC-1α is associated with impaired mitochondrial biology in heart diseases and energy expenditure (30). PGC-1α is also considered as a vital regulator of the scavenging of ROS. There is research reporting that ROS accelerates the deposition of collagen through the activation of p53, which results in severe fibrosis (31). In this study, ROS levels were increased in WT mice after AngII infusion, which has been proved to be associated with inhibition of PGC-1α-activated catalase expression (32). Our data showed a slight increase in PGC-1α expression in the heart of WT mice after treatment with AngII. More importantly, AngII failed to enhance PGC-1α expression in the heart of SP mice, which suggested that AngII-induced the PGC-1α upregulation in whole heart tissue which might be attributed to the impact of CF on other cells. Hence, we proposed that the absence of PGC-1α in CFs exerts impact on other cells in the heart, leading to the aggravation of cardiac remodeling. In addition, PGC-1α is an essential component of inflammatory response. Overexpression of PGC-1α inhibits the production of pro-inflammatory cytokines and promotes the secretion of anti-inflammatory cytokines in the heart, preventing the heart from getting damaged (33–35). In our study, CF-specific PGC-1α knockdown promoted the expression of pro-inflammatory cytokines in the heart, which indicated that PGC-1α in CFs took part in the inflammatory response. Previous report has demonstrated that pro-inflammatory cytokines facilitated the transition of CFs to myofibroblasts (8). According to the research, there are only ~2% activated CFs in the adult heart (36). Our data shows that in CF-specific PGC-1α KO mice, plenty of activated CFs convert into myofibroblasts even without the stimulation of AngII by detecting the high expression of fibrosis markers and cardiac hypertrophy markers. All these data show that PGC-1α in CFs, as a versatile factor, plays a vital role in regulating cardiac remodeling. On the contrary, several researches demonstrate that overexpression of PGC-1α beyond physiological content leads to mitochondrial proliferation and myofibrillar displacement, which finally contributes to cardiac failure (30, 37). Thus, maintaining PGC-1α in a physiological stage is crucial for cardiovascular health. Our results exhibited that both AngII and PGC-1α KO have an influence on cardiac remodeling, which may indicate that PGC-1α and AngII perform through an overlapping pathway. The aforesaid SIRT1 is an essential protein in regulating the fibrosis-related pathway in many organs through regulating gene transcription (38, 39). AngII-induced cardiovascular remodeling is reported to be closely related to the reduction of SIRT1. On the other hand, overexpression of SIRT1 suppresses the ROS-induced p38/mitogen-activated protein kinase (MAPK) pathway, which promotes the activation of CFs (40, 41). Moreover, as mentioned before, PGC-1α plays a protective role through cooperating with the activated SIRT1 (29). AngII and PGC-1α might affect the function of SIRT1, leading to the activation of the p38/MAPK pathway and the transition of CFs. There are some limitations in our study. It remains uncertain whether overexpression of PGC-1α could improve cardiac remodeling. Furthermore, the underlying mechanism that CF-specific knockout of PGC-1α participates in cardiac remodeling remains unclear, which still needs further study.

In conclusion, we have discovered the PGC-1α-mediated pathology of cardiac remodeling, especially cardiac fibrosis. We propose that the absence of PGC-1α in CFs impairs the balance of the synthesis and degeneration of collagen through regulating ROS production and inflammation, leading to deposition of collagens and cardiac remodeling. Our findings reveal that PGC-1α is critical for the cardiac fibrosis by multiple fibrogenic pathways.

AUTHOR CONTRIBUTIONS

X-xP and C-cR designed the study. H-jC performed the experiments, analyzed the data, and wrote the manuscript. L-l-qD conducted the *in vitro* experiments. All authors contributed to the article and approved the submitted version.

REFERENCES

1. Berk BC, Fujiwara K, Lehoux S. ECM remodeling in hypertensive heart disease. *J Clin Invest.* (2007) 117:568–75. doi: 10.1172/JCI31044
2. Drazner MH. The progression of hypertensive heart disease. *Circulation.* (2011) 123:327–34. doi: 10.1161/CIRCULATIONAHA.108.845792
3. Campbell SE, Katwa LC. Angiotensin II stimulated expression of transforming growth factor-beta1 in cardiac fibroblasts and myofibroblasts. *J Mol Cell*

Cardiol. (1997) 29:1947–58. doi: 10.1006/jmcc.1997.0435

4. Medugorac I. Characterization of intramuscular collagen in mammalian left ventricle. *Basic Res Cardiol.* (1982) 77:589–98. doi: 10.1007/BF01908312
5. Brown RD, Ambler SK, Mitchell MD, Long CS. The cardiac fibroblast: therapeutic target in myocardial remodeling and failure. *Annu Rev Pharmacol Toxicol.* (2005) 45:657–87. doi: 10.1146/annurev.pharmtox.45.120403.095802
6. Cleutjens JP, Blankesteijn WM, Daemen MJ, Smits JF. The infarcted myocardium: simply dead tissue, or a lively target for therapeutic interventions. *Cardiovasc Res.* (1999) 44:232–41. doi: 10.1016/S0008-6363(99)00212-6
7. van den Borne SW, Diez J, Blankesteijn WM, Verjans J, Hofstra L, Narula J. Myocardial remodeling after infarction: the role of myofibroblasts. *Nat Rev Cardiol.* (2010) 7:30–7. doi: 10.1038/nrcardio.2009.199
8. Porter KE, Turner NA. Cardiac fibroblasts: at the heart of myocardial remodeling. *Pharmacol Ther.* (2009) 123:255–78. doi: 10.1016/j.pharmthera.2009.05.002
9. Kalluri R, Neilson EG. Epithelial-mesenchymal transition and its implications for fibrosis. *J Clin Invest.* (2003) 112:1776–84. doi: 10.1172/JCI200320530
10. Zeisberg EM, Tarnavski O, Zeisberg M, Dorfman AL, McMullen JR, et al. Endothelial-to-mesenchymal transition contributes to cardiac fibrosis. *Nat Med.* (2007) 13:952–61. doi: 10.1038/nm1613
11. Foo IT, Naylor IL, Timmons MJ, Trejdosiewicz LK. Intracellular actin as a marker for myofibroblasts in vitro. *Lab Invest.* (1992) 67:727–33.
12. Rönty MJ, Leivonen SK, Hinz B, Rachlin A, Otey CA, Kähäri VM, et al. Isoform-specific regulation of the actin-organizing protein palladin during TGF-beta1-induced myofibroblast differentiation. *J Invest Dermatol.* (2006) 126:2387–96. doi: 10.1038/sj.jid.5700427
13. Pho M, Lee W, Watt DR, Laschinger C, Simmons CA, McCulloch CA. Cofilin is a marker of myofibroblast differentiation in cells from porcine aortic cardiac valves. *Am J Physiol Heart Circ Physiol.* (2008) 294:H1767–78. doi: 10.1152/ajpheart.01305.2007
14. Kuncio GS, Neilson EG, Haverty T. Mechanisms of tubulointerstitial fibrosis. *Kidney Int.* (1991) 39:550–6. doi: 10.1038/ki.1991.63
15. Handschin C, Spiegelman BM. Peroxisome proliferator-activated receptor gamma coactivator 1 coactivators, energy homeostasis, and metabolism. *Endocr Rev.* (2006) 27:728–35. doi: 10.1210/er.2006-0037
16. Puigserver P, Wu Z, Park CW, Graves R, Wright M, Spiegelman BM. A cold-inducible coactivator of nuclear receptors linked to adaptive thermogenesis. *Cell.* (1998) 92:829–39. doi: 10.1016/S0092-8674(00)81410-5
17. Wu Z, Puigserver P, Andersson U, Zhang C, Adelmant G, Mootha V, et al. Mechanisms controlling mitochondrial biogenesis and respiration through the thermogenic coactivator PGC-1. *Cell.* (1999) 98:115–24. doi: 10.1016/S0092-8674(00)80611-X
18. Sterbauer H, Oberkofler H, Krempler F, Patsch W. Human peroxisome proliferator activated receptor gamma coactivator 1 (PPARGC1) gene: cDNA sequence, genomic organization, chromosomal localization, and tissue expression. *Genomics.* (1999) 62:98–102. doi: 10.1006/geno.1999.5977
19. Knutti D, Kaul A, Kralli A. A tissue-specific coactivator of steroid receptors, identified in a functional genetic screen. *Mol Cell Biol.* (2000) 20:2411–22. doi: 10.1128/MCB.20.7.2411-2422.2000
20. Huss JM, Kelly DP. Nuclear receptor signaling and cardiac energetics. *Circ Res.* (2004) 95:568–78. doi: 10.1161/01.RES.0000141774.29937.e3
21. Huss JM, Kelly DP. Mitochondrial energy metabolism in heart failure: a question of balance. *J Clin Invest.* (2005) 115:547–55. doi: 10.1172/JCI24405
22. Besse-Patin A, Léveillé M, Oropeza D, Nguyen BN, Prat A, Estall JL. Estrogen signals through peroxisome proliferator-activated receptor-γ coactivator 1α to reduce oxidative damage associated with diet-induced fatty liver disease. *Gastroenterology.* (2017) 152:243–56. doi: 10.1053/j.gastro.2016.09.017
23. Leone TC, Lehman JJ, Finck BN, Schaeffer PJ, Wende AR, Boudina S, et al. PGC-1alpha deficiency causes multi-system energy metabolic derangements: muscle dysfunction, abnormal weight control and hepatic steatosis. *PLoS Biol.* (2005) 3:e101. doi: 10.1371/journal.pbio.0030101
24. Arany Z, Novikov M, Chin S, Ma Y, Rosenzweig A, Spiegelman BM. Transverse aortic constriction leads to accelerated heart failure in mice lacking PPAR-gamma coactivator 1alpha. *Proc Natl Acad Sci USA.* (2006) 103:10086–91. doi: 10.1073/pnas.0603615103
25. Dubey RK, Gillespie DG, Jackson EK. Adenosine inhibits collagen and protein synthesis in cardiac fibroblasts: role of A2B receptors. *Hypertension.* (1998) 31:943–8. doi: 10.1161/01.HYP.31.4.943
26. Marmolino D, Manto M, Acquaviva F, Vergara P, Ravella A, Monticelli A, et al. PGC-1alpha down-regulation affects the antioxidant response in Friedreich's ataxia. *PLoS ONE.* (2010) 5:e10025. doi: 10.1371/journal.pone.0010025
27. Leask A, Abraham DJ. TGF-beta signaling and the fibrotic response. *FASEB J.* (2004) 18:816–27. doi: 10.1096/fj.03-1273rev
28. Lagouge M, Argmann C, Gerhart-Hines Z, Meziane H, Lerin C, Daussin F, et al. Resveratrol improves mitochondrial function and protects against metabolic disease by activating SIRT1 and PGC-1alpha. *Cell.* (2006) 127:1109–22. doi: 10.1016/j.cell.2006.11.013
29. Waldman M, Cohen K, Yadin D, Nudelman V, Gorfil D, Laniado-Schwartzman M, et al. Regulation of diabetic cardiomyopathy by caloric restriction is mediated by intracellular signaling pathways involving 'SIRT1 and PGC-1α'. *Cardiovasc Diabetol.* (2018) 17:111. doi: 10.1186/s12933-018-0757-1
30. Lehman JJ, Barger PM, Kovacs A, Saffitz JE, Medeiros DM, Kelly DP. Peroxisome proliferator-activated receptor gamma coactivator-1 promotes cardiac mitochondrial biogenesis. *J Clin Invest.* (2000) 106:847–56. doi: 10.1172/JCI10268
31. Al-Ani B, Alzamil NM, Hewett PW, Al-Hashem F, Bin-Jaliah I, Shatoor AS, et al. Metformin ameliorates ROS-p53-collagen axis of fibrosis and dyslipidemia in type 2 diabetes mellitus-induced left ventricular injury. *Arch Physiol Biochem.* (2021) 13:1–7. doi: 10.1080/13813455.2020.1869265
32. Xiong S, Salazar G, San Martin A, Ahmad M, Patrushev N, Hilenski L, et al. PGC-1 alpha serine 570 phosphorylation and GCN5-mediated acetylation by angiotensin II drive catalase down-regulation and vascular hypertrophy. *J Biol Chem.* (2010) 285:2474–87. doi: 10.1074/jbc.M109.065235
33. Sczelecki S, Besse-Patin A, Abboud A, Kleiner S, Laznik-Bogoslavski D, Wrann CD, et al. Loss of Pgc-1α expression in aging mouse muscle potentiates glucose intolerance and systemic inflammation. *Am J Physiol Endocrinol Metab.* (2014) 306:E157–67. doi: 10.1152/ajpendo.00578.2013
34. Eisele PS, Furrer R, Beer M, Handschin C. The PGC-1 coactivators promote an anti-inflammatory environment in skeletal muscle *in vivo*. *Biochem Biophys Res Commun.* (2015) 464:692–7. doi: 10.1016/j.bbrc.2015.06.166
35. Buler M, Aatsinki SM, Skoumal R, Komka Z, Tóth M, Kerkelä R, et al. Energy-sensing factors coactivator peroxisome proliferator-activated receptor γ coactivator 1-α (PGC-1α) and AMP-activated protein kinase control expression of inflammatory mediators in liver: induction of interleukin 1 receptor antagonist. *J Biol Chem.* (2012) 287:1847–60. doi: 10.1074/jbc.M111.302356
36. Wu R, Ma F, Tosevska A, Farrell C, Pellegrini M, Deb A. Cardiac fibroblast proliferation rates and collagen expression mature early and are unaltered with advancing age. *JCI Insight.* (2020) 5:140628. doi: 10.1172/jci.insight.140628
37. Russell LK, Mansfield CM, Lehman JJ, Kovacs A, Courtois M, Saffitz JE, et al. Cardiac-specific induction of the transcriptional coactivator peroxisome proliferator-activated receptor gamma coactivator-1alpha promotes mitochondrial biogenesis and reversible cardiomyopathy in a developmental stage-dependent manner. *Circ Res.* (2004) 94:525–33. doi: 10.1161/01.RES.0000117088.36577.EB
38. Li XZ, Cheng LZ, Yan YM, Liu BH, Cheng YX. SIRT1 inhibitory compounds from the roots of Codonopsis pilosula. *J Asian Nat Prod Res.* (2019) 21:25–32. doi: 10.1080/10286020.2017.1422491
39. Hwang JS, Kang ES, Han SG, Lim DS, Paek KS, Lee CH, et al. Formononetin inhibits lipopolysaccharide-induced release of high mobility group box 1 by upregulating SIRT1 in a PPARδ-dependent manner. *PeerJ.* (2018) 6:e4208. doi: 10.7717/peerj.4208
40. Burke RM, Dirkx RA Jr, Quijada P, Lighthouse JK, Mohan A, O'Brien M, et al. Prevention of fibrosis and pathological cardiac remodeling by salinomycin. *Circ Res.* (2021) 128:1663–78. doi: 10.1161/CIRCRESAHA.120.317791
41. Zhou L, Zhang S, Bolor-Erdene E, Wang L, Tian D, Mei Y. NAMPT/SIRT1 attenuate Ang II-induced vascular remodeling and vulnerability to hypertension by inhibiting the ROS/MAPK pathway. *Oxid Med Cell Longev.* (2020) 2020:1974265. doi: 10.1155/2020/1974265

11

Inhibition of Peptidyl Arginine Deiminase 4-Dependent Neutrophil Extracellular Trap Formation Reduces Angiotensin II-Induced Abdominal Aortic Aneurysm Rupture in Mice

Ming Wei[1,2], *Xia Wang*[1,2], *Yanting Song*[1,2], *Di Zhu*[3], *Dan Qi*[1,2], *Shiyu Jiao*[1,2], *Guomin Xie*[1,2], *Ye Liu*[1,2], *Baoqi Yu*[1,2], *Jie Du*[1,4,5], *Yuji Wang*[3]* and *Aijuan Qu*[1,2]*

[1] Department of Physiology and Pathophysiology, School of Basic Medical Sciences, Capital Medical University, Beijing, China, [2] Key Laboratory of Remodeling-Related Cardiovascular Diseases, Ministry of Education, Beijing, China, [3] School of Pharmaceutical Sciences, Capital Medical University, Beijing, China, [4] Beijing Institute of Heart, Lung and Blood Vessel Diseases, Beijing, China, [5] Beijing Anzhen Hospital, Capital Medical University, Beijing, China

***Correspondence:**
Yuji Wang
wangyuji@ccmu.edu.cn
Aijuan Qu
aijuanqu@ccmu.edu.cn

Objective: Neutrophil infiltration plays an important role in the initiation and development of abdominal aortic aneurysm (AAA). Recent studies suggested that neutrophils could release neutrophil extracellular traps (NETs), leading to tissue injury in cardiovascular diseases. However, the role of NETs in AAA is elusive. This study aimed to investigate the role and underlying mechanism of NETs in AAA development.

Methods and Results: An angiotensin II (Ang II) infusion-induced AAA model was established to investigate the role of NETs during AAA development. Immunofluorescence staining showed that citrullinated histone 3 (citH3), myeloperoxidase (MPO), and neutrophil elastase (NE) (NET marker) expressions were significantly increased in Ang II-infused $ApoE^{-/-}$ mice. The circulating double-stranded DNA (dsDNA) level was also elevated, indicating the increased NET formation during AAA. PAD4 inhibitor YW3-56 inhibited Ang II-induced NET formation. Disruption of NET formation by YW3-56 markedly reduced Ang II-induced AAA rupture, as revealed by decreased aortic diameter, vascular smooth muscle cell (VSMC) apoptosis, and elastin degradation. Apoptosis of VSMC was evaluated by TUNEL staining and Annexin V-FITC/PI staining through flow cytometry. Western blot and inhibition experiments revealed that NETs induced VSMC apoptosis *via* p38/JNK pathway, indicating that PAD4-dependent NET formation played an important role in AAA.

Conclusions: This study suggests that PAD4-dependent NET formation is critical for AAA rupture, which provides a novel potential therapeutic strategy for AAA disease.

Keywords: abdominal aortic aneurysm, neutrophil extracellular traps, vascular smooth muscle cells, apoptosis, peptidyl arginine deiminase 4

INTRODUCTION

Abdominal aortic aneurysm (AAA) is clinically defined as the increase of aortic diameter by at least 50% compared with the regular diameter. AAA is common in men aged over 65 years (1). In general, aneurysms remain asymptomatic until rupture. AAA rupture leads to a 30-day mortality rate up to 70% (2). Nowadays, surgical treatment is the most important strategy for treating AAA (3). However, the risk of surgery is high and long-term survival is still dissatisfactory (4, 5). Looking for more effective treatments for AAA requires a better understanding of its pathological process.

During AAA formation, major pathological changes include vascular smooth muscle cell (VSMC) apoptosis, extracellular matrix degradation, and inflammatory cell infiltration in aortic media and adventitia (6, 7). As the first line of innate immunity, neutrophils are quickly recruited to the location of inflammation (8). Neutrophils were associated with oxidative stress in mice and humans (9, 10). Neutrophil deficiency alleviated AAA (11). Therefore, neutrophils play an important role in AAA development.

In addition to phagocytosis and degranulation, neutrophils have also been found to form NETs in response to inflammatory stimuli. The extracellular structures of NETs are formed by DNA, decondensed chromatin, nuclear proteins, and cytoplasmic proteins (12, 13). NETosis is a program for the formation of NETs since it was initially shown that NET formation was accompanied by cell death (14). It is characterized by the release of decondensed chromatin associated with modification histone and granule components into the cytosol. Currently, different forms of NETosis have been described. Classical or suicidal NETosis leads to cell death. Vital NETosis releases NETs in the form of vesicles (15). In the formation of NETs, peptidyl arginine deiminase 4 (PAD4) mediates chromatin decondensation by citrullinating histones. Histone mixed with granule proteins is released from the neutrophil (16). As cytoplasmic proteins, NE and MPO can be transported into the nucleus to degrade linker histones, accelerating the process of chromatin decondensation (13, 17). Intensive investigations on NETs over the last years revealed a potential involvement of the NETs in immune diseases. NETs accelerated local pathological inflammatory response by increasing the infiltration of inflammatory factors and inducing the lytic cell death of VSMCs (18–20). The role of NETs in vascular diseases like thrombosis and atherosclerosis has been found. However, its role in AAA has been scarcely analyzed. It is important to clarify the underlying mechanism of NETs and find a more effective drug therapy to slow down the rupture process in AAA. Therefore, this study aims to investigate (1) the main mechanism of NETs in regulating the pathological process of AAA and (2) whether the AAA process can be inhibited by the administration of PAD4 inhibitor YW3-56.

In the current study, NET formation can be induced by Ang II. NETs induced the apoptosis of VSMCs *via* p38/JNK pathway. Furthermore, PAD4 inhibitor YW3-56 ameliorated AAA rupture by inhibiting NET formation. These results suggest that inhibition of the NET formation may provide a potential treatment method for AAA.

Abbreviations: AAA, Abdominal aortic aneurysm; Ang II, Angiotensin II; *ApoE*, Apolipoprotein E; citH3, Citrullinated histones3; MPO, Myeloperoxidase; NETs, Neutrophil extracellular traps; NE, Neutrophil elastase; PAD4, Peptidyl arginine deiminase 4; PBS, Phosphate-buffered saline; VSMCs, Vascular smooth muscle cells; IL Interleukin; TF, Tissue factor; MMP, Matrix metalloproteinases; TUNEL, TdT-mediated dUTP nick end labeling; qPCR, Quantitative-polymerase chain reaction; PBS, Phosphate-buffered saline; H&E, Hematoxylin and eosin staining; FBS, Fetal bovine serum; DAPI, 4′,6-diamidino-2-phenylindole; SM22α Smooth Muscle 22 alpha; GAPDH, Glyceraldehyde-3phosphate dehydrogenase; JNK, Jun N-terminal kinase.

METHODS AND MATERIALS

Mouse Model of Ang II-Induced AAA

ApoE$^{-/-}$ mice on C57BL/6J background were purchased from the Jackson Laboratory (Bar Harbor, ME, USA). Mice were housed in temperature-controlled (20–22°C) and light-controlled (12-h light/dark cycle) rooms with free access to water and food. To establish the Ang II-induced AAA model, 10–12-week-old male mice were used for experiments. All mouse genotypes were identified by tail clip samples on PCR. Primers are listed in **Supplementary Table 1**. All animal studies were carried out in accordance with guidelines and approved by the Capital Medical University Animal Care and Use Committee. Experiments were performed under a project license (AEEI-2018-127) granted by the ethics board of Capital Medical University.

The Ang II-induced AAA model was generated as follows. Micro-osmotic pumps (ALZET DURECT 1004, Durect Corp, Cupertino, CA, USA) loaded with saline or angiotensin II (A9525, Sigma-Aldrich, St. Louis, MO, USA) were subcutaneously implanted in 10–12-week-old male *ApoE*$^{-/-}$ mice at a delivery rate of 1,000 ng/kg/min for 28 days (21).

For NET inhibition *in vivo*, PAD4 inhibitor YW3-56 was synthesized as previously described (22). YW3-56 (10 mL/kg) or vehicle was administered intravenously every other day from 1 day before Ang II infusion. An equal amount of DMSO was used as the control group.

Blood Pressure Measurements

Blood pressure was monitored every other day after Ang II infusion by the tail-cuff method (BP2000, Visitech Systems, Apex, NC, USA) to confirm the efficiency of Ang II as described previously (23).

Vascular Ultrasonic Studies

Echocardiography assessment was performed to analyze the diameter of vessels in mice infused with Ang II after 28 days using a Vevo 2100 console (Visual Sonics Vevo 2100, FUJIFILM, Bothell, WA, USA). B-mode ultrasound data were acquired for the aorta in the diastole cardiac cycle. The transducer with a central frequency of 40 MHz and a focal length of 7 mm (MS 550D) was used. Images of the abdominal aorta of the mouse were acquired. The maximal dilated portion of the suprarenal aorta diameters was measured in internal diameter by ultrasonic statistical software analysis. The increase in the outer

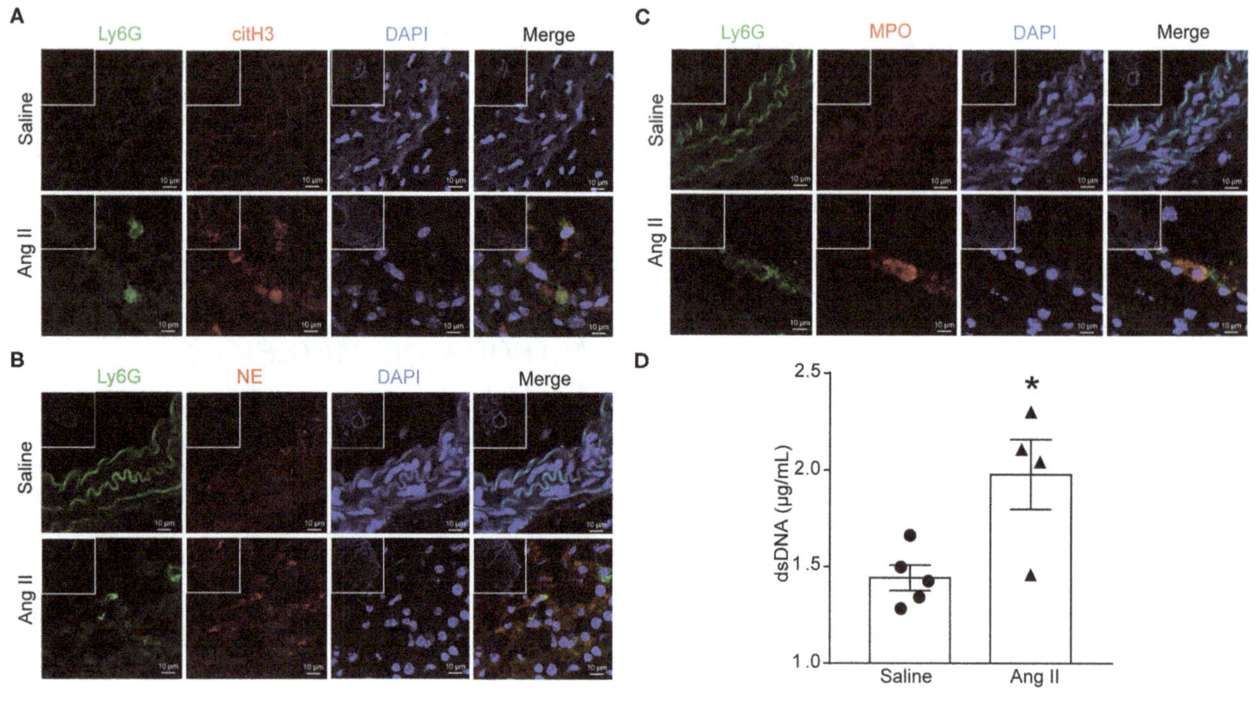

FIGURE 1 | Ang II induced NET formation *in vivo*. *ApoE*$^{-/-}$ mice were infused with saline or 1,000 ng/kg/min Ang II for 28 days. **(A–C)** Immunofluorescence analysis of mouse abdominal aortas for NET markers citH3 (red), NE (red), and MPO (red) with neutrophil marker Ly6G (green). Nuclei were stained with DAPI. **(D)** Measurement of dsDNA in the serum from saline or Ang II (1,000 ng/kg/min) infused *ApoE*$^{-/-}$ mice. $n = 5$/saline group, $n = 4$/Ang II group, $^*p < 0.05$. Statistical significance was analyzed by the unpaired *t*-test.

width of the suprarenal aorta by at least 50% was identified as aneurysm formation.

Histological Analysis

All mice were sacrificed with inhaled isoflurane (1% in O_2) at the end of the experiment, and the blood was collected before the mice were flushed with 20 mL saline-EDTA. Aortas were exposed under a dissecting microscope and photographed after the peri-adventitial tissue was removed. Subsequently, the abdominal aortas were obtained, fixed with 4% paraformaldehyde (PFA), and embedded in OCT. Aortas were sectioned into 7 μm for further analysis. Frozen aortic sections of *ApoE*$^{-/-}$ mice were stained with hematoxylin (RY-ICH001a, Roby, Beijing, China) and eosin (RY-ICH002a, Roby, Beijing, China) (H&E) as described previously (23). Aortic sections were stained using the Gomori Aldehyde-Fuchsin Kit (MST-8047, Maixin Bio, Fuzhou, China) for elastin assessment as described previously. Elastin degradation was graded as (1) no degradation with a well-organized elastic layer; (2) mild degradation with some interruptions and fractures; (3) severe degradation with fragmentation and loss; and (4) rupture (24). At least five fields for each section were captured for elastic fiber content.

Immunohistochemical Staining

After being washed by PBS three times, the frozen aortic sections were fixed with 4% PFA for 15 min and permeabilized with 0.1% Triton X-100 (T9284, Sigma, St.Louis, MO, USA) for 10 min. Samples were incubated with 3% hydrogen peroxide for 10 min followed by goat serum blocking (ZLI-9056, ZsBio, Beijing, China). The sections were incubated with the specific antibody for MPO (1:200, ab65871, Abcam, Cambridge, MA, USA) overnight at 4°C. After being washed with PBS three times the next day, the sections were incubated with goat anti-rabbit IgG secondary antibody (ZF-0136, ZsBio, Beijing, China) at room temperature for 30 min. The positive-stained cells were detected with diaminobenzidine (DAB) (GK600505, GeneTech, Shanghai, China).

Immunofluorescence Staining

For immunofluorescence analysis, cells grown on fibronectin-coated glass coverslips or frozen aortic sections were fixed with 4% PFA for 15 min, permeabilized with 0.1% Triton X-100, and blocked with 10% goat serum at room temperature for 1 h. Samples were incubated with anti-rabbit citH3 antibody (for citrulline R2, R8, and R17; 1:200, ab5103, Abcam, USA), anti-rat Ly6G (1:200, ab25377, Abcam, USA), anti-rabbit-NE antibody (1:200, ab21595, Abcam, USA), and anti-rabbit-MPO antibody (1:200, ab65871, Abcam, USA) at 4°C overnight. On the 2nd day, slides were incubated with goat anti-rabbit/rat TRITC/FITC secondary antibody for 1 h at room temperature and mounted with DAPI (4′,6-diamidino-2-phenylindole, Vector, ZsBio, Beijing, China). Images were obtained using a confocal microscope. At least five fields for each

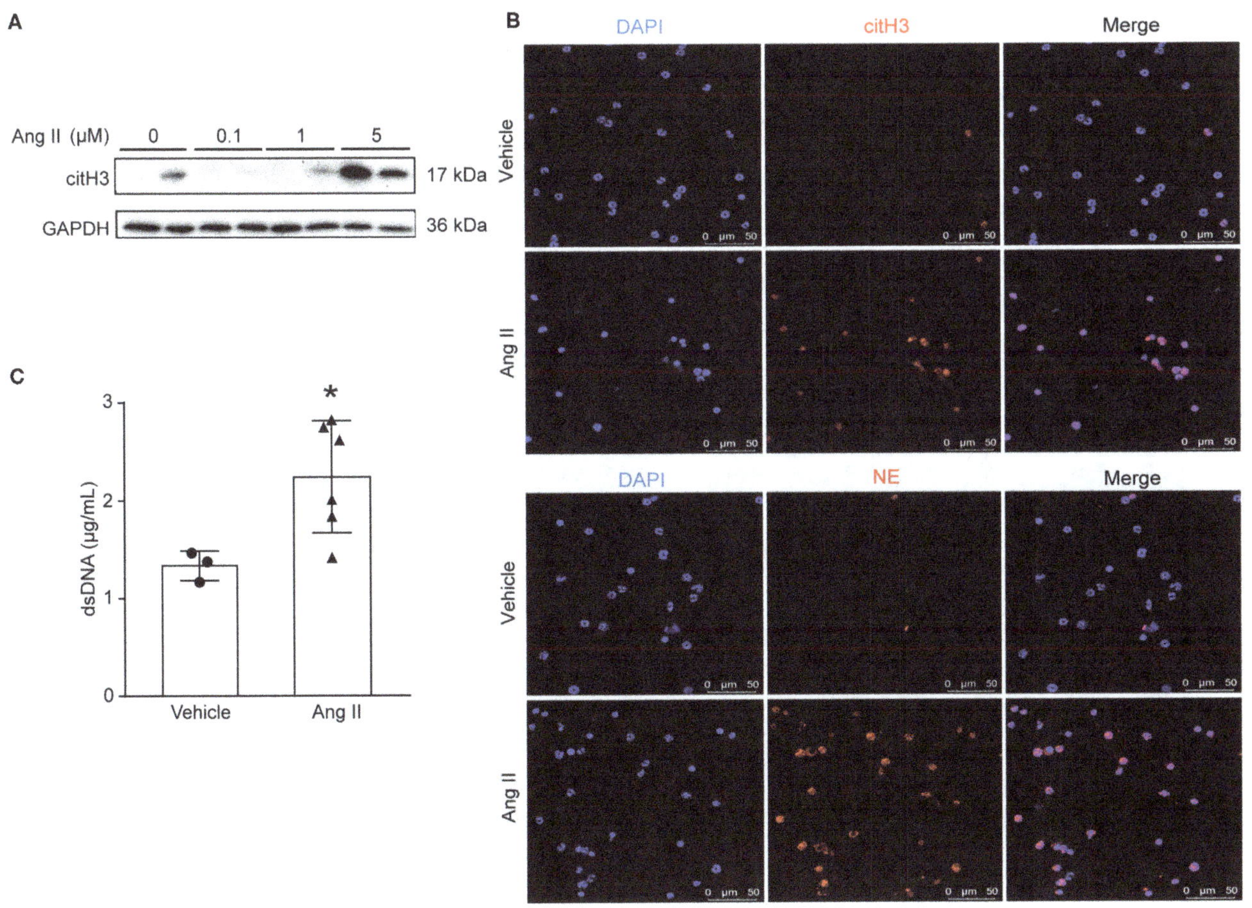

FIGURE 2 | Ang II induced NET formation *in vitro*. Neutrophils were isolated from $ApoE^{-/-}$ mice and treated with Ang II for 4 h. **(A)** Western blot for citH3 in different concentrations of Ang II (0, 100 nM, 1 μM, and 5 μM)-treated neutrophils. **(B)** Immunofluorescence analysis of Ang II (5 μM)-treated bone marrow-derived neutrophils for citH3 (red) or NE (red). Nuclei were stained with DAPI. **(C)** Measurement of dsDNA in Ang II-treated neutrophils. $n = 3$/vehicle group, $n = 6$/Ang II group, $^*p < 0.05$. Statistical significance was analyzed by the unpaired *t*-test.

coverslip were captured. The image analysis was performed with ImageJ (NIH, Bethesda, MD, USA).

TUNEL Staining

After rinsing twice with PBS, the samples were fixed with 4% PFA and permeabilized in 0.1% Triton X-100 for 10 min. After being washed with PBS, the samples were blocked by goat serum for 30 min at room temperature. A TUNEL reaction mixture (about 10 μL) (12156792910, Roche, Balsai, Switzerland) was added to the samples. After being incubated at 37°C for 1.5 h, samples were incubated with anti-SM22α antibody (1:200, ab7817, Abcam, USA) at 4°C overnight. Samples were incubated with goat anti-rabbit FITC secondary antibody for 1 h at room temperature the next day and sealed with DAPI.

Neutrophil Isolation

Bone marrow-derived neutrophils were isolated from $ApoE^{-/-}$ mice. Bone marrow cells were collected by flushing the femur with PBS and filtering through a sterile 70-μm nylon cell strainer. Cell suspension was layered in a ratio of 1 to 3 on top of Histopaque-1077 (10771, Sigma-Aldrich, MO, USA). After centrifugation, cell precipitation was resuspended with PBS. Cell suspension was layered in a ratio of 1 to 2 on top of Histopaque-1119 (11191, Sigma-Aldrich, MO, USA). Neutrophils were separated on the top of Histopaque-1119 after centrifugation. Neutrophils were resuspended in RPMI 1640 medium after being washed with PBS (18). Neutrophil purity was checked by immunofluorescence. In addition, 1×10^5 cells/well were seeded in 2% fibronectin-treated coverslips to perform the immunofluorescence staining. Cells were incubated for 4 h at 37°C.

Preparation for NETs

Mouse bone marrow neutrophils were stimulated with Ang II (5 μM) for 4 h to induce NETs. After confirmation of NET formation by visualization of extracellular DNA with DAPI, the culture medium was removed and neutrophils were washed and incubated for 1 h with RPMI 1640 medium. Supernatants were collected and centrifuged (10 min, 400 g). Neutrophils and cell debris were pelleted at the bottom. Supernatant was spun

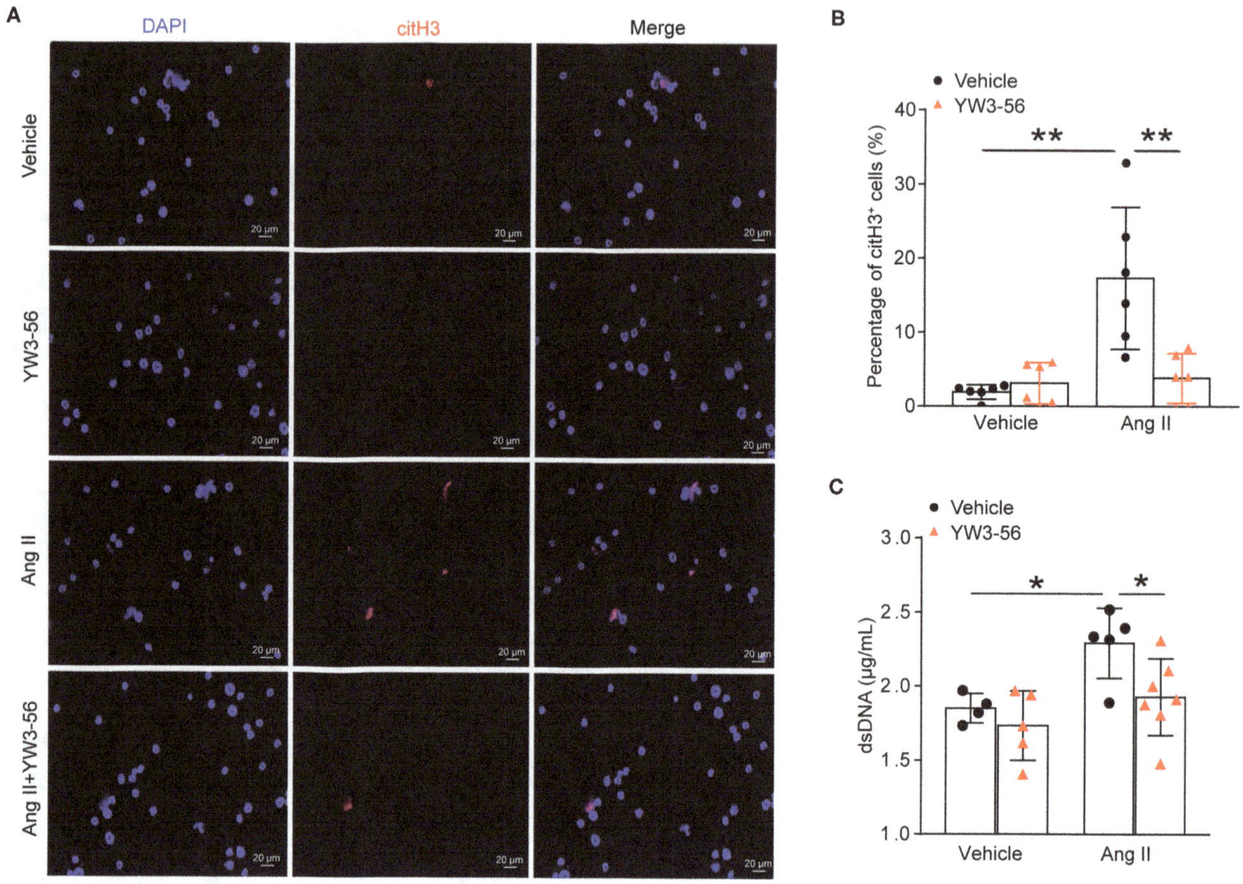

FIGURE 3 | PAD4 inhibitor YW3-56 suppressed Ang II-induced NET formation *in vitro*. Bone marrow-derived neutrophils from $ApoE^{-/-}$ mice were treated with vehicle or 5 μM Ang II for 4 h in the presence of vehicle or YW3-56. **(A)** Immunofluorescence analysis for citH3 (red). Nuclei were stained with DAPI. **(B)** Measurement of the percentage of citH3-positive cells. $n = 6$ per group, $^{**}p < 0.01$. **(C)** Measurement of dsDNA in vehicle or Ang II-stimulated neutrophils with or without YW3-56 treatment. $n = 4$/vehicle group, $n = 5$/YW3-56 group, $n = 5$/Ang II group, $n = 7$/Ang II+YW3-56 group, $^{*}p < 0.05$. Statistical significance was determined by one-way ANOVA test followed by the unpaired *t*-test.

(10 min, 17,000 g) at 4°C. Pellets were resuspended and obtained together in ice-cold PBS. Quant-iT PicoGreen dsDNA Assay Kit (Thermo Fisher Scientific, Waltham, MA, USA) was used to measure the concentration according to the manufacturer's instructions, and NETs were either used immediately or stored at −80°C (25).

Mouse Primary VSMC Isolation

Primary VSMCs were isolated from aortas of 10- to 12-week-old male $ApoE^{-/-}$ mice as previously described (23). Mice were killed by inhaled isoflurane (1% in O_2). The whole aortic portions were dissected and then digested with 347 U/mg type II collagenase (Worthington, Lakewood, NJ, USA) at 37°C for 30 min. The adventitia was carefully removed. A sterile cotton-tipped applicator was used to remove the endothelium by gently rubbing the intima. The aortas were minced into small pieces and digested with a mixture of 347 U/mg collagenase II and 6 U/mg elastase IV (Sigma-Aldrich) for 30 min at 37°C. Cells were then cultured with SMCM (ScienCell, CA, USA) supplemented with 10% fetal bovine serum (FBS), 1% smooth muscle growth supplement, and 1% penicillin streptomycin. VSMCs from passages 3 to 9 were used for all *in vitro* experiments. VSMCs were treated with 10 μg NETs for 24 h before starvation (1% FBS) for 8 h (26). To determine whether p38 inhibitor SB203580 or JNK inhibitor SP600125 could reverse NET-induced VSMC apoptosis, p38 inhibitor SB203580 (S1076, Selleckchem, Houston, TX, USA) or JNK inhibitor SP600125 (S1876, Beyotime, Shanghai, China) was preincubated in primary VSMC.

Annexin V/PI Assay

Annexin V/PI apoptosis detection kit (556547, BD Biosciences, San Jose, CA, USA) was used to detect apoptosis according to the manufacturer's instructions. The cell culture medium of the primary VSMCs was carefully collected into a centrifuge tube. Then, the VSMCs were digested with EDTA-free trypsin and collected in the centrifuge tube again, and centrifuged at 1,000 rpm for 5 min. Cells were washed with PBS and resuspended with 1× binding buffer. Annexin V/Alexa Fluor 488 of 5 μl was added into the cell suspension and mixed well. After being kept

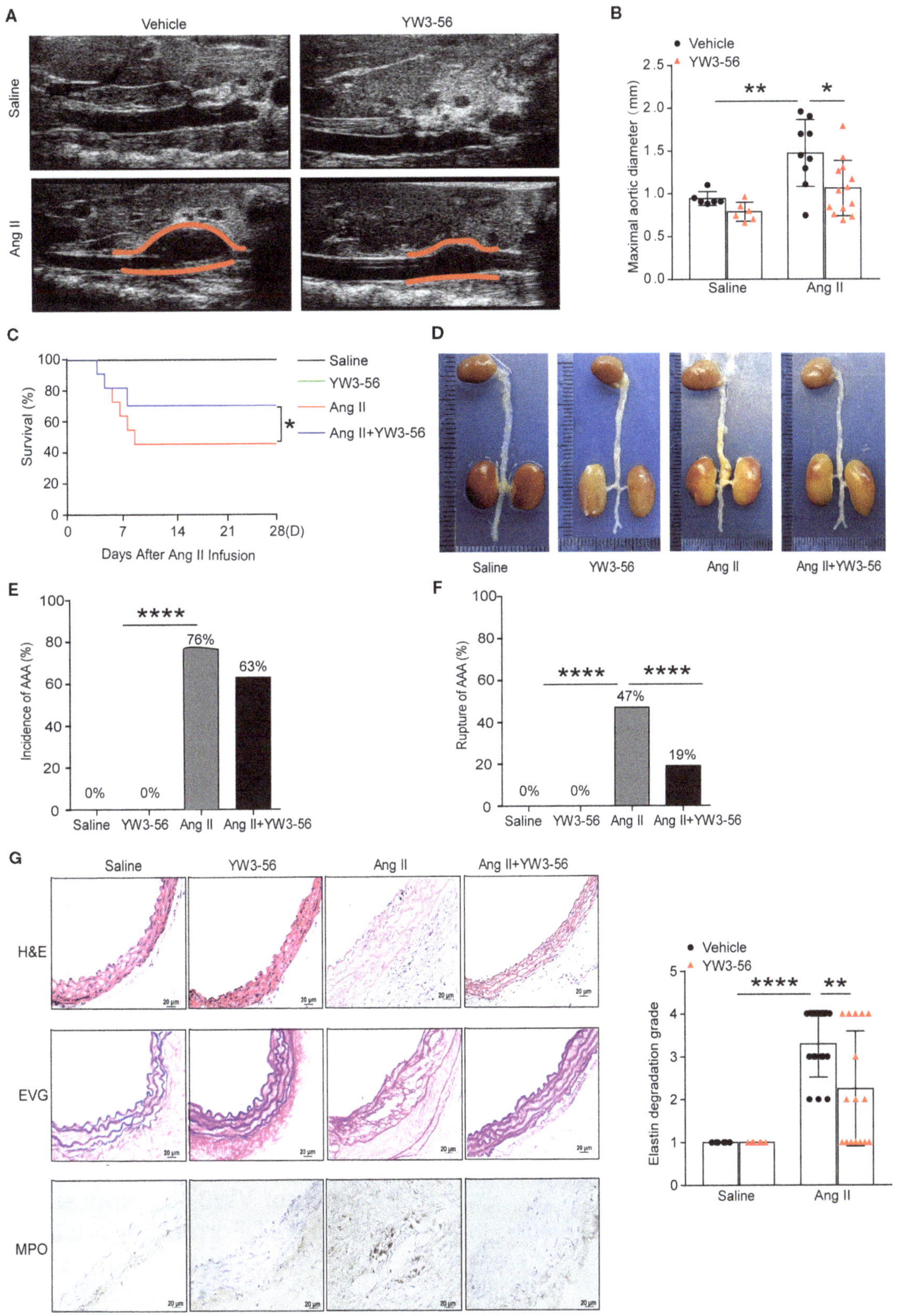

FIGURE 4 | PAD4 inhibitor YW3-56 reduced Ang II-induced AAA rupture. *ApoE*$^{-/-}$ mice were infused with saline or 1,000 ng/kg/min Ang II for 28 days in the presence of vehicle or YW3-56. **(A)** B-mode ultrasound of abdominal aortas and **(B)** statistical analysis of maximal aortic diameter. $n = 6$/saline group, $n = 6$/YW3-56

(Continued)

FIGURE 4 | group, $n = 9$/Ang II group, $n = 13$/Ang II+YW3-56 group, $^{*}p < 0.05$, $^{**}p < 0.01$. Statistical significance was determined by one-way ANOVA test followed by the unpaired *t*-test. **(C)** The survival rate of Ang II-induced AAA in $ApoE^{-/-}$ mice in the presence of vehicle or YW3-56. $^{*}p < 0.05$, significance was determined by the log-rank (Mantel–Cox) test. **(D)** Representative photos for aortas from the above mice. **(E)** The incidence rate of AAA from the above mice. $n = 6$–17, $^{****}p < 0.0001$. Statistical significance was determined by Fisher exact test. **(F)** The rupture rate of AAA from the above mice. $n = 6$–17, $^{****}p < 0.0001$. Statistical significance was determined by Fisher exact test. **(G)** Representative images of H&E, EVG, and MPO staining for the abdominal aortas from the above mice. $n = 6$–17, $^{**}p < 0.01$, $^{****}p < 0.0001$. Statistical significance was determined by one-way ANOVA test followed by the unpaired *t*-test.

at room temperature for 5 min, PI (5 μL) was added and mixed with cell suspension. The mixtures were analyzed immediately using flow cytometry.

Real-Time Quantitative PCR

Total RNA was extracted from the whole aortic portion of mice using TRIzol reagent (15596018, Invitrogen, Carlsbad, CA, USA). Retro-transcription in cDNA was synthesized from 2 μg of RNA and performed with GoScript™ Reverse Transcription System (A5001, Promega, Mannheim, Germany). Real-time quantitative PCR was performed with SYBR Green PCR Kit (420A, Takara, Shiga, Japan) with the CFX Connect Real-Time System (Bio-Rad, Hercules, CA, USA). Results were analyzed, and fold change over *Actb* was calculated by the comparative cycle method ($2^{-\Delta\Delta Ct}$). All primer sequences are shown in **Supplementary Table 2**.

Western Blot

Whole-cell lysate was extracted from VSMCs or neutrophils using RIPA Lysis Buffer (C1053, Applygen, Beijing, China). The protein concentration of the samples was measured by Pierce™ BCA Protein Assay Kit (23209, Thermo Fisher Scientific, Waltham, MA, USA). An equal amount of protein per sample and molecular weight markers was subjected to SDS-polyacrylamide gel electrophoresis (SDS-PAGE). Membranes were blocked and probed for primary antibodies against citH3 (1:1000 dilution; ab5103, Abcam, USA), GAPDH (1:2000 dilution; 10494-1-AP, Proteintech, Chicago, IL, USA), p38 (1:1000 dilution; 8690s, CST, Danvers, MA, USA), p-p38 (Thr180/Tyr182) (1:1000 dilution; 4511s, CST, USA), JNK (1:1000 dilution; 9252s, CST, USA), and p-JNK (Thr183/Tyr185) (1:1000 dilution; 4668s, CST, USA) overnight at 4°C. Anti-mouse (1:2000, 7076S; Cell Signaling, MA, USA) and anti-rabbit secondary antibody (1:2000, 7074S; Cell Signaling, MA, USA) conjugated with horseradish peroxidase for 1 h at room temperature. Chemiluminescence HRP Substrate Kit (Millipore, Bedford, MA, USA) was used to perform immunodetection analysis. The mean band intensity was measured with ImageJ.

Statistical Analysis

All data are shown as the means ± S.E.M. Two-tailed unpaired Student's *t*-test was used to compare two groups. Comparisons among more than two independent groups were analyzed by one-way or two-way analysis of variance (ANOVA). Differences among multiple groups with one variable were determined using one-way analysis of variance (one-way ANOVA) followed by Bonferroni's *post-hoc* test. Two-way ANOVA followed by Bonferroni's *post-hoc* test was used to compare multiple groups with more than one variable. The Fisher exact test was used to compare the incidence and rupture rate of AAA. The log-rank (Mantel–Cox) test was used to analyze the survival percentage of Ang II-infused mice. Statistical analysis was performed with Prism 7 software (GraphPad Software, San Diego, CA, USA). $p < 0.05$ was considered statistically significant.

RESULTS

Ang II Induced NET Formation *in vivo*

To determine the formation of NETs in Ang II-induced AAA, $ApoE^{-/-}$ mice were infused with saline or 1,000 ng/kg/min Ang II for 28 days to establish the Ang II-induced AAA. PAD4-mediated decondensation of chromatin to form citrullinated histones is a key step in the formation of NETs. Therefore, the presence of citH3 is a marker of NETs (27). Cytoplasmic proteins NE and MPO were also used as NET markers. Immunofluorescence results showed that citH3 (red), neutrophil elastase (red), or MPO (red) colocalized with DAPI in Ly6G (green)-marked neutrophils in the Ang II-treated AAA (**Figures 1A–C**). dsDNA release associated with the formation of NETs (28) and was used as one of the detection indicators for NETs (26). The dsDNA level was also increased in Ang II-infused mice compared with the saline-treated group (**Figure 1D**). These results showed that NET formation is increased in Ang II-induced AAA in $ApoE^{-/-}$ mice.

Ang II Induced NET Formation *in vitro*

To examine whether Ang II could induce NET formation *in vitro*, bone marrow-derived neutrophils were isolated by density gradient centrifugation from $ApoE^{-/-}$ mice and stimulated with Ang II with dosages of 0, 100 nM, 1 μM, and 5 μM *in vitro*. The expression of citH3 was detected by Western blot (**Figure 2A**). The results showed that citH3 expression was significantly increased after 5 μM Ang II stimulation in neutrophils. Immunofluorescence staining results also showed that Ang II significantly increased the expression of citH3 and NE compared with the vehicle group (**Figure 2B**). The dsDNA level was also increased in Ang II stimulated bone-marrow neutrophils (**Figure 2C**). These results demonstrated that Ang II induced NET formation *in vitro*.

PAD4 Inhibitor YW3-56 Suppressed Ang II-Induced NET Formation *in vitro*

NET formation was increased in AAA. PAD4-mediated histone citrullination and chromatin decondensation are essential steps in NET formation. Cl-amidine is a known PAD pan-inhibitor. To develop more potent inhibitors of PAD4, the N-terminus and C-terminus of Cl-amidine were modified. The activity of the synthetic compound YW3-56 was evaluated. YW3-56 as a Cl-amidine analog has improved the bioavailability

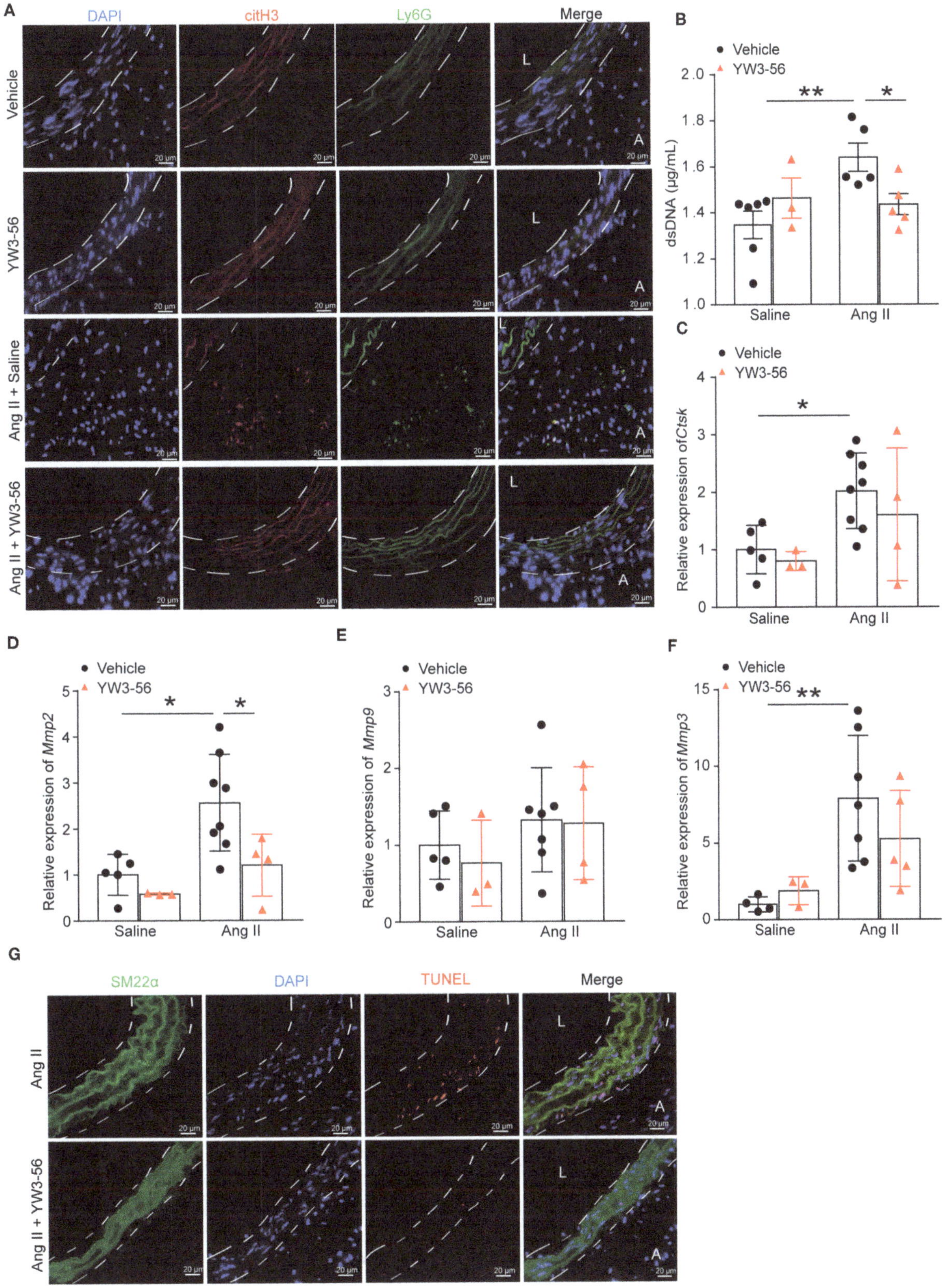

FIGURE 5 | PAD4 inhibitor YW3-56 reduced NET formation and VSMC apoptosis in Ang II-induced AAA. *ApoE*$^{-/-}$ mice were infused with saline or 1,000 ng/kg/min Ang II for 28 days in the presence of vehicle or YW3-56. **(A)** Immunofluorescence analysis for citH3 (red) and Ly6G (green) in the abdominal aortas. Nuclei were

(Continued)

FIGURE 5 | stained with DAPI. L: lumen, A: adventitia. **(B)** Measurement of dsDNA in the serum of Ang II-induced *ApoE*$^{-/-}$ mice with or without YW3-56. n = 6/saline group, n = 3/YW3-56 group, n = 5/Ang II group, n = 5/Ang II+YW3-56 group, $^{*}p < 0.05$, $^{**}p < 0.01$. **(C–F)** Aortic *Mmp2/3/9* and *Ctsk* mRNAs were measured by RT-qPCR. n = 3–8, $^{*}p < 0.05$, $^{**}p < 0.01$. **(G)** TUNEL staining for apoptosis cells (red). VSMCs were stained with SM22α. Nuclei were stained with DAPI. Statistical significance was determined by one-way ANOVA test followed by the unpaired t-test.

and increased the permeability. Moreover, subsequent trials showed that YW3-56 exerted an antitumor effect (22). To investigate whether YW3-56 could inhibit the formation of NETs, immunofluorescence staining was performed in bone marrow-derived neutrophils with Ang II stimulation. The results showed that Ang II significantly increased the expression of citH3, whereas this effect was decreased by YW3-56 treatment (**Figures 3A,B**). Nevertheless, YW3-56 slightly reduced the dsDNA level stimulated by Ang II in bone marrow-derived neutrophils (**Figure 3C**). The above results showed that YW3-56 reduced the formation of NETs in mouse bone marrow-derived neutrophils induced by Ang II.

PAD4 Inhibitor YW3-56 Reduced Ang II-Induced AAA Rupture

To validate the effect of YW3-56 in Ang II-induced AAA of *ApoE*$^{-/-}$ mice, YW3-56 (10 mL/kg) was intraperitoneally injected every other day from 1 day before Ang II infusion. Ultrasound results showed that Ang II significantly increased the blood vessel diameter leading to the formation of AAA, while YW3-56 restricted the blood vessel diameter dilation and reduced the formation of AAA induced by Ang II (**Figures 4A,B**). YW3-56 also reduced the mortality induced by Ang II in *ApoE*$^{-/-}$ mice (**Figure 4C**). Morphological results showed that YW3-56 attenuated the Ang II-induced increase of the vessel diameter (**Figure 4D**). The incidence rate of AAA in Ang II infused mice with or without YW3-56 showed no significant difference (**Figure 4E**). The rupture rate with YW3-56 treatment in Ang II infused mice was significantly decreased compared with Ang II infused mice (**Figure 4F**). These data suggested that PAD4 inhibitor YW3-56 inhibited AAA rupture but has little effect on AAA initiation/formation. Morphologically, H&E staining of the abdominal aorta of *ApoE*$^{-/-}$ mice showed that YW3-56 mitigated the blood vessel diameter and inflammatory cell infiltration increase caused by Ang II. Gomori Aldehyde-Fuchsin results showed that Ang II significantly increased the fracture of the elastic lamina, which can be significantly alleviated by YW3-56. MPO immunohistochemistry showed that YW3-56 reduced neutrophil infiltration caused by Ang II perfusion (**Figure 4G**). These results showed that PAD4 inhibitor YW3-56 mainly reduced the blood vessel diameter, inflammation, and elastin degradation induced by Ang II. It emphasized the important role of YW3-56 in suppressing AAA rupture.

PAD4 Inhibitor YW3-56 Decreased NET Formation and VSMC Apoptosis in Ang II-Induced AAA

To further clarify whether YW3-56 reduced the rupture of AAA by inhibiting the formation of NETs, immunofluorescence staining was performed. The results showed that YW3-56 reduced the citH3 level in Ang II-induced aneurysm (**Figure 5A**). YW3-56 also decreased the dsDNA level induced by Ang II (**Figure 5B**). RT-qRCR results showed that Ang II infusion increased the level of *Ctsk*, *Mmp2*, *Mmp9*, and *Mmp3*, while YW3-56 attenuated the *Mmp2* expression induced by Ang II (**Figures 5C–F**). Immunofluorescence staining also showed that YW3-56 decreased the apoptosis of VSMCs induced by Ang II (**Figure 5G**). These results showed that YW3-56 reduced VSMC apoptosis and further decreased AAA rupture by suppression of NET formation.

NET Induced VSMC Apoptosis *via* p38/JNK Pathway

VSMC apoptosis leads to massive loss of contractile cells and dilation of the abdominal aortic wall (29). To explore whether NETs induced by Ang II affected the apoptosis of VSMCs, NETs were used to stimulate VSMCs for 24 h. TUNEL staining showed that NETs significantly increased the apoptosis of VSMCs (**Figure 6A**). Furthermore, Annexin V-FITC/PI staining flow cytometry analysis results also demonstrated that NET treatment increased VSMC apoptosis (**Figure 6B**). Mitogen-activated protein kinases are widely expressed serine/tyrosine kinases that play an important role in a variety of signal transduction pathways in mammalian cells (30). The p38 signaling pathway is an important branch of the MAPK pathway which is essential in various physiological and pathological processes such as apoptosis, inflammation, cell stress, and cell cycle and growth (30). To study whether NETs induced VSMC apoptosis *via* the MAPK signaling pathway, Western blot was performed on VSMCs after NET stimulation. The results showed that the phosphorylation levels of p38 and JNK were significantly higher after NET administration (**Figure 6C**), suggesting that NETs induced VSMC apoptosis *via* p38/JNK pathway.

Inhibition p38/JNK Pathway Suppressed NET-Induced VSMC Apoptosis

To verify whether NETs induced VSMC apoptosis *via* p38/JNK pathway, VSMCs were preincubated with p38 inhibitor SB203580 or JNK inhibitor SP600125 for 30 min before NET treatment. TUNEL staining showed that the inhibitor of p38/JNK could decrease NET-induced VSMC apoptosis (**Figure 7A**). These results suggested that NETs accelerated the apoptosis of VSMCs through p38 and JNK signaling pathway.

DISCUSSION

In summary, this work provided several new findings as follows: (1). NETs accelerated VSMC apoptosis *via* p38/JNK pathway; (2). PAD4 inhibitor YW3-56 inhibited NET formation and then reduced Ang II-induced aortic diameter increase and elastin

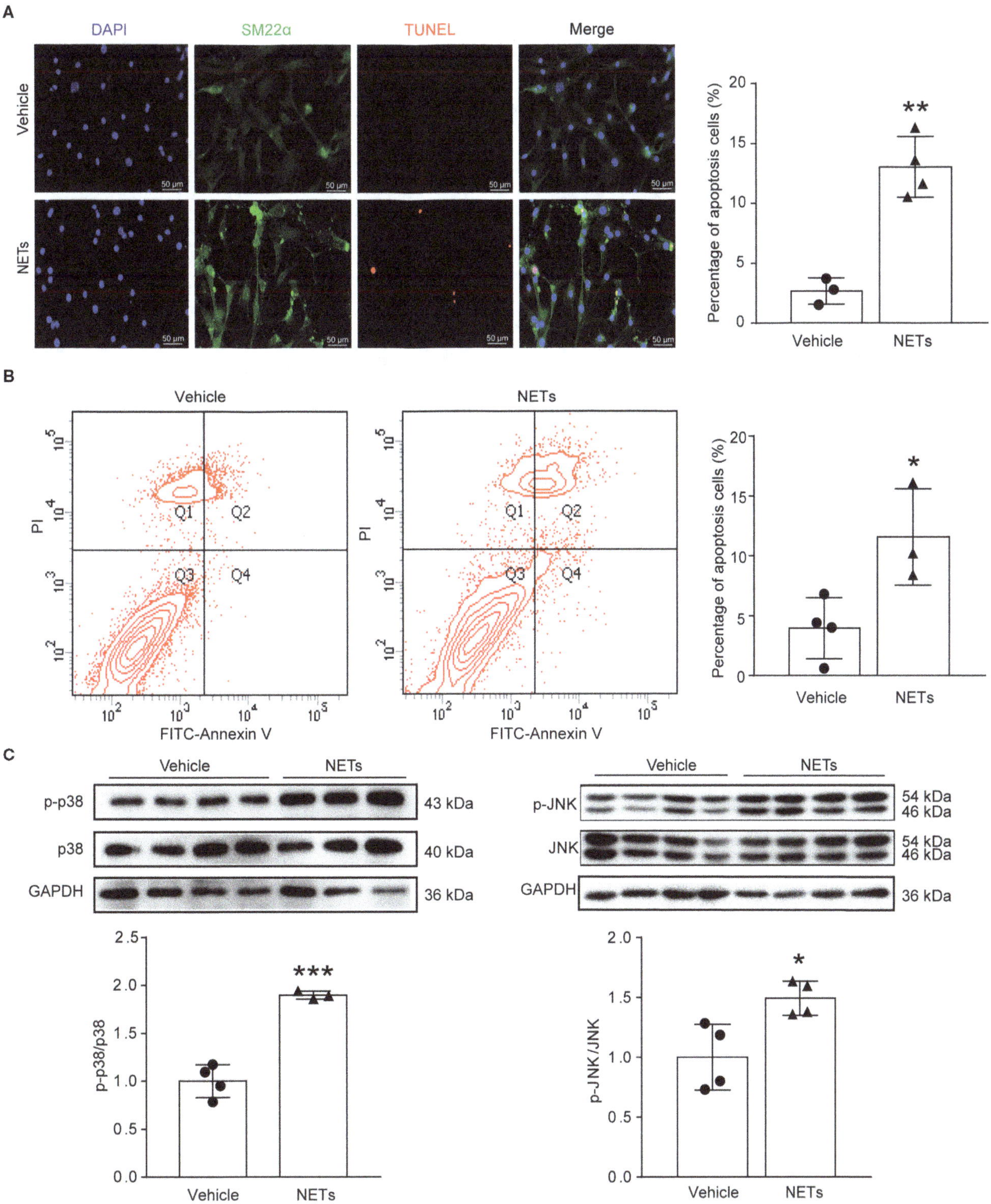

FIGURE 6 | NETs induced VSMC apoptosis *via* p38/JNK pathway. Primary VSMCs isolated from aortas of $ApoE^{-/-}$ mice were treated with vehicle or 10 μg NETs for 24 h. **(A)** TUNEL staining for apoptosis cells (red). The percentage of apoptosis cells was analyzed. VSMCs were stained with SM22α. Nuclei were stained with DAPI. $n = 3$/vehicle group, $n = 4$/NET group, $^{**}p < 0.01$. Statistical significance was analyzed by the unpaired t-test. **(B)** Annexin V-FITC/PI staining for VSMC apoptosis. $n = 4$/vehicle group, $n = 3$/NET group, $^{*}p < 0.05$. Statistical significance was analyzed by the unpaired t-test. **(C)** Western blot for p38/JNK level. $n = 3$–4, $^{*}p < 0.05$, $^{***}p < 0.001$. Statistical significance was analyzed by the unpaired t-test.

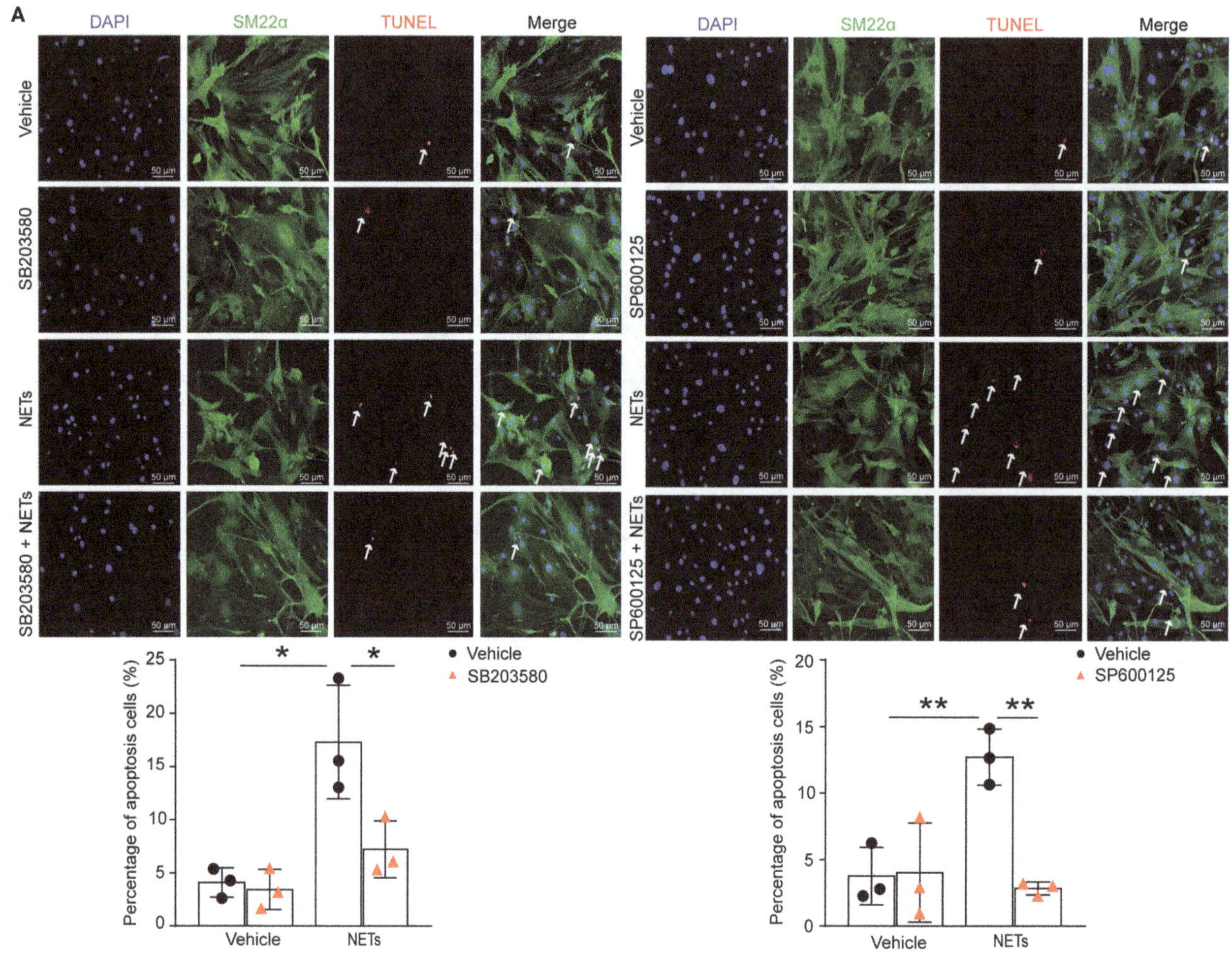

FIGURE 7 | Inhibition p38/JNK pathway suppressed NETs induced VSMC apoptosis. Primary VSMCs isolated from aortas of *ApoE*$^{-/-}$ mice were preincubated with p38 inhibitor SB203580 or JNK inhibitor SP600125 for 30 min before NET treatment for 24 h. **(A)** TUNEL staining for apoptosis cells (red) and the percentage of apoptosis cells were analyzed. VSMCs were stained with SM22α. Nuclei were stained with DAPI. $n = 3$ per group, $^{*}p < 0.05$, $^{**}p < 0.01$. Statistical significance was determined by one-way ANOVA test followed by the unpaired *t*-test.

degradation. It is important to note that PAD4 inhibitor YW3-56 significantly alleviates Ang II-induced AAA rupture. Inhibition of NET formation or p38/JNK pathway may therefore be a potential therapeutic strategy for treating AAA.

AAA rupture is thought to occur when the hemodynamics generated by pulsating blood flow exceeds the strength of the AAA wall. The process involves several pathological processes, including infiltration of inflammatory cells, ECM degradation, and VSMC apoptosis. Neutrophils contribute to the pathological mechanisms of AAA, such as proteolysis, oxidative stress, and adventitia immune inflammatory processes driving aortic wall remodeling (31). NETs are considered not only an important defense tool of neutrophils but also an indispensable participant to exacerbate a variety of cardiovascular diseases, such as atherosclerosis and atherothrombosis (32). NETs were associated with AAA development in the elastase-induced AAA model. DNAse I premature treatment suppressed AAA development, suggesting the involvement of NETs in AAA formation (19). Pretreatment with ceramide synthesis fumonisin inhibitor decreased IL-1β-induced ceramide synthesis and IL-1β-induced NETosis, indicating that ceramide synthesis is involved in NETosis in AAA (18). In this study, Ang II treatment significantly increased the formation of NETs. This is consistent with a previous report that levels of citH3 increased in the Ang II-induced AAA model (33). However, the mechanism by which NET affect AAA processes is not clear.

It is well-established that VSMCs play an important role in the development of AAA (34). miR-106a promoted VSMC apoptosis and MMP production. Therefore, the development of AAA was accelerated (35). In this study, TUNEL staining and Annexin V-FITC/PI analysis results also demonstrated that NET treatment increased VSMC apoptosis *via* p38/JNK pathway. ECM degradation causes elastin degradation, thereby impairing aortic strength and elasticity (36). MMPs contain several members implicated in AAA formation. MMPs are capable of degrading elastin type I and type III collagen which are predominant types found in the aortic wall. MMP overexpression was also responsible for aneurysmal degeneration and rupture in experimental studies in rats (37, 38). NET formation increased the level of MMP2/9 in this study. Targeting ECM degradation, VSMC apoptosis, and inflammation may be a potential therapeutic approach for AAA pathogenesis.

PAD4 plays an important role in NET formation by catalyzing histone citrullination (16). PAD inhibitor Cl-amidine reduced NET formation in atherosclerosis induced by high-cholesterol diet (39). Therefore, reducing NET formation by inhibiting PAD4 is a way to treat AAA. PAD4 inhibitor YW3-56 reduced Ang II-induced aortic diameter increase and elastin degradation. PAD4 inhibitor YW3-56 significantly alleviates Ang II-induced AAA rupture.

Of note, Wolf Eilenberg et al. (40) demonstrated that histone citrullination is a novel biomarker in AAA and PAD4 inhibitor GSK484 attenuated Ang II-induced AAA. However, how the NETs affected AAA was unexplored. In our study, NETs increased apoptosis of VSMCs *via* p38/JNK pathway. In addition, PAD4 inhibitor YW3-56 as a Cl-amidine analog has improved the bioavailability and increased the permeability. YW3-56 suppressed cancer cell growth significantly (22). Inhibition of NET formation by YW3-56 reduced the rupture of AAA. It provided in-depth knowledge of a new PAD4 inhibitor YW3-56 in decreasing NET formation.

In conclusion, this study showed that NET formation was increased in Ang II-induced AAA. Inhibition of NET formation by YW3-56 ameliorated Ang II-induced AAA rupture. Clarifying the role of NETs in AAA may contribute to a better understanding of the pathophysiology of AAA, which also provides a new idea for the prevention and treatment in AAA.

AUTHOR CONTRIBUTIONS

MW performed the experiments and wrote the manuscript. XW guided the drawing. YS, DZ, and DQ discussed the results. YW generously provided PAD4 inhibitor YW3-56. AQ designed the experiments and wrote the manuscript. All the authors read and modified the final version of the manuscript.

REFERENCES

1. Keisler B, Carter C. Abdominal aortic aneurysm. *Am Fam Physician.* (2015) 91:538–43.
2. Tchana-Sato V, Sakalihasan N, Defraigne JO. Ruptured abdominal aortic aneurysm. *Rev Med Liege.* (2018) 73:296–9. doi: 10.3238/arztebl.2012.0727
3. Lindeman JH, Matsumura JS. Pharmacologic management of aneurysms. *Circ Res.* (2019) 124:631–46. doi: 10.1161/CIRCRESAHA.118.312439
4. O'Driscoll JM, Bahia SS, Gravina A, Di Fino S, Thompson MM, Karthikesalingam A, et al. Transthoracic echocardiography provides important long-term prognostic information in selected patients undergoing endovascular abdominal aortic repair. *Circ Cardiovasc Imaging.* (2016) 9:e003557. doi: 10.1161/CIRCIMAGING.115.003557
5. Buck DB, van Herwaarden JA, Schermerhorn ML, Moll FL. Endovascular treatment of abdominal aortic aneurysms. *Nat Rev Cardiol.* (2014) 11:112–23. doi: 10.1038/nrcardio.2013.196
6. Nordon M, Hinchliffe RJ, Loftus IM, Thompson MM. Pathophysiology and epidemiology of abdominal aortic aneurysms. *Nat Rev Cardiol.* (2011) 8:92–102. doi: 10.1038/nrcardio.2010.180
7. Raaz U, Toh R, Maegdefessel L, Adam M, Nakagami F, Emrich FC, et al. Hemodynamic regulation of reactive oxygen species: implications for vascular diseases. *Antioxid Redox Signal.* (2014) 20:914–28. doi: 10.1089/ars.2013.5507
8. Weber C, Zernecke A, Libby P. The multifaceted contributions of leukocyte subsets to atherosclerosis: lessons from mouse models. *Nat Rev Immunol.* (2008) 8:802–15. doi: 10.1038/nri2415
9. Pagano MB, Zhou HF, Ennis TL, Wu X, Lambris JD, Atkinson JP, et al. Complement-dependent neutrophil recruitment is critical for the development of elastase-induced abdominal aortic aneurysm. *Circulation.* (2009) 119:1805–13. doi: 10.1161/CIRCULATIONAHA.108.832972
10. Houard X, Touat Z, Ollivier V, Louedec L, Philippe M, Sebbag U, et al. Mediators of neutrophil recruitment in human abdominal aortic aneurysms. *Cardiovasc Res.* (2009) 82:532–41. doi: 10.1093/cvr/cvp048
11. Eliason JL, Hannawa KK, Ailawadi G, Sinha I, Ford JW, Deogracias MP, et al. Neutrophil depletion inhibits experimental abdominal aortic aneurysm formation. *Circulation.* (2005) 112:232–40. doi: 10.1161/CIRCULATIONAHA.104.517391
12. Brinkmann V, Reichard U, Goosmann C, Fauler B, Uhlemann Y, Weiss DS, et al. Neutrophil extracellular traps kill bacteria. *Science.* (2004) 303:1532–5. doi: 10.1126/science.1092385
13. Vorobjeva NV, Pinegin BV. Neutrophil extracellular traps: mechanisms of formation and role in health and disease. *Biochemistry (Mosc).* (2014) 79:1286–96. doi: 10.1134/S0006297914120025
14. Steinberg BE, Grinstein S. Unconventional roles of the NADPH oxidase: signaling, ion homeostasis, cell death. *Sci STKE.* (2007) 2007:pe11. doi: 10.1126/stke.3792007pe11
15. de Bont CM, Boelens WC, Pruijn GJM. NETosis, complement, and coagulation: a triangular relationship. *Cell Mol Immunol.* (2019) 16:19–27. doi: 10.1038/s41423-018-0024-0
16. Neeli I, Dwivedi N, Khan S, Radic M. Regulation of extracellular chromatin release from neutrophils. *J Innate Immun.* (2009) 1:194–201. doi: 10.1159/000206974
17. Karlsson A, Dahlgren C. Assembly and activation of the neutrophil NADPH oxidase in granule membranes. *Antioxid Redox Signal.* (2002) 4:49–60. doi: 10.1089/152308602753625852
18. Meher K, Spinosa M, Davis JP, Pope N, Laubach VE, Su G, et al. Novel role of IL (Interleukin)-1beta in neutrophil extracellular trap formation and abdominal aortic aneurysms. *Arterioscler Thromb Vasc Biol.* (2018) 38:843–53. doi: 10.1161/ATVBAHA.117.309897
19. Yan H, Zhou HF, Akk A, Hu Y, Springer LE, Ennis TL, et al. Neutrophil proteases promote experimental abdominal aortic aneurysm *via* extracellular trap release and plasmacytoid dendritic cell activation. *Arterioscler Thromb Vasc Biol.* (2016) 36:1660–9. doi: 10.1161/ATVBAHA.116.307786
20. Silvestre-Roig C, Braster Q, Wichapong K, Lee EY, Teulon JM, Berrebeh N, et al. Externalized histone H4 orchestrates chronic inflammation by inducing lytic cell death. *Nature.* (2019) 569:236–40. doi: 10.1038/s41586-019-1167-6
21. Qin Y, Cao X, Guo J, Zhang Y, Pan L, Zhang H, et al. Deficiency of cathepsin S attenuates angiotensin II-induced abdominal aortic aneurysm formation in apolipoprotein E-deficient mice. *Cardiovasc Res.* (2012) 96:401–10. doi: 10.1093/cvr/cvs263
22. Wang Y, Li P, Wang S, Hu J, Chen XA, Wu J, et al. Anticancer peptidylarginine deiminase (PAD) inhibitors regulate the autophagy flux and the mammalian target of rapamycin complex 1 activity. *J Biol Chem.* (2012) 287:25941–53. doi: 10.1074/jbc.M112.375725

23. Qi, Wei M, Jiao S, Song Y, Wang X, Xie G, et al. Hypoxia inducible factor 1alpha in vascular smooth muscle cells promotes angiotensin II-induced vascular remodeling *via* activation of CCL7-mediated macrophage recruitment. *Cell Death Dis.* (2019) 10:544. doi: 10.1038/s41419-019-1757-0
24. Chen HZ, Wang F, Gao P, Pei JF, Liu Y, Xu TT, et al. Age-associated sirtuin 1 reduction in vascular smooth muscle links vascular senescence and inflammation to abdominal aortic aneurysm. *Circ Res.* (2016) 119: 1076–88. doi: 10.1161/CIRCRESAHA.116.308895
25. Najmeh S, Cools-Lartigue J, Giannias B, Spicer J, Ferri LE. Simplified human neutrophil extracellular traps (NETs) isolation and handling. *J Vis Exp.* (2015) 98:52687. doi: 10.3791/52687
26. Li L, Yu X, Liu J, Wang Z, Li C, Shi J, et al. Neutrophil extracellular traps promote aberrant macrophages activation in behcet's disease. *Front Immunol.* (2020) 11:590622. doi: 10.3389/fimmu.2020.590622
27. Du M, Yang W, Schmull S, Gu J, Xue S. Inhibition of peptidyl arginine deiminase-4 protects against myocardial infarction induced cardiac dysfunction. *Int Immunopharmacol.* (2020) 78:106055. doi: 10.1016/j.intimp.2019.106055
28. Toussaint M, Jackson DJ, Swieboda D, Guedan A, Tsourouktsoglou TD, Ching YM, et al. Host DNA released by NETosis promotes rhinovirus-induced type-2 allergic asthma exacerbation. *Nat Med.* (2017) 23:681–91. doi: 10.1038/nm.4332
29. Zhang Z, Zou G, Chen X, Lu W, Liu J, Zhai S, et al. Knockdown of lncRNA PVT1 inhibits vascular smooth muscle cell apoptosis and extracellular matrix disruption in a murine abdominal aortic aneurysm model. *Mol Cells.* (2019) 42:218–27. doi: 10.14348/molcells.2018.0162
30. Sun Y, Liu WZ, Liu T, Feng X, Yang N, Zhou HF. Signaling pathway of MAPK/ERK in cell proliferation, differentiation, migration, senescence and apoptosis. *J Recept Signal Transduct Res.* (2015) 35:600–4. doi: 10.3109/10799893.2015.1030412
31. Kim HW, Blomkalns AL, Ogbi M, Thomas M, Gavrila D, Neltner BS, et al. Role of myeloperoxidase in abdominal aortic aneurysm formation: mitigation by taurine. *Am J Physiol Heart Circ Physiol.* (2017) 313:H1168–79. doi: 10.1152/ajpheart.00296.2017
32. Doring Y, Soehnlein O, Weber C. Neutrophil extracellular traps in atherosclerosis and atherothrombosis. *Circ Res.* (2017) 120:736–43. doi: 10.1161/CIRCRESAHA.116.309692
33. Spinosa M, Su G, Salmon MD, Lu G, Cullen JM, Fashandi AZ, et al. Resolvin D1 decreases abdominal aortic aneurysm formation by inhibiting NETosis in a mouse model. *J Vasc Surg.* (2018) 68:93S–103S. doi: 10.1016/j.jvs.2018.05.253
34. Kawai T, Takayanagi T, Forrester SJ, Preston KJ, Obama T, Tsuji T, et al. Vascular ADAM17 (a Disintegrin and Metalloproteinase Domain 17) is required for angiotensin II/beta-aminopropionitrile-induced abdominal aortic aneurysm. *Hypertension.* (2017) 70:959–63. doi: 10.1161/HYPERTENSIONAHA.117.09822
35. Han ZL, Wang HQ, Zhang TS, He YX, Zhou H. Up-regulation of exosomal miR-106a may play a significant role in abdominal aortic aneurysm by inducing vascular smooth muscle cell apoptosis and targeting TIMP-2, an inhibitor of metallopeptidases that suppresses extracellular matrix degradation. *Eur Rev Med Pharmacol Sci.* (2020) 24:8087–95. doi: 10.26355/eurrev_202008_22493
36. Krishna SM, Morton SK, Li J, Golledge J. Risk factors and mouse models of abdominal aortic aneurysm rupture. *Int J Mol Sci.* (2020) 21:7250. doi: 10.3390/ijms21197250
37. Rabkin SW. The role matrix metalloproteinases in the production of aortic aneurysm. *Prog Mol Biol Transl Sci.* (2017) 147:239–65. doi: 10.1016/bs.pmbts.2017.02.002
38. Maguire M, Pearce SWA, Xiao R, Oo AY, Xiao Q. Matrix metalloproteinase in abdominal aortic aneurysm and aortic dissection. *Pharmaceuticals (Basel).* (2019) 12:118. doi: 10.3390/ph12030118
39. Knight JS, Luo W, O'Dell AA, Yalavarthi S, Zhao W, Subramanian V, et al. Peptidylarginine deiminase inhibition reduces vascular damage and modulates innate immune responses in murine models of atherosclerosis. *Circ Res.* (2017) 114:947–56. doi: 10.1161/CIRCRESAHA.114.303312
40. Eilenberg W, Zagrapan B, Bleichert S, Ibrahim N, Knobl V, Brandau A, et al. Histone citrullination as a novel biomarker and target to inhibit progression of abdominal aortic aneurysms. *Transl Res.* (2021) 233:32–46. doi: 10.1016/j.trsl.2021.02.003

12

Arrhythmogenic Hearts in PKD2 Mutant Mice are Characterized by Cardiac Fibrosis, Systolic and Diastolic Dysfunctions

*Farideh Amirrad [1,2], Rajasekharreddy Pala [1], Kiumars Shamloo [1], Brian S. Muntean [3] and Surya M. Nauli [1,2]**

[1] Department of Biomedical and Pharmaceutical Sciences, Chapman University, Irvine, CA, United States, [2] Department of Medicine, University of California, Irvine, Orange, CA, United States, [3] Department of Pharmacology and Toxicology, Medical College of Georgia, Augusta University, Augusta, GA, United States

***Correspondence:**
Surya M. Nauli
nauli@chapman.edu;
snauli@uci.edu

Autosomal dominant polycystic kidney disease (PKD) is a hereditary disorder affecting multiple organs, including the heart. PKD has been associated with many cardiac abnormalities including the arrhythmogenic remodeling in clinical evaluations. In our current study, we hypothesized that *Pkd2* gene mutation results in structural and functional defects in the myocardium. The structural and functional changes of *Pkd2* mutant hearts were analyzed in the myocardial-specific *Pkd2* knockout (KO) mouse. We further assessed a potential role of TGF-b_1 signaling in the pathology of *Pkd2*-KO hearts. Hearts from age-matched 6-month-old *MyH6•Pkd2*$^{wt/wt}$ (control or wild-type) and *MyH6•Pkd2*$^{flox/flox}$ (mutant or *Pkd2*-KO) mice were used to study differential heart structure and function. Cardiac histology was used to study structure, and the "isolated working heart" system was adapted to mount and perfuse mouse heart to measure different cardiac parameters. We found that macrophage1 (M1) and macrophage 2 (M2) infiltration, transforming growth factor (TGF-b_1) and TGF-b_1 receptor expressions were significantly higher in *Pkd2*-KO, compared to wild-type hearts. The increase in the extracellular matrix in *Pkd2*-KO myocardium led to cardiac hypertrophy, interstitial and conduction system fibrosis, causing cardiac dysfunction with a predisposition to arrhythmia. Left ventricular (LV) expansion or compliance and LV filling were impaired in fibrotic *Pkd2*-KO hearts, resulted in diastolic dysfunction. LV systolic contractility and elastance decreased in fibrotic *Pkd2*-KO hearts, resulted in systolic dysfunction. Compared to wild-type hearts, *Pkd2*-KO hearts were less responsive to the pharmacological stress-test and changes in preload. In conclusion, *Pkd2*-KO mice had systolic and diastolic dysfunction with arrhythmogenic hearts.

Keywords: polycystic kidney disease, cardiovascular, fibrosis, cardiac function, inflammation

INTRODUCTION

Autosomal dominant polycystic kidney disease (PKD) is the most common hereditary renal disorder that affects 1 in 800 live births. Mutations in the *Pkd1* and *Pkd2* genes that encode membrane-associated polycystin-1 and polycystin-2, respectively, contribute to the development of cystic kidneys, which are characterized with severe renal fibrosis (1–3). Polycystin-1 is an eleven-transmembrane protein interacting with polycystin-2, a member of the transient receptor potential (TRP) protein family that forms a calcium-permeable cation channel. Polycystin-2 is a non-selective cation channel with high calcium (Ca^{2+}) permeability. The genetic mutation eventually causes kidney enlargement, deformation, renal failure, and various extra-renal manifestations (4–6).

Cardiovascular complications are a major cause of morbidity and mortality in PKD patients. Cardiovascular manifestations in PKD include hypertension (7, 8), left ventricular hypertrophy (7, 9), valvular heart disease (10), intracranial and extracranial aneurysms (11), and atrial fibrillation (11). Hypertension occurs in 50–70% of patients before any significant depletion in the glomerular filtration rate, and it occurs at an earlier age in PKD patients compared to the general population (8). Hypertension is a main early finding of PKD prior to any renal dysfunction, which can accelerate end-stage kidney disease in about 60 percent of PKD patients (12, 13).

The cardiovascular complications in PKD, including hypertension and cardiac dysfunction, are thought to be secondary to polycystic kidneys. However, recent studies indicate that alterations in the polycystins expression directly affect the cardiomyocyte, endothelial and vascular smooth muscles functions, which could be responsible for cardiovascular disease (14). Polycystin-1 and–2 have been proposed to function as pressure sensors within the cardiovascular system (15). Polycystin-1 and–2 function as mechanosensory proteins in the cardiomyocytes to govern cardiomyocyte contractility (16–18). Both polycystins play a role in intracellular calcium homeostasis by interacting with the ryanodine receptor, which induces calcium release from the endoplasmic reticulum in the heart (19).

Left ventricular hypertrophy (LVH) is another cardiovascular complication commonly measured in clinical studies using echocardiography in PKD patients (9, 20). LVH is a significant and independent risk factor for cardiovascular morbidity and mortality, and it is associated with poor prognosis in PKD patients. The presence of LVH affects clinical outcomes, with increased risk of atrial or ventricular arrhythmia (21), systolic and diastolic dysfunction (22, 23), congestive heart failure (24), cardiovascular mortality (21), and sudden cardiac death (21). LVH has a high prevalence in PKD patients with hypertension (7) or even in non-hypertensive PKD patients (25). In extensive echocardiographic analyses, LVH is predicted to be associated with left ventricular fibrosis (9, 26). Cardiac fibrosis is a scarring process in the cardiac muscle with collagen deposition, fibroblast activation, and fibroblasts differentiation to myofibroblasts (27).

Our current studies examined the hypothesis that *Pkd2* gene mutation resulted in structural and functional heart defects. We studied fibrosis and fibrotic pathways in the cardiac tissues of *Pkd2* mutant mouse model, and the effect of *Pkd2* gene mutation on cardiac function was studied using an isolated working heart apparatus.

RESULTS

To identify any abnormality in the structure and function of PKD hearts, transgenic heart-specific mice were used throughout the studies unless indicated. The *MyH6•Pkd2 mutant*$^{wt/wt}$ mice were used as control or wild-type (WT), and *MyH6•Pkd2 mutant*$^{flox/flox}$ was designated as mutant (*Pkd2*-KO).

The *Pkd2*-KO Hearts Were Characterized With Hypertrophy, Cardiac Fibrosis, and Fibrotic Conduction System

The most apparent phenotype in the *Pkd2*-KO hearts was hypertrophy and interstitial fibrosis. The *Pkd2*-KO left ventricular (LV) myocardial thickness (**Figures 1A,B**) and heart-to-body-weight ratio (**Figure 1C**) were significantly increased in *Pkd2*-KO compared to control WT hearts. The extensive diffuse and reactive interstitial fibrosis of LV were significantly higher in *Pkd2*-KO, compared to WT hearts (**Figures 1D,E**). The size of LV myocardiocytes was significantly larger in *Pkd2*-KO than WT hearts (**Figures 1F,G**), supporting the myocyte hypertrophy in *Pkd2*-KO hearts. The sinoatrial node (SAN) and atrioventricular node (AVN) were also studied to examine fibrosis in the cardiac conduction system in *Pkd2*-KO mice. Upregulation of fatty and fibrotic tissues was observed in SAN and surrounding tissues in *Pkd2*-KO mice (**Figure 2A**). Although significant fibrosis was detected in SAN, fibrosis was not statistically significant in AVN between *Pkd2*-KO and WT hearts (**Figure 2B**). Because no significant fibrosis was found in AVN, cell numbers were further analyzed (**Figure 3**). AVN was identified by both its position within the heart and localization of hyperpolarization-activated cyclic nucleotide-gated channel 4 (HCN4), which is known to localize in heart conduction systems. AVN significantly had a lower cell number in *Pkd2*-KO than WT hearts.

Because heart conduction systems including SAN and AVN have an important role in electro-cardiac propagation (28, 29), electrocardiac properties were further analyzed in *Pkd2*-KO mice. The heart rate based on the *in vivo* electrocardiogram (ECG) was 583 ± 5 beats per minute for the WT mice and 625 ± 10 beats per minute for *Pkd2*-KO mice; we did not observe an apparent irregularity in ECG (**Figure 4A**). In order to evaluate the electrical activity of the heart in the absence of neurohumoral effects, we obtained an *ex vivo* ECG from isolated hearts (**Figure 4B**). Without neurohumoral effects, WT hearts showed a regular rhythm with 125 ± 20 beats per minute, and the *Pkd2*-KO hearts had arrhythmic heart rate of 127 ± 22 beats per minute evidence from atrial fibrillation or atrioventricular block characterized by irregular R-R intervals. Cardiac arrhythmia was also evidence in *Pkd2*-KO hearts at higher preloads.

Based on these analyses, our studies indicated that the *Pkd2*-KO hearts were hypertrophied with interstitial fibrosis and abnormal SAN and AVN. The impact of cardiac and conduction system fibrosis might thus result in arrhythmogenic hearts in *Pkd2*-KO mice.

The *Pkd2*-KO Hearts Had Abnormal Systolic and Diastolic Functions

The heart-specific *Pkd2* mutant knockout did not show any behavior issue, at least not within the end-point of our studies at 6-months of age. However, because these mice had cardiac hypertrophy and fibrosis (**Figure 1**), heart functions were

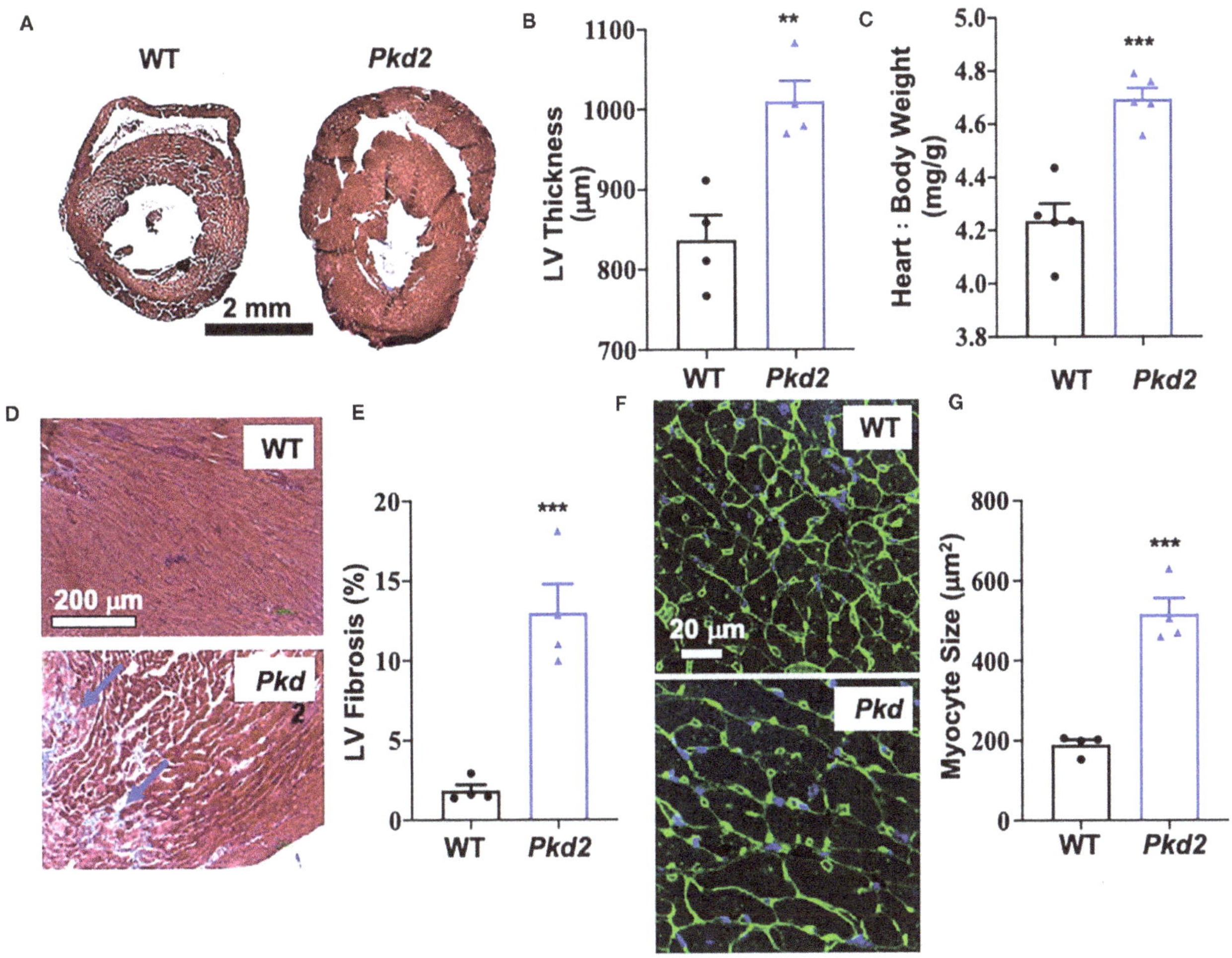

FIGURE 1 | The hearts from *Pkd2*-KO mice are characterized with hypertrophy and fibrosis. **(A–C)** Masson's trichrome staining was used to analyzed hearts from wild-type (WT) and *Pkd2*-KO (*Pkd2*) mice. Representative of left ventricular thickness (hypertrophy) is shown **(A)** and quantified **(B,C)**. **(D,E)** Left ventricular (LV) fibrosis is analyzed; arrows indicate fibrosis **(D)**. LV fibrosis was quantified **(E)**. Data show a significant increase in LV myocardial hypertrophy and fibrosis in *Pkd2*-KO compared to WT mice. Fibrosis revealed by trichrome cooperation in the tissue was quantified with binary masking of the blue-color image **(D,E)**. WGA staining was used for cell surface staining and cell size measurement. Representative of LV cardiomyocyte size (hypertrophy) is shown **(F)** and quantified **(G)**. $N = 4$ mice for each WT and *Pkd2*-KO group at age matched of 6 months old. $^{**}p < 0.01$; $^{***}p < 0.001$.

evaluated independently from the autonomic neuronal system by analyzing the left ventricular pressure-volume relationship (PV loop). PV loop allows a more precise analysis of heart functions by plotting the changes in left ventricular pressure and volume during each cardiac cycle. In order to quantify the changes in heart functions during physiologic stresses, LV parameters in both WT and *Pkd2*-KO were further evaluated in response to adrenaline (4 μg/L) or diltiazem (0.08 μg/L; **Figure 5A**). As expected, while adrenaline increased heart rate and contractility via β_1-receptors, diltiazem had a negative inotropic and negative chronotropic effects in both WT and *Pkd2*-KO hearts (**Supplementary Table 1**). The end-systolic pressure volume relationship (ESPVR) is a relationship between LV pressure (LVP) and volume (LVV) at the end of the systole, and the ESPVR is considered a marker for LV systolic contractile function and elastance (30–32). Our results demonstrated that the LV ESPVR, stroke volume (SV), and ejection fraction (EF) didn't change significantly after adrenaline or diltiazem in *Pkd2*-KO hearts (**Figure 5B**), which could be a result of decreased heart muscle contractility due to fibrosis and systolic dysfunction of LV. Despite no changes in the ESPVR, SV, and EF in *Pkd2*-KO hearts, the cardiac output (CO) was significantly altered by adrenaline or diltiazem. Importantly, the CO in responses to the pharmacological agents was significantly less in *Pkd2*-KO than WT hearts primarily due to contractility dysfunction in *Pkd2*-KO hearts. The LV Pmax (maximum pressure) and LV ESP (end-systolic pressure) were higher in *Pkd2*-KO hearts before and after adrenaline and diltiazem, which could be due to LV fibrosis, stiffness, structural changes, and narrow LV chamber (**Supplementary Table 1**).

Preload is used to express EDV (end-diastolic volume); therefore, the higher the preload is, the greater the EDV is.

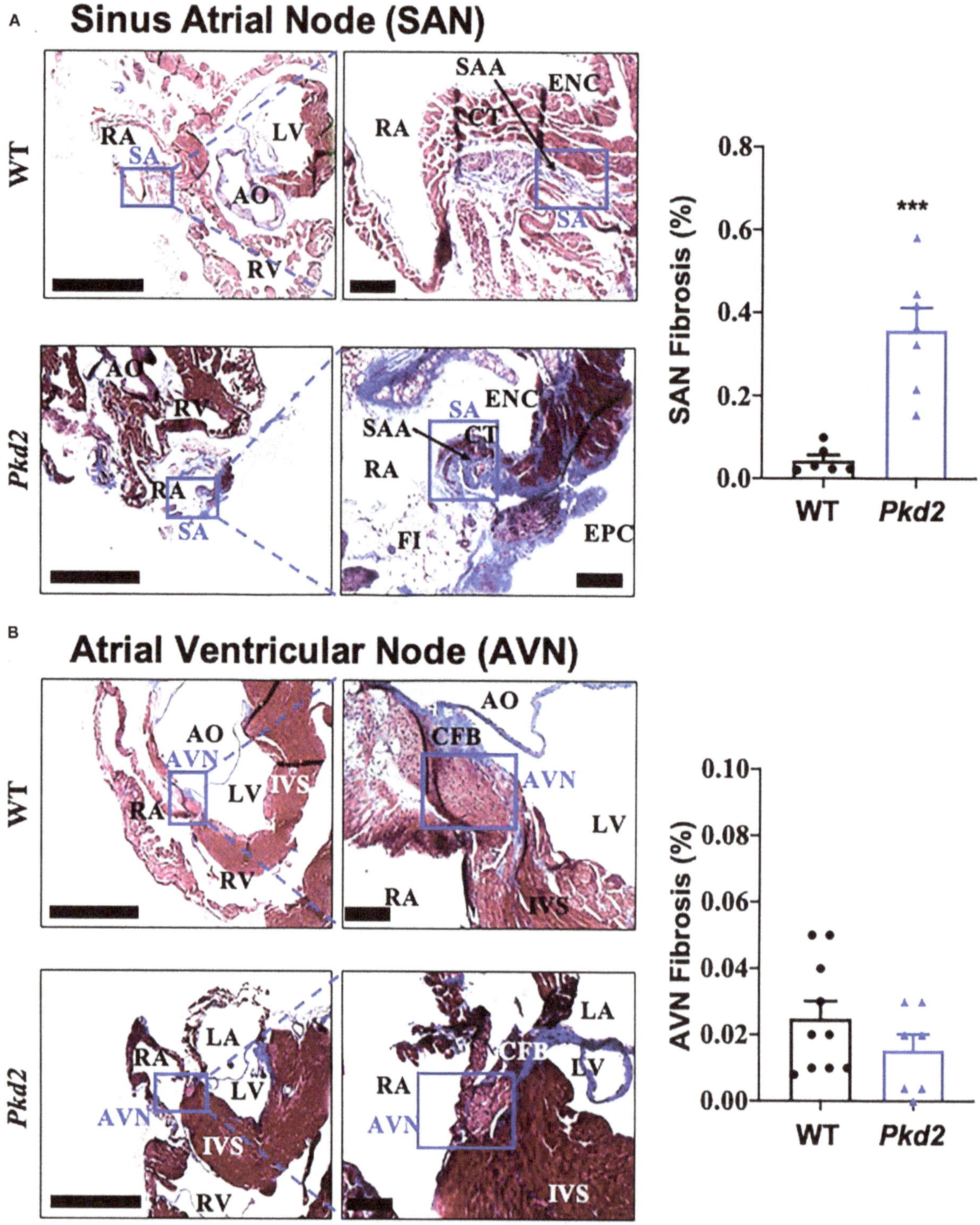

FIGURE 2 | The sinoatrial node (SAN) *Pkd2*-KO mice are characterized with fibrosis and fatty infiltration. Masson's trichrome staining was performed in wild-type (WT) and *Pkd2*-KO (*Pkd2*) mouse hearts. **(A)** A significant increase of fibrotic tissue is seen in SAN of right atrium in PKD mouse compared to WT. Boxes indicated SAN, and the left panel is further magnified and shown in the right panel. **(B)** No significant difference of fibrotic tissue is detected in AVN of right atrium in *Pkd2*-KO mouse. Boxes indicated AVN, and the left panel is further magnified and shown in the right panel. AO, aorta; AVN, atrioventricular node; CFB, central fibrous body; CT, Crista terminalis; ENC, endocardium; EPC, epicardium; FI, fatty infiltration; IVS, interventricular septum; LV, left ventricle; RA, right atrium; RV, right ventricle; SA, sinoatrial node; SAA, sinoatrial artery. Scale Bar = 20 mm. *N* = 6–10 mice for each WT and *Pkd2*-KO group at age matched of 6 months old. $^{***}p < 0.001$.

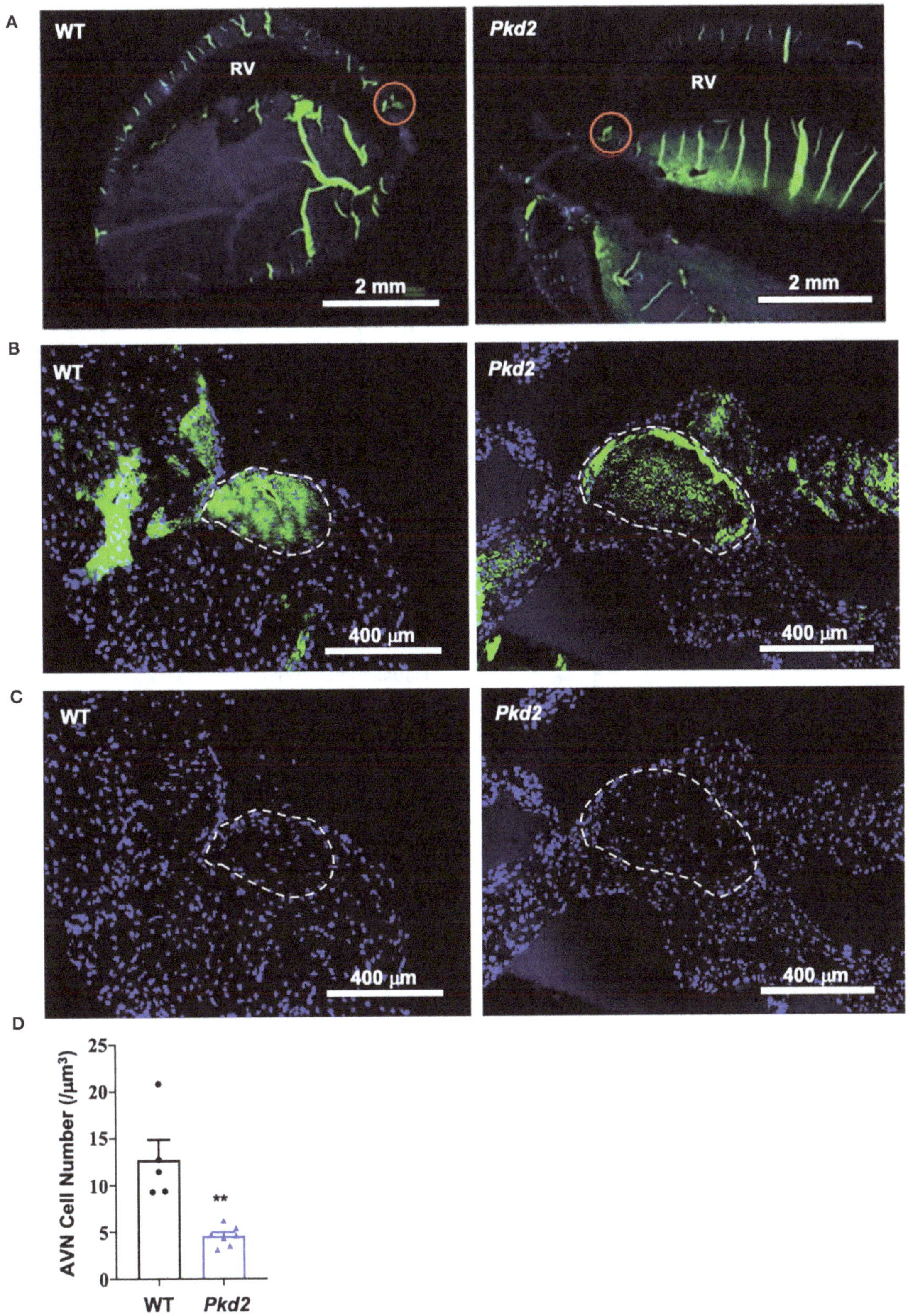

FIGURE 3 | Cell number is decreased in *Pkd2*-KO mouse atrioventricular node. **(A)** Heart tissues were stained with anti-HCN4 antibody used as a marker for the myocardial conduction system (green staining). Atrioventricular node (AVN) is identified by both location and HCN4-postive staining indicated by the red circles; RV, right ventricle. **(B)** The AVN is next identified as region of interest. **(C)** Number of cell nucleus (DAPI; blue staining) is counted. **(D)** Data reveal a significantly lower number of cells in AVN of *Pkd2*-KO mouse hearts. $N = 5$ mice for each WT and *Pkd2*-KO group at age matched of 6 months old. $^{**}p < 0.01$.

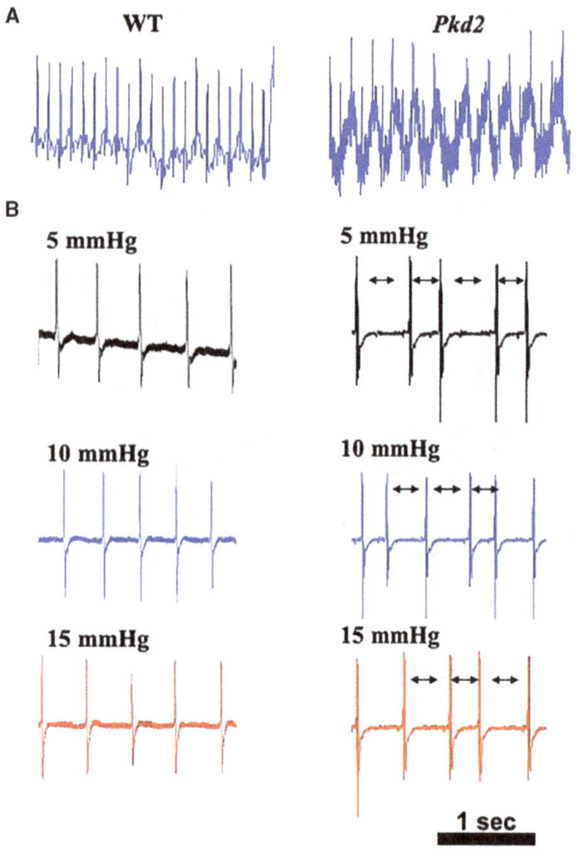

FIGURE 4 | The hearts from *Pkd2*-KO mice with no autonomic input have irregular beats. **(A)** Representatives of *in vivo* electrocardiogram (ECG) are shown with averaged frequency of 540–600 beats/min in wild-type (WT) and *Pkd2*-KO (*Pkd2*) mice. **(B)** Representatives of *ex vivo* ECG with no autonomic input are shown with different preloads of 5, 10, and 15 mmHg. The *Pkd2*-KO heart ECG shows irregular heartbeat with normal QRS shape. All ECG from *Pkd2*-KO showed irregular R-R intervals (arrows). N = 3–4 mice for each WT and *Pkd2*-KO age-matched 6 months old.

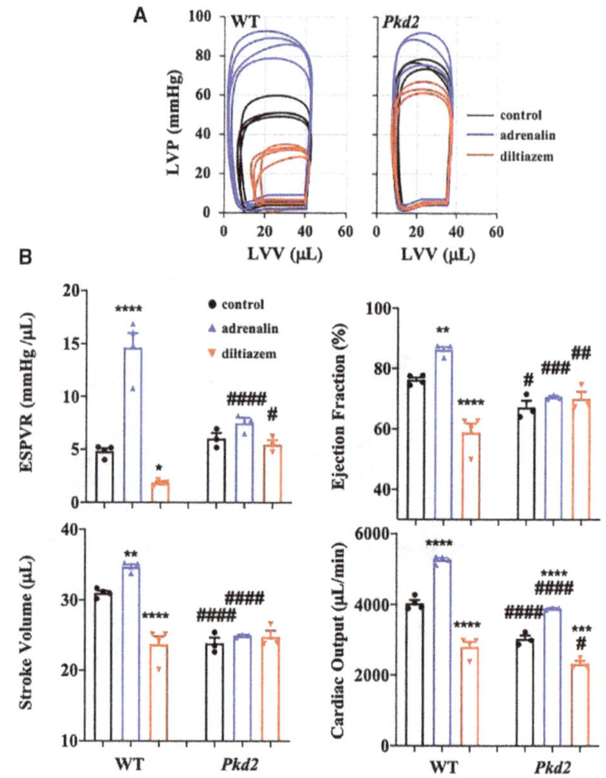

FIGURE 5 | The cardiac function of *Pkd2*-KO mice is not responsive on changes in cardiac stresses. **(A)** Individual graphs of the relationship between left ventricle pressure (LVP) and left ventricle volume (LVV) heart function are shown before and after injection of adrenaline (4 mg/L) and diltiazem (0.08 mg/L) in wild-type (WT) and *Pkd2*-KO (Pkd2) hearts. **(B)** End-systolic-pressure-volume relationship (ESPVR, an index of systolic contractility function), stroke volume, ejection fraction, and cardiac output are used to evaluate the heart responses on positive-stress (adrenaline) and negative-stress (diltiazem). N = 3–4 mice for each WT and *Pkd2*-KO age-matched 6 months old. Statistical significance between control and treatment is indicated with asterisk (*) sign; between genotypes in hash (#). *$p < 0.05$; **$p < 0.01$; ***$p < 0.001$; ****$p < 0.0001$ compared to control within the same genotype. #$p < 0.05$; ###$p < 0.001$; ####$p < 0.0001$ compared to the corresponding WT.

EDV depends on left ventricular compliance during diastole. The 5, 10, and 15 mmHg preload pressures were therefore used to study EDV and other cardiac functions (**Figure 6A**). In *Pkd2*-KO mice, the EDV decreased and did not change with increasing preload due to abnormal LV expansion or compliance and filling impairment in the fibrotic hearts (**Supplementary Table 2**). Decreased EDV subsequently led to decrease in SV and CO significantly in *Pkd2*-KO compared to WT hearts (**Figure 6B**). Furthermore, dP/dt_{min} which is a valuable marker for diastolic function (25) was significantly decreased in *Pkd2*-KO than WT hearts, indicating *Pkd2*-KO hearts had a diastolic failure due to compliance and filling impairment. Finally, the ESPVR was significantly higher in *Pkd2*-KO than the WT hearts in all preloads (**Figure 6B**). The steep and leftward of ESPVR slope was most likely not due to the improved myocardial function, but it was due to a narrow chamber in the hypertrophic and fibrotic LV. In *Pkd2*-KO hearts, the EF could not compensate in response to different preloads due to abnormal contractility in the fibrotic LV. Higher preload did not affect *ex vivo* ECG in either rhythmic WT or arrhythmic *Pkd2*-KO hearts. The *ex vivo* heart rate was also not significantly altered by higher preloads in both mice (**Figure 4B, Supplementary Table 1**).

The *Pkd1* mutant myocytes have been previously shown to have abnormal contractile calcium (16, 33). To investigate if it was also the case in our *Pkd2* mutant, we used lentivirus shRNA knockdown system to examine the effects of *Pkd2* knockdown (KD) in contractility and calcium. The contractile efficacy in myocytes was calculated by measuring the changes in muscle displacement (cell shortening) for each myocyte beat. The infection and blocking efficiencies of different *Pkd2* shRNAs were first verified in a kidney cell line and were further examined in primary cultured myocytes (**Supplementary Figure 1**). The *Pkd2* shRNA-D was selected and used, because it

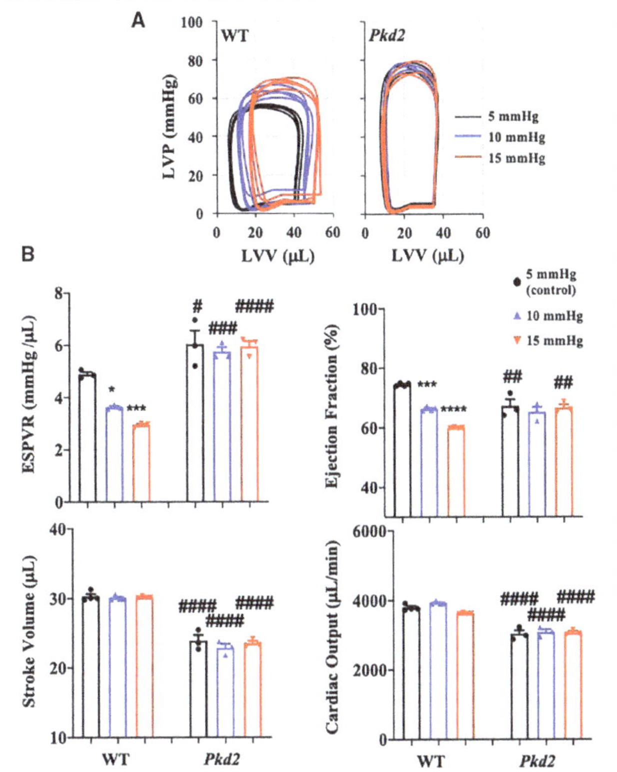

FIGURE 6 | The cardiac function of *Pkd2*-KO mice is not responsive on changes in preloads. **(A)** Individual graphs of pressure-volume loop show effects of different preloads of 5, 10, and 15 mmHg on heart function. **(B)** End-systolic-pressure-volume relationship (ESPVR, an index of systolic contractility function), stroke volume, ejection fraction, and cardiac output are used to measure heart functions in response to different pre-load levels. *N* =3–4 mice for each WT and PKD age-matched 6 months old. Statistical significance between control and treatment is indicated with asterisk (*) sign; between genotypes in hash (#). $^{*}p < 0.05$; $^{***}p < 0.001$; $^{****}p < 0.0001$; $^{\#}p < 0.05$; $^{\#\#}p < 0.01$; $^{\#\#\#}p < 0.001$; $^{\#\#\#\#}p < 0.0001$.

showed the highest knockdown efficiency. The myocyte contractions and calcium oscillations in *Pkd2* knockdown myocytes occurred more frequently than in control myocytes (**Supplementary Figure 2; Supplementary Videos 1, 2**). Further, the intracellular contractile calcium levels from *Pkd2*-KD myocytes were significantly lower than those from the control. The *Pkd2*-KD myocytes consistently and significantly showed a decrease in contractility. We also confirmed the knockdown studies in cardiomyocytes using a mouse model with complete *Pkd2* knockout (**Supplementary Figure 3; Supplementary Videos 3, 4**). Mouse *Pkd2* knockout cardiomyocytes were characterized by increased contractile oscillation frequency, decreased contractile calcium and dampened contractile strength.

Fibrotic Pathways Were Activated in Macrophage Infiltrated *Pkd2* Mutant Hearts

The contractile calcium and contractility were abnormal in single *Pkd2*-KO myocytes (**Supplementary Figures 2, 3**), and the ESPVR and SV among others were functionally impaired in *Pkd2*-KO hearts (**Figures 4–6**). Together with the arrhythmogenic characterization of *Pkd2*-KO hearts (**Figure 4**), we speculated that interstitial and SAN fibrosis together with hypertrophy and abnormal contractile calcium could play important roles in *Pkd2*-KO hearts, leading to impaired cardiac functions (**Figures 1, 2**).

To examine if/how fibrosis pathways were activated, TGF-β_1 expression in the circulating plasma and heart itself was analyzed with ELISA. While no difference was observed in the plasma level of TGF-β_1, ELISA quantifications showed a significant increase of TGF-β_1 in *Pkd2*-KO compared to WT hearts (**Figure 7A**). ELISA result was further supported by the Western blot data, which showed a significant increase in TGF-β_1 expression level in *Pkd2*-KO compared to WT hearts (**Figure 7B**). We subsequently evaluated TGF-β_1 receptor expression in the WT and *Pkd2*-KO hearts. The expression level of TGF-β_1 receptor was significantly higher in *Pkd2*-KO than WT hearts (**Figure 7C**). To study the downstream effect of TGF-β_1, we also evaluated phosphorylated-Smad3 (pSmad3), total-Smad3 (tSmad3), and β-catenin expression levels in the hearts. Our results showed higher expressions of pSmad3, tSmad3, and β-catenin in WT compared to *Pkd2*-KO hearts (**Figures 7D,E, Supplementary Figure 4**). While pSmad3 and tSmad3 were higher in WT hearts, the fractionation study showed that pSmad3 and tSmad3 were localized in nuclear fraction of *Pkd2*-KO myocytes (**Supplementary Figure 5**).

To confirm the Western blot data, immunohistochemistry studies were performed to evaluate TGF-β_1 and TGF-β_1 receptor expressions. Consistent to our immunoblot results, expressions of both TGF-β_1 and TGF-β_1 receptors were significantly higher in *Pkd2*-KO compared to WT hearts (**Figures 8A,B**). The expression levels of pSmad3 and β-catenin were also analyzed with immunofluorescence studies. Consistent with our Western blot data, expressions of both pSmad3 and β-catenin in cytosol were significantly lower in *Pkd2*-KO compared to WT hearts (**Figures 9A,B**). The nucleus-to-cytosol ratio of both pSmad3 and β-catenin were significantly higher in *Pkd2*-KO than WT hearts, indicating greater the nuclear localizations of pSmad3 and β-catenin in *Pkd2*-KO hearts.

Because the *Pkd2*-KO hearts are characterized with a higher TGF-β_1 expression, we next analyzed a potential inflammation in the *Pkd2*-KO hearts. We investigated potential infiltration in heart tissues by macrophage M1 and M2, which is known to be a local source for TGF-β_1 (34). The immunofluorescence analyses revealed that macrophage M1 and M2 infiltration was significantly higher in the mouse *Pkd2*-KO compared to WT hearts (**Figures 10A,B**).

DISCUSSIONS

Cardiovascular complications remain a major cause of mortality and morbidity in patients with autosomal dominant polycystic kidney disease (PKD) (21), but the etiopathogenesis behind the complications is not completely understood. Our current

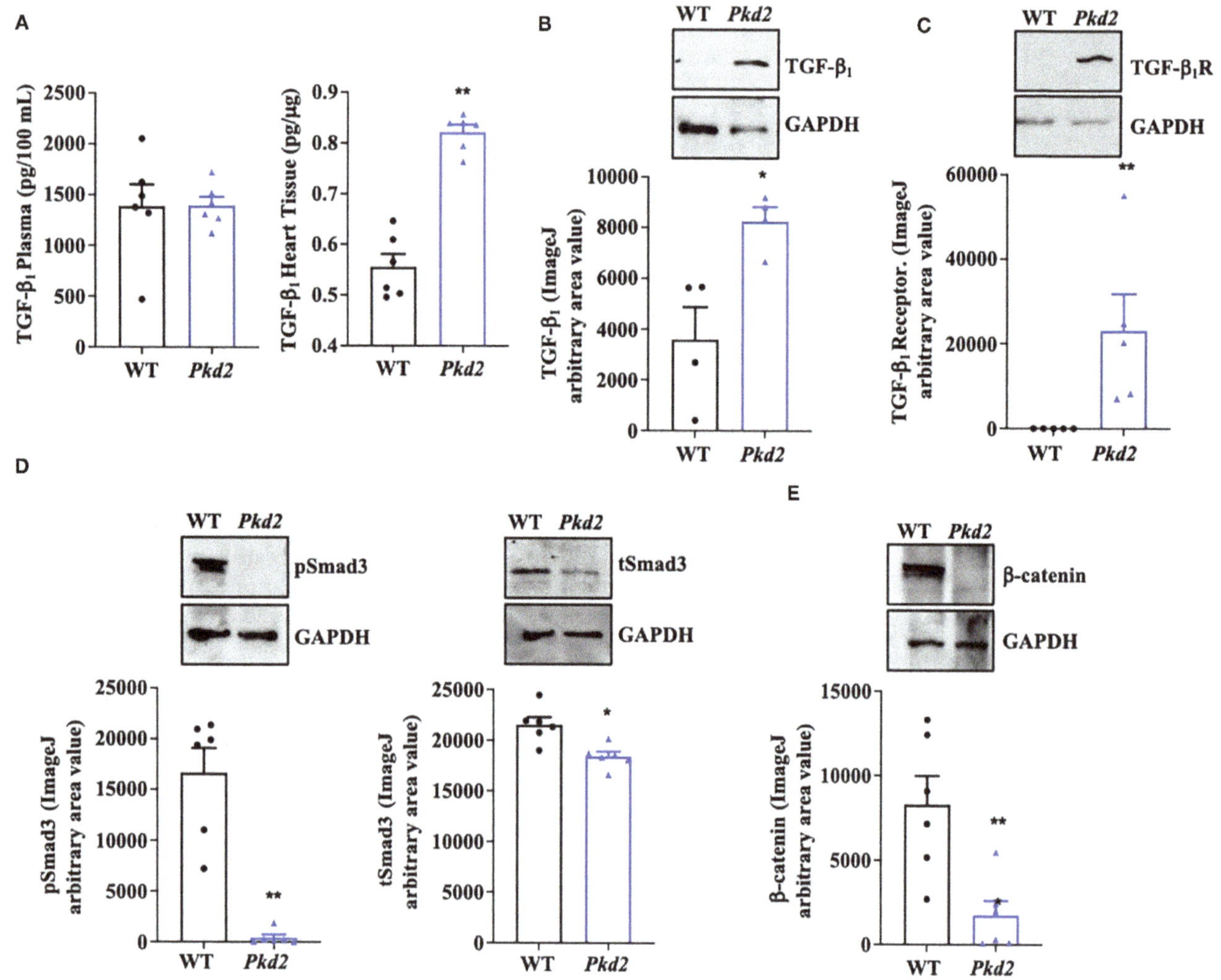

FIGURE 7 | The hearts from *Pkd2*-KO mice demonstrate abnormal fibrotic pathways. **(A)** ELISA measurements of TGF-β_1 were done in circulating plasma (left panel) and heart tissues (right panel). **(B,C)** Western blot analyses of mouse tissues show significantly higher expressions of TGF-β_1 and TGF-β_1 receptors in *Pkd2*-KO (*Pkd2*) compared to WT mice. **(D,E)** Western blot analyses of mouse tissues show significantly higher expressions of tSMAD3, pSmad3, and β-catenin in WT compared to *Pkd2*-KO mice. $N = 4$–6 mice for each WT and PKD age-matched 6 months old. $^*p < 0.05$; $^{**}p < 0.01$.

research focused mainly on the impact of *Pkd2* gene mutation on heart tissues and functions. Based on the structural changes in the heart tissues, we showed clear evidence of cardiac remodeling, including LV hypertrophy, and interstitial fibrosis. The *Pkd2*-KO hearts showed a scarring process and cardiac muscle fibrosis with the fatty fibrotic changes in the sinoatrial node (SAN), which could serve as the underlying risk factor for cardiac arrhythmia in PKD patients. This tissue remodeling was thus associated with arrhythmogenic heart, systolic, and diastolic dysfunctions. Our studies also pointed to the involvement of macrophages, secreting anti-inflammatory TGF-β_1, and TGF-β_1 receptor expression in the *Pkd2*-KO heart tissues, and subsequently activating SMAD and β-catenin pathways in *Pkd2*-KO hearts (**Figure 11**).

A common event in all myocardial fibrotic remodeling involves either mechanical or chemical loading in the heart (35), although fibroblast cilia have also been recently shown to involve in the process (36). The chemical loading-induced fibrosis is usually associated with activation of immune cells and inflammation, leading to the increased extracellular matrix (36). Among the inflammatory cells, the macrophages play the most extensive role in secreting factors associated with inflammation. Our data showed that the macrophage M1 and M2 significantly infiltrated *Pkd2*-KO hearts. This suggested that M1 plays an essential role in cardiac inflammation, and it might play a role in the onset or progression of fibrosis in *Pkd2*-KO hearts (37). On the other hand, M2 may involve in matrix deposition and tissue remodeling in *Pkd2*-KO hearts (37). This suggested that our *Pkd2*-KO hearts were still undergoing the inflammation process and progressing toward fibrosis, although fibrosis and remodeling could be detected and confirmed in histochemistry analyses.

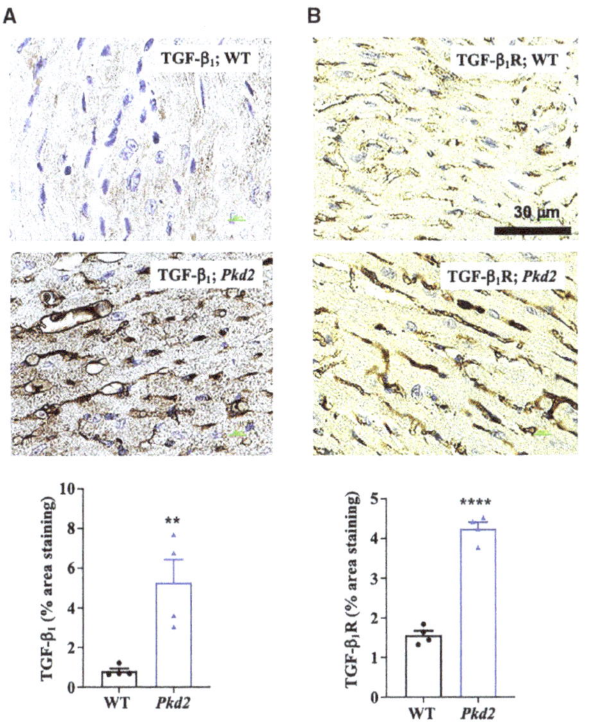

FIGURE 8 | The hearts from *Pkd2*-KO mice are characterized with upregulated fibrotic pathways. **(A,B)** Immunohistochemistry staining demonstrated a significant increase of TGF-β_1 and TGF-β_1 receptor (dark brown color) in *Pkd2*-KO (*Pkd2*) hearts compared to the wild-type (WT). A total of 8 independent slides were used for each mouse. $^{**}p < 0.01$; $^{****}p < 0.0001$.

The roles of mediators TGF-β_1, Smad, and β-catenin were next examined because they are generally known signaling pathways leading to cardiac fibrosis (35, 38–40). At least in the *Pkd2*-KO mouse model, circulating TGF-β_1 did not seem to be increased, indicating that TGF-β_1 might be restricted and localized within cardiac tissues. Of note is that not only TGF-β_1 but also its receptor had increased in expressions and might have critical roles in the cardiac fibrosis. These studies were supported by immunoblotting, ELISA, and immunohistology studies. Both pSmad3 and β-catenin were significantly localized in the nucleus of *Pkd2*-KO myocytes, indicating a significant nuclear translocation and fibrotic signaling activation (38, 41). Immunofluorescent studies and immunoblots in mouse tissues indicated a lower total expression of pSmad3, tSMAD3, or β-catenin in *Pkd2*-KO hearts in cytosol. We further evaluated tSMAD3 and pSMAD3 expressions in the nucleus. Results indicated a higher nuclear localization of pSMAD3 in the *Pkd2*-KO compared to WT hearts. Because of the low cytosolic expression of pSmad3 or β-catenin in *Pkd2*-KO hearts, we further speculated that this might be a compensatory mechanism by the cardiac tissues to slow down the fibrotic process in *Pkd2*-KO tissues.

Given a strong pathogenesis association between cardiac fibrosis and myocardial dysfunction (42), we decided to study the heart functions using the *Pkd2*-KO mouse model (**Supplementary Tables 1, 2**). An isolated working heart system is commonly used to gather precise LV pressure-volume relations (PV loop) independent of systemic neuronal effect. PV loop is a powerful tool that provides us qualitative and quantitative measurements of the heart functions. PV loop provides many hemodynamic parameters that are not measurable by other methods, including elastance, contractility, and stroke work. The *Pkd2*-KO fibrotic hearts negatively affected expansion, compliance, and filling of LV as indicated by the end-diastolic volume (EDV). With less volume in the heart at the end of diastole (EDV), the stroke volume (SV) and cardiac output (CO) also decreased significantly. On the other hand, dP/dt_{min}, a valuable marker for diastolic function, decreased in *Pkd2*-KO hearts. Based on these results, *Pkd2*-KO hearts were further confirmed to have diastolic failure due to compliance and filling impairment. It is known that oxygen extraction during diastole is higher than during systolic interval (43); perivascular fibrosis can therefore restrict the oxygen diffusion during diastole, which may further worsen diastolic function (43).

The end-systolic pressure-volume relationship (ESPVR) is considered a marker for left ventricular contractility and elastance (30–32). In *Pkd2*-KO hearts, the LV ESPVR did not change significantly after adrenaline and diltiazem injection due to fibrosis, decreased heart muscle contractility and systolic dysfunction of the LV. This was also supported by the results from the LV end-systolic volume (ESV), stroke volume (SV), and ejection fraction (EF). Moreover, the ESPVR was also analyzed in different preloads. The ESPVR with steep and leftward slope was significantly higher in *Pkd2*-KO hearts in all preloads, indicating a narrow chamber in the hypertrophic and fibrotic ventricle. In addition, the contractile calcium was significantly lower, resulting in weak contraction in *Pkd2* mutant myocytes (18).

Fibrotic tissue forms a barrier between cardiomyocytes, which can result not only in systolic dysfunction but also in electric conduction impairment (43). Increased fibrosis within and around SAN can cause structural destruction and dysfunction, leading to arrhythmia (44, 45). While no apparent arrhythmia was observed in the *Pkd2*-KO mouse model *in vivo*, the *Pkd2*-KO hearts were susceptible to arrhythmia when hearts were isolated away from neuronal input in the *ex vivo* studies. Atrial fibrillation (AF) or AV block was seen in isolated *Pkd2*-KO hearts. While the role of cardiac fibrosis is well-known in both atrial and ventricular arrhythmias, SAN dysfunction is a common finding in AF patients, particularly with advanced atrial fibrosis with SAN involvement (44). We also looked at HCN4, an ion channel responsible for the slow Na^+ current in the heart conduction system. HCN-positive nodal cells were significantly decreased in the atria-ventricular node of *Pkd2*-KO hearts. Of note is that HCN4 channels are required for generating slow current, which is responsible for spontaneous depolarization of the specialized myocytes of the heart pacemaker (46).

In conclusion, our studies indicated fibrosis in *Pkd2*-KO hearts. Fibrosis in the conduction system might results in arrhythmia, and thus the PKD patients might be susceptible to atrial fibrillation (12) and potential arrhythmia-induced sudden cardiac death (47). Our studies implicated that cardiac fibrosis was also contributed to systolic and diastolic dysfunctions,

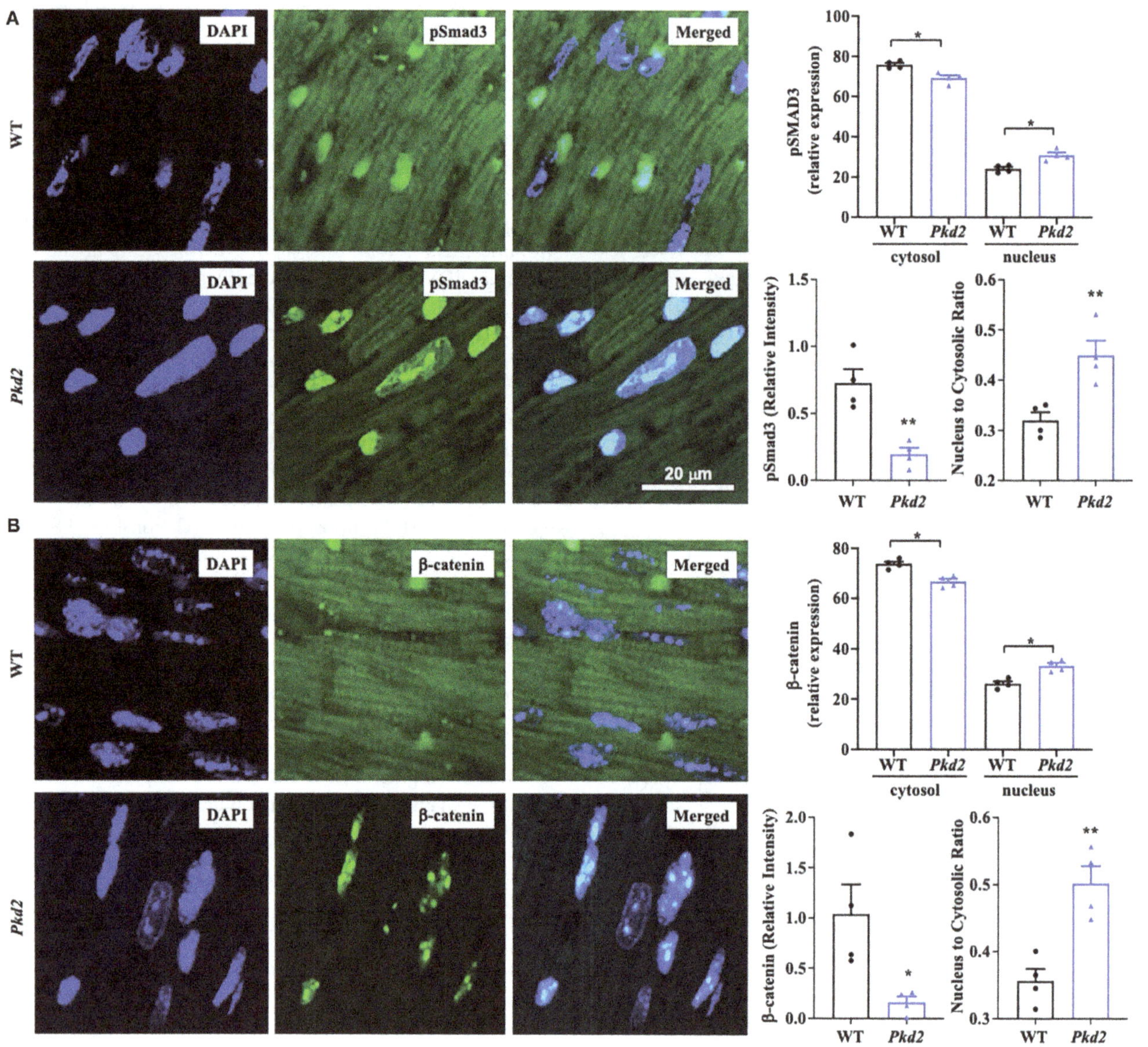

FIGURE 9 | The hearts from *Pkd2*-KO mice are characterized with a significant increase in nuclear localization of pSMAD3 and β-catenin. **(A,B)** Immunofluorescence staining of pSmad3 **(A)** or β-catenin **(B)** revealed a significant increase in nuclear localization and nucleus to cytoplasm ratio of pSmad3 or β-catenin in *Pkd2*-KO (*Pkd2*) compared to wild-type (WT) hearts. $N = 4$ mice for each group. A total of 8 independent slides were used for each mouse. $^*p < 0.05$; $^{**}p < 0.01$.

which are seen in PKD patients (48). A potential prospect for therapeutic manipulation might therefore involve cardiac inflammation induced by TGF-b1.

MATERIALS AND METHODS

Throughout our studies, mice were used to examine the structural and functional changes of the heart. Our animal studies were approved by the Chapman University Institutional Animal Care and Use Committee (IACUC# 2020-1132 and PHS# D17-00960). The *Pkd2*$^{flox/flox}$ mice were previously given from Dr. Jing Zhou's laboratory at Harvard Medical School (49, 50); these mice were bred with heart-specific transgenic mice *MyH6* (Jackson Laboratory; stock#011038). *MyH6•Pkd2*$^{wt/wt}$ mouse is denoted as wild-type (WT; control), and *MyH6•Pkd*$^{flox/flox}$ is designated as mutant or *Pkd2*-KO. Heart structure, function and electrocardiogram (ECG) were examined and measured at 6-months-old of age. Both male and female mice were used, and sex was identified to be an independent covariate to heart functions.

Masson's Trichrome Staining

To evaluate myocadiac fibrosis and hypertrophy, heart tissues were collected and fixed in 10% formalin. The tissues were dehydrated in ethanol and xylene, embedded in liquid paraffin, and cut with a thickness of 5 μm. Cut sections were stained with

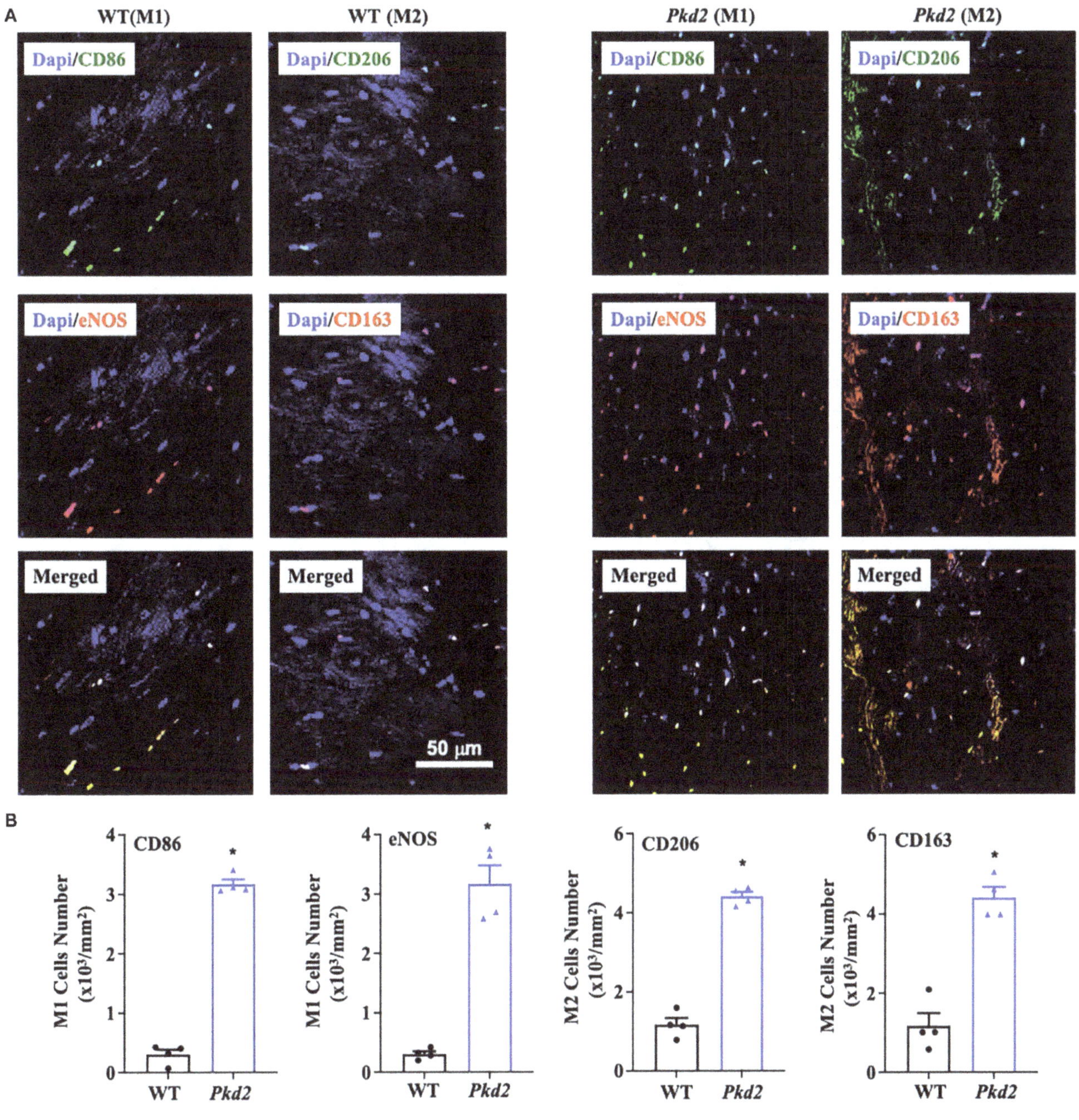

FIGURE 10 | The hearts from *Pkd2*-KO mice are significantly infiltrated by macrophages. **(A,B)** Immunofluorescence staining revealed a significant higher number of macrophages M1 and M2. Image was quantified by binary masking of the red or green fluorescence image. $N = 4$ mice for each WT and *Pkd2*-KO age-matched 6 months old. $^*p < 0.05$.

Masson's trichrome kit (Cat# 25088-1; *Polysciences, Inc.*), and images were visualized and captured using KEYENCE BZ-X710 or Nikon Eclipse Ti microscope.

Immunofluorescence Studies

To examine protein localization and expression, the formalin-fixed tissues were de-paraffinized. After deparaffinization and dehydration of paraffin sections, heat-induced epitope retrieval was performed using a pressure cooker and sodium citrate buffer (10 mM sodium citrate, 0.05% tween-20, pH 6.0). Once boiled, slides were transferred from phosphate-buffered saline (PBS) to the sodium citrate buffer in pressure cooker for 10 min, and then cooled to room temperature for 30 min. To permeabilize the tissues, slides were washed with permeabilization buffer containing 0.3% triton-100 in PBS for 10 min. After permeabilization, slides were blocked with 5% bovine serum albumin and 0.1% triton-100 in PBS solution and subsequently processed to detect specific

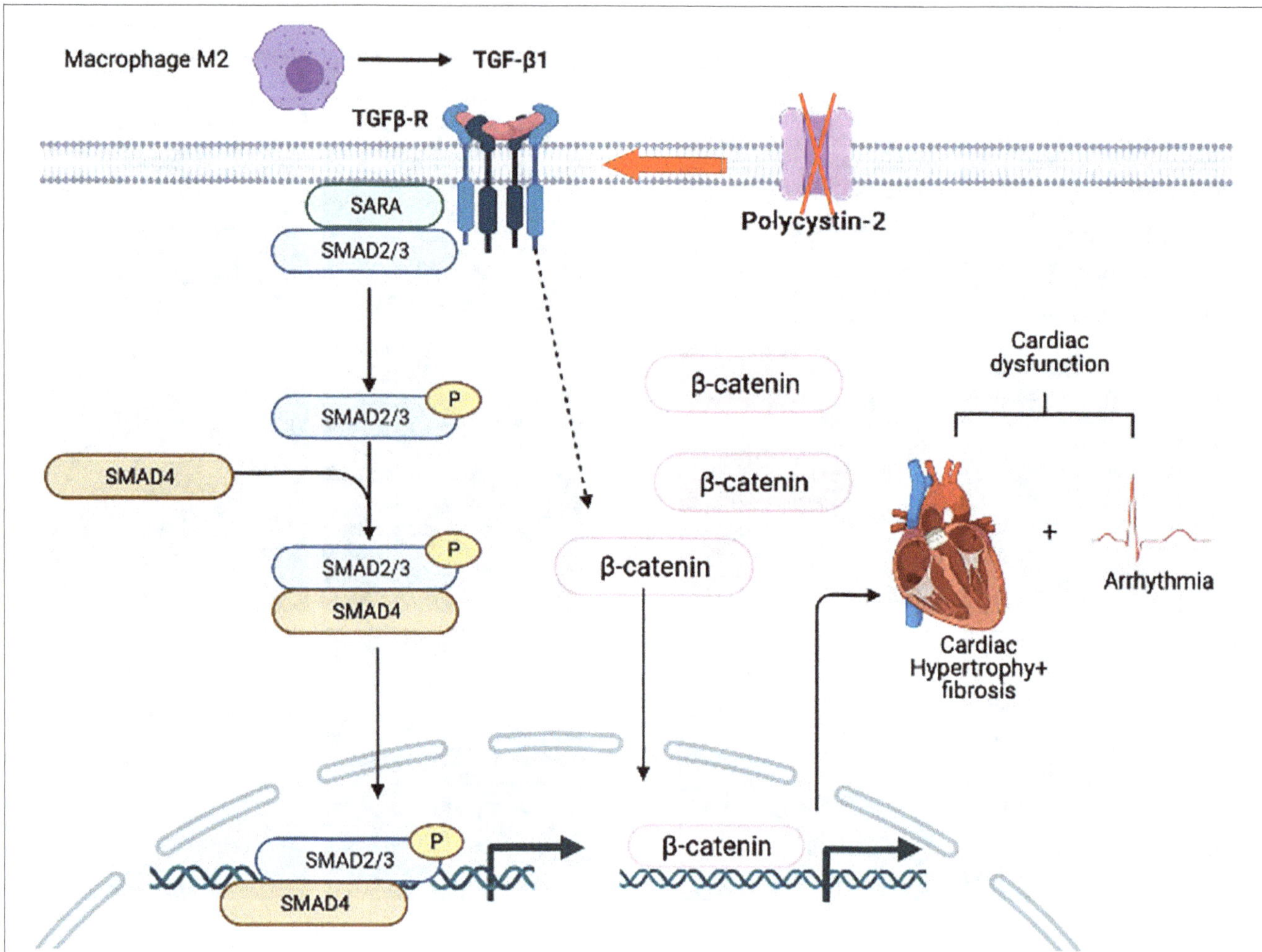

FIGURE 11 | Hypothetical diagram summarizes the pathogeneses of PKD hearts. We hypothesize that hearts from *Pkd2*-KO mice are characterized by the overexpression of TGF-β_1 receptor. Local TGF-β_1 secretion by infiltrating macrophages further exacerbates the activation of fibrotic pathways resulting in hypertrophy and interstitial fibrosis. Subsequent activation of TGF-β_1 receptor results in the activation of pSMAD3 and b-catenin in the myocytes. The fibrosis in the sinoatrial node and surrounding tissue can results in arrhythmogenic heart. All of which will cause systolic and diastolic cardiac dysfunction.

proteins. All washing steps were done three times with PBS-T (tween-20, 0.05%).

For cell surface staining and cell size measurement, tissue slides were incubated with wheat germ agglutinin (WGA) (1:1,000; Cat# FL-1021; Vectorlabs) for 20 min. To detect specialized conduction cells in the atrioventricular node, tissues were incubated with rat anti-HCN4 antibody (1:1,000; Cat# ab32675; *Abcam, Inc.*) overnight at 4°C in a humidified chamber followed with AlexaFluor-488 goat anti-rat fluorescence secondary antibody (1:500; Cat# ab6840; *Abcam, Inc*). To study fibrotic pathways, anti-β-catenin (1:50; Cat# sc-133240; *Santa Cruz, Inc.*) and anti-pSMAD3 (1:1,000; Cat# sc-517575; *Santa Cruz, Inc*) antibodies were used in the same manner as anti-HCN4 antibody followed with AlexaFluor-488 secondary goat anti-mouse antibody (1:1,000; Cat# ab150113; *Abcam, Inc*). To evaluate macrophages infiltration, tissues were stained with anti-NOS2 antibody (1:50; Cat# sc-7271; *Santa Cruz, Inc*), and anti-CD-86 (1:50; Cat# sc-52448; *Santa Cruz, Inc*) for macrophages M1detection, anti-CD163 antibody (1:50; sc-20066; *Santa Cruz, Inc*), and anti-CD-206 (1:100; Cat# ab91992; *Signaling, Inc*) antibodies for macrophages M2 detection, followed with horse anti-mouse antibody Texas Red (1:1,000; Cat# NC9634446; *Thermo Fisher Scientific*), and AlexaFluor-488 goat anti-rat fluorescence secondary antibody (1:500; Cat# ab6840; *Abcam, Inc*), AlexaFluor-488 secondary goat anti-mouse antibody (1:1,000; Cat# ab150113; *Abcam, Inc*), and AlexaFluor-488 goat anti-rabbit fluorescence secondary antibody (1:500; Cat# ab91992; *Signaling, Inc*). In all cases, we used 4′,6-diamidino-2-phenylindole (DAPI) as a nuclear binding dye. All images were taken with the confocal A1R$^+$ Nikon microscope (Version 4.30).

Immunohistology

To examine protein localization and expression, the formalin-fixed tissues were de-paraffinized. After deparaffinization and dehydration of paraffin sections, heat-induced epitope retrieval was performed using a pressure cooker and sodium citrate buffer

(10 mM sodium citrate, 0.05% tween-20, pH 6.0). Once boiled, slides were transferred from PBS to the sodium citrate buffer in pressure cooker for 10 min. Slides were then cooled to room temperature for 30 min, and permeabilized with permeabilization buffer containing 0.3% triton-100 in PBS for 10 min. To block endogenous peroxidase activity, slides were incubated in 3% hydrogen peroxide for 10 min and blocked with animal-free blocking solution (Cat# 15019; *Cell Signaling, Inc.*). After blocking, slides were incubated overnight at 4°C with mouse monoclonal anti-TGF-β_1 (1:50; Cat# sc-130348; *Santa Cruz, Inc.*) or rabbit polyclonal anti-TGF-β_1 receptor (1:100; Cat# ab235178; *Abcam, Inc.*) and subsequently incubated with SignalStain Boost Detection Reagent (HRP mouse; Cat# 8125; or HRP Rabbit; Cat# 8114; *Cell Signaling, Inc.*) for 30 min at room temperature. Slides were then incubated for 2–10 min with SignalStain DAB (Cat# 8059; *Cell Signaling, Inc.*), immersed in distilled H_2O, stained with hematoxylin (Cat# 14166; *Cell Signaling, Inc.*) and mounted with coverslips. All washing steps were done three times with PBS-T (tween-20, 0.05%).

Western Blot Analyses

To evaluate protein expressions, proteins were extracted from the tissues using radioimmunoprecipitation assay (RIPA) lysis buffer (Cat# 89901, *Thermo Fisher, Inc.*) containing Halt protease inhibitor cocktail (Cat# 78425, *Thermo Fisher, Inc.*). Total protein was quantified using the Bradford assay. Extracted proteins (25–50 μg) were loaded into 10% sodium dodecyl sulfate-polyacrylamide gel electrophoresis (SDS-PAGE) gel and transferred onto nitrocellulose membrane afterward. For nuclear fractionation, immunoprecipitation with anti-Histone H3 was used and loaded to the gels. The membrane was then blocked with 5% dry milk and subsequently processed to detect specific proteins using a standard method.

We used the following primary antibodies: rabbit polyclonal anti-TGF-β_1 (1:1,000; Cat# ab92486; *Abcam, Inc.*), rabbit polyclonal anti-TGF-β_1 receptor (1:1,000; Cat# ab31013; *Abcam, Inc.*), mouse monoclonal anti-β-catenin (1:100; Cat# sc-133240; *Santa Cruz, Inc.*), rabbit monoclonal pSmad3 (1:1,000; Cat# 9520s; *Cell Signaling, Inc.*), rabbit monoclonal Smad3 (1:1,000; Cat# 9523s; *Cell Signaling, Inc.*), rabbit polyclonal histone H3 (1:1,000; Cat# 9715s; *Cell Signaling, Inc.*), and anti-GAPDH (1:100; Cat# sc-365062; *Santa Cruz, Inc.*). Except for anti-GAPDH antibody which was already tagged with horseradish peroxidase (HRP), HRP-tagged secondary antibodies were used accordingly, followed with chemiluminescent substrate (Cat# 34577; *Thermo Fisher Scientific, Inc.*). Protein detection was carried out with Bio-Rad imager (ChemiDoc™ XRS+ System with Image Lab™ Software; Cat# 1708265; *Bio-Rad, Inc.*).

ShRNA Knockdown

Lentiviral vectors containing shRNA to *Pkd2* knockdown (*Origene*; pGFP-C-shLenti clone ID: TL310397) were transfected into HEK293T cells. Viral supernatants were collected and pooled at 24- and 48-h post-transfection. Primary mouse myocytes were then incubated with pseudoviral particles and 8 μg/ml polybrene for 48 h prior to analysis. Transduction efficiency was observed via GFP reporter fluorescence, and *Pkd2* knockdown was verified through Western blot analysis. The shRNA sequences used in our experiments are shown below.

Descriptions	Sequences
scrambled control	5′-TGA CCA CCC TGA CCT ACG GCG TGC AGT GC-3′
Pkd2 A	5′-TTG TGC ATC TTG ACC TAC GGC ATG ATG AG-3′
Pkd2 B	5′-TAC GGC ATG ATG AGC TCC AAT GTG TAC TA-3′
Pkd2 C	5′-TTT GAT TTC TTC CTG GCA GCC TGT GAG AT-3′
Pkd2 D	5′-GTC TGG ATT AAG CTC TTC AAA TTC ATC AA-3′

Cytosolic Calcium Measurements

To observe cytosolic calcium in cultured cardiomyocytes, cells were incubated with 10 μM fura-2AM (Invitrogen) and protected from light for 30 min. Calcium was measured by comparing fura-2 excitation at 340 nm (bound calcium) and 380 nm (free calcium). After each experiment, free cytosolic calcium was determined by perfusing ionomycin (10 μM final concentration) to obtain the maximum calcium signal followed by the addition of EGTA (2 mM final concentration) to observe the minimum calcium signal. All experiments were performed at 37°C in a heated microscope chamber.

Enzyme-Linked Immunosorbent Assay (ELISA)

To detect TGF-β_1 in the circulating plasma, blood was collected from a submandibular vein (cheek punch) using a heparinized tube. Within 30 min of collection, blood was centrifuged for 15 min at 1000 × g at 4 °C, and supernatant was collected for the ELISA assay. To detect TGF-β_1 in the heart, the heart tissues were collected and homogenized in RIPA buffer containing Halt protease inhibitor cocktail, and total protein was quantified with Bradford assay from a commercially available kit (Cat# PI23227; *ThermoFisher Scientific, Inc.*).

The TGF-β_1 level was measured using a commercially available mouse TGF-β_1 ELISA kit (Cat# LS-F5184, *LSBio, Inc.*). The assay was based on the sandwich ELISA method. Each well had been pre-coated with TGF-β_1 antibody. Tissue lysate samples were added to the wells, and the target antigen (TGF-β_1) was bound to the antibody. The unbounded proteins were washed away, and biotin-conjugated detection antibody was added, which bound to the captured antigen. Avidin-tagged HRP conjugate was added to bind with biotin. The TMB (3,3′,5,5′-tetramethylbenzidine) detection substrate was added to react with the HRP enzyme leading to color development, which was proportional to total TGF-β1 bound. A stop solution (sulfuric acid) was added to terminate the color development reaction, and the optical density of each well was measured at a wavelength of 450 nm.

Electrocardiogram (ECG) and Heart Functions

To study isolated heart functions, the 6-month-old mouse was injected with heparin (100 units; IP) to prevent blood coagulation and anesthetized with ketamine 8–10 min later (200-350 mg/kg; IP). Mouse's chest was wiped clean with water, dried, and shaved to obtain *in vivo* ECG. The ultrasonic gel was warmed to 37°C to reduce stress to the mouse. The electrodes were then placed onto the mouse's chest. One electrode was placed around the xiphoid process of the left side of (the) sternum, and the other electrode at the 4th or 5th intercostal space on the right side. The ECG reading was taken at 5-s interval.

Immediately after obtaining *in vivo* ECG, an incision was made in the mid-abdomen toward the diaphragm. The diaphragm was opened, the thoracic cage was cut bilaterally, and the heart was dissected out. Immediately after the heart dissection, the aorta was cannulated and perfused with Krebs-Ringer solution (125 mM NaCl, 2.5 mM KCl, 1.25 mM NaH2PO4, 2 mM CaCl2, 1 mM $MgCl_2$, 25 mM $NaHCO_3$, and 25 mM glucose), which was continuously bubbled with carbogen (95% O_2 and 5% CO_2) to reach a pH of 7.4 at 38.0°C.

The *ex-vivo* perfusion of the mouse's heart was performed, the left atrium was cannulated, and cardiac function parameters were recorded using the working heart system (**Supplementary Video 5**; *Emka Technology, Inc.*). This approach provided quantitative measurements and heart functions that other methods cannot measure, including elastance, contractility, and stroke work. For evaluation of cardiac electrical activity in the absence of neurohumoral factors, an *ex vivo* ECG was obtained from the software after placing ECG electrodes on the right atrium and apex of the heart. Other cardiac parameters, including left ventricle pressure (LVP), left atrial pressure (LAP), aortic pressure (AP), and aortic flow (AoF) were obtained from the software. The preload and afterload were adjusted manually as needed.

The heart's responses to the external stresses were examined with a pharmacological stress test. The stress test was performed by using epinephrine (4 μg/L) or diltiazem (0.08 μg/L). *End-systolic pressure-volume relationship* (ESPVR), left ventricle pressure maximum (LVP max), and end-systolic pressure (ESP), left ventricle end-systolic volume (LV ESV), stroke volume (SV), and ejection fraction (EF) were obtained from the software or pressure-volume analysis. In some cases, preload was adjusted from 5 mmHg to either 10 or 15 mmHg. We used preload to indicate end-diastolic volume (EDV); therefore, the higher the preload was, the greater the EDV was. Preload was changed manually on the preload reservoir graduated cylinder, located on the isolated working heart system. After increasing the preload, LV pressure max (LV Pmax), end-systolic pressure (ESP), end-diastolic pressure (EDP), end-systolic volume (ESV), end-diastolic volume (EDV), stroke volume (SV), and ejection fraction (EF) were obtained from the software data and pressure-volume analysis.

Data and Statistical Analysis

Image analyses were performed in Nikon NIS-Element for Advanced Research software (Version 4.51). This software was also used for image capture, segmentation, 3D object reconstruction, and automatic object recognition. A Photometric Coolsnap EZ CCD Monochrome Digital Camera was used to capture images with a 1392 × 1040 imaging array to resolve fine details of the images. Binary masking was used to calculate cell size, fibrosis, ventricular thickness, and image intensity for protein expression and localization based on granularity, shape, size, and pixel intensity. Quantitation of Western blots was done with the NIH Fiji ImageJ (Version 2.1). After a box of the intended proteins was drawn using the "gel" analysis function, the area under the curve was measured for the intensity of each protein band. All images were finalized on a six-core Mac Pro, 3.9 GHz to facilitate complete data extraction. Scale bars are provided in all figures and videos to indicate the actual image size.

A list of heart functions was measured or calculated using *Emka Technology* software. The software captured and recorded real-time data for electrical heart propagation, cardiac contractility, heart rate, left ventricle pressure and volume, preload, afterload, aortic pressure, and aortic outflow. These data were further used to calculate stroke volume, cardiac output, end-diastolic/systolic volume, and left atrial pressure rise and fall. Additional analyses were performed in Microsoft Excel for macOS (Version 16.48).

Our statistical analyses were performed using GraphPad Prism for macOS (Version 9.1). To compare two groups of unpaired datasets, a non-parametric student *t*-test was used with two-tail assuming no Gaussian distribution. For comparison within 3 or more groups with no matching datasets, we used non-parametric or mixed ordinary one-way ANOVA. The mean of each group was then compared with the mean of every other group using Tukey *post-hoc* multiple comparison test with multiplicity adjusted *P*-value for each comparison. $P < 0.05$ was considered significant in our studies. A more precise *P*-value was reported separately in the graphs. The total measurements and N values were also reported independently in each figure legend.

AUTHOR CONTRIBUTIONS

FA collected, analyzed data, drafted the manuscript, and oversaw the experimental progress. RP bred mice and served as a double-blind operator. KS assisted in tissue processing, working heart system, and served as another double-blind operator. BM performed calcium imaging studies. SN drafted the manuscript, designed research, and oversaw the study. All authors were participating in finalizing the manuscript.

REFERENCES

1. Zhang Y, Dai Y, Raman A, Daniel E, Metcalf J, Reif G, et al. Overexpression of TGF-beta1 induces renal fibrosis and accelerates the decline in kidney function in polycystic kidney disease. *Am J Physiol Renal Physiol.* (2020) 319:F1135–48. doi: 10.1152/ajprenal.00366.2020
2. Norman J. Fibrosis and progression of autosomal dominant polycystic kidney disease (ADPKD). *Biochim Biophys Acta.* (2011) 1812:1327–36. doi: 10.1016/j.bbadis.2011.06.012
3. Ratnam S, Nauli SM. Hypertension in autosomal dominant polycystic kidney disease: a clinical and basic science perspective. *Int J Nephrol Urol.* (2010) 2:294–308.
4. Menezes LF, Germino GG. The pathobiology of polycystic kidney disease from a metabolic viewpoint. *Nat Rev Nephrol.* (2019) 15:735–49. doi: 10.1038/s41581-019-0183-y
5. Torres VE, Harris PC. Progress in the understanding of polycystic kidney disease. *Nat Rev Nephrol.* (2019) 15:70–2. doi: 10.1038/s41581-018-0108-1
6. Bergmann C, Guay-Woodford LM, Harris PC, Horie S, Peters DJM, Torres VE. Polycystic kidney disease. *Nat Rev Dis Primers.* (2018) 4:50. doi: 10.1038/s41572-018-0047-y
7. Chapman AB, Johnson AM, Rainguet S, Hossack K, Gabow P, Schrier RW. Left ventricular hypertrophy in autosomal dominant polycystic kidney disease. *J Am Soc Nephrol.* (1997) 8:1292–7. doi: 10.1681/ASN.V881292
8. Gabow PA, Johnson AM, Kaehny WD, Kimberling WJ, Lezotte DC, Duley IT, et al. Factors affecting the progression of renal disease in autosomal-dominant polycystic kidney disease. *Kidney Int.* (1992) 41:1311–9. doi: 10.1038/ki.1992.195
9. Suwa Y, Higo S, Nakamoto K, Sera F, Kunimatsu S, Masumura Y, et al. Old-Age onset progressive cardiac contractile dysfunction in a patient with polycystic kidney disease harboring a PKD1 frameshift mutation. *Int Heart J.* (2019) 60:220–5. doi: 10.1536/ihj.18-184
10. Leier CV, Baker PB, Kilman JW, Wooley CF. Cardiovascular abnormalities associated with adult polycystic kidney disease. *Ann Intern Med.* (1984) 100:683–8. doi: 10.7326/0003-4819-100-5-683
11. Pirson Y, Chauveau D, Torres V. Management of cerebral aneurysms in autosomal dominant polycystic kidney disease. *J Am Soc Nephrol.* (2002) 13:269–76. doi: 10.1681/ASN.V131269
12. Yu TM, Chuang YW, Yu MC, Huang ST, Chou CY, Lin CL, et al. New-onset atrial fibrillation is associated with polycystic kidney disease: a nationwide population-based Cohort Study. *Medicine.* (2016) 95:e2623. doi: 10.1097/MD.0000000000002623
13. Romao EA, Moyses Neto M, Teixeira SR, Muglia VF, Vieira-Neto OM, Dantas M. Renal and extrarenal manifestations of autosomal dominant polycystic kidney disease. *Braz J Med Biol Res.* (2006) 39:533–8. doi: 10.1590/S0100-879X2006000400014
14. Chapman AB, Stepniakowski K, Rahbari-Oskoui F. Hypertension in autosomal dominant polycystic kidney disease. *Adv Chronic Kidney Dis.* (2010) 17:153–63. doi: 10.1053/j.ackd.2010.01.001
15. Sharif-Naeini R, Folgering JH, Bichet D, Duprat F, Lauritzen I, Arhatte M, et al. Polycystin-1 and–2 dosage regulates pressure sensing. *Cell.* (2009) 139:587–96. doi: 10.1016/j.cell.2009.08.045
16. Altamirano F, Schiattarella GG, French KM, Kim SY, Engelberger F, Kyrychenko S, et al. Polycystin-1 assembles with Kv channels to govern cardiomyocyte repolarization and contractility. *Circulation.* (2019) 140:921–36. doi: 10.1161/CIRCULATIONAHA.118.034731
17. Criollo A, Altamirano F, Pedrozo Z, Schiattarella GG, Li DL, Rivera-Mejias P, et al. Polycystin-2-dependent control of cardiomyocyte autophagy. *J Mol Cell Cardiol.* (2018) 118:110–21. doi: 10.1016/j.yjmcc.2018.03.002
18. Pedrozo Z, Criollo A, Battiprolu PK, Morales CR, Contreras-Ferrat A, Fernandez C, et al. Polycystin-1 is a cardiomyocyte mechanosensor that governs L-type Ca2+ channel protein stability. *Circulation.* (2015) 131:2131–42. doi: 10.1161/CIRCULATIONAHA.114.013537
19. Anyatonwu GI, Estrada M, Tian X, Somlo S, Ehrlich BE. Regulation of ryanodine receptor-dependent calcium signaling by polycystin-2. *Proc Natl Acad Sci USA.* (2007) 104:6454–9. doi: 10.1073/pnas.0610324104
20. Morita H. Secondary cardiomyopathy in polycystic kidney disease syndrome. *Int Heart J.* (2019) 60:10–11. doi: 10.1536/ihj.18-514
21. Fick GM, Johnson AM, Hammond WS, Gabow PA. Causes of death in autosomal dominant polycystic kidney disease. *J Am Soc Nephrol.* (1995) 5:2048–56. doi: 10.1681/ASN.V5122048
22. Kang YR, Ahn JH, Kim KH, Choi YM, Choi J, Park JR. Multiple cardiovascular manifestations in a patient with autosomal dominant polycystic kidney disease. *J Cardiovasc Ultrasound.* (2014) 22:144–7. doi: 10.4250/jcu.2014.22.3.144
23. Bardaji A, Vea AM, Gutierrez C, Ridao C, Richart C, Oliver JA. Left ventricular mass and diastolic function in normotensive young adults with autosomal dominant polycystic kidney disease. *Am J Kidney Dis.* (1998) 32:970–5. doi: 10.1016/S0272-6386(98)70071-X
24. de Chickera S, Akbari A, Levin A, Tang M, Brown P, Djurdev O, et al. The risk of adverse events in patients with polycystic kidney disease with advanced chronic kidney disease. *Can J Kidney Health Dis.* (2018) 5:2054358118774537. doi: 10.1177/2054358118774537
25. Schrier RW. Renal volume, renin-angiotensin-aldosterone system, hypertension, and left ventricular hypertrophy in patients with autosomal dominant polycystic kidney disease. *J Am Soc Nephrol.* (2009) 20:1888–93. doi: 10.1681/ASN.2008080882
26. Saito M, Okayama H, Yoshii T, Higashi H, Morioka H, Hiasa G, et al. Clinical significance of global two-dimensional strain as a surrogate parameter of myocardial fibrosis and cardiac events in patients with hypertrophic cardiomyopathy. *Eur Heart J Cardiovasc Imaging.* (2012) 13:617–23. doi: 10.1093/ejechocard/jer318
27. Travers JG, Kamal FA, Robbins J, Yutzey KE, Blaxall BC. Cardiac fibrosis: the fibroblast awakens. *Circ Res.* (2016) 118:1021–40. doi: 10.1161/CIRCRESAHA.115.306565
28. Bartos DC, Grandi E, Ripplinger CM. Ion channels in the heart. *Compr Physiol.* (2015) 5:1423–64. doi: 10.1002/cphy.c140069
29. Moorman AF, de Jong F, Denyn MM, Lamers WH. Development of the cardiac conduction system. *Circ Res.* (1998) 82:629–44. doi: 10.1161/01.RES.82.6.629
30. Walley KR. Left ventricular function: time-varying elastance and left ventricular aortic coupling. *Crit Care.* (2016) 20:270. doi: 10.1186/s13054-016-1439-6
31. Aghajani E, Muller S, Kjorstad KE, Korvald C, Nordhaug D, Revhaugand A, et al. The pressure-volume loop revisited: is the search for a cardiac contractility index a futile cycle? *Shock.* (2006) 25:370–6. doi: 10.1097/01.shk.0000209521.20496.7a
32. Kass DA, Beyar R, Lankford E, Heard M, Maughan WL, Sagawa K. Influence of contractile state on curvilinearity of in situ end-systolic pressure-volume relations. *Circulation.* (1989) 79:167–78. doi: 10.1161/01.CIR.79.1.167
33. Lee JJ, Cheng SJ, Huang CY, Chen CY, Feng L, Hwang DY, et al. Primary cardiac manifestation of autosomal dominant polycystic kidney disease revealed by patient induced pluripotent stem cell-derived cardiomyocytes. *EBioMedicine.* (2019) 40:675–84. doi: 10.1016/j.ebiom.2019.01.011
34. Wang Y, Zhang L, Wu GR, Zhou Q, Yue H, Rao LZ, et al. MBD2 serves as a viable target against pulmonary fibrosis by inhibiting macrophage M2 program. *Sci Adv.* (2021) 7:eabb6075. doi: 10.1126/sciadv.abb6075
35. Yan W, Wang P, Zhao CX, Tang J, Xiao X, Wang DW. Decorin gene delivery inhibits cardiac fibrosis in spontaneously hypertensive rats by modulation of transforming growth factor-beta/Smad and p38 mitogen-activated protein kinase signaling pathways. *Hum Gene Ther.* (2009) 20:1190–200. doi: 10.1089/hum.2008.204
36. Villalobos E, Criollo A, Schiattarella GG, Altamirano F, French KM, May HI, et al. Fibroblast primary cilia are required for cardiac fibrosis. *Circulation.* (2019) 139:2342–57. doi: 10.1161/CIRCULATIONAHA.117.028752
37. Atri C, Guerfali FZ, Laouini D. Role of human macrophage polarization in inflammation during infectious diseases. *Int J Mol Sci.* (2018) 19:1801. doi: 10.3390/ijms19061801
38. Xiang FL, Fang M, Yutzey KE. Loss of beta-catenin in resident cardiac fibroblasts attenuates fibrosis induced by pressure overload in mice. *Nat Commun.* (2017) 8:712. doi: 10.1038/s41467-017-00840-w

39. Ma F, Li Y, Jia L, Han Y, Cheng J, Li H, et al. Macrophage-stimulated cardiac fibroblast production of IL-6 is essential for TGF beta/Smad activation and cardiac fibrosis induced by angiotensin II *PLoS ONE.* (2012) 7:e35144. doi: 10.1371/journal.pone.0035144
40. Attaran S, Sherwood R, Dastidar MG, El-Gamel A. Identification of low circulatory transforming growth factor beta-1 in patients with degenerative heart valve disease. *Interact Cardiovasc Thorac Surg.* (2010) 11:791–3. doi: 10.1510/icvts.2010.244384
41. Venkatesan N, Pini L, Ludwig MS. Changes in Smad expression and subcellular localization in bleomycin-induced pulmonary fibrosis. *Am J Physiol Lung Cell Mol Physiol.* (2004) 287:L1342–7. doi: 10.1152/ajplung.00035.2004
42. Webber M, Jackson SP, Moon JC, Captur G. Myocardial fibrosis in heart failure: anti-fibrotic therapies and the role of cardiovascular magnetic resonance in drug trials. *Cardiol Ther.* (2020) 9:363–76. doi: 10.1007/s40119-020-00199-y
43. Piek A, de Boer RA, Sillje HH. The fibrosis-cell death axis in heart failure. *Heart Fail Rev.* (2016) 21:199–211. doi: 10.1007/s10741-016-9536-9
44. Csepe TA, Kalyanasundaram A, Hansen BJ, Zhao J, Fedorov VV. Fibrosis: a structural modulator of sinoatrial node physiology and dysfunction. *Front Physiol.* (2015) 6:37. doi: 10.3389/fphys.2015.00037
45. Akoum N, McGann C, Vergara G, Badger T, Ranjan R, Mahnkopf C, et al. Atrial fibrosis quantified using late gadolinium enhancement MRI is associated with sinus node dysfunction requiring pacemaker implant. *J Cardiovasc Electrophysiol.* (2012) 23:44–50. doi: 10.1111/j.1540-8167.2011.02140.x
46. DiFrancesco D. The role of the funny current in pacemaker activity. *Circ Res.* (2010) 106:434–46. doi: 10.1161/CIRCRESAHA.109.208041
47. Yang B, Wang Q, Wang R, Xu T. Clinical manifestation, management and prognosis of acute myocardial infarction in autosomal dominant polycystic kidney disease. *Kidney Blood Press Res.* (2018) 43:1806–12. doi: 10.1159/000495638
48. Huebener P, Abou-Khamis T, Zymek P, Bujak M, Ying X, Chatila K, et al. CD44 is critically involved in infarct healing by regulating the inflammatory and fibrotic response. *J Immunol.* (2008) 180:2625–33. doi: 10.4049/jimmunol.180.4.2625
49. Pala R, Mohieldin AM, Sherpa RT, Kathem SH, Shamloo K, Luan Z, et al. Ciliotherapy: remote control of primary cilia movement and function by magnetic nanoparticles. *ACS Nano.* (2019) 13:3555–72. doi: 10.1021/acsnano.9b00033
50. Pala R, Mohieldin AM, Shamloo K, Sherpa RT, Kathem SH, Zhou J, et al. Personalized nanotherapy by specifically targeting cell organelles to improve vascular hypertension. *Nano Lett.* (2019) 19:904–14. doi: 10.1021/acs.nanolett.8b04138

13

Cardiac Fibrosis in the Pressure Overloaded Left and Right Ventricle as a Therapeutic Target

*Katharina Schimmel[1,2,3], Kenzo Ichimura[1,2,3], Sushma Reddy[3,4], Francois Haddad[2,3,5] and Edda Spiekerkoetter[1,2,3]**

[1] Division Pulmonary, Allergy and Critical Care Medicine, Department of Medicine, Stanford University School of Medicine, Stanford, CA, United States, [2] Vera Moulton Wall Center for Pulmonary Vascular Disease, Stanford University, Stanford, CA, United States, [3] Stanford Cardiovascular Institute, Stanford University, Stanford, CA, United States, [4] Pediatric Cardiology, Stanford University, Stanford, CA, United States, [5] Cardiovascular Medicine, Stanford University, Stanford, CA, United States

***Correspondence:**
Edda Spiekerkoetter
eddas@stanford.edu

Myocardial fibrosis is a remodeling process of the extracellular matrix (ECM) following cardiac stress. “Replacement fibrosis” is a term used to describe wound healing in the acute phase of an injury, such as myocardial infarction. In striking contrast, ECM remodeling following chronic pressure overload insidiously develops over time as “reactive fibrosis” leading to diffuse interstitial and perivascular collagen deposition that continuously perturbs the function of the left (L) or the right ventricle (RV). Examples for pressure-overload conditions resulting in reactive fibrosis in the LV are systemic hypertension or aortic stenosis, whereas pulmonary arterial hypertension (PAH) or congenital heart disease with right sided obstructive lesions such as pulmonary stenosis result in RV reactive fibrosis. In-depth phenotyping of cardiac fibrosis has made it increasingly clear that both forms, replacement and reactive fibrosis co-exist in various etiologies of heart failure. While the role of fibrosis in the pathogenesis of RV heart failure needs further assessment, reactive fibrosis in the LV is a pathological hallmark of adverse cardiac remodeling that is correlated with or potentially might even drive both development and progression of heart failure (HF). Further, LV reactive fibrosis predicts adverse outcome in various myocardial diseases and contributes to arrhythmias. The ability to effectively block pathological ECM remodeling of the LV is therefore an important medical need. At a cellular level, the cardiac fibroblast takes center stage in reactive fibrotic remodeling of the heart. Activation and proliferation of endogenous fibroblast populations are the major source of synthesis, secretion, and deposition of collagens in response to a variety of stimuli. Enzymes residing in the ECM are responsible for collagen maturation and cross-linking. Highly cross-linked type I collagen stiffens the ventricles and predominates over more elastic type III collagen in pressure-overloaded conditions. Research has attempted to identify pro-fibrotic drivers causing fibrotic remodeling. Single key factors such as Transforming Growth Factor β (TGFβ) have been described and subsequently targeted to test their usefulness in inhibiting fibrosis in cultured fibroblasts of the ventricles, and in animal models of cardiac fibrosis. More recently, modulation of phenotypic behaviors like inhibition of proliferating fibroblasts has emerged as a strategy to reduce pathogenic cardiac fibroblast numbers in the heart. Some studies targeting LV reactive fibrosis as outlined above have successfully led to improvements of cardiac structure and function in relevant animal models. For the RV, fibrosis research is needed to better understand the evolution and roles of fibrosis in RV failure. RV fibrosis is seen as an integral part of RV remodeling and presents at varying degrees in patients with PAH and animal models replicating the disease of RV afterload. The extent to which ECM remodeling impacts RV function and thus patient survival is less clear. In this review, we describe differences as well as common characteristics and key players in ECM remodeling of the LV vs. the RV in response to pressure overload. We review pre-clinical studies assessing the effect of anti-fibrotic drug candidates on LV and RV function and their premise for clinical testing. Finally, we discuss the mode of action, safety and efficacy of anti-fibrotic drugs currently tested for the treatment of left HF in clinical trials, which might guide development of new approaches to target right heart failure. We touch upon important considerations and knowledge gaps to be addressed for future clinical testing of anti-fibrotic cardiac therapies.

Keywords: fibrosis, extracellular matrix, cardiac fibroblast, cardiac function, left ventricle, right ventricle, pressure-overload, hypertension

INTRODUCTION

Reactive fibrosis is a process that accompanies cardiac remodeling in a wide range of heart diseases. Fibrotic remodeling of the heart affects the extracellular matrix (ECM), which is a three-dimensional elastic network of collagen fibers and non-structural proteins that embeds cardiomyocytes, vessels, cardiac fibroblasts, and immune cells, and represents the scaffold of the healthy heart. Depending on the etiology and pathological context, ECM remodeling can primarily affect the left or the right ventricle, respective atria, or all chambers of the heart at once.

Historically, cardiac fibrosis has been broadly categorized into two types: reparative, also called replacement fibrosis, and reactive fibrosis, also called diffuse myocardial fibrosis, given the fact that it manifests as excessive and diffuse deposition of ECM components in interstitial and perivascular areas (**Figure 1**). Replacement fibrosis is the result of a healing process after acute myocardial infarction (MI), or cardiomyocyte death of other causes. It is visible as a fibrotic scar triggered by ischemic cell death. Inhibition of this type of fibrosis in the acute phase of injury leads to local rupture of the ventricular wall and increased mortality (1–4). Reactive fibrosis on the other hand describes the diffuse deposition and cross-linking of collagens in interstitial and perivascular areas that occur in chronic cardiac conditions, as observed after MI in the remote zone of the remodeling myocardium, or in many non-ischemic heart conditions. An example resulting in reactive fibrosis would be HF associated with pressure overload due to long-standing hypertension or stenosis.

The notion that changes in the ECM of the human heart occur in cardiac disease is based on a very old idea and was first interrogated in 1957 (5). Even though this study documented no increase in collagen concentration in the LV in various conditions such as atherosclerosis, hypertrophy, and coronary occlusion, the hypothesis that the ECM might be affected in a way that disrupts cardiac function has been revisited time and again ever since and feeds a line of research that has been proliferative until today (3, 6–11). Over time, it became increasingly clear that not only ECM quantity (12–16), but also ECM quality should be taken into consideration. First, different collagen types occur in the heart that have different biophysical and physiochemical properties (17–19). Type I collagen represents approximately 85% of the total collagen proteins and builds thick, highly cross-linked fibers that are important for strength, whereas type III collagen confers elasticity to the interstitial network by forming flexible, thin fibers (6, 17, 19). In human hearts, both aging and pressure overload due to hypertension or aortic stenosis lead to an excess of the stiffer type I collagen over the more elastic type III collagen in the left ventricle (7, 9, 20, 21). Second, the degree of collagen cross-linking, which can be measured by taking the ratio of stiff insoluble to soluble collagen, rather than collagen amounts has been found to associate with LV stiffness in hypertensive patients with symptomatic (stage C) heart failure (22). Increased collagen cross-linking has also been found in endocardial biopsies from patients presenting with heart failure with preserved (HFpEF) or reduced (HFrEF) ejection fraction, and to correlate with increased myocardial stiffness (8, 23–25). Of note, increased collagen cross-linking by lysyl oxidase was found to be normalized after using the diuretic torsemide in a small number of patients with chronic HF (26) and resulted in normalization of LV chamber stiffness. Even though these effects might be collateral and a direct action of torsemide on cardiac fibrosis needs to be established, these data are suggestive of adverse ECM remodeling that might be taken into consideration as a potential candidate for direct therapeutic targeting.

In 1988, the cardiac fibroblast was identified to be the major source of collagen fibers, and the predominant type I collagen producing cell in the heart (27, 28). A line of extensive research uncovered the critical role of cardiac fibroblasts in initiation, modulation, and execution of ECM remodeling (29–31). It comes

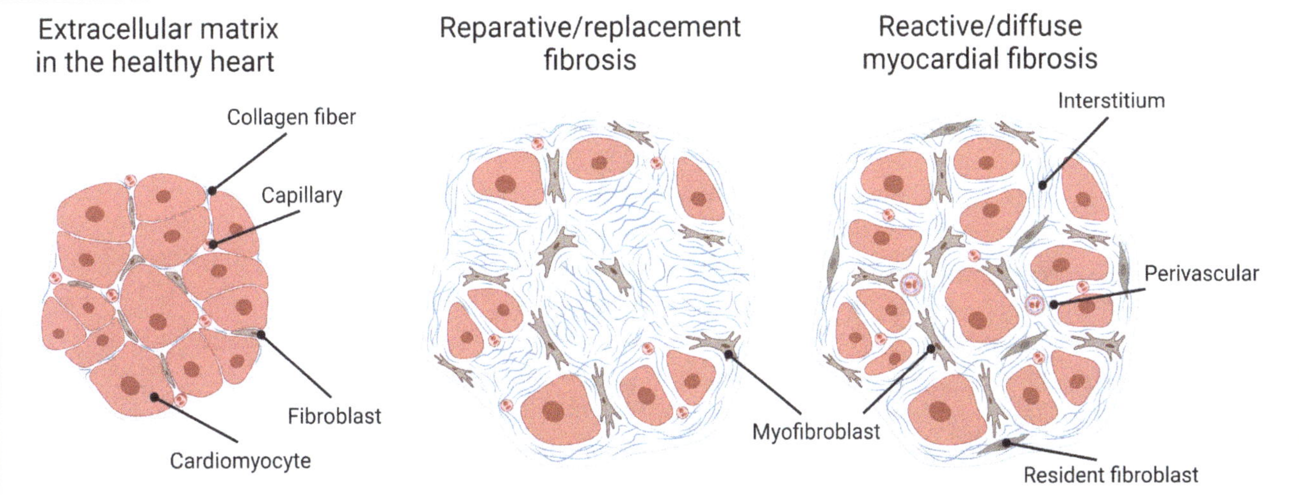

FIGURE 1 | Types of cardiac fibrosis. The extracellular matrix in the healthy heart **(left)** is a three-dimensional network of collagen fibers that embeds cardiac cells such as cardiomyocytes, capillaries, and fibroblasts. "Replacement/reparative fibrosis" **(middle)** is visible as a collagen-based scar that is formed during a healing process and replaces dying cardiomyocytes after ischemic insults. "Reactive/diffuse myocardial fibrosis" **(right)** accompanies heart failure due to pressure overload and manifests as diffuse deposition of cross-linked collagens in interstitial and perivascular areas. Both patterns of fibrous deposits can be observed in patients with heart failure with reactive fibrosis, due to the formation of micro scars related to smaller foci of replacement fibrosis that are reflective of a loss of small numbers of cardiomyocytes.

as no surprise that the cardiac fibroblast has been extensively studied as a potential target for ECM remodeling in the heart.

In this review, we focus on reactive fibrosis affecting the LV and the RV in chronic cardiac conditions and discuss the phenotypic and clinical consequences of adverse ECM remodeling in the pressure- overloaded heart. We reflect on therapeutic approaches aimed at improving detrimental effects of the fibrotic program of reactive fibrosis, and the potential relevance of preserving required functions of fibrosis. To facilitate anti-fibrotic drug development in the future, we identify open questions to be addressed by research, and potential considerations for clinical trial design.

THE THERAPEUTIC VALUE OF TARGETING FIBROTIC REMODELING IN FAILURE OF THE LEFT OR THE RIGHT HEART

Despite extensive research, the exact role of cardiac fibrosis in heart diseases remains largely elusive. The extent to which fibrosis is a causal, contributing or an adaptive mechanism in the pathogenesis of cardiac conditions is likely context dependent, or co-exists, considering its heterogeneous nature as well as functional and phenotypic diversity (**Figure 1**). Reparative fibrosis, which locally replaces dying cardiomyocytes, might potentially be necessary to maintain the integrity of the heart (4, 29). Reactive cardiac fibrosis is hypothesized to be the result of an adaptive process that increases structural support to a higher workload for the heart. Accumulating evidence though suggests that reactive fibrosis correlates with changes in architecture, physiology, and function of the heart (7, 10, 11, 13, 30, 31), as well as disease severity and worse clinical outcome of patients with HF of various etiologies (32–35). Of note, it has been shown that fibrosis may precede the development of HFpEF (35), which might make a causative relation more plausible and warrants further investigations. In the following section, we therefore review existing evidence of the variable contribution of reactive fibrosis on left and right ventricular dysfunction, with a focus on pressure overloaded conditions (**Figure 2**). These observations might support the rationale for anti-fibrotic interventions to improve cardiac function and clinical outcomes in patients with reactive fibrosis.

Extracellular Matrix Remodeling Impairs Left Ventricular Function and Physiology in Pressure Overloaded Conditions

HF is characterized by a progressive deterioration of LV function. Reactive fibrosis in the LV develops in chronic pressure overloaded conditions, such as hypertensive heart disease or aortic stenosis (**Figure 2**). Considering the importance of collagen cross-linking and accumulation of highly cross-linked collagen type I in myocardial stiffening, addressing the relationship between ECM remodeling and LV function and detailed phenotyping of these qualities was a major focus in fibrosis research during the past two decades. Collagen cross-linking determines the reversibility of experimental fibrosis (36), the stiffness of collagen fibers, and their resistance to degradation by matrix metalloproteinases (37). It can be measured in human myocardial biopsies or autopsies as well as experimental animal tissue by colorimetric and enzymatic assays, and after correcting the concentration of each form of collagen by the total amount of protein, collagen cross-linking is calculated as the ratio between insoluble and soluble collagen (38, 39). Mounting evidence

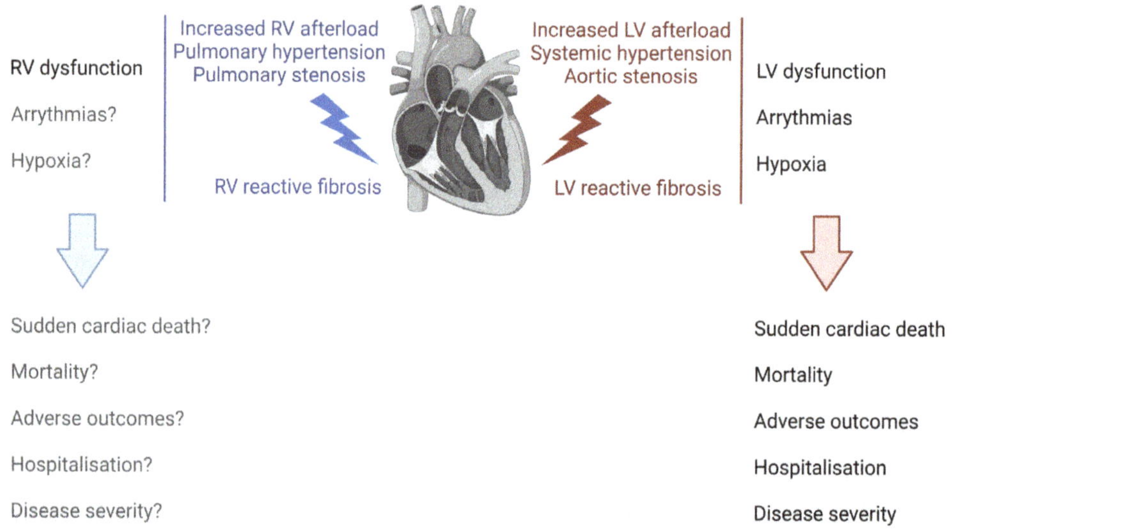

FIGURE 2 | The impact of right and left ventricular reactive fibrosis on cardiac function, physiology, and clinical outcome. Increased LV afterload induces LV reactive fibrosis **(right)** that correlates with LV dysfunction, and increases the risk for arrythmias and for hypoxic conditions in the LV. Together, these changes in the LV increase the risk for sudden cardiac death, increase patient mortality, and associate with adverse outcomes, hospitalization, and disease severity. RV reactive fibrosis **(left)** following an increased RV afterload leads to increased RV stiffness and dysfunction. However, the role of fibrosis in the development of RV failure is not fully understood.

suggests that the degree of collagen cross-linking, and an increase in the ratio of insoluble to soluble collagen, correlates with LV stiffness and diastolic dysfunction in hypertensive heart disease (8, 22, 23, 25) and aortic stenosis (40). Of note, therapeutic interventions for chronic HF such as the use of loop diuretic torsemide have been associated with an improvement in collagen cross-linking in the remodeled myocardium. In 2004, López et al. sought to determine if torsemide has anti-fibrotic effects on the failing heart beyond its effect on diuresis (41). Compared to furosemide, torsemide was able to improve LV diastolic function in chronic HF patients (42) and showed a lower mortality in the TORIC study (43), despite exerting similar renal effects (44, 45). These superior clinical effects of torsemide in patients with New York Heart Association functional class II to IV chronic HF were associated with lower collagen volume fractions (CVF) in myocardial biopsies and circulating carboxy-terminal peptide of procollagen type I (PIP), a biomarker for collagen type I synthesis (41). Based on these findings, the authors concluded that torsemide was able to reverse reactive fibrosis. In a pilot follow-up study, they demonstrated that torsemide modified collagen cross-linking by the enzyme lysyl oxidase (LOX) in patients with severe chronic HF that resulted in improvement of LV chamber stiffness that was more pronounced than in the furosemide treated group (26). Regardless of whether torsemide exerts a direct effect on the fibrotic responses or whether the observed effect is secondary to an improved heart failure management, these studies are evidence that reactive cardiac fibrosis can regress, along with improvement of LV function, which has important clinical implications for patients with HF. It should be noted that many of above studies have analyzed relatively small patient sample numbers. However, the collectivity of the resulting data might imply that interventions leading to regression of established reactive fibrosis could be successful in improving LV stiffness and dysfunction.

In addition to its impact on LV function, reactive fibrosis increases the risk of ventricular arrhythmias (46) (**Figure 2**). As such, all histological forms of cardiac fibrosis, diffuse interstitial fibrosis as characteristic for reactive fibrosis, patchy collagen deposition, or dense scars resulting from local healing processes provide substrate for arrhythmogenesis. Myocardial electrophysiologic consequences range from slower action potential propagation, re-entry initiation, promotion of after-depolarizations, to increased ectopic automaticity, and are greatly dependent on the architecture of fibrosis (47). Of note, reactive fibrosis is associated with ventricular arrhythmias independent of LV function in hypertensive heart disease (30). Anti-fibrotic therapies are therefore expected to have beneficial effects on ventricular arrhythmias in addition to beneficial effects on LV function.

Perivascular fibrosis, specifically, in addition to diffuse interstitial fibrosis, has implications for ischemia in the heart (**Figure 2**). For example, in patients with non-ischemic HF of various etiologies, coronary perivascular fibrosis associated with the impairment of coronary blood flow independently of interstitial fibrosis or cardiac function (48). Even though this was an observational study with a relatively small number of patients, these data might imply compromised coronary microcirculation and supply of nutrients and oxygen to the heart muscle in HF. Coronary microvascular rarefaction and fibrosis were also described in patients with HFpEF (49).

The hypothesis that reactive fibrosis might lead to hypoxic and dysfunctional collagen-encircled cardiomyocytes, was first tested 1995 in dogs with chronic HF induced by sequential intracoronary microembolizations (50). Even though confirming studies are required, results of previous work showed that reactive interstitial fibrosis in viable myocardium was inversely correlated to capillary density (capillary/fiber ratio), and positively correlated with an increased oxygen diffusion distance, suggesting that cardiomyocytes in LV regions with severe reactive interstitial fibrosis might be subjected to chronic hypoxia. Increased hypoxia in cardiomyocytes would eventually lead to more cell death, which would feed a vicious cycle in which dying cardiomyocytes were replaced by even more collagens in form of a reparative fibrotic process, leading to a further decline of LV function. In human studies, fibrosis and microvascular remodeling was assessed in 30 hearts with end-stage hypertrophic cardiomyopathy. Topological association of arteriolar abnormalities such as tunica media hypertrophy and intimal hyperplasia and severity of fibrosis was characterized in different areas (51). Further studies addressing the role of reactive fibrosis in generating a hypoxic environment for cardiomyocytes under pressure overloaded conditions are warranted.

As described above, reactive fibrosis is associated with distorted myocardial architecture, physiology, and cardiac function, and as such might play a critical role in the development of pressure-overload induced HF and adverse clinical outcomes in patients (**Figure 2**). Reactive LV fibrosis is implicated in the clinical course of HF in the following ways:

(*i*) *Reactive fibrosis plays a prognostic role in HF.* The severity of fibrosis assessed with cardiac magnetic resonance imaging (CMRI) correlates with a risk for sudden cardiac death, as well as cardiac and all-cause mortality in patients with non-high-risk hypertrophic cardiomyopathy (HCM) (33). Moreover, extracellular volume (ECV) associates with markers of disease severity in patients with HFpEF (32). It should be mentioned, however, that in terms of outcome, ECV did associate with outcome among CMR parameters, but only without adjustment for important clinical and invasive hemodynamic parameters in this study (32). However, a similar study found that fibrosis quantified by ECV CMR measures is prevalent in the LV of patients with HFpEF and associated with disease severity and adverse outcomes (35). In hypertensive heart disease, cardiac fibrosis associated with poor outcome and hospitalization with HF (52, 53). As such, reactive fibrosis was suggested to be a risk factor for sudden arrhythmic death in patients with heart disease of various etiologies (30, 46, 54, 55).

(*ii*) *Reactive fibrosis defines the response to treatment modalities in HF.* Weidemann et al. showed a correlation of severity of reactive fibrosis at the time of surgery and parameters of longitudinal systolic function with clinical outcome post-surgery by assessing standard and tissue Doppler echocardiography and late-enhancement cardiac magnetic resonance imaging (CMRI) at baseline and 9 months after aortic valve replacement in patients with severe aortic stenosis, as well as endomyocardial biopsies obtained during valve replacement surgery (56). These results are supported by Azevedo et al. who quantified fibrosis and LV function in patients with severe aortic stenosis by Gadolinium-enhanced MRI [contrast-enhanced (ce)-MRI] and picrosirius red staining of myocardial samples obtained at the time of aortic valve replacement, and a repeat ce-MRI 27 ± 22 months after surgery (34). To evaluate long-term survival, patients were followed for 52 ± 17 months. The amount of fibrosis inversely correlated with the extent of LV functional improvement, and directly associated with all-cause mortality post-surgery (34), suggesting that the degree of fibrosis predicts clinical outcome and long-term recovery after aortic valve replacement.

Although reactive fibrosis in the LV plays a prognostic role in HF and defines the response to treatment modalities, it represents one of many factors that change in adverse cardiac remodeling of the pressure overloaded heart. The extent to which reactive fibrosis contributes to the progression of HF compared to other possible key-players that can impact LV function, such as cardiomyocyte stiffness (57), or biomechanical LV wall stress (58, 59), remains to be addressed.

Extracellular Matrix Remodeling Correlates With Right Ventricular Dysfunction in the Pressure Overloaded Right Ventricle

RV function is a key prognostic factor for patients with not only pulmonary arterial hypertension (PAH) (60) but also other subtypes of pulmonary hypertension (PH), such as group 2 PH (PH due to left heart disease) (61), group 3 PH (PH due to lung disease) (62), and also group 4 PH (chronic thromboembolic pulmonary hypertension) (63) (**Figure 2**). In fact, RV failure is the leading cause of death of patients with PAH (64). The development of fibrosis in the RV is a hallmark of RV failure and generally considered as a key player in the maladaptive process.

Several histology studies have reported mild but significant increase in RV fibrosis in patients with PAH (65, 66). CMRI studies reported that the volume of RV fibrosis strongly correlates with RV function, such as RVEF (67–69). Furthermore, increased biomarkers of collagen metabolism such as matrix metalloproteinase 9 (MMP-9) and tissue inhibitors of matrix metalloproteinase 1 (TIMP-1) are associated with disease severity in PAH (70). Nonetheless, the role of fibrosis in the development of RV failure and how that affects the RV function is not fully understood.

There is some evidence showing that RV fibrosis is related to end-diastolic wall stress (71). Using RV trabecular strips of pulmonary artery-banded (PAB) rodent models, Rain et al. showed that fibrosis-mediated stiffness was increased in animals with severe RV dysfunction and the ratio of collagen I/III expression was elevated (72). Kusakari et al. further reported that active tension and Ca^{2+} responsiveness was lower compared to sham animals in the RV papillary muscles (73).

However, it is still not clear whether targeting RV fibrosis is an ideal therapeutic target. A certain degree of RV fibrosis might be protective against mechanical stress by preventing excess RV dilatation and preserving the ventricular shape as it has been shown in the LV. Although RV stiffness is related to disease severity in PAH patients (65, 74), not only the amount of fibrosis but also the cardiomyocyte stiffness contributes significantly to RV stiffness particularly in the early stage of RV failure (72). Furthermore, RV functional recovery after mechanical unloading by lung transplantation has been reported, however, whether the functional recovery of the RV is related to reduced RV fibrosis

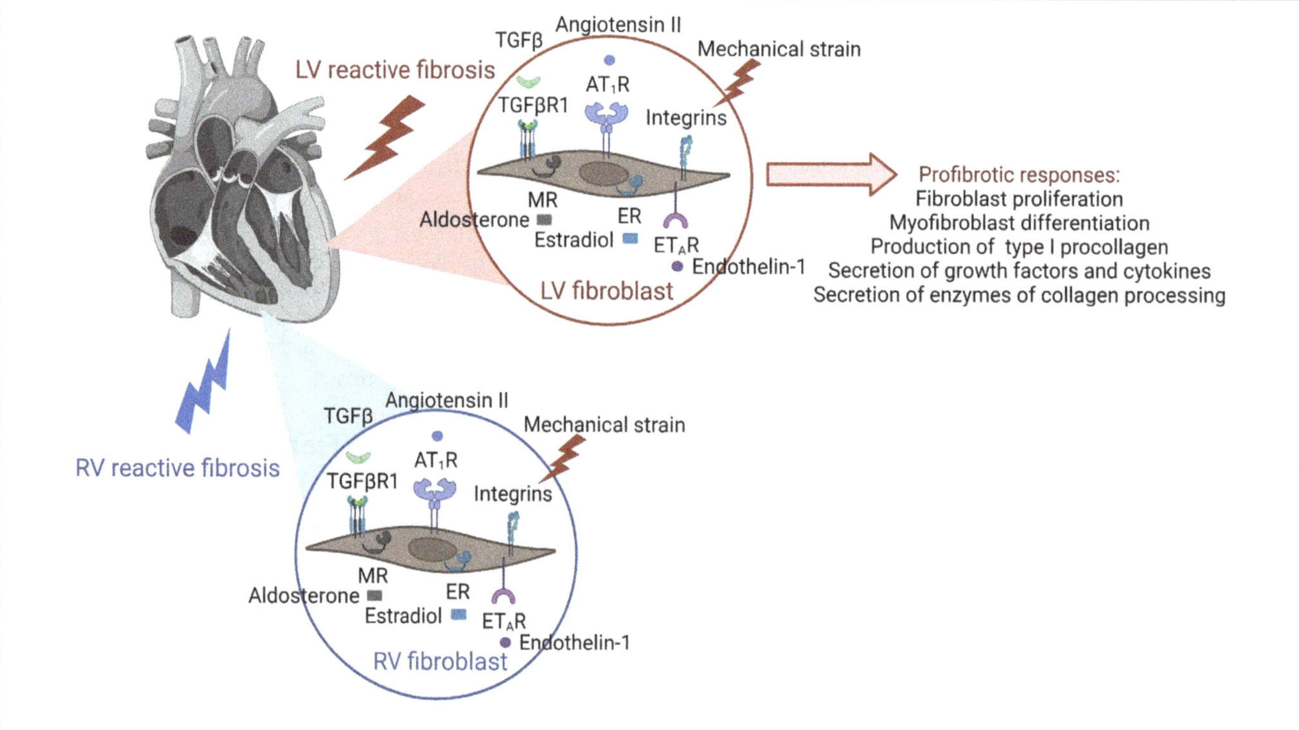

FIGURE 3 | Receptor activation of cardiac fibroblasts leads to pro-fibrotic cellular behaviors. The same receptors of fibroblast activation are present in the fibroblasts of both ventricles, but involvement of signaling pathways and functional outcome of fibroblast responses have been mostly studied in the LV.

is unknown. Studies in mice showed that cardiac fibrosis is in principle reversible once the RV afterload is normalized in a novel de-banding model where pulmonary arterial banding is reversed by using self-absorbable sutures (75).

As myocardial fibrosis both in the LV and the RV appears to be a useful indicator for long-term survival, it has implications not only as an important therapeutic target in the failing heart but also as a biomarker that could be assessed using a combination of biopsies, non-invasive imaging modalities, and circulating biomarkers.

THE CARDIAC FIBROBLAST IN LEFT AND RIGHT VENTRICULAR FIBROSIS

The cell biology of reactive fibrosis including mechanisms and pathways underlying fibroblast activation were most recently reviewed in great detail (76). We therefore provide a brief overview of newest insights on fundamental processes and key steps resulting in fibroblast behaviors that are responsible for an excessive deposition of collagens in the overloaded myocardium (**Figure 3**). Different stages of fibroblast activation have been described: Activation of resting cardiac fibroblasts to so called "activated fibroblasts" is accompanied by a high proliferation activity, periostin expression as well as secretion of collagen. Further differentiation of these activated fibroblasts into "myofibroblasts" changes the behavior and expression pattern of the cells which now express α-smooth muscle actin (α-SMA), less periostin, but more collagen than activated fibroblasts (77). A robust classification of fibroblast populations and activation stages requires the experimental ability to identify heterogeneous fibroblasts. With emerging technologies such as single-cell RNA sequencing (scRNAseq) we start to appreciate fibroblast heterogeneity present after pressure overload (78). However, it is currently unknown how and when different fibroblast populations or activation stages contribute to reactive fibrosis. Mechanisms of fibroblast activation described below are mostly derived from results generated before the advent of scRNA seq.

In the healthy adult mammalian heart, cardiac fibroblasts comprise around 20% of non-myocyte cells, without any significant changes in cell numbers or proliferative activities (79–81). Overloaded conditions lead to an accumulation of collagens, which might be due to the differentiation of activated fibroblasts to myofibroblasts, as well as an increase of cardiac fibroblast numbers in the heart. Historically, the latter event was thought to be dependent on endothelial-to-mesenchymal transition (EndoMT) and the recruitment of circulating hematopoietic progenitors to the diseased myocardium in various fibrotic heart conditions (82–84). This paradigm was revisited in 2014 by an in-depth analysis using refined fibroblast-lineage-tracing and demonstrated that accumulation of activated fibroblasts upon pressure overloaded conditions is neither attributed to EndoMT, nor the recruitment of hematopoietic progenitors, but to proliferation of activated resident fibroblast populations in the LV (81). Of note, the same study also found that αSMA, a marker of myofibroblasts, was only expressed by 15% of collagen1a1-labeled fibroblasts following pressure overload induction by TAC. These findings suggest that the accumulation of collagens seen in reactive fibrosis due to pressure overload might be the result of enhanced proliferation of activated resident fibroblasts, in addition to differentiation of activated fibroblasts to αSMA positive myofibroblasts.

The origin of fibroblasts in the RV during development differs from LV and RV. RV fibroblasts are derived exclusively from the epicardium *via* epicardium-to-mesenchymal transition, whereas fibroblasts in the LV are derived from both epicardium but also from endocardium *via* endothelial-to-mesenchymal transition (81). While fibroblasts in the LV under pressure overload have been studied extensively and shown to be derived by proliferation of resident fibroblasts (81), this has not yet been confirmed in the RV.

Myofibroblasts most recently have been shown to have protective effects in the pressure-overloaded LV (85). In the pressure overloaded LV after TAC, TGF-β/Smad3-activated cardiac myofibroblasts played an important protective role by preserving the ECM network, suppressing macrophage-driven inflammation, and attenuating cardiomyocyte injury. The protective actions of the myofibroblasts were mediated, at least in part, through Smad-dependent suppression of matrix-degrading proteases. It was suggested previously that a myofibroblast-mediated scar forms following cardiomyocyte death, resulting in microscopic scars when individual myocytes are lost (29). Indeed, myofibroblasts can engulf dead cells (86). This might imply that myofibroblasts may be the main effector cell responsible for reparative fibrosis not only following MI, but also in conditions of chronic overload. Further research is required to understand the exact contribution of different activation stages of resident cardiac fibroblasts to reactive fibrosis development and progression.

Collectively, this might result in new concepts supporting the rationale that targeting proliferation of activated resident cardiac fibroblasts in pressure-overloaded conditions rather than EndoMT, or the recruitment of hematopoietic progenitors might provide novel therapeutic opportunities, which warrant further investigations.

Factors driving pro-fibrotic behaviors that lead to the formation of diffuse myocardial fibrosis, such as increased fibroblast proliferation rates as well as collagen synthesis and secretion, are numerous in the diseased heart, and it can be anticipated that many of them occur at the same time. Cardiac fibroblasts have many receptors to respond to various stimuli (**Figure 3**).

Mechanical stress as occurring in pressure overload due to hypertensive heart disease and aortic stenosis can be sensed by cardiac fibroblasts by 2 classes of cell surface receptors, integrins, and discoidin domain receptors (87, 88). These receptors also mediate fibroblast interactions with the ECM and stimulate various cellular responses, such as fibroblast migration and proliferation, as well as differentiation into myofibroblasts.

Angiotensin II is not only expressed by the liver but can also be expressed by myofibroblasts. It can stimulate myofibroblasts in an autocrine manner, as well as most likely also other fibroblast populations in the heart, *via* binding to the G protein-coupled AT1 receptor (29, 89–91). This binding promotes fibroblast proliferative as well as procollagen I and III synthesis and secretion activities (29, 92, 93). Cardiac fibroblast proliferation is induced *via* mitogen-activated protein (MAP) kinases and the extracellular signal-regulated kinase (ERK) 1/2 that is activated by angiotensin II (93, 94). Procollagen I and III synthesis and secretion are mediated in this case by augmenting TGF-β/SMAD signaling pathways (29, 95). Of note, the profibrotic angiotensin II/AT1 receptor axis, has a counter-regulatory, fibro lytic axis in the myofibroblast and potentially also other fibroblasts in the heart, known as the ACE2-angiotensin (1–7)-Mas signaling axis (29). Angiotensin converting enzyme 2 (ACE2) is a homolog of ACE that is insensitive to ACE inhibitors and can hydrolyze angiotensin II into angiotensin (1–7) which binds to a Mas receptor to induce myofibroblast apoptosis through inhibition of antiapoptotic proteins (29).

TGF-β can signal through canonical, SMAD-dependent pathways, and non-canonical pathways. TGF-β-Smad2/3 signaling in activated resident cardiac fibroblasts has been identified as a key mediator of the fibrotic response in the pressure-overloaded LV (96). The canonical, SMAD-dependent pathway is mediated by the formation of a hetero-tetrameric complex between TGF-βRII and TGF-βRI molecules induced by TGF-β binding. The receptor complex then phosphorylates SMAD2 and SMAD3, which form a complex with SMAD4 in the cytoplasm (97, 98). The SMAD complex translocates to the nucleus and binds to SMAD binding elements to act as a transcription factor that leads to expression of collagen, CTGF, myofibroblast-associated proteins such as smooth muscle actin, periostin and IL11 (76, 99–102). In addition, TGFβ1 can trigger non-canonical, SMAD-independent signaling, that is mediated by TGFβ-activated kinase 1 (TAK1), mitogen-activated protein kinases (MAPKs) and Rho A (76). Importantly, in cultivated myofibroblasts isolated from hearts of patients with end-stage HF, inhibition of TGFβR1 kinase activity induced a dedifferentiation of myofibroblasts and a reduction of expression of profibrotic proteins, suggesting a certain plasticity of these cells (103).

Endothelin-1 (ET-1) is a vasoactive factor predominantly secreted by endothelial cells, but also by fibroblasts, cardiomyocytes, and macrophages. ET-1 can bind to ET receptors that are present on cardiac fibroblasts (104), thereby contributing to the development of myocardial fibrosis. Among many heart-independent functions, such as regulation of blood pressure through synergistic interactions with angiotensin II, proliferative effects of ET-1 in connective tissue disorders have increasingly been recognized (105).

Finally, it should be noted that both age and sex are factors that seem to mediate diffuse myocardial fibrosis (20, 106–111). With aging, increases in the production of fibrillar collagen were seen both in cardiac tissue of animals and human biopsies (110). In addition, collagen processing and maturation are altered, while collagen cross-linking due to advanced glycation end products (AGEs) increases, and collagen degradation becomes less effective. Molecular mechanisms associated with cardiac aging are inflammatory pathways (111), mitochondrial oxidative stress, insulin/insulin-like growth factor/PI3K pathway, adrenergic and renin angiotensin II signaling (RAAS), and

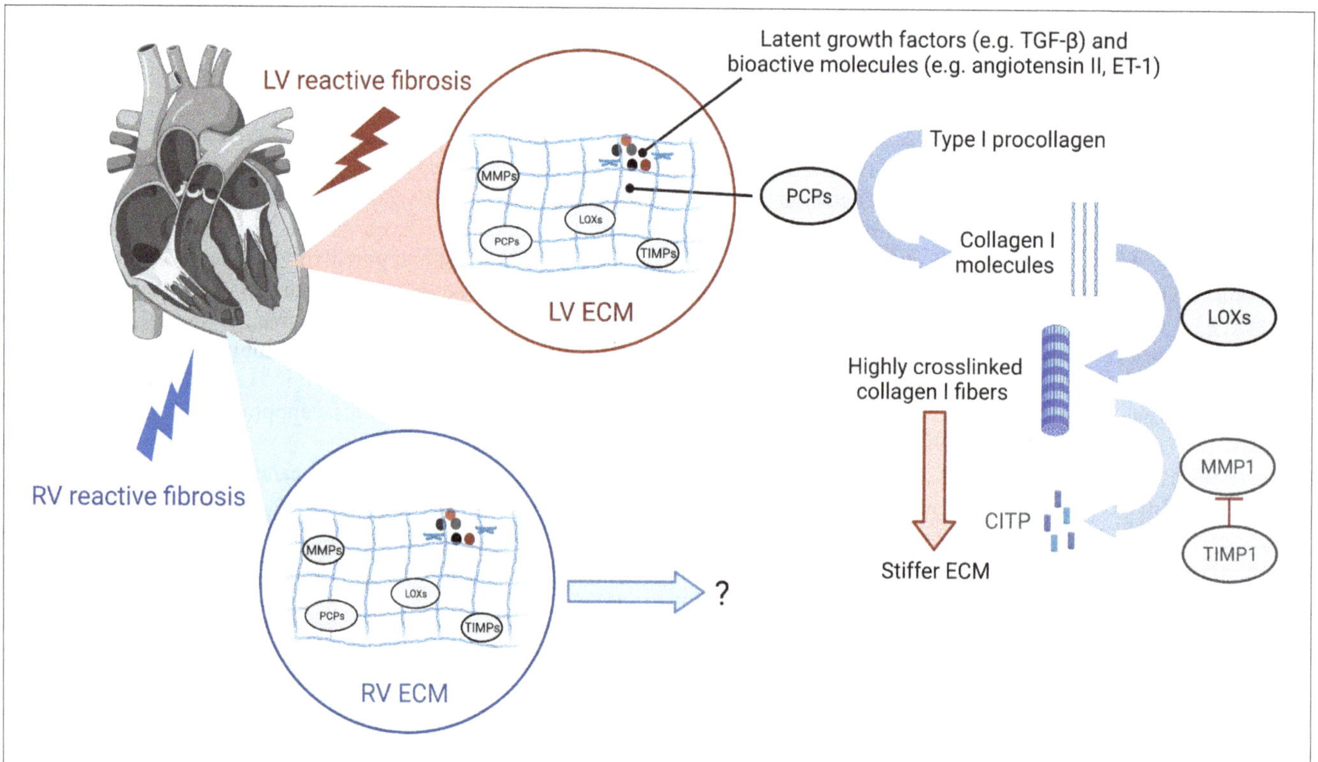

FIGURE 4 | Changes of the extracellular matrix during reactive fibrosis leading to left ventricular stiffening. Enzymes responsible for collagen turnover are induced in both LV and RV reactive fibrosis. While studies show that collagen I cross-linking and deposition of highly cross-linked collagen I fibers impact LV function by stiffening the ECM, research is needed to understand ECM remodeling of the RV and functional consequences. Type I procollagen secreted by cardiac fibroblasts is processed to type I collagen molecules by procollagen carboxy-terminal proteinases (PCPs). Lysyl oxidases (LOXs) are enzymes that cross-link adjacent type I collagen molecules to highly cross-linked type I collagen fibers that stiffen the LV and have increased resistance to degradation by matrix metalloproteinase 1 (MMP1). MMPs, along with their inhibitors TIMPs, are responsible for ECM degradation to the carboxy-terminal telopeptide of type I collagen (CITP). While the same enzymes involved in collagen-turnover are induced in the pressure-overloaded RV, the dynamics of ECM deposition and maturation, and the extent of collagen cross-linking contributing to the severity of RV stiffness require further research.

nutrient signaling (112), all of which might directly act on the cardiac fibroblast to perpetuate reactive fibrosis. Female sex up to a certain age seems to have cardio-protective effects that might be explained by 17β-Estradiol-mediated differential estrogen receptor (ERα and ERβ) signaling in cardiac fibroblasts which regulate collagen I and III expression in the heart (113). In line, upon pressure-overload due to aortic stenosis, cardiac tissue of male patients was found to have higher expression of collagen types I and III than of female patients (106, 107).

In addition it should be noted that non-fibroblast cardiac cells such as cardiomyocytes, inflammatory, smooth muscle and endothelial cells present in both ventricles can also modulate cardiac fibroblasts by secreting factors directly impacting on fibroblast behaviors (76, 114–118).

EXTRACELLULAR MATRIX REMODELING IN THE LEFT VS. RIGHT VENTRICLE

The cardiac ECM provides a three-dimensional scaffold that is paramount for the healthy architecture, structure, mechanics, myocyte orientation, and transmission of contractile force of the heart (119–121). The ECM consists mostly of the structural type I and type III collagens that build the dynamic fibrillar network (122). In addition, it contains a wide range of glycoproteins, glycosaminoglycans, and proteoglycans, stored latent growth factors such as transforming growth factor-β (TGF-β) (123), bioactive molecules such as angiotensin II (124, 125) and endothelin (ET)-1 (126, 127), and enzymes catalyzing collagen maturation, processing, and degradation (128) (**Figure 4**). Pathologic remodeling of the ECM as occurring in reactive fibrosis is associated with changes in quantities, the composition of ECM components, and ECM quality such as collagen cross-linking. These quantitative and qualitative changes of the ECM can physically impair cardiomyocyte contractility and relaxation, and disturb electrical conductivity, as well as regional nutrient and oxygen diffusion. Outcomes of approaches that target some of the key modulators of these ECM changes, mostly tested for their effect on reactive fibrosis in the LV in experimental animals or patients, are discussed in section "Anti-fibrotic Therapies and Their Impact on Left or Right Ventricular Function in Animal Studies" and "Anti-fibrotic Drugs in Clinical Testing for Left Ventricle and Right Ventricle Heart Failure." We here describe the role of important ECM modifiers in early development, progression, and degradation of diffuse myocardial fibrosis in the overloaded heart.

Excessive deposition of thick, highly cross-linked collagen type I fibers as seen for example in pressure-overloaded conditions (7, 9, 21) is the end-result of a highly complex process with many factors involved. Collagen synthesis by cardiac fibroblasts can be stimulated by mechanical strain, connective tissue growth factor (CTGF), TGF-β (31, 129), or angiotensin II (92). The cardiac fibroblast processes pro-collagen α-chains into triple helical pro-collagen, after a hydroxylation step of proline residues that takes place during the polypeptide elongation (128). The resulting 4-Hydroxyproline is a prerequisite for the triple helix formation and essential for its stability. Once collagen precursor type I procollagen is secreted by cardiac fibroblasts and myofibroblasts, enzymes called procollagen carboxy-terminal proteinases (PCPs), also produced by cardiac fibroblasts, convert these precursors into the mature collagen, type I collagen-forming microfibril molecules (130) (**Figure 4**). These molecules are then stabilized by inter-molecular covalent cross-links between polypeptide chains of adjacent fibrils that are catalyzed by the enzyme lysil oxidase (LOX). Resulting deposition of highly cross-linked collagen fibers leads to a stiffer ECM, which can activate cardiac fibroblasts and ensue a vicious cycle that promotes further progression of reactive fibrosis (87, 88). Elevated myocardial expression of PCPs, PCP enhancer 1 (PCPE1) which is a positive regulator of PCP, LOXs, and lysyl oxidase homolog 2 (LOXL2) has been observed in patients with HFpEF or HFrEF due to pressure overload, and associated with the severity of diffuse myocardial fibrosis determined by collagen deposition or collagen cross-linking (22, 23, 26, 131, 132).

Enzymes that degrade collagen fibers, such as matrix metalloproteinases (MMPs), and their inhibitors, tissue inhibitors of metalloproteinases (TIMPs) (**Figure 4**) have been proposed to play opposing roles in diffuse myocardial fibrosis (133). Clinical data are mixed and conflicting, which might be partly attributed to the fact that in some cases, mRNA or protein expression was measured without determination of actual enzymatic activities. A study analyzing the ratio between MMP-1 and its inhibitor TIMP-1 in cardiac tissue of patients with hypertensive HF by western blot and immunohistochemistry found that probands presenting with HFrEF had an excess of MMP1 relative to TIMP1, while the ratio in patients presenting with HFpEF was comparable with healthy individuals (10). On a histological level, patients with HFrEF had regionally diminished collagen deposits, but more perivascular and replacement fibrosis than their HFpEF counterparts. In addition, the MMP-1 to TIMP-1 ratio measured *via* enzyme-linked immunosorbent assay (ELISA) in serum was inversely correlated with the ejection fraction (EF) and directly correlated with LV end-diastolic diameter (LVEDD). Another interesting finding was that patients with aortic stenosis and HFrEF had higher levels of MMP1 and other MMPs and a lower level of TIMPs in the myocardium as compared to patients with HFpEF with the same etiology (134). The degree of collagen I deposition correlated with increased expression levels of MMPs, TIMP-1 and -2, and a decreased expression of TIMP-4 in this study, with the highest MMP expression levels together with gelatinolytic activities of MMP-2 as measured by zymography in the patient group with the lowest EF. The authors concluded that during the progression from compensated hypertrophy to HF, ECM turnover is characterized by the upregulation of MMPs and their inadequate inhibition by TIMPs (134). It was proposed that systolic dysfunction in patients with HFrEF due to hypertension or aortic stenosis might be caused by disruption of the mysial collagen scaffold that may facilitate cardiomyocyte slippage and loss of synchrony and synergy of cardiomyocyte contraction (135).

With in-depth reviews of the role of MMPs and TIMPs in cardiac extracellular matrix remodeling already existent in the literature (136), it should be noted that a consensus on whether reduced collagen degradation, or rather increased deposition might be the major contributor to overall collagen accumulation in the pressure-overloaded heart, has yet to be reached.

Although the role and composition of the ECM in the RV are considered to be similar to that of LV, few studies have investigated the difference between the LV and RV. A study using autopsy samples from patients who died of a non-cardiac cause showed that normal RV has higher collagen content than the LV: 7.4% in RV vs. 5.5% in LV (5). Another study using explanted donor hearts from patients with end-stage dilated cardiomyopathy and ischemic cardiomyopathy showed that the distribution of ECM proteins, such as laminin, fibronectin, and collagen I and IV, as well as MMPs differed between LV and RV (137). These differences are thought to be related to the fact that LV and RV have different embryological origin (138). Also, it could be related to the fact that the RV undergoes significant regression after switching from fetal circulation to postnatal circulation. Another striking fact is that the RV may be exposed to a fivefold increase in afterload, such as in the case of PAH, whereas the afterload increase the LV faces is usually less than twofold even in the most severe case of aortic stenosis. A study comparing the response of the RV and LV using PAB and transverse aortic constriction (TAC) mice models showed that several transcripts were differentially increased only in the pressure-overloaded RV (139). Studies like these are required to delineate potential differences between RV vs. LV reactive fibrosis due to pressure overload. However, limitations of this approach are that the relative pressure increase for a healthy RV after PAB is much higher than the relative pressure increase for a healthy LV after TAC, given that the healthy pulmonary circulation is a low-pressure system, which could lead to a differential gene expression. In general, most of our knowledge about the mechanism of RV fibrosis is extrapolated from LV research (140).

ANTI-FIBROTIC THERAPIES AND THEIR IMPACT ON LEFT OR RIGHT VENTRICULAR FUNCTION IN ANIMAL STUDIES

As research uncovers the mechanisms involved in reactive fibrosis, new targets and strategies are identified. We here briefly highlight preclinical studies modulating some of the most relevant targets involving extracellular collagen turnover, and cardiac fibroblast responses in the LV and the RV.

Although numerous preclinical studies using animal models of PH (i.e., hypoxia-induced PH mouse model, monocrotaline rat PH model, and Sugen/hypoxia rat PH model) have shown a reduction of RV fibrosis in response to therapeutic interventions, most of these interventions also attenuated the pulmonary vasculopathy and decreased the pulmonary arterial pressure. Thus, it is not clear whether these interventions directly or indirectly reduced fibrosis by decreasing the RV afterload in these animal models. In this section, we will only discuss preclinical studies done in the pure RV pressure overload model (PAB) and the interventions aimed to directly target the RV.

Angiotensin and Aldosterone

Systemic infusion of the pro-hypertensive hormone angiotensin II is a well-established and widely used *in vivo* preclinical model of LV reactive fibrosis due to pressure-overload mimicking systemic hypertension in patients (141). Given the gradual increase in pressure overload imposed on the heart of the animal as compared to models based on aortic banding, a relatively slowly progressing ECM remodeling can be achieved, which recapitulates human chronic disease (142). This led to a frequent use of this model of cardiac fibrosis, far beyond pre-clinical testing of Renin-Angiotensin-Aldosterone-System (RAAS) modulators. Interestingly, the profibrotic effect of angiotensin II could be seen upon chronic infusion of a low-dose angiotensin II, which did not increase systemic arterial blood pressures (143), and might therefore be mediated by direct effects of angiotensin II on cardiac fibroblasts (92, 93). Both Angiotensin 1 Receptor (AT1R) antagonists as well as Angiotensin Converting Enzyme (ACE) inhibitors have improved cardiac remodeling of the ECM and hypertrophy, together with reduction of arrhythmias, in pre-clinical testing (144–146).

Inhibition of the aldosterone pathway using mineralocorticoid receptor (MR) antagonists led to attenuated angiotensin II-induced fibrosis without affecting the blood pressure level in the mouse, halted progression of cardiac fibrosis and ameliorated myocardial global longitudinal strain in the hypertensive rat (147, 148).

As activation of the neurohormonal system has been also proposed as a key player in maladaptive RV failure, inhibition of the renin-angiotensin-aldosterone system by angiotensin receptor blockers (ARB) losartan (149) and Neprilysin inhibitor/ARB sacubitril/valsartan (150) has been tested and shown to reduce RV fibrosis without modifying RV afterload.

Extracellular Collagen Processing

Considering the strong correlation between the extent of collagen cross-linking with impairment of cardiac function and with a poor prognosis in HF patients, the enzymes catalyzing covalent cross-links between polypeptide chains of adjacent fibrils, lysyl oxidase (LOX), and lysyl oxidase homolog 2 (LOXL2), could be of major interest as therapeutic target. However, it was suggested that on the one hand a healthy degree of collagen cross-linking is needed for the adequate formation of collagen fibers and on the other hand that a stable ECM might be beneficial in overloaded conditions. Reducing excessive LOX expression or restoring the balance in LOX activity might therefore be superior to the irreversible blockage of LOX enzymatic activity (151).

Direct inhibition of LOXL2 by specific neutralizing monoclonal antibodies in mice with cardiac hypertrophy 2 weeks after TAC-surgery led to the elimination of cardiac fibrosis progression and major improvements of LV function without impacting hypertrophy (132). Direct inhibition of LOX in a volume-overloaded rat model prevented LV dysfunction and improved profiles of collagen and MMPs/TIMPs (152).

Presumably indirect effects on LOX modulation were observed upon chronic blockade of the TGF-β type III receptor beta glycan using the peptide P144 in spontaneously hypertensive rats which led to a reduced expression of LOX and a decrease in collagen cross-linking (153).

In human TGF-β1-stimulated fibroblasts, EXP3179, a non-antihypertensive metabolite of angiotensin II antagonist losartan, reduced over-expression and enhanced activity of LOX (154). *In vivo*, chronic treatment with EXP3179 prevented LOX upregulation and collagen cross-linking without impacting the systemic blood pressure in a rat hypertensive model. Taken together, collagen cross-linking enzymes might be used as therapeutic targets of anti-fibrotic drugs.

Transforming Growth Factor-β1

The role of the pro-fibrotic cytokine TGF-β1 was determined in animal studies using genetic and pharmacological interventions. TGF-β1 belongs to the TGF-β family of proteins, which have been described as the "master regulators" of fibrosis (155). Mice with inducible TGF-β receptor type R1/2 or SMAD3 deletions under the promotor of the myofibroblast marker periostin are protected against cardiac fibrosis and diastolic dysfunction in response to TAC (96). However, inducible overexpression of an inactive TGF-β type II receptor under the control of a metallothionein-derived promoter resulted in profound LV dilation and dysfunction in the pressure-overloaded mouse heart (156). Interestingly, cardiomyocyte-specific deletion of SMAD4, a central intracellular downstream mediator of TGF-β1 signaling, led to disturbances of systolic function in adult mice under basal conditions. Of note, canonical TGF-β signaling plays an important role in survival and contractility for cardiomyocytes during cell stress. In addition, TGF-β signaling can confer cardio protection not only in the pressure-overloaded (85), but also the infarcted myocardium (101). Therefore, caution is warranted when inhibiting this pathway therapeutically, in particular for long-term applications. On the other hand, heterozygous loss of TGF-β1 was shown to ameliorate myocardial fibrosis and LV compliance in aging mice, which explains their increased survival over the life span compared to wildtype control mice (157). Blocking of non-canonical TGF-β signaling by MAPK pathway inhibitors reduced ECM production in the renal fibroblast (158).

The TGF-β1 inhibitor pirfenidone, which is an approved drug for the treatment of idiopathic pulmonary fibrosis, showed anti-fibrotic effects in pre-clinical animal models of fibrosis across organs, namely lung, liver, LV, RV, and kidney (159). Pirfenidone not only inhibits synthesis and secretion of TGF-β1 by cardiac fibroblasts, but also their proliferation and migration activities, as well as differentiation into myofibroblasts (160). In various pre-clinical models of cardiac pressure-overload, pirfenidone improved LV function and fibrosis (161–163).

Reduction of RV fibrosis by pirfenidone has also been reported in the PAB animal model of RV pressure overload. Crnkovic et al. demonstrated a significant reduction of RV fibrosis by treating the animals with pirfenidone after RV fibrosis was established (i.e., 1 week after PAB); however, they did not observe an improvement in RV function (140). The authors speculated that this disconnection between reduction of RV fibrosis and RV dysfunction could be associated with the fact that RV dysfunction is not only driven by fibrosis but also strongly by the sarcomere impairment of the cardiomyocytes. On the other hand, Boehm et al. showed in the same animal model that activation of Bone Morphogenetic Protein signaling, a member of TGF-β superfamily, with FK506 was associated with reduction of fibrosis and improvement of RV function (164). They showed that FK506 reduced fibroblast proliferation and collagen production in a BMP-dependent fashion. Of note, the RV function of pirfenidone-treated animals were assessed after 3 weeks of treatment, while animals treated with FK506 were assessed after 7 weeks of treatment. This might suggest that the effect of fibrosis on RV function may differ during the development of pressure-overload induced RV failure. Further study is needed to elucidate the timing and duration of the therapeutic interventions in RV failure.

Endothelin-1

ET-1 has been shown to be compartmentalized in the myocardial interstitium, and ET-1 uptake was enhanced in a swine model of chronic HF (127). Angiotensin II-induced cardiac hypertrophy, interstitial and perivascular fibrosis were found to be dependent on ET-1, independently from blood pressure (165), suggesting that ET-1 plays an important role in fibrosis development in hypertensive conditions.

The Endothelin receptor antagonist macitentan was shown to have anti-fibrotic effect in PAB rabbit model (165).

Fibroblast Phenotypic Behavior

Newest approaches aimed at inhibiting pro-fibrotic responses of activated cardiac fibroblasts in a non-cellular-target-specific fashion. Discovery screens were based on the impact of drug candidates on proliferation rates (166, 167) and collagen type I expression of cardiac fibroblasts (167). Prominent anti-fibrotic effects of lead compounds identified correlated with improved LV function in two pressure-overloaded animal models with first promising safety data.

Other Mechanisms Studied in the Right Ventricle

With the presumption that growth factor plays an important role in fibroblast proliferation, receptor tyrosine kinase inhibitors sunitinib and sorafenib have been examined in PAB rat model and have shown to reduce RV fibrosis (168).

Several other factors that been suggested to influence the RV adaptation. Activation of the nitric oxide (NO)/soluble guanylyl cyclase (sGC)/cyclic guanosine 3'5'-monophosphate (cGMP) pathway by the phosphodiesterase type 5 (PDE-5) inhibitor sildenafil (169) and the soluble guanylate cyclase activator riociguat (170) as well as activation of the prostacyclin pathway by iloprost (171) were first examined in PH animal models. When being tested in PAB models of isolated RV afterload, they were shown to reduce RV fibrosis suggesting an anti-fibrotic effect beyond their vasodilatory effect. The role of sex hormones, especially the protective role of estrogen and deleterious effect of androgen on RV function, has been proposed and castration (removal of testis) reduced RV fibrosis in PAB male mice (172). Another hallmark of maladaptive RV failure is a metabolic shift from glucose oxidation to glycolysis in the RV myocardium. Partial inhibition of fatty acid oxidation by trimetazidine and ranolazine reduced the collagen content in the RV of PAB rats (173). Another hallmark of RV failure, inflammation and oxidative stress was been targeted by a Nuclear factor kappa B (NF-kB) inhibitor (174), the antioxidant protandim (175), an apoptosis signal-regulating kinase 1 (ASK1) inhibitor (176), and p38 mitogen-activated protein kinase (MAPK) inhibitor (177) which resulted in a reduction of RV fibrosis, emphasizing the important but understudied interplay between inflammation and fibrosis—the immune system and cardiac fibroblasts.

ANTI-FIBROTIC DRUGS IN CLINICAL TESTING FOR LEFT AND RIGHT VENTRICULAR HEART FAILURE

As discussed above, research efforts aimed at understanding the initiation and progression of adverse ECM remodeling have generated awareness of a panel of responsible key-players, some of which have subsequently been tested as therapeutic targets in humans. It should be noted that most anti-fibrotic therapies for the heart that seemed promising in experimental models have not been evaluated in patients, while the ones that underwent clinical testing mostly amounted to data that are limited or conflicting. We here discuss clinical testing of drugs that target extracellular collagen processing and/or cellular responses of the cardiac fibroblast (**Figures 3, 4** and **Table 1**). No antifibrotic drug designed to specifically target ECM remodeling has reached clinical practice yet. However, some routinely used LV HF therapies have shown beneficial effects in this context, as outlined below in section "Renin–Angiotensin–Aldosterone System Inhibitors" and "Modulators of Extracellular Collagen Processing."

Clinical Trials Targeting Fibrosis in Left Ventricular Heart Failure

Renin–Angiotensin–Aldosterone System Inhibitors

Clinical evidence indicates that the mainstay therapy for LV systolic HF, inhibiting the RAAS axis, targets diffuse myocardial fibrosis. As outlined in section "Extracellular Matrix Remodeling in the Left vs. Right Ventricle," cardiac fibroblasts express an AT1 receptor and respond to angiotensin II binding by ECM production and cellular proliferation (90, 92, 93, 124). In line, the ACE inhibitor lisinopril or the ARB losartan were associated with

TABLE 1 | HF therapies and agents with the potential to modulate receptors present on cardiac fibroblasts or extracellular collagen processing in clinical testing for LV and RV overloaded conditions.

Cardiac condition	Target	Study	Agent	Patients (*n*)	Findings
LV overload	RAAS	(178)	ACE inhibitor lisinopril	35	Administration of lisinopril, but not hydrochlorothiazide for 6 months decreased CVF in endomyocardial biopsies of hypertensive patients
		(179)	ARB losartan	19	Administration of losartan for 12 months decreased CVF in endomyocardial biopsies of hypertensive patients with severe fibrosis, but not in patients with non-severe fibrosis
		(226)	ARB losartan	37	Administration of losartan but not amlodipine for 12 months decreased CVF in endomyocardial biopsies and serum biomarker PIP in patients with hypertensive heart disease
		RAAM-PEF	Aldosterone antagonist eplerenone	44	Administration of eplerenone for 6 months reduced biomarkers of collagen turnover in HFpEF patients with a history of hypertension
		Aldo-DHF	MR antagonist spironolactone	422	Administration of spironolactone for 12 months improved diastolic function but did not improve HF symptoms in HFpEF patients, mostly with a history of hypertension
		TOPCAT	MR antagonist spironolactone	3,445	Administration of spironolactone for 3.3 years decreased hospitalization for HF, but not death from cardiovascular causes, aborted cardiac arrest, or hospitalization for any reason in HFpEF patients, mostly with a history of hypertension
		(186)	MR antagonist spironolactone	40	Administration of spironolactone for 6 months decreased the rate of extracellular expansion but did not change myocardial extracellular volume measured by MRI in HFpEF patients
	Extracellular collagen processing	(26)	Diuretic torsemide	20	Administration of torsemide but not furosemide for 8 months decreased LOX protein expression and collagen cross-linking in endomyocardial biopsies of chronic HF patients
		(41)	Diuretic torsemide	36	Administration of torsemide but not furosemide for 8 months decreased CVF in endomyocardial biopsies and serum biomarker PIP of class II to IV chronic HF patients
		(131)	Diuretic torsemide	22	Administration of torsemide but not furosemide for 8 months decreased CVF and PCP activation in endomyocardial biopsies and serum biomarker PICP of chronic HF patients
		TORAFIC	Diuretic torsemide	155	Administration of torsemide or furosemide for 8 months had no effect on serum biomarker PICP in hypertensive patients with mild chronic HF
	TGFβ inhibitors	PIROUETTE	TGFβ inhibitor pirfenidone	80	Administration of pirfenidone for 52 weeks decreased ECV measured by MRI in HFpEF patients, mostly with hypertension
	ET-1 inhibitors	(205)	Dual ET A/B receptor antagonist enrasentan	72	Administration of enrasentan for 6 months increased LV-EDVI in asymptomatic patients with LV dysfunction
		EARTH	ET antagonist darusentan	485	Administration of darusentan for 6 months did not change LV-ESV at, measured by MRI in patients with LV systolic dysfunction
RV overload	RAAS	STAR-HF	MR antagonist spironolactone	30 estimated	Ongoing; administration of spironolactone for 12 weeks will be assessed by biomarkers of fibrosis and T1 weighted MRI in patients with right HF

ACE, angiotensin converting enzyme; CVF, collagen volume fraction; ARB, angiotensin receptor blocker; HFpEF, Heart Failure with preserved ejection fraction; MR, mineralocorticoid receptor; MRI, magnetic resonance imaging; LOX, lysil oxidase; PIP/PICP, procollagen type I carboxy-terminal peptide (biomarker of collagen type I fiber synthesis); TGFβ, Transforming Growth Factor-β1; ET, endothelin-1; LV-EDVI, left ventricular end diastolic volume index; LV-ESV left ventricular end-systolic volume.

reducing the extent of reactive fibrosis together with LV stiffness, and improving LV diastolic dysfunction, when given to small cohorts of patients with hypertensive heart disease (178, 179).

Mineralocorticoid receptor (MR) antagonists are another class of established drugs for the treatment of LV systolic HF. Aldosterone can augment angiotensin II signaling, and also induce cardiac fibroblast proliferation independently of angiotensin II signaling, when binding to the MR *via* upregulation of MAPK pathways (180, 181). The double–blind clinical trial TOPCAT (Aldosterone Antagonist Therapy for Adults With Heart Failure and Preserved Systolic Function) testing the MR antagonist spironolactone in 3,445 HFpEF patients, did not significantly reduce the incidence of death from cardiovascular causes, cardiac arrest, or hospitalization (182). However, a subgroup of selected patients, many with atrial fibrillation and elevated heart failure biomarkers, showed a clinical benefit of spironolactone administration (183). While the rationale for this trial was based on the potential of MR antagonists to reduce fibrosis, cardiac fibrosis was not a studied end-point. In addition, aldosterone or MR antagonists led to improved tissue relaxation and positive changes in markers of collagen turnover in patients with HFpEF (184, 185). Recent studies applying CMR–derived measures of diffuse myocardial fibrosis as a primary end point demonstrated spironolactone-mediated decrease in the rate of extracellular expansion, with a decrease in the masses of cellular and extracellular myocardial compartments, in patients with HFpEF (186). Above therapies are safely used in the clinic and have the ability to target the AT1 or the MR axis in cardiac fibroblasts. However, some fibrotic burden still remains upon treatment, and given the prognostic role of fibrosis, this might contribute to the lack of a mortality benefit or reduction in hospitalization within HFpEF patients.

Modulators of Extracellular Collagen Processing

Diuretics are in clinical use to unload the heart. In small studies with patients with hypertensive HF, addition of the loop diuretic torsemide to conventional HF therapy led to beneficial modulation of extracellular collagen processing that associated with improvements in ECM quality and LV function (26, 41, 131). A decreased activity of the mature collagen type I-forming enzyme PCP and therefore less collagen deposition, as well as decreased expression of the collagen cross-linking catalyzing enzyme LOX and therefore less collagen cross-linking was observed after torsemide treatment. This was true only for the loop diuretic torsemide, but not furosemide. However, in a multicenter study of 155 hypertensive patients with chronic HF, the TORAFIC study, there were no significant differences between torsemide or furosemide groups in terms of changes in the serum procollagen type I carboxyterminal peptide (PICP), a biochemical marker of collagen type I fibers synthesis and deposition (187). It should be noted that the TORAFIC study did not assess fibrosis with histological or imaging modalities. In addition, the patient population had less severe HF compared to the preceding studies in smaller cohorts of hypertensive HF patients. Further studies are required to assess if it would be beneficial to select patients who might benefit from treatment with torsemide over furosemide. Nevertheless, long-term administration (around 10 years) of loop diuretics seemed to be safe.

Collectively, even though exact mechanistic studies are missing, modulation of ECM quality *per se* might represent a promising avenue for fibrosis treatment in the future and should be tested in large randomized controlled clinical trials. Of note, inhibition of LOXL-2 using the humanized monoclonal antibody simtuzumab has already been tested in phase II clinical trials in patients with hepatic or pulmonary fibrosis, demonstrating the feasibility direct targeting of collagen cross-linking (188, 189).

Transforming Growth Factor-β1 Inhibitors

Myocardial and serum levels of the profibrotic cytokine TGF-β1 are elevated in patients with HF due to hypertension or aortic stenosis (190, 191). The small molecule pirfenidone is orally bioavailable, and one of the most extensively studied inhibitors of the profibrotic cytokine TGF-β1. Pirfenidone reduces the synthesis and release of TGF-β1 in cardiac fibroblasts *in vitro*, as well as expression of TNF-α and PDGF, and is licensed for the treatment of idiopathic pulmonary fibrosis (160, 192, 193). In patients with pulmonary fibrosis, pirfenidone was shown to be safe and well tolerated, with infrequent and mild gastrointestinal and skin-related adverse events (194–197). Pirfenidone recently underwent a randomized, double-blind, placebo-controlled phase II PIROUETTE (Pirfenidone in patients with heart failure and preserved left ventricular ejection fraction) trial for HF, with CMR-assessed diffuse myocardial fibrosis as one of the study endpoints (198). Of note, patients with HFpEF were stratified based on fibrosis burden at baseline using ECV on CMR, based on the histologically-backed observation that regression of myocardial fibrosis was most pronounced in patients with the greatest burden of fibrosis at baseline (178, 179, 199). Given the fact that pirfenidone does not have any hemodynamic effects, results from the PIROUETTE trial might be of great interest also from a mechanistic perspective. First modest beneficial results were presented by Dr. Christopher Miller at the American College of Cardiology Virtual Annual Scientific Session (200), May 17, 2021. Pirfenidone led to a modest reduction in myocardial fibrosis without impacting diastolic function or 6-min walk distance (201). Potential deleterious effects, especially for long-term treatment regimens using pirfenidone, could arise due to the cardio protective side of TGF-β signaling described in section "Transforming Growth Factor-β1," and should be closely monitored for in future studies.

Endothelin-1 Inhibitors

While the dual endothelin receptor subtype A and B antagonist bosentan prevented fibrosis of various organs in animal models (202), the majority of clinical studies show that inhibition of the vasoconstrictor peptide endothelin-1 might not be the ideal anti-fibrotic strategy for the heart. For the treatment of pulmonary hypertension, the dual endothelin (ET) A and B inhibitors bosentan and macitentan, as well as the mono ET A inhibitor ambrisentan, are FDA approved. Initially, a small study in 36 men with severe HF showed promising results on systemic and pulmonary hemodynamics upon additional administration of bosentan (203). However, subsequent clinical testing of various endothelin receptor antagonists were neutral or showed harmful effects (204, 205). For example, administration of enrasentan resulted in adverse cardiac remodeling assessed by CMR parameters of LV end-diastolic volumes in 72 patients with asymptomatic LV systolic dysfunction (205). In a double-blind, placebo-controlled trial testing five different doses of darusentan, no improvement in cardiac remodeling, clinical symptoms or outcomes based on CMRI endpoints was shown in 642 patients with chronic HF (204). The general conclusion drawn was that endothelin-1 blockade might not be useful as an add-on treatment.

Clinical Trials Targeting Fibrosis in Right Ventricular Failure

Currently, there is only one clinical trial (STAR-HF: NCT03344159) assessing RV fibrosis as one of the outcomes. This trial is a phase 4 clinical trial investigating the effect of the mineralocorticoid receptor antagonist spironolactone in patients with chronic RV failure caused by either PH or cardiomyopathy. RV fibrosis will be assessed *via* T1 weighted MRI and serum biomarkers. There are no clinical trials that are directly targeting RV fibrosis or are examining the feasibility of anti-fibrotic therapy in RV failure.

FUTURE DIRECTIONS

Despite pre-clinical successes, clinical testing of anti-fibrotic compounds has been unsuccessful. Endeavors to develop therapeutic approaches for reactive myocardial fibrosis go hand in hand with fundamental questions, such as (*i*) *Should therapeutic strategies block chronic maladaptive forms of fibrosis, while preserving its adaptive function to confer chamber stability, or locally replace dying cardiomyocytes upon overloaded conditions?* (*ii*) *Is established reactive myocardial fibrosis reversible?* To aid in the development of effective and safe therapeutic strategies, we are discussing these important considerations in the following section.

The Potential Necessity to Preserve Adaptive While Targeting Maladaptive Functions of Fibrosis in the Overloaded Heart

Myocardial fibrosis in pressure overloaded conditions is very complex and given its heterogeneity in functional profiles, there is a call for a better definition, phenotyping, and quantification of the different types of fibrosis that exist in HF (206) (**Figure 1**). Toward this end, studies using invasive biopsy and non-invasive imaging show that in severe aortic stenosis, three main subtypes of fibrosis co-exist in the LV: pronounced fibrotic endocardial thickening, micro scars in the sub-endo myocardium resulting from reparative fibrosis, and diffuse interstitial fibrosis corresponding to reactive fibrosis (207). In other words, reparative fibrosis seems to take place locally to replace dying cardiomyocytes, whereas at the same time reactive fibrosis leads to adverse remodeling resulting in worse LV function and clinical outcome for the patient. This raises the question whether long-term antifibrotic intervention that also targets the potentially required reparative fibrosis in form of micro scars might be beneficial. Pre-clinical studies indicate that early stages of ECM remodeling of the pressure-overloaded, hypertrophied non-human primate heart are accompanied by reactive fibrosis without cardiomyocyte death, while in later stages a certain degree of reparative fibrosis is present (208). If this timeline was translatable to human ECM remodeling, clinical trials testing new anti-fibrotic therapies would need to be designed with optimal timing in mind. In a small systematic histological and histometric study of 30 hearts with end-stage hypertrophic cardiomyopathy, harvested at time of transplant, replacement fibrosis was the most prevalent form of fibrosis which in total occupied almost over a third of the LV (51). Antifibrotic therapy therefore might not necessarily be beneficial in end-stage heart failure when replacement fibrosis instead of reactive fibrosis is most prevalent. Taking into consideration that reactive fibrosis might lead to hypoxic conditions that favor cardiomyocyte death, anti-fibrotic interventions at earlier timepoints might be indicated. This would help prevent local replacement fibrosis and micro scar development, a known substrate for arrhythmias. As reactive fibrosis initially might be an important adaptive mechanism to add to chamber stability and prevent dilation of the ventricle, it is important to characterize at which time-point and which amount of reactive fibrosis becomes maladaptive. In general, any additional management of underlying etiologies to reduce the cardiac afterload would be paramount.

How Do We Assess and Quantify Fibrosis in Humans Longitudinally With Therapeutic Intervention

A combination of imaging techniques and circulating biomarkers indicating activity of reactive myocardial fibrosis in real-time would be useful to guide timing of anti-fibrotic interventions, and to monitor efficacy. Latest imaging techniques employ CMRI as a non-invasive assessment tool not only of cardiac structure and function, but also of tissue characteristics. CMRI allows direct detection of fibrotic patches as seen in large post-infarct scars *via* late-gadolinium enhancement (LGE), and indirect assessment of diffuse interstitial fibrosis by T1 mapping of the myocardial wall, including native T1 differentiating normal from infarcted myocardium, post-contrast T1, and extracellular volume fraction (ECV) (209). However, clinical studies validating ECV measurements with quantification of histological collagen deposition in biopsies seem conflicting (207, 210, 211). In addition, LGE techniques are qualitative and not able to visualize replacement fibrosis occurring in the overloaded heart, which can occupy very small regions and is not associated with a large scar as present following myocardial infarction. Further limitations of CMRI-based assessments are a lack of sensitivity in detecting early stage disease, as well as of the ability to capture active fibrogenesis of reactive fibrosis. As such, molecular imaging of cardiac fibrosis could have the potential to overcome all these obstacles (212), both for the LV as well as the RV. Molecular imaging can sensitively quantify specific fibrotic pathways by using small molecules, peptides, or antibodies that are tagged with an imaging reporter, and that bind to a protein, receptor, or fibrotic process of interest (213). The molecular imaging probes can then be visualized with positron emission tomography (PET), single-photon emission computed tomography (SPECT), or MRI. Molecular imaging has already successfully reached the clinics for applications related to various fibrotic lung diseases, thanks to pioneering studies conducted within the last two decades (214–216). For the fibrotic heart, development of this technology is lagging behind and until now it has been used to demonstrate focal scarring after myocardial infarction in pre-clinical (217–220) and preliminary clinical studies (221) by tracing myofibroblasts, or collagen type I. Recent advances demonstrated feasibility of detecting diffuse interstitial myocardial fibrosis using specific collagen probes in the β2-AR (β-2-adrenergic receptor) overexpressing mouse model *in vivo*, and in ischemic human heart specimens (222). Importantly, specific tracers directed toward molecular targets that allow for a differentiation of pro-fibrotic responses associated with the different stages of a wound healing processes, and other fibrotic processes that also occur in a pressure-overloaded condition, such as ECM accumulation and cross-linking, do exist (212, 213). Further research to validate their usefulness in the overloaded heart is warranted.

Evidence of Reversibility of Reactive Cardiac Fibrosis

Pre-clinical and clinical histological evidence suggests that in general, established reactive myocardial fibrosis is able to regress in the pressure-overloaded LV, even at later stages (178, 179, 223–225). Regression of fibrosis was evident in these cases after unloading the heart by treating underlying hypertension. Experimental models of hypertensive cardiac fibrosis include the angiotensin II infused mouse, with normalization of blood pressure achieved by cessation of angiotensin II infusion that led to an incomplete resolution of myocardial fibrosis with concomitant improvement of cardiac function (223). In Sprague-Dawley and in spontaneously hypertensive rats, regression of collagen deposition occurred after treatment with angiotensin-converting enzyme (ACE) inhibitors, and in cases that included cardiac functional measurements, fibrosis regression was seen together with an improvement of abnormal myocardial diastolic stiffness (224, 225). In a study using a small number of patients with hypertensive heart disease, ACE inhibition with lisinopril regressed myocardial fibrosis on endomyocardial biopsy that was accompanied by improved LV diastolic function (178). Interestingly, the ARB losartan induced regression of myocardial fibrosis that was associated with a reduction of myocardial stiffness in hypertensive patients with severe fibrosis, but not with non-severe fibrosis, as assessed by collagen volume fraction (CVF) quantification in endomyocardial biopsies in a small study (179). This finding might imply that patients with hypertension might benefit from treatment stratification that includes assessment of their fibrotic status. Of note, normalization of blood pressure did not prove to be effective in reversing established cardiac fibrosis in all cases. For example, normalization of blood pressure using the calcium channel blocker amlodipine failed to reduce CVF in endomyocardial biopsies, and serum levels of PIP in hypertensive patients (226). *In vitro* studies using rat cardiac fibroblasts demonstrated that cardiac fibroblasts expressed an angiotensin II receptor that controls proliferative activities and is sensitive to the antagonist losartan (91, 93), suggesting that fibrosis regression by ACE inhibitors and ARBs might at least in part be mediated by direct actions on cardiac fibroblasts.

Clinical data on the reversibility of reactive fibrosis after unloading the LV from pressure by replacing the aortic valve in the setting of aortic stenosis seem reaffirming. In a study utilizing CMRI and CVF assessment in biopsies in patients with severe aortic stenosis, aortic valve replacement led to regression of reactive fibrosis, but not replacement fibrosis, that was accompanied by structural improvements and amelioration of diastolic dysfunction after 1-year post-surgery follow-up (227). In line, a study that included asymptomatic mild, moderate, and severe aortic stenosis patients, as well as symptomatic patients who underwent aortic valve replacement, showed that reactive myocardial fibrosis regressed, while midwall LGE was irreversible post valve replacement (228). It should be noted that a third study concluded that myocardial fibrosis is not reversible 9 months after aortic valve replacement (56). However, histology was only assessed at time of surgery, and CMRI included LGE for assessment of reparative fibrosis but not T1 mapping and ECV for reactive fibrosis. The results of this study might be congruent with subsequent studies as noted above, concluding that replacement fibrosis might not be reversible. In contrast, reactive fibrosis can regress in the LV upon unloading of pressure-overload due to aortic stenosis.

In other settings, cardiac fibrosis might be not reversible. For example, mechanical volume and pressure unloading of the heart by left ventricular assist devices (LVAD) as a means to bridge time until a heart transplant becomes available, or as a final treatment option for end-stage HF, sometimes is followed by cardiac recovery so that the LVAD can be weaned off in some cases. Interestingly, pre-clinical studies demonstrated that replicating mechanical unloading in a rat model of TAC by heterotopic heart transplantation led to complete regression of cardiomyocyte hypertrophy, while fibrotic remodeling was significantly exacerbated (229). The authors concluded that this result might explain the low rates of LVAD removal in the clinics. As a matter of fact, reports describing LVAD explantation after successful myocardial recovery under LVAD therapy are rare (230, 231). Moreover, clinical data using a small number of patients showed persistence of cardiac fibrosis after 8 months of unloading using a LVAD (232). Conflicting results suggested that reduced MMP activity diminished damage to the ECM and contribute to LV functional recovery after LVAD support (39). Further studies with larger patient numbers might be required to reach conclusive results.

Mechanistically, reversal of reactive cardiac fibrosis likely includes degradation or modification of the fibrotic extracellular matrix, and changes in cellular behaviors of activated fibroblasts and myofibroblasts such as proliferation and collagen I synthesis, apoptosis, senescence, dedifferentiation, and reprogramming. Further research would be needed to understand mechanisms of fibrosis resolution, which might benefit from newest technical developments, such as single cell RNA sequencing (scRNAseq), or molecular imaging techniques.

Even though regression of reactive myocardial fibrosis is possible in some scenarios as mentioned above, complete fibrosis resolution and regaining of healthy state levels have never been achieved in humans. This observation supports the notion that further regression would require the development of additional fibrosis-resolving treatments. However, as reactive fibrosis develops in response to a mechanical stimulus such as pressure-overload it may play additional important adaptive roles by providing structural stability. Unless there is evidence of ongoing, unrestrained, and non-beneficial fibrosis at some point in the cardiac remodeling process, there might be therefore also potential negative consequences of inhibiting fibrosis. In any case, treating the underlying condition in parallel by for example reducing RV pressure-overload or aortic stenosis would be paramount.

CONCLUSION

Reactive fibrosis in the pressure overloaded LV and RV accompanies cardiac remodeling that leads to heart failure. Most studies aimed at understanding the impact of reactive fibrosis on cardiac function, physiology and patient outcomes have been conducted in the LV. A limitation of probably all human correlational studies is the small patient number and occasional inconsistencies in readouts that range from histology, imaging modalities to fibrosis-biomarkers. In addition, up to one-third of HFpEF patients have normal measures of myocardial fibrosis, which might call for stratification for individuals that might benefit from anti-fibrotic therapies. Lastly, timing of anti-fibrotic drug administration might be an important factor to be considered for clinical trial designs to optimize efficacy and safety. Non-invasive imaging could be used to guide optimal timing and monitor treatment response. CMRI can be used to determine reactive fibrosis *via* T1 mapping and ECV assessment and captures existing ECM deposits in the heart. Molecular imaging would additionally enable visualization of active fibrogenesis of reactive fibrosis occurring in real-time. In addition, T1 mapping would allow reactive fibrosis to be graded, and the question if there is a point of no return for reversal of reactive fibrosis could be answered.

Fibrosis research has been hampered by technical limitations affecting both *in vitro* and *in vivo* experiments. The mayor limitation of *in vitro* studies is the lack of healthy fibroblasts in a culture dish due to immediate differentiation into myofibroblasts that is induced by the strain of the plastic surface. This imposes difficulties not only in understanding differences in the healthy vs. activated fibroblast, but also dissecting the role of myofibroblasts vs. proliferating resident fibroblasts in myocardial remodeling. Cardiac fibroblast markers used *in vivo* mostly lack specificity and for that reason, cardiac fibroblast-specific ablation of factors of interest remains challenging. However, it should be noted that emerging newer technologies, such as scRNA seq, might help in these quests. Most recently, a vast heterogeneity in cardiac fibroblast populations has been uncovered using scRNAseq (86), and differences in their functions need to be addressed in future studies. Time-dependent changes in fibroblast populations or states in the pressure-overloaded LV or RV and their functional contributions to reactive fibrosis development, progression or regression should be determined. In addition, other cell types involved in these processes might be uncovered. This will be helpful in guiding drug development, and timing of administration.

Most of our perception on reactive fibrosis stems from studies focused on the LV. Further research is needed to understand the contribution of reactive fibrosis in the RV with regards to RV dysfunction, arrhythmias, and creation of hypoxic conditions. In addition, RV fibrosis as predictor of survival of patients is currently unknown. RV biopsies of the RV free wall would put patients at risk for perforation, therefore the use of non-invasive imaging and biomarkers to assess reactive fibrosis in addition to the meticulous study of human heart tissue at the time of transplant or surgery, would be the first-line modalities to address these questions.

Despite all the above-mentioned challenges in fibrosis research, the observation that fibrosis regression is possible, is promising and a fascinating area to study. Understudied research areas include the process of intracellular collagen degradation, namely phagocytosis of macrophages and cardiac fibroblasts (233) as well as the modulation of collagen cross-linking, as a means to reverse fibrosis. Given the structural stability conferred to the heart by reactive fibrosis, therapeutic strategies that induce fibrosis resolution should be accompanied by management of the underlying etiology, such as interventions that relieve the afterload. Collaborative efforts across disciplines including cell biology, mouse genetics, imaging, cardiology, and pharmacology will be required to help unveil mechanisms and dynamics of reactive fibrosis and translate them into therapeutic approaches that can be tested and ultimately used in clinical practice.

AUTHOR CONTRIBUTIONS

KS and ES conceptualized the review. KS and KI wrote the manuscript. KS created the figures and table. ES, SR, and FH critically reviewed and provided feedback and guidance. All authors contributed to the article and approved the submitted version.

ACKNOWLEDGMENTS

All figures were created with BioRender.com.

REFERENCES

1. Omiya S, Omori Y, Taneike M, Protti A, Yamaguchi O, Akira S, et al. Toll-like receptor 9 prevents cardiac rupture after myocardial infarction in mice independently of inflammation. *Am J Physiol Heart Circ Physiol.* (2016) 311:H1485–97. doi: 10.1152/ajpheart.00481.2016
2. Nagai T, Honda S, Sugano Y, Matsuyama T, Ohta–Ogo K, Asaumi Y, et al. Decreased myocardial dendritic cells is associated with impaired reparative fibrosis and development of cardiac rupture after myocardial infarction in humans. *J Am Heart Assoc.* (2014) 3:e000839. doi: 10.1161/JAHA.114.000839
3. Ushakov A, Ivanchenko V, Gagarina A. Regulation of myocardial extracellular matrix dynamic changes in myocardial infarction and

postinfarct remodeling. *Curr Cardiol Rev.* (2020) 16:11–24. doi: 10.2174/1573403X15666190509090832

4. Kanisicak O, Khalil H, Ivey MJ, Karch J, Maliken BD, Correll RN, et al. Genetic lineage tracing defines myofibroblast origin and function in the injured heart. *Nat Commun.* (2016) 7:12260. doi: 10.1038/ncomms12260
5. Oken DE, Boucek RJ. Quantitation of collagen in human myocardium. *Circ Res.* (1957) 5:357–61. doi: 10.1161/01.res.5.4.357
6. Weber KT. Cardiac interstitium in health and disease: the fibrillar collagen network. *J Am Coll Cardiol.* (1989) 13:1637–52. doi: 10.1016/0735-1097(89)90360-4
7. Echegaray K, Andreu I, Lazkano A, Villanueva I, Sáenz A, Elizalde MR, et al. Role of myocardial collagen in severe aortic stenosis with preserved ejection fraction and symptoms of heart failure. *Rev Espanola Cardiol Engl Ed.* (2017) 70:832–40. doi: 10.1016/j.rec.2016.12.038
8. Zile MR, Baicu CF, Ikonomidis JS, Stroud RE, Nietert PJ, Bradshaw AD, et al. Myocardial stiffness in patients with heart failure and a preserved ejection fraction: contributions of collagen and titin. *Circulation.* (2015) 131:1247–59. doi: 10.1161/circulationaha.114.013215
9. Querejeta R, López B, González A, Sánchez E, Larman M, Martínez Ubago JL, et al. Increased collagen Type I synthesis in patients with heart failure of hypertensive origin. *Circulation.* (2004) 110:1263–8. doi: 10.1161/01.CIR.0000140973.60992.9A
10. López B, González A, Querejeta R, Larman M, Díez J. Alterations in the pattern of collagen deposition may contribute to the deterioration of systolic function in hypertensive patients with heart failure. *J Am Coll Cardiol.* (2006) 48:89–96. doi: 10.1016/j.jacc.2006.01.077
11. Brower GL, Gardner JD, Forman MF, Murray DB, Voloshenyuk T, Levick SP, et al. The relationship between myocardial extracellular matrix remodeling and ventricular function. *Eur J Cardio-Thorac Surg Off J Eur Assoc Cardio Thorac Surg.* (2006) 30:604–10. doi: 10.1016/j.ejcts.2006.07.006
12. Pearlman ES, Weber KT, Janicki JS, Pietra GG, Fishman AP. Muscle fiber orientation and connective tissue content in the hypertrophied human heart. *Lab Investig J Tech Methods Pathol.* (1982) 46:158–64.
13. Rossi MA. Pathologic fibrosis and connective tissue matrix in left ventricular hypertrophy due to chronic arterial hypertension in humans. *J Hypertens.* (1998) 16:1031–41. doi: 10.1097/00004872-199816070-00018
14. Bartosová D, Chvapil M, Koreckı B, Poupa O, Rakusan K, Turek Z, et al. The growth of the muscular and collagenous parts of the rat heart in various forms of cardiomegaly. *J Physiol.* (1969) 200:285–95. doi: 10.1113/jphysiol.1969.sp008693
15. Anderson KR, Sutton MG, Lie JT. Histopathological types of cardiac fibrosis in myocardial disease. *J Pathol.* (1979) 128:79–85. doi: 10.1002/path.1711280205
16. Huysman JA, Vliegen HW, Van der Laarse A, Eulderink F. Changes in nonmyocyte tissue composition associated with pressure overload of hypertrophic human hearts. *Pathol Res Pract.* (1989) 184:577–81. doi: 10.1016/S0344-0338(89)80162-1
17. Collier P, Watson CJ, van Es MH, Phelan D, McGorrian C, Tolan M, et al. Getting to the heart of cardiac remodeling; how collagen subtypes may contribute to phenotype. *J Mol Cell Cardiol.* (2012) 52:148–53. doi: 10.1016/j.yjmcc.2011.10.002
18. Weber KT, Pick R, Jalil JE, Janicki JS, Carroll EP. Patterns of myocardial fibrosis. *J Mol Cell Cardiol.* (1989) 21(Suppl 5):121–31. doi: 10.1016/0022-2828(89)90778-5
19. Eghbali M, Weber KT. Collagen and the myocardium: fibrillar structure, biosynthesis and degradation in relation to hypertrophy and its regression. *Mol Cell Biochem.* (1990) 96:1–14. doi: 10.1007/BF00228448
20. Gazoti Debessa CR, Mesiano Maifrino LB, Rodrigues de Souza R. Age related changes of the collagen network of the human heart. *Mech Ageing Dev.* (2001) 122:1049–58. doi: 10.1016/s0047-6374(01)00238-x
21. López B, González A, Querejeta R, Larman M, Rábago G, Díez J. Association of cardiotrophin-1 with myocardial fibrosis in hypertensive patients with heart failure. *Hypertens Dallas Tex 1979.* (2014) 63:483–9. doi: 10.1161/HYPERTENSIONAHA.113.02654
22. López B, Querejeta R, González A, Larman M, Díez J. Collagen cross-linking but not collagen amount associates with elevated filling pressures in hypertensive patients with stage C heart failure: potential role of lysyl oxidase. *Hypertens Dallas Tex 1979.* (2012) 60:677–83. doi: 10.1161/HYPERTENSIONAHA.112.196113
23. Kasner M, Westermann D, Lopez B, Gaub R, Escher F, Kühl U, et al. Diastolic tissue Doppler indexes correlate with the degree of collagen expression and cross-linking in heart failure and normal ejection fraction. *J Am Coll Cardiol.* (2011) 57:977–85. doi: 10.1016/j.jacc.2010.10.024
24. Pérez del Villar C, Savvatis K, López B, Kasner M, Martinez-Legazpi P, Yotti R, et al. Impact of acute hypertension transients on diastolic function in patients with heart failure with preserved ejection fraction. *Cardiovasc Res.* (2017) 113:906–14. doi: 10.1093/cvr/cvx047
25. López B, González A, Lindner D, Westermann D, Ravassa S, Beaumont J, et al. Osteopontin-mediated myocardial fibrosis in heart failure: a role for lysyl oxidase? *Cardiovasc Res.* (2013) 99:111–20. doi: 10.1093/cvr/cvt100
26. López B, Querejeta R, González A, Beaumont J, Larman M, Díez J. Impact of treatment on myocardial lysyl oxidase expression and collagen cross-linking in patients with heart failure. *Hypertens Dallas Tex 1979.* (2009) 53:236–42. doi: 10.1161/HYPERTENSIONAHA.108.125278
27. Eghbali M, Czaja MJ, Zeydel M, Weiner FR, Zern MA, Seifter S, et al. Collagen chain mRNAs in isolated heart cells from young and adult rats. *J Mol Cell Cardiol.* (1988) 20:267–76. doi: 10.1016/s0022-2828(88)80059-2
28. Eghbali M, Blumenfeld OO, Seifter S, Buttrick PM, Leinwand LA, Robinson TF, et al. Localization of types I, III and IV collagen mRNAs in rat heart cells by in situ hybridization. *J Mol Cell Cardiol.* (1989) 21:103–13. doi: 10.1016/0022-2828(89)91498-3
29. Bomb R, Heckle MR, Sun Y, Mancarella S, Guntaka RV, Gerling IC, et al. Myofibroblast secretome and its auto-/paracrine signaling. *Expert Rev Cardiovasc Ther.* (2016) 14:591–8. doi: 10.1586/14779072.2016.1147348
30. McLenachan JM, Dargie HJ. Ventricular arrhythmias in hypertensive left ventricular hypertrophy. Relationship to coronary artery disease, left ventricular dysfunction, and myocardial fibrosis. *Am J Hypertens.* (1990) 3:735–40. doi: 10.1093/ajh/3.10.735
31. MacKenna D, Summerour SR, Villarreal FJ. Role of mechanical factors in modulating cardiac fibroblast function and extracellular matrix synthesis. *Cardiovasc Res.* (2000) 46:257–63. doi: 10.1016/s0008-6363(00)00030-4
32. Duca F, Kammerlander AA, Zotter-Tufaro C, Aschauer S, Schwaiger ML, Marzluf BA, et al. Interstitial fibrosis, functional status, and outcomes in heart failure with preserved ejection fraction: insights from a prospective cardiac magnetic resonance imaging study. *Circ Cardiovasc Imaging.* (2016) 9:e005277. doi: 10.1161/CIRCIMAGING.116.005277
33. Briasoulis A, Mallikethi-Reddy S, Palla M, Alesh I, Afonso L. Myocardial fibrosis on cardiac magnetic resonance and cardiac outcomes in hypertrophic cardiomyopathy: a meta-analysis. *Heart Br Card Soc.* (2015) 101:1406–11. doi: 10.1136/heartjnl-2015-307682
34. Azevedo CF, Nigri M, Higuchi ML, Pomerantzeff PM, Spina GS, Sampaio RO, et al. Prognostic significance of myocardial fibrosis quantification by histopathology and magnetic resonance imaging in patients with severe aortic valve disease. *J Am Coll Cardiol.* (2010) 56:278–87. doi: 10.1016/j.jacc.2009.12.074
35. Schelbert EB, Fridman Y, Wong TC, Abu Daya H, Piehler KM, Kadakkal A, et al. Temporal relation between myocardial fibrosis and heart failure with preserved ejection fraction: association with baseline disease severity and subsequent outcome. *JAMA Cardiol.* (2017) 2:995–1006. doi: 10.1001/jamacardio.2017.2511
36. van der Slot-Verhoeven AJ, van Dura EA, Attema J, Blauw B, Degroot J, Huizinga TWJ, et al. The type of collagen cross-link determines the reversibility of experimental skin fibrosis. *Biochim Biophys Acta.* (2005) 1740:60–7. doi: 10.1016/j.bbadis.2005.02.007
37. Robins SP. Biochemistry and functional significance of collagen cross-linking. *Biochem Soc Trans.* (2007) 35:849–52. doi: 10.1042/BST0350849
38. López-De León A, Rojkind M. A simple micromethod for collagen and total protein determination in formalin-fixed paraffin-embedded sections. *J Histochem Cytochem.* (1985) 33:737–43. doi: 10.1177/33.8.2410480
39. Li YY, Feng Y, McTiernan CF, Pei W, Moravec CS, Wang P, et al. Downregulation of matrix metalloproteinases and reduction in collagen damage in the failing human heart after support with left ventricular assist devices. *Circulation.* (2001) 104:1147–52. doi: 10.1161/hc3501.095215
40. Beaumont J, López B, Ravassa S, Hermida N, San José G, Gallego I, et al. MicroRNA-19b is a potential biomarker of increased myocardial collagen

cross-linking in patients with aortic stenosis and heart failure. *Sci Rep.* (2017) 7:40696.

41. López B, Querejeta R, González A, Sánchez E, Larman M, Díez J. Effects of loop diuretics on myocardial fibrosis and collagen type I turnover in chronic heart failure. *J Am Coll Cardiol.* (2004) 43:2028–35. doi: 10.1016/j.jacc.2003.12.052
42. Yamato M, Sasaki T, Honda K, Fukuda M, Akutagawa O, Okamoto M, et al. Effects of torasemide on left ventricular function and neurohumoral factors in patients with chronic heart failure. *Circ J Off J Jpn Circ Soc.* (2003) 67:384–90. doi: 10.1253/circj.67.384
43. Cosín J, Díez J, Toric investigators. Torasemide in chronic heart failure: results of the TORIC study. *Eur J Heart Fail.* (2002) 4:507–13. doi: 10.1016/s1388-9842(02)00122-8
44. Murray MD, Deer MM, Ferguson JA, Dexter PR, Bennett SJ, Perkins SM, et al. Open-label randomized trial of torsemide compared with furosemide therapy for patients with heart failure. *Am J Med.* (2001) 111:513–20. doi: 10.1016/s0002-9343(01)00903-2
45. Broekhuysen J, Deger F, Douchamps J, Ducarne H, Herchuelz A. Torasemide, a new potent diuretic. Double-blind comparison with furosemide. *Eur J Clin Pharmacol.* (1986) 31:29–34. doi: 10.1007/BF00541464
46. Nguyen M-N, Kiriazis H, Gao X-M, Du X-J. Cardiac fibrosis and arrhythmogenesis. *Compr Physiol.* (2017) 7:1009–49. doi: 10.1002/cphy.c160046
47. Kawara T, Derksen R, de Groot JR, Coronel R, Tasseron S, Linnenbank AC, et al. Activation delay after premature stimulation in chronically diseased human myocardium relates to the architecture of interstitial fibrosis. *Circulation.* (2001) 104:3069–75. doi: 10.1161/hc5001.100833
48. Dai Z, Aoki T, Fukumoto Y, Shimokawa H. Coronary perivascular fibrosis is associated with impairment of coronary blood flow in patients with non-ischemic heart failure. *J Cardiol.* (2012) 60:416–21. doi: 10.1016/j.jjcc.2012.06.009
49. Mohammed SF, Hussain S, Mirzoyev SA, Edwards WD, Maleszewski JJ, Redfield MM. Coronary microvascular rarefaction and myocardial fibrosis in heart failure with preserved ejection fraction. *Circulation.* (2015) 131:550–9. doi: 10.1161/circulationaha.114.009625
50. Sabbah HN, Sharov VG, Lesch M, Goldstein S. Progression of heart failure: a role for interstitial fibrosis. *Mol Cell Biochem.* (1995) 147:29–34. doi: 10.1007/BF00944780
51. Galati G, Leone O, Pasquale F, Olivotto I, Biagini E, Grigioni F, et al. Histological and histometric characterization of myocardial fibrosis in end-stage hypertrophic cardiomyopathy: a clinical-pathological study of 30 explanted hearts. *Circ Heart Fail.* (2016) 9:e003090. doi: 10.1161/CIRCHEARTFAILURE.116.003090
52. Ravassa S, López B, Querejeta R, Echegaray K, San José G, Moreno MU, et al. Phenotyping of myocardial fibrosis in hypertensive patients with heart failure. Influence on clinical outcome. *J Hypertens.* (2017) 35:853–61. doi: 10.1097/HJH.0000000000001258
53. López B, Ravassa S, González A, Zubillaga E, Bonavila C, Bergés M, et al. Myocardial collagen cross-linking is associated with heart failure hospitalization in patients with hypertensive heart failure. *J Am Coll Cardiol.* (2016) 67:251–60. doi: 10.1016/j.jacc.2015.10.063
54. Tin LL, Beevers DG, Lip GYH. Hypertension, left ventricular hypertrophy, and sudden death. *Curr Cardiol Rep.* (2002) 4:449–57. doi: 10.1007/s11886-002-0105-6
55. Gulati A, Jabbour A, Ismail TF, Guha K, Khwaja J, Raza S, et al. Association of fibrosis with mortality and sudden cardiac death in patients with nonischemic dilated cardiomyopathy. *JAMA.* (2013) 309:896–908. doi: 10.1001/jama.2013.1363
56. Weidemann F, Herrmann S, Störk S, Niemann M, Frantz S, Lange V, et al. Impact of myocardial fibrosis in patients with symptomatic severe aortic stenosis. *Circulation.* (2009) 120:577–84. doi: 10.1161/CIRCULATIONAHA.108.847772
57. Borbély A, van der Velden J, Papp Z, Bronzwaer JGF, Edes I, Stienen GJM, et al. Cardiomyocyte stiffness in diastolic heart failure. *Circulation.* (2005) 111:774–81. doi: 10.1161/01.CIR.0000155257.33485.6D
58. Liu W, Wang Z. Current understanding of the biomechanics of ventricular tissues in heart failure. *Bioengineering.* (2019) 7:2. doi: 10.3390/bioengineering7010002
59. Voorhees AP, Han H-C. Biomechanics of cardiac function. *Compr Physiol.* (2015) 5:1623–44. doi: 10.1002/cphy.c140070
60. van de Veerdonk MC, Kind T, Marcus JT, Mauritz G-J, Heymans MW, Bogaard H-J, et al. Progressive right ventricular dysfunction in patients with pulmonary arterial hypertension responding to therapy. *J Am Coll Cardiol.* (2011) 58:2511–9. doi: 10.1016/j.jacc.2011.06.068
61. Ghio S, Gavazzi A, Campana C, Inserra C, Klersy C, Sebastiani R, et al. Independent and additive prognostic value of right ventricular systolic function and pulmonary artery pressure in patients with chronic heart failure. *J Am Coll Cardiol.* (2001) 37:183–8. doi: 10.1016/s0735-1097(00)01102-5
62. Amano M, Izumi C, Baba M, Abe R, Matsutani H, Inao T, et al. Progression of right ventricular dysfunction and predictors of mortality in patients with idiopathic interstitial pneumonias. *J Cardiol.* (2020) 75:242–9. doi: 10.1016/j.jjcc.2019.08.010
63. Li Y, Liang L, Guo D, Yang Y, Gong J, Zhang X, et al. Right ventricular function predicts adverse clinical outcomes in patients with chronic thromboembolic pulmonary hypertension: a three-dimensional echocardiographic study. *Front Med.* (2021) 8:697396. doi: 10.3389/fmed.2021.697396
64. Tonelli AR, Arelli V, Minai OA, Newman J, Bair N, Heresi GA, et al. Causes and circumstances of death in pulmonary arterial hypertension. *Am J Respir Crit Care Med.* (2013) 188:365–9. doi: 10.1164/rccm.201209-1640OC
65. Rain S, Handoko ML, Trip P, Gan CTJ, Westerhof N, Stienen GJ, et al. Right ventricular diastolic impairment in patients with pulmonary arterial hypertension. *Circulation.* (2013) 128:2016–25. doi: 10.1161/CIRCULATIONAHA.113.001873
66. van der Bruggen CE, Happé CM, Dorfmüller P, Trip P, Spruijt OA, Rol N, et al. Bone morphogenetic protein receptor Type 2 mutation in pulmonary arterial hypertension: a view on the right ventricle. *Circulation.* (2016) 133:1747–60.
67. Freed BH, Gomberg-Maitland M, Chandra S, Mor-Avi V, Rich S, Archer SL, et al. Late gadolinium enhancement cardiovascular magnetic resonance predicts clinical worsening in patients with pulmonary hypertension. *J Cardiovasc Magn Reson.* (2012) 14:11. doi: 10.1186/1532-429X-14-11
68. Roller FC, Wiedenroth C, Breithecker A, Liebetrau C, Mayer E, Schneider C, et al. Native T1 mapping and extracellular volume fraction measurement for assessment of right ventricular insertion point and septal fibrosis in chronic thromboembolic pulmonary hypertension. *Eur Radiol.* (2017) 27:1980–91. doi: 10.1007/s00330-016-4585-y
69. Mehta BB, Auger DA, Gonzalez JA, Workman V, Chen X, Chow K, et al. Detection of elevated right ventricular extracellular volume in pulmonary hypertension using Accelerated and Navigator-Gated Look-Locker Imaging for Cardiac T1 Estimation (ANGIE) cardiovascular magnetic resonance. *J Cardiovasc Magn Reson.* (2015) 17:110. doi: 10.1186/s12968-015-0209-y
70. Safdar Z, Tamez E, Chan W, Arya B, Ge Y, Deswal A, et al. Circulating collagen biomarkers as indicators of disease severity in pulmonary arterial hypertension. *JACC Heart Fail.* (2014) 2:412–21. doi: 10.1016/j.jchf.2014.03.013
71. Gold J, Akazawa Y, Sun M, Hunter KS, Friedberg MK. Relation between right ventricular wall stress, fibrosis, and function in right ventricular pressure loading. *Am J Physiol-Heart Circ Physiol.* (2020) 318:H366–77. doi: 10.1152/ajpheart.00343.2019
72. Rain S, Andersen S, Najafi A, Gammelgaard Schultz J, da Silva Gonçalves Bós D, Handoko ML, et al. Right ventricular myocardial stiffness in experimental pulmonary arterial hypertension: relative contribution of fibrosis and myofibril stiffness. *Circ Heart Fail.* (2016) 9:e002636. doi: 10.1161/CIRCHEARTFAILURE.115.002636
73. Kusakari Y, Urashima T, Shimura D, Amemiya E, Miyasaka G, Yokota S, et al. Impairment of excitation-contraction coupling in right ventricular hypertrophied muscle with fibrosis induced by pulmonary artery banding. *PLoS One.* (2017) 12:e0169564. doi: 10.1371/journal.pone.0169564
74. Trip P, Rain S, Handoko ML, van der Bruggen C, Bogaard HJ, Marcus JT, et al. Clinical relevance of right ventricular diastolic stiffness in pulmonary hypertension. *Eur Respir J.* (2015) 45:1603–12. doi: 10.1183/09031936.00156714
75. Boehm M, Tian X, Mao Y, Ichimura K, Dufva MJ, Ali K, et al. Delineating the molecular and histological events that govern right ventricular recovery using a novel mouse model of pulmonary artery de-banding. *Cardiovasc Res.* (2020) 116:1700–9. doi: 10.1093/cvr/cvz310

76. Frangogiannis NG. Cardiac fibrosis. *Cardiovasc Res.* (2021) 117:1450–88.
77. Tallquist MD, Molkentin JD. Redefining the identity of cardiac fibroblasts. *Nat Rev Cardiol.* (2017) 14:484–91. doi: 10.1038/nrcardio.2017.57
78. Ren Z, Yu P, Li D, Li Z, Liao Y, Wang Y, et al. Single-cell reconstruction of progression trajectory reveals intervention principles in pathological cardiac hypertrophy. *Circulation.* (2020) 141:1704–19. doi: 10.1161/CIRCULATIONAHA.119.043053
79. Pinto AR, Ilinykh A, Ivey MJ, Kuwabara JT, D'Antoni ML, Debuque R, et al. Revisiting cardiac cellular composition. *Circ Res.* (2016) 118:400–9. doi: 10.1161/CIRCRESAHA.115.307778
80. Bergmann O, Zdunek S, Felker A, Salehpour M, Alkass K, Bernard S, et al. Dynamics of cell generation and turnover in the human heart. *Cell.* (2015) 161:1566–75. doi: 10.1016/j.cell.2015.05.026
81. Moore-Morris T, Guimarães-Camboa N, Banerjee I, Zambon AC, Kisseleva T, Velayoudon A, et al. Resident fibroblast lineages mediate pressure overload-induced cardiac fibrosis. *J Clin Invest.* (2014) 124:2921–34. doi: 10.1172/JCI74783
82. Zeisberg EM, Tarnavski O, Zeisberg M, Dorfman AL, McMullen JR, Gustafsson E, et al. Endothelial-to-mesenchymal transition contributes to cardiac fibrosis. *Nat Med.* (2007) 13:952–61.
83. Widyantoro B, Emoto N, Nakayama K, Anggrahini DW, Adiarto S, Iwasa N, et al. Endothelial cell-derived endothelin-1 promotes cardiac fibrosis in diabetic hearts through stimulation of endothelial-to-mesenchymal transition. *Circulation.* (2010) 121:2407–18. doi: 10.1161/CIRCULATIONAHA.110.938217
84. van Amerongen MJ, Bou-Gharios G, Popa E, van Ark J, Petersen AH, van Dam GM, et al. Bone marrow-derived myofibroblasts contribute functionally to scar formation after myocardial infarction. *J Pathol.* (2008) 214:377–86. doi: 10.1002/path.2281
85. Russo I, Cavalera M, Huang S, Su Y, Hanna A, Chen B, et al. Protective effects of activated myofibroblasts in the pressure-overloaded myocardium are mediated through smad-dependent activation of a matrix-preserving program. *Circ Res.* (2019) 124:1214–27. doi: 10.1161/CIRCRESAHA.118.314438
86. Kurose H. Cardiac fibrosis and fibroblasts. *Cells.* (2021) 10:1716. doi: 10.3390/cells10071716
87. Herum KM, Lunde IG, McCulloch AD, Christensen G. The Soft- and hard-heartedness of cardiac fibroblasts: mechanotransduction signaling pathways in fibrosis of the heart. *J Clin Med.* (2017) 6:E53. doi: 10.3390/jcm6050053
88. Goldsmith EC, Bradshaw AD, Zile MR, Spinale FG. Myocardial fibroblast-matrix interactions and potential therapeutic targets. *J Mol Cell Cardiol.* (2014) 70:92–9. doi: 10.1016/j.yjmcc.2014.01.008
89. Katwa LC, Tyagi SC, Campbell SE, Lee SJ, Cicila GT, Weber KT. Valvular interstitial cells express angiotensinogen and cathepsin D, and generate angiotensin peptides. *Int J Biochem Cell Biol.* (1996) 28:807–21. doi: 10.1016/1357-2725(96)00012-x
90. Katwa LC, Campbell SE, Tyagi SC, Lee SJ, Cicila GT, Weber KT. Cultured myofibroblasts generate angiotensin peptides de novo. *J Mol Cell Cardiol.* (1997) 29:1375–86. doi: 10.1006/jmcc.1997.0376
91. Villarreal FJ, Kim NN, Ungab GD, Printz MP, Dillmann WH. Identification of functional angiotensin II receptors on rat cardiac fibroblasts. *Circulation.* (1993) 88:2849–61. doi: 10.1161/01.cir.88.6.2849
92. Brilla CG, Zhou G, Matsubara L, Weber KT. Collagen metabolism in cultured adult rat cardiac fibroblasts: response to angiotensin II and aldosterone. *J Mol Cell Cardiol.* (1994) 26:809–20. doi: 10.1006/jmcc.1994.1098
93. Schorb W, Booz GW, Dostal DE, Conrad KM, Chang KC, Baker KM. Angiotensin II is mitogenic in neonatal rat cardiac fibroblasts. *Circ Res.* (1993) 72:1245–54. doi: 10.1161/01.res.72.6.1245
94. Olson ER, Shamhart PE, Naugle JE, Meszaros JG. Angiotensin II-induced extracellular signal-regulated kinase 1/2 activation is mediated by protein kinase Cdelta and intracellular calcium in adult rat cardiac fibroblasts. *Hypertens Dallas Tex 1979.* (2008) 51:704–11. doi: 10.1161/HYPERTENSIONAHA.107.098459
95. Wang W, Huang XR, Canlas E, Oka K, Truong LD, Deng C, et al. Essential role of Smad3 in angiotensin II-induced vascular fibrosis. *Circ Res.* (2006) 98:1032–9. doi: 10.1161/01.RES.0000218782.52610.dc
96. Khalil H, Kanisicak O, Prasad V, Correll RN, Fu X, Schips T, et al. Fibroblast-specific TGF-β-Smad2/3 signaling underlies cardiac fibrosis. *J Clin Invest.* (2017) 127:3770–83. doi: 10.1172/JCI94753
97. Wells RG, Gilboa L, Sun Y, Liu X, Henis YI, Lodish HF. Transforming growth factor-beta induces formation of a dithiothreitol-resistant type I/Type II receptor complex in live cells. *J Biol Chem.* (1999) 274:5716–22. doi: 10.1074/jbc.274.9.5716
98. Derynck R, Zhang YE. Smad-dependent and Smad-independent pathways in TGF-beta family signalling. *Nature.* (2003) 425:577–84. doi: 10.1038/nature02006
99. Travers JG, Kamal FA, Robbins J, Yutzey KE, Blaxall BC. Cardiac fibrosis: the fibroblast awakens. *Circ Res.* (2016) 118:1021–40. doi: 10.1161/CIRCRESAHA.115.306565
100. Daniels A, van Bilsen M, Goldschmeding R, van der Vusse GJ, van Nieuwenhoven FA. Connective tissue growth factor and cardiac fibrosis. *Acta Physiol Oxf Engl.* (2009) 195:321–38. doi: 10.1111/j.1748-1716.2008.01936.x
101. Hanna A, Frangogiannis NG. The role of the TGF-β superfamily in myocardial infarction. *Front Cardiovasc Med.* (2019) 6:140. doi: 10.3389/fcvm.2019.00140
102. Schafer S, Viswanathan S, Widjaja AA, Lim W-W, Moreno-Moral A, DeLaughter DM, et al. IL-11 is a crucial determinant of cardiovascular fibrosis. *Nature.* (2017) 552:110–5. doi: 10.1038/nature24676
103. Nagaraju CK, Robinson EL, Abdesselem M, Trenson S, Dries E, Gilbert G, et al. Myofibroblast phenotype and reversibility of fibrosis in patients with end-stage heart failure. *J Am Coll Cardiol.* (2019) 73:2267–82. doi: 10.1016/j.jacc.2019.02.049
104. Katwa LC, Guarda E, Weber KT. Endothelin receptors in cultured adult rat cardiac fibroblasts. *Cardiovasc Res.* (1993) 27:2125–9. doi: 10.1093/cvr/27.12.2125
105. Dashwood MR, Abraham D. Endothelin: from bench to bedside and back. *Pharmacol Res.* (2011) 63:445–7. doi: 10.1016/j.phrs.2011.04.005
106. Villari B, Campbell SE, Schneider J, Vassalli G, Chiariello M, Hess OM. Sex-dependent differences in left ventricular function and structure in chronic pressure overload. *Eur Heart J.* (1995) 16:1410–9. doi: 10.1093/oxfordjournals.eurheartj.a060749
107. Kararigas G, Dworatzek E, Petrov G, Summer H, Schulze TM, Baczko I, et al. Sex-dependent regulation of fibrosis and inflammation in human left ventricular remodelling under pressure overload. *Eur J Heart Fail.* (2014) 16:1160–7. doi: 10.1002/ejhf.171
108. Singh A, Musa TA, Treibel TA, Vassiliou VS, Captur G, Chin C, et al. Sex differences in left ventricular remodelling, myocardial fibrosis and mortality after aortic valve replacement. *Heart Br Card Soc.* (2019) 105:1818–24. doi: 10.1136/heartjnl-2019-314987
109. Tastet L, Kwiecinski J, Pibarot P, Capoulade R, Everett RJ, Newby DE, et al. Sex-Related differences in the extent of myocardial fibrosis in patients with aortic valve stenosis. *JACC Cardiovasc Imaging.* (2020) 13:699–711. doi: 10.1016/j.jcmg.2019.06.014
110. Horn MA, Trafford AW. Aging and the cardiac collagen matrix: novel mediators of fibrotic remodelling. *J Mol Cell Cardiol.* (2016) 93:175–85. doi: 10.1016/j.yjmcc.2015.11.005
111. Chen W, Frangogiannis NG. The role of inflammatory and fibrogenic pathways in heart failure associated with aging. *Heart Fail Rev.* (2010) 15:415–22. doi: 10.1007/s10741-010-9161-y
112. Dai D-F, Chen T, Johnson SC, Szeto H, Rabinovitch PS. Cardiac aging: from molecular mechanisms to significance in human health and disease. *Antioxid Redox Signal.* (2012) 16:1492–526. doi: 10.1089/ars.2011.4179
113. Dworatzek E, Mahmoodzadeh S, Schriever C, Kusumoto K, Kramer L, Santos G, et al. Sex-specific regulation of collagen I and III expression by 17β-Estradiol in cardiac fibroblasts: role of estrogen receptors. *Cardiovasc Res.* (2019) 115:315–27. doi: 10.1093/cvr/cvy185
114. Kong P, Christia P, Frangogiannis NG. The pathogenesis of cardiac fibrosis. *Cell Mol Life Sci CMLS.* (2014) 71:549–74. doi: 10.1007/s00018-013-1349-6
115. Dewachter C, Belhaj A, Rondelet B, Vercruyssen M, Schraufnagel DP, Remmelink M, et al. Myocardial inflammation in experimental acute right ventricular failure: effects of prostacyclin therapy. *J Heart Lung Transplant Off Publ Int Soc Heart Transplant.* (2015) 34:1334–45. doi: 10.1016/j.healun.2015.05.004
116. Overbeek MJ, Mouchaers KTB, Niessen HM, Hadi AM, Kupreishvili K, Boonstra A, et al. Characteristics of interstitial fibrosis and inflammatory cell infiltration in right ventricles of systemic sclerosis-associated pulmonary arterial hypertension. *Int J Rheumatol.* (2010) 2010:604615. doi: 10.1155/2010/604615

117. Luitel H, Sydykov A, Schymura Y, Mamazhakypov A, Janssen W, Pradhan K, et al. Pressure overload leads to an increased accumulation and activity of mast cells in the right ventricle. *Physiol Rep.* (2017) 5:e13146. doi: 10.14814/phy2.13146
118. Nergui S, Fukumoto Y, Do EZ, Nakajima S, Shimizu T, Ikeda S, et al. Role of endothelial nitric oxide synthase and collagen metabolism in right ventricular remodeling due to pulmonary hypertension. *Circ J Off J Jpn Circ Soc.* (2014) 78:1465–74. doi: 10.1253/circj.cj-13-1586
119. Streeter DD, Spotnitz HM, Patel DP, Ross J, Sonnenblick EH. Fiber orientation in the canine left ventricle during diastole and systole. *Circ Res.* (1969) 24:339–47. doi: 10.1161/01.res.24.3.339
120. Streeter DD Jr., Bassett DL. An engineering analysis of myocardial fiber orientation in pig's left ventricle in systole. *Anat Rec.* (1966) 155:503–11. doi: 10.1002/ar.1091550403
121. Borg TK, Caulfield JB. The collagen matrix of the heart. *Fed Proc.* (1981) 40:2037–41.
122. Robinson TF, Cohen-Gould L, Factor SM, Eghbali M, Blumenfeld OO. Structure and function of connective tissue in cardiac muscle: collagen types I and III in endomysial struts and pericellular fibers. *Scanning Microsc.* (1988) 2:1005–15.
123. Horiguchi M, Todorovic V, Hadjiolova K, Weiskirchen R, Rifkin DB. Abrogation of both short and long forms of latent transforming growth factor-β binding protein-1 causes defective cardiovascular development and is perinatally lethal. *Matrix Biol.* (2015) 43:61–70. doi: 10.1016/j.matbio.2015.03.006
124. Dell'Italia LJ, Meng QC, Balcells E, Wei CC, Palmer R, Hageman GR, et al. Compartmentalization of angiotensin II generation in the dog heart. Evidence for independent mechanisms in intravascular and interstitial spaces. *J Clin Invest.* (1997) 100:253–8. doi: 10.1172/JCI119529
125. Wei C-C, Meng QC, Palmer R, Hageman GR, Durand J, Bradley WE, et al. Evidence for angiotensin-converting enzyme- and chymase-mediated angiotensin II formation in the interstitial fluid space of the Dog heart in vivo. *Circulation.* (1999) 99:2583–9. doi: 10.1161/01.cir.99.19.2583
126. Multani MM, Ikonomidis JS, Kim PY, Miller EA, Payne KJ, Mukherjee R, et al. Dynamic and differential changes in myocardial and plasma endothelin in patients undergoing cardiopulmonary bypass. *J Thorac Cardiovasc Surg.* (2005) 129:584–90. doi: 10.1016/j.jtcvs.2004.07.018
127. Ergul A, Walker CA, Goldberg A, Baicu SC, Hendrick JW, King MK, et al. ET-1 in the myocardial interstitium: relation to myocyte ECE activity and expression. *Am J Physiol-Heart Circ Physiol.* (2000) 278:H2050–6. doi: 10.1152/ajpheart.2000.278.6.H2050
128. Bishop JE, Laurent GJ. Collagen turnover and its regulation in the normal and hypertrophying heart. *Eur Heart J.* (1995) 16(Suppl C):38–44. doi: 10.1093/eurheartj/16.suppl_c.38
129. Chen MM, Lam A, Abraham JA, Schreiner GF, Joly AH. CTGF expression is induced by TGF- beta in cardiac fibroblasts and cardiac myocytes: a potential role in heart fibrosis. *J Mol Cell Cardiol.* (2000) 32:1805–19. doi: 10.1006/jmcc.2000.1215
130. Kessler E, Takahara K, Biniaminov L, Brusel M, Greenspan DS. Bone morphogenetic protein-1: the type I procollagen C-proteinase. *Science.* (1996) 271:360–2. doi: 10.1126/science.271.5247.360
131. López B, González A, Beaumont J, Querejeta R, Larman M, Díez J. Identification of a potential cardiac antifibrotic mechanism of torasemide in patients with chronic heart failure. *J Am Coll Cardiol.* (2007) 50:859–67. doi: 10.1016/j.jacc.2007.04.080
132. Yang J, Savvatis K, Kang JS, Fan P, Zhong H, Schwartz K, et al. Targeting LOXL2 for cardiac interstitial fibrosis and heart failure treatment. *Nat Commun.* (2016) 7:13710. doi: 10.1038/ncomms13710
133. Fan D, Takawale A, Lee J, Kassiri Z. Cardiac fibroblasts, fibrosis and extracellular matrix remodeling in heart disease. *Fibrogenesis Tissue Repair.* (2012) 5:15. doi: 10.1186/1755-1536-5-15
134. Polyakova V, Hein S, Kostin S, Ziegelhoeffer T, Schaper J. Matrix metalloproteinases and their tissue inhibitors in pressure-overloaded human myocardium during heart failure progression. *J Am Coll Cardiol.* (2004) 44:1609–18. doi: 10.1016/j.jacc.2004.07.023
135. López B, Ravassa S, Moreno MU, José GS, Beaumont J, González A, et al. Diffuse myocardial fibrosis: mechanisms, diagnosis and therapeutic approaches. *Nat Rev Cardiol.* (2021) 18:479–98. doi: 10.1038/s41569-020-00504-1
136. Spinale FG. Myocardial matrix remodeling and the matrix metalloproteinases: influence on cardiac form and function. *Physiol Rev.* (2007) 87:1285–342. doi: 10.1152/physrev.00012.2007
137. Herpel E, Singer S, Flechtenmacher C, Pritsch M, Sack F-U, Hagl S, et al. Extracellular matrix proteins and matrix metalloproteinases differ between various right and left ventricular sites in end-stage cardiomyopathies. *Virchows Arch.* (2005) 446:369–78. doi: 10.1007/s00428-004-1177-z
138. Zaffran S, Kelly RG, Meilhac SM, Buckingham ME, Brown NA. Right ventricular myocardium derives from the anterior heart field. *Circ Res.* (2004) 95:261–8. doi: 10.1161/01.RES.0000136815.73623.BE
139. Urashima T, Zhao M, Wagner R, Fajardo G, Farahani S, Quertermous T, et al. Molecular and physiological characterization of RV remodeling in a murine model of pulmonary stenosis. *Am J Physiol-Heart Circ Physiol.* (2008) 295:H1351–68. doi: 10.1152/ajpheart.91526.2007
140. Crnkovic S, Egemnazarov B, Damico R, Marsh LM, Nagy BM, Douschan P, et al. Disconnect between fibrotic response and right ventricular dysfunction. *Am J Respir Crit Care Med.* (2019) 199:1550–60. doi: 10.1164/rccm.201809-1737OC
141. Sun Y, Ramires FJ, Weber KT. Fibrosis of atria and great vessels in response to angiotensin II or aldosterone infusion. *Cardiovasc Res.* (1997) 35:138–47. doi: 10.1016/s0008-6363(97)00097-7
142. Conceição G, Heinonen I, Lourenço AP, Duncker DJ, Falcão-Pires I. Animal models of heart failure with preserved ejection fraction. *Neth Heart J Mon J Neth Soc Cardiol Neth Heart Found.* (2016) 24:275–86.
143. Regan JA, Mauro AG, Carbone S, Marchetti C, Gill R, Mezzaroma E, et al. A mouse model of heart failure with preserved ejection fraction due to chronic infusion of a low subpressor dose of angiotensin II. *Am J Physiol Heart Circ Physiol.* (2015) 309:H771–8. doi: 10.1152/ajpheart.00282.2015
144. Pahor M, Bernabei R, Sgadari A, Gambassi G, Lo Giudice P, Pacifici L, et al. Enalapril prevents cardiac fibrosis and arrhythmias in hypertensive rats. *Hypertension.* (1991) 18:148–57. doi: 10.1161/01.hyp.18.2.148
145. Ham O, Jin W, Lei L, Huang HH, Tsuji K, Huang M, et al. Pathological cardiac remodeling occurs early in CKD mice from unilateral urinary obstruction, and is attenuated by Enalapril. *Sci Rep.* (2018) 8:16087. doi: 10.1038/s41598-018-34216-x
146. Burke RM, Lighthouse JK, Mickelsen DM, Small EM. Sacubitril/Valsartan decreases cardiac fibrosis in left ventricle pressure overload by restoring PKG signaling in cardiac fibroblasts. *Circ Heart Fail.* (2019) 12:e005565. doi: 10.1161/CIRCHEARTFAILURE.118.005565
147. Nishioka T, Suzuki M, Onishi K, Takakura N, Inada H, Yoshida T, et al. Eplerenone attenuates myocardial fibrosis in the angiotensin II-induced hypertensive mouse: involvement of tenascin-C induced by aldosterone-mediated inflammation. *J Cardiovasc Pharmacol.* (2007) 49:261–8. doi: 10.1097/FJC.0b013e318033dfd4
148. Leader CJ, Moharram M, Coffey S, Sammut IA, Wilkins GW, Walker RJ. Myocardial global longitudinal strain: an early indicator of cardiac interstitial fibrosis modified by spironolactone, in a unique hypertensive rat model. *PLoS One.* (2019) 14:e0220837. doi: 10.1371/journal.pone.0220837
149. Friedberg MK, Cho M-Y, Li J, Assad RS, Sun M, Rohailla S, et al. Adverse biventricular remodeling in isolated right ventricular hypertension is mediated by increased transforming growth Factor-β1 signaling and is abrogated by angiotensin receptor blockade. *Am J Respir Cell Mol Biol.* (2013) 49:1019–28. doi: 10.1165/rcmb.2013-0149OC
150. Sharifi Kia D, Benza E, Bachman TN, Tushak C, Kim K, Simon MA. Angiotensin receptor—neprilysin inhibition attenuates right ventricular remodeling in pulmonary hypertension. *J Am Heart Assoc.* (2020) 9:e015708. doi: 10.1161/JAHA.119.015708
151. González A, López B, Ravassa S, San José G, Díez J. The complex dynamics of myocardial interstitial fibrosis in heart failure. Focus on collagen cross-linking. *Biochim Biophys Acta BBA Mol Cell Res.* (2019) 1866:1421–32. doi: 10.1016/j.bbamcr.2019.06.001
152. El Hajj EC, El Hajj MC, Ninh VK, Gardner JD. Inhibitor of lysyl oxidase improves cardiac function and the collagen/MMP profile in response to volume overload. *Am J Physiol Heart Circ Physiol.* (2018) 315:H463–73. doi: 10.1152/ajpheart.00086.2018

153. Hermida N, López B, González A, Dotor J, Lasarte JJ, Sarobe P, et al. A synthetic peptide from transforming growth factor-beta1 type III receptor prevents myocardial fibrosis in spontaneously hypertensive rats. *Cardiovasc Res.* (2009) 81:601–9. doi: 10.1093/cvr/cvn315
154. Miguel-Carrasco JL, Beaumont J, San José G, Moreno MU, López B, González A, et al. Mechanisms underlying the cardiac antifibrotic effects of losartan metabolites. *Sci Rep.* (2017) 7:41865. doi: 10.1038/srep41865
155. Meng X, Nikolic-Paterson DJ, Lan HY. TGF-β: the master regulator of fibrosis. *Nat Rev Nephrol.* (2016) 12:325–38. doi: 10.1038/nrneph.2016.48
156. Lucas JA, Zhang Y, Li P, Gong K, Miller AP, Hassan E, et al. Inhibition of transforming growth factor-beta signaling induces left ventricular dilation and dysfunction in the pressure-overloaded heart. *Am J Physiol Heart Circ Physiol.* (2010) 298:H424–32. doi: 10.1152/ajpheart.00529.2009
157. Brooks WW, Conrad CH. Myocardial fibrosis in transforming growth factor β1Heterozygous mice. *J Mol Cell Cardiol.* (2000) 32:187–95. doi: 10.1006/jmcc.1999.1065
158. Gao X, Wu G, Gu X, Fu L, Mei C. Kruppel-like factor 15 modulates renal interstitial fibrosis by ERK/MAPK and JNK/MAPK pathways regulation. *Kidney Blood Press Res.* (2013) 37:631–40. doi: 10.1159/000355743
159. Schaefer CJ, Ruhrmund DW, Pan L, Seiwert SD, Kossen K. Antifibrotic activities of pirfenidone in animal models. *Eur Respir Rev Off J Eur Respir Soc.* (2011) 20:85–97. doi: 10.1183/09059180.00001111
160. Shi Q, Liu X, Bai Y, Cui C, Li J, Li Y, et al. In vitro effects of pirfenidone on cardiac fibroblasts: proliferation, myofibroblast differentiation, migration and cytokine secretion. *PLoS One.* (2011) 6:e28134. doi: 10.1371/journal.pone.0028134
161. Yamazaki T, Yamashita N, Izumi Y, Nakamura Y, Shiota M, Hanatani A, et al. The antifibrotic agent pirfenidone inhibits angiotensin II-induced cardiac hypertrophy in mice. *Hypertens Res Off J Jpn Soc Hypertens.* (2012) 35:34–40. doi: 10.1038/hr.2011.139
162. Wang Y, Wu Y, Chen J, Zhao S, Li H. Pirfenidone attenuates cardiac fibrosis in a mouse model of TAC-Induced left ventricular remodeling by suppressing NLRP3 inflammasome formation. *Cardiology.* (2013) 126:1–11. doi: 10.1159/000351179
163. Mirkovic S, Seymour A-ML, Fenning A, Strachan A, Margolin SB, Taylor SM, et al. Attenuation of cardiac fibrosis by pirfenidone and amiloride in DOCA-salt hypertensive rats. *Br J Pharmacol.* (2002) 135:961–8. doi: 10.1038/sj.bjp.0704539
164. Boehm M, Tian X, Ali MK, Mao Y, Ichimura K, Zhao M, et al. Improving right ventricular function by increasing BMP signaling with FK506. *Am J Respir Cell Mol Biol.* (2021) 65:272–87. doi: 10.1165/rcmb.2020-0528OC
165. Adiarto S, Heiden S, Vignon-Zellweger N, Nakayama K, Yagi K, Yanagisawa M, et al. ET-1 from endothelial cells is required for complete angiotensin II-induced cardiac fibrosis and hypertrophy. *Life Sci.* (2012) 91:651–7. doi: 10.1016/j.lfs.2012.02.006
166. Schimmel K, Stojanović SD, Huang C-K, Jung M, Meyer MH, Xiao K, et al. Combined high-throughput library screening and next generation RNA sequencing uncover microRNAs controlling human cardiac fibroblast biology. *J Mol Cell Cardiol.* (2021) 150:91–100. doi: 10.1016/j.yjmcc.2020.10.008
167. Schimmel K, Jung M, Foinquinos A, José GS, Beaumont J, Bock K, et al. Natural compound library screening identifies new molecules for the treatment of cardiac fibrosis and diastolic dysfunction. *Circulation.* (2020) 141:751–67. doi: 10.1161/CIRCULATIONAHA.119.042559
168. Kojonazarov B, Sydykov A, Pullamsetti SS, Luitel H, Dahal BK, Kosanovic D, et al. Effects of multikinase inhibitors on pressure overload-induced right ventricular remodeling. *Int J Cardiol.* (2013) 167:2630–7. doi: 10.1016/j.ijcard.2012.06.129
169. Borgdorff MA, Bartelds B, Dickinson MG, van Wiechen MPH, Steendijk P, de Vroomen M, et al. Sildenafil treatment in established right ventricular dysfunction improves diastolic function and attenuates interstitial fibrosis independent from afterload. *Am J Physiol Heart Circ Physiol.* (2014) 307:H361–9. doi: 10.1152/ajpheart.00843.2013
170. Rai N, Veeroju S, Schymura Y, Janssen W, Wietelmann A, Kojonazarov B, et al. Effect of riociguat and sildenafil on right heart remodeling and function in pressure overload induced model of pulmonary arterial banding. *BioMed Res Int.* (2018) 2018:1–9. doi: 10.1155/2018/6593682
171. Gomez-Arroyo J, Sakagami M, Syed AA, Farkas L, Van Tassell B, Kraskauskas D, et al. Iloprost reverses established fibrosis in experimental right ventricular failure. *Eur Respir J.* (2015) 45:449–62. doi: 10.1183/09031936.00188013
172. Hemnes AR, Maynard KB, Champion HC, Gleaves L, Penner N, West J, et al. Testosterone negatively regulates right ventricular load stress responses in mice. *Pulm Circ.* (2012) 2:352–8. doi: 10.4103/2045-8932.101647
173. Fang Y-H, Piao L, Hong Z, Toth PT, Marsboom G, Bache-Wiig P, et al. Therapeutic inhibition of fatty acid oxidation in right ventricular hypertrophy: exploiting Randle's cycle. *J Mol Med.* (2012) 90:31–43. doi: 10.1007/s00109-011-0804-9
174. Yoshida K, Abe K, Ishikawa M, Saku K, Shinoda-Sakamoto M, Ishikawa T, et al. Inhibition of TLR9-NF-κB-mediated sterile inflammation improves pressure overload-induced right ventricular dysfunction in rats. *Cardiovasc Res.* (2019) 115:658–68. doi: 10.1093/cvr/cvy209
175. Bogaard HJ, Natarajan R, Henderson SC, Long CS, Kraskauskas D, Smithson L, et al. Chronic pulmonary artery pressure elevation is insufficient to explain right heart failure. *Circulation.* (2009) 120:1951–60. doi: 10.1161/CIRCULATIONAHA.109.883843
176. Budas GR, Boehm M, Kojonazarov B, Viswanathan G, Tian X, Veeroju S, et al. ASK1 inhibition halts disease progression in preclinical models of pulmonary arterial hypertension. *Am J Respir Crit Care Med.* (2018) 197:373–85. doi: 10.1164/rccm.201703-0502OC
177. Kojonazarov B, Novoyatleva T, Boehm M, Happe C, Sibinska Z, Tian X, et al. p38 MAPK inhibition improves heart function in pressure-loaded right ventricular hypertrophy. *Am J Respir Cell Mol Biol.* (2017) 57:603–14. doi: 10.1165/rcmb.2016-0374OC
178. Brilla CG, Funck RC, Rupp H. Lisinopril-mediated regression of myocardial fibrosis in patients with hypertensive heart disease. *Circulation.* (2000) 102:1388–93. doi: 10.1161/01.cir.102.12.1388
179. Díez J, Querejeta R, López B, González A, Larman M, Martínez Ubago JL. Losartan-dependent regression of myocardial fibrosis is associated with reduction of left ventricular chamber stiffness in hypertensive patients. *Circulation.* (2002) 105:2512–7. doi: 10.1161/01.cir.0000017264.66561.3d
180. Lemarié CA, Simeone SMC, Nikonova A, Ebrahimian T, Deschênes M-E, Coffman TM, et al. Aldosterone-induced activation of signaling pathways requires activity of angiotensin type 1a receptors. *Circ Res.* (2009) 105:852–9. doi: 10.1161/CIRCRESAHA.109.196576
181. Stockand JD, Meszaros JG. Aldosterone stimulates proliferation of cardiac fibroblasts by activating Ki-RasA and MAPK1/2 signaling. *Am J Physiol Heart Circ Physiol.* (2003) 284:H176–84. doi: 10.1152/ajpheart.00421.2002
182. Pfeffer MA, Pitt B, McKinlay SM. Spironolactone for heart failure with preserved ejection fraction. *N Engl J Med.* (2014) 371:181–2.
183. Pfeffer MA, Claggett B, Assmann SF, Boineau R, Anand IS, Clausell N, et al. Regional variation in patients and outcomes in the treatment of preserved cardiac function heart failure with an aldosterone antagonist (TOPCAT) trial. *Circulation.* (2015) 131:34–42. doi: 10.1161/CIRCULATIONAHA.114.013255
184. Deswal A, Richardson P, Bozkurt B, Mann DL. Results of the randomized aldosterone antagonism in heart failure with preserved ejection fraction trial (RAAM-PEF). *J Card Fail.* (2011) 17:634–42. doi: 10.1016/j.cardfail.2011.04.007
185. Edelmann F, Wachter R, Schmidt AG, Kraigher-Krainer E, Colantonio C, Kamke W, et al. Effect of spironolactone on diastolic function and exercise capacity in patients with heart failure with preserved ejection fraction: the Aldo-DHF randomized controlled trial. *JAMA.* (2013) 309:781–91. doi: 10.1001/jama.2013.905
186. McDiarmid AK, Swoboda PP, Erhayiem B, Bounford KA, Bijsterveld P, Tyndall K, et al. Myocardial effects of aldosterone antagonism in heart failure with preserved ejection fraction. *J Am Heart Assoc.* (2020) 9:e011521. doi: 10.1161/JAHA.118.011521
187. Torafic Investigators Group. Effects of prolonged-release torasemide versus furosemide on myocardial fibrosis in hypertensive patients with chronic heart failure: a randomized, blinded-end point, active-controlled study. *Clin Ther.* (2011) 33:1204–13.e3. doi: 10.1016/j.clinthera.2011.08.006
188. Muir AJ, Levy C, Janssen HLA, Montano-Loza AJ, Shiffman ML, Caldwell S, et al. Simtuzumab for primary sclerosing cholangitis: phase 2 study results with insights on the natural history of the disease. *Hepatol Baltim Md.* (2019) 69:684–98. doi: 10.1002/hep.30237

189. Raghu G, Brown KK, Collard HR, Cottin V, Gibson KF, Kaner RJ, et al. Efficacy of simtuzumab versus placebo in patients with idiopathic pulmonary fibrosis: a randomised, double-blind, controlled, phase 2 trial. *Lancet Respir Med.* (2017) 5:22–32. doi: 10.1016/S2213-2600(16)30421-0
190. Almendral JL, Shick V, Rosendorff C, Atlas SA. Association between transforming growth factor-beta(1) and left ventricular mass and diameter in hypertensive patients. *J Am Soc Hypertens JASH.* (2010) 4:135–41. doi: 10.1016/j.jash.2010.02.007
191. Hein S, Arnon E, Kostin S, Schönburg M, Elsässer A, Polyakova V, et al. Progression from compensated hypertrophy to failure in the pressure-overloaded human heart: structural deterioration and compensatory mechanisms. *Circulation.* (2003) 107:984–91. doi: 10.1161/01.cir.0000051865.66123.b7
192. Lopez-de la Mora DA, Sanchez-Roque C, Montoya-Buelna M, Sanchez-Enriquez S, Lucano-Landeros S, Macias-Barragan J, et al. Role and new insights of pirfenidone in fibrotic diseases. *Int J Med Sci.* (2015) 12:840–7. doi: 10.7150/ijms.11579
193. Martin J, Kelly DJ, Mifsud SA, Zhang Y, Cox AJ, See F, et al. Tranilast attenuates cardiac matrix deposition in experimental diabetes: role of transforming growth factor-β. *Cardiovasc Res.* (2005) 65:694–701. doi: 10.1016/j.cardiores.2004.10.041
194. Taniguchi H, Ebina M, Kondoh Y, Ogura T, Azuma A, Suga M, et al. Pirfenidone in idiopathic pulmonary fibrosis. *Eur Respir J.* (2010) 35:821–9.
195. Noble PW, Albera C, Bradford WZ, Costabel U, Glassberg MK, Kardatzke D, et al. Pirfenidone in patients with idiopathic pulmonary fibrosis (CAPACITY): two randomised trials. *Lancet Lond Engl.* (2011) 377:1760–9. doi: 10.1016/S0140-6736(11)60405-4
196. King TE, Bradford WZ, Castro-Bernardini S, Fagan EA, Glaspole I, Glassberg MK, et al. A Phase 3 trial of pirfenidone in patients with idiopathic pulmonary fibrosis. *N Engl J Med.* (2014) 370:2083–92.
197. Ogura T, Azuma A, Inoue Y, Taniguchi H, Chida K, Bando M, et al. All-case post-marketing surveillance of 1371 patients treated with pirfenidone for idiopathic pulmonary fibrosis. *Respir Investig.* (2015) 53:232–41. doi: 10.1016/j.resinv.2015.06.001
198. Lewis GA, Schelbert EB, Naish JH, Bedson E, Dodd S, Eccleson H, et al. Pirfenidone in heart failure with preserved ejection fraction-rationale and design of the PIROUETTE trial. *Cardiovasc Drugs Ther.* (2019) 33:461–70. doi: 10.1007/s10557-019-06876-y
199. Izawa H, Murohara T, Nagata K, Isobe S, Asano H, Amano T, et al. Mineralocorticoid receptor antagonism ameliorates left ventricular diastolic dysfunction and myocardial fibrosis in mildly symptomatic patients with idiopathic dilated cardiomyopathy: a pilot study. *Circulation.* (2005) 112:2940–5. doi: 10.1161/CIRCULATIONAHA.105.571653
200. ACC. *Pirfenidone in Heart Failure With Preserved Ejection Fraction - PIROUTTE.* (2021). Available online at: https://www.acc.org/latest-in-cardiology/clinical-trials/2021/05/14/19/52/pirouette#references-for-article (accessed May 17, 2021).
201. Lewis GA, Dodd S, Clayton D, Bedson E, Eccleson H, Schelbert EB, et al. Pirfenidone in heart failure with preserved ejection fraction: a randomized phase 2 trial. *Nat Med.* (2021) 27:1477–82. doi: 10.1038/s41591-021-01452-0
202. Clozel M, Salloukh H. Role of endothelin in fibrosis and anti-fibrotic potential of bosentan. *Ann Med.* (2005) 37:2–12. doi: 10.1080/07853890410018925
203. Sütsch G, Kiowski W, Yan X-W, Hunziker P, Christen S, Strobel W, et al. Short-Term oral endothelin-receptor antagonist therapy in conventionally treated patients with symptomatic severe chronic heart failure. *Circulation.* (1998) 98:2262–8. doi: 10.1161/01.cir.98.21.2262
204. Anand I, McMurray J, Cohn JN, Konstam MA, Notter T, Quitzau K, et al. Long-term effects of darusentan on left-ventricular remodelling and clinical outcomes in the EndothelinA Receptor Antagonist Trial in Heart Failure (EARTH): randomised, double-blind, placebo-controlled trial. *Lancet Lond Engl.* (2004) 364:347–54. doi: 10.1016/S0140-6736(04)16723-8
205. Prasad SK, Dargie HJ, Smith GC, Barlow MM, Grothues F, Groenning BA, et al. Comparison of the dual receptor endothelin antagonist enrasentan with enalapril in asymptomatic left ventricular systolic dysfunction: a cardiovascular magnetic resonance study. *Heart Br Card Soc.* (2006) 92:798–803. doi: 10.1136/hrt.2004.049734
206. de Boer RA, De Keulenaer G, Bauersachs J, Brutsaert D, Cleland JG, Diez J, et al. Towards better definition, quantification and treatment of fibrosis in heart failure. A scientific roadmap by the Committee of Translational Research of the Heart Failure Association (HFA) of the European Society of Cardiology. *Eur J Heart Fail.* (2019) 21:272–85. doi: 10.1002/ejhf.1406
207. Treibel TA, López B, González A, Menacho K, Schofield RS, Ravassa S, et al. Reappraising myocardial fibrosis in severe aortic stenosis: an invasive and non-invasive study in 133 patients. *Eur Heart J.* (2018) 39:699–709. doi: 10.1093/eurheartj/ehx353
208. Weber KT, Janicki JS, Shroff SG, Pick R, Chen RM, Bashey RI. Collagen remodeling of the pressure-overloaded, hypertrophied nonhuman primate myocardium. *Circ Res.* (1988) 62:757–65. doi: 10.1161/01.res.62.4.757
209. Mewton N, Liu CY, Croisille P, Bluemke D, Lima JAC. Assessment of myocardial fibrosis with cardiovascular magnetic resonance. *J Am Coll Cardiol.* (2011) 57:891–903.
210. Diao K-Y, Yang Z-G, Xu H-Y, Liu X, Zhang Q, Shi K, et al. Histologic validation of myocardial fibrosis measured by T1 mapping: a systematic review and meta-analysis. *J Cardiovasc Magn Reson Off J Soc Cardiovasc Magn Reson.* (2016) 18:92. doi: 10.1186/s12968-016-0313-7
211. Everett RJ, Stirrat CG, Semple SIR, Newby DE, Dweck MR, Mirsadraee S. Assessment of myocardial fibrosis with T1 mapping MRI. *Clin Radiol.* (2016) 71:768–78. doi: 10.1016/j.crad.2016.02.013
212. Montesi SB, Désogère P, Fuchs BC, Caravan P. Molecular imaging of fibrosis: recent advances and future directions. *J Clin Invest.* (2019) 129:24–33. doi: 10.1172/JCI122132
213. Désogère P, Montesi SB, Caravan P. Molecular probes for imaging fibrosis and fibrogenesis. *Chem Eur J.* (2019) 25:1128–41. doi: 10.1002/chem.201801578
214. Lebtahi R, Moreau S, Marchand-Adam S, Debray M-P, Brauner M, Soler P, et al. Increased uptake of 111In-octreotide in idiopathic pulmonary fibrosis. *J Nucl Med Off Publ Soc Nucl Med.* (2006) 47:1281–7.
215. Carbone R, Filiberti R, Grosso M, Paredi P, Peano L, Cantalupi D, et al. Octreoscan perspectives in sarcoidosis and idiopathic interstitial pneumonia. *Eur Rev Med Pharmacol Sci.* (2003) 7:97–105.
216. Ambrosini V, Zompatori M, Luca FD, Antonia D, Allegri V, Nanni C, et al. 68Ga-DOTANOC PET/CT allows somatostatin receptor imaging in idiopathic pulmonary fibrosis: preliminary results. *J Nucl Med.* (2010) 51:1950–5. doi: 10.2967/jnumed.110.079962
217. van den Borne SWM, Isobe S, Verjans JW, Petrov A, Lovhaug D, Li P, et al. Molecular imaging of interstitial alterations in remodeling myocardium after myocardial infarction. *J Am Coll Cardiol.* (2008) 52:2017–28. doi: 10.1016/j.jacc.2008.07.067
218. van den Borne SWM, Isobe S, Zandbergen HR, Li P, Petrov A, Wong ND, et al. Molecular imaging for efficacy of pharmacologic intervention in myocardial remodeling. *JACC Cardiovasc Imaging.* (2009) 2:187–98. doi: 10.1016/j.jcmg.2008.11.011
219. Caravan P, Das B, Dumas S, Epstein FH, Helm PA, Jacques V, et al. Collagen-Targeted MRI contrast agent for molecular imaging of fibrosis. *Angew Chem Int Ed.* (2007) 46:8171–3. doi: 10.1002/anie.200700700
220. Helm PA, Caravan P, French BA, Jacques V, Shen L, Xu Y, et al. Postinfarction myocardial scarring in mice: molecular MR imaging with use of a collagen-targeting contrast agent. *Radiology.* (2008) 247:788–96. doi: 10.1148/radiol.2473070975
221. Verjans J, Wolters S, Laufer W, Schellings M, Lax M, Lovhaug D, et al. Early molecular imaging of interstitial changes in patients after myocardial infarction: comparison with delayed contrast-enhanced magnetic resonance imaging. *J Nucl Cardiol.* (2010) 17:1065–72. doi: 10.1007/s12350-010-9268-5
222. Ezeani M, Noor A, Alt K, Lal S, Donnelly PS, Hagemeyer CE, et al. Collagen–targeted peptides for molecular imaging of diffuse cardiac fibrosis. *J Am Heart Assoc Cardiovasc Cerebrovasc Dis.* (2021) 10:e022139. doi: 10.1161/JAHA.121.022139
223. Kwiecinski J, Lennen RJ, Gray GA, Borthwick G, Boswell L, Baker AH, et al. Progression and regression of left ventricular hypertrophy and myocardial fibrosis in a mouse model of hypertension and concomitant cardiomyopathy. *J Cardiovasc Magn Reson.* (2020) 22:57. doi: 10.1186/s12968-020-00655-7
224. Brilla CG, Matsubara L, Weber KT. Advanced hypertensive heart disease in spontaneously hypertensive rats. Lisinopril-mediated regression of

myocardial fibrosis. *Hypertens Dallas Tex 1979.* (1996) 28:269–75. doi: 10.1161/01.hyp.28.2.269

225. Brilla CG. Regression of myocardial fibrosis in hypertensive heart disease: diverse effects of various antihypertensive drugs. *Cardiovasc Res.* (2000) 46:324–31. doi: 10.1016/s0008-6363(99)00432-0
226. López B, Querejeta R, Varo N, González A, Larman M, Martínez Ubago JL, et al. Usefulness of serum carboxy-terminal propeptide of procollagen type I in assessment of the cardioreparative ability of antihypertensive treatment in hypertensive patients. *Circulation.* (2001) 104:286–91. doi: 10.1161/01.cir.104.3.286
227. Treibel TA, Kozor R, Schofield R, Benedetti G, Fontana M, Bhuva AN, et al. Reverse myocardial remodeling following valve replacement in patients with aortic stenosis. *J Am Coll Cardiol.* (2018) 71:860–71. doi: 10.1016/j.jacc.2017.12.035
228. Everett RJ, Tastet L, Clavel M-A, Chin CWL, Capoulade R, Vassiliou VS, et al. Progression of hypertrophy and myocardial fibrosis in aortic stenosis: a multicenter cardiac magnetic resonance study. *Circ Cardiovasc Imaging.* (2018) 11:e007451. doi: 10.1161/CIRCIMAGING.117.007451
229. Schaefer A, Schneeberger Y, Schulz S, Krasemann S, Werner T, Piasecki A, et al. Analysis of fibrosis in control or pressure overloaded rat hearts after mechanical unloading by heterotopic heart transplantation. *Sci Rep.* (2019) 9:5710. doi: 10.1038/s41598-019-42263-1
230. Frazier OH, Baldwin ACW, Demirozu ZT, Segura AM, Hernandez R, Taegtmeyer H, et al. Ventricular reconditioning and pump explantation in patients supported by continuous-flow left ventricular assist devices. *J Heart Lung Transplant.* (2015) 34:766–72. doi: 10.1016/j.healun.2014.09.015
231. Drakos SG, Mehra MR. Clinical myocardial recovery during long-term mechanical support in advanced heart failure: insights into moving the field forward. *J Heart Lung Transplant.* (2016) 35:413–20. doi: 10.1016/j.healun.2016.01.001
232. Farris SD, Don C, Helterline D, Costa C, Plummer T, Steffes S, et al. Cell-specific pathways supporting persistent fibrosis in heart failure. *J Am Coll Cardiol.* (2017) 70:344–54. doi: 10.1016/j.jacc.2017.05.040
233. McKleroy W, Lee T-H, Atabai K. Always cleave up your mess: targeting collagen degradation to treat tissue fibrosis. *Am J Physiol Lung Cell Mol Physiol.* (2013) 304:L709–21. doi: 10.1152/ajplung.00418.2012

Permissions

All chapters in this book were first published by Frontiers; hereby published with permission under the Creative Commons Attribution License or equivalent. Every chapter published in this book has been scrutinized by our experts. Their significance has been extensively debated. The topics covered herein carry significant findings which will fuel the growth of the discipline. They may even be implemented as practical applications or may be referred to as a beginning point for another development.

The contributors of this book come from diverse backgrounds, making this book a truly international effort. This book will bring forth new frontiers with its revolutionizing research information and detailed analysis of the nascent developments around the world.

We would like to thank all the contributing authors for lending their expertise to make the book truly unique. They have played a crucial role in the development of this book. Without their invaluable contributions this book wouldn't have been possible. They have made vital efforts to compile up to date information on the varied aspects of this subject to make this book a valuable addition to the collection of many professionals and students.

This book was conceptualized with the vision of imparting up-to-date information and advanced data in this field. To ensure the same, a matchless editorial board was set up. Every individual on the board went through rigorous rounds of assessment to prove their worth. After which they invested a large part of their time researching and compiling the most relevant data for our readers.

The editorial board has been involved in producing this book since its inception. They have spent rigorous hours researching and exploring the diverse topics which have resulted in the successful publishing of this book. They have passed on their knowledge of decades through this book. To expedite this challenging task, the publisher supported the team at every step. A small team of assistant editors was also appointed to further simplify the editing procedure and attain best results for the readers.

Apart from the editorial board, the designing team has also invested a significant amount of their time in understanding the subject and creating the most relevant covers. They scrutinized every image to scout for the most suitable representation of the subject and create an appropriate cover for the book.

The publishing team has been an ardent support to the editorial, designing and production team. Their endless efforts to recruit the best for this project, has resulted in the accomplishment of this book. They are a veteran in the field of academics and their pool of knowledge is as vast as their experience in printing. Their expertise and guidance has proved useful at every step. Their uncompromising quality standards have made this book an exceptional effort. Their encouragement from time to time has been an inspiration for everyone.

The publisher and the editorial board hope that this book will prove to be a valuable piece of knowledge for researchers, students, practitioners and scholars across the globe.

List of Contributors

Weijiang Tan, Xiang Li, Shuang Zheng and Honghua Chen
Guangdong Provincial Key Laboratory of Laboratory Animals, Guangdong Laboratory Animals Monitoring Institute, Guangzhou, China

Feng Hua Yang
Guangdong Provincial Key Laboratory of Laboratory Animals, Guangdong Laboratory Animals Monitoring Institute, Guangzhou, China
Department of Cardiovascular Surgery, The First Affiliated Hospital, Jinan University, Guangzhou, China

Xiaohui Li and Xiaoshen Zhang
Department of Cardiovascular Surgery, The First Affiliated Hospital, Jinan University, Guangzhou, China

W. Glen Pyle
Department of Biomedical Sciences, University of Guelph, Guelph, ON, Canada

Jian Wu and Yunzeng Zou
Shanghai Institute of Cardiovascular Diseases, Zhongshan Hospital and Institutes of Biomedical Sciences, Fudan University, Shanghai, China

Huan Sun
Cardiology Department, China-Japan Union Hospital of Jilin University, Changchun, China

Peter H. Backx
Department of Biology, York University, Toronto, ON, Canada
Department of Physiology, University of Toronto, Toronto, ON, Canada

Lingfang Zhuang, Zizhu Liu, Chenni Li, Qi Jin, Lin Lu, Rong Tao, Xiaoxiang Yan and Kang Chen
Department of Vascular and Cardiology, Ruijin Hospital, Shanghai Jiao Tong University School of Medicine, Shanghai, China
Institute of Cardiovascular Diseases, Shanghai Jiao Tong University School of Medicine, Shanghai, China

Ye Mao
Department of Health Management Center, Ruijin Hospital Lu Wan Branch, Shanghai Jiao Tong University School of Medicine, Shanghai, China

Bo Liang and Rui Li
Nanjing University of Chinese Medicine, Nanjing, China

Yi Liang
Southwest Medical University, Luzhou, China

Ning Gu
Nanjing Hospital of Chinese Medicine Affiliated to Nanjing University of Chinese Medicine, Nanjing, China

Eleni Vasilopoulos
Centers for Cardiovascular Research, Lewis Katz School of Medicine at Temple University, Philadelphia, PA, United States

Li Li
Department of Cell Biology and Genetics, School of Basic Medical Science, Shanxi Medical University, Taiyuan, China

Ming Liu
Centers for Cardiovascular Research, Lewis Katz School of Medicine at Temple University, Philadelphia, PA, United States
Department of Cell Biology and Genetics, School of Basic Medical Science, Shanxi Medical University, Taiyuan, China

Na Wu and Haitao Shen
Departments of Endocrinology and Emergency Medicine, Shengjing Hospital of China Medical University, Shenyang, China

Ruijing Zhang
Centers for Cardiovascular Research, Lewis Katz School of Medicine at Temple University, Philadelphia, PA, United States
Department of Nephrology, The Affiliated People's Hospital of Shanxi Medical University, Taiyuan, China

Jirong Wang
Centers for Cardiovascular Research, Lewis Katz School of Medicine at Temple University, Philadelphia, PA, United States
Department of Cardiology, The Affiliated People's Hospital of Shanxi Medical University, Taiyuan, China

William Y. Yang
Rutgers University, New Brunswick, NJ, United States

Xiaohua Jiang and Xiaofeng Yang
Centers for Cardiovascular Research, Lewis Katz School of Medicine at Temple University, Philadelphia, PA, United States
Metabolic Disease Research, Inflammation, Translational & Clinical Lung Research, Thrombosis Research, Lewis Katz School of Medicine at Temple University, Philadelphia, PA, United States
Centers of Cardiovascular Research, Inflammation and Lung Research, Philadelphia, PA, United States
Departments of Cardiovascular Sciences, Metabolic Disease Research, Thrombosis Research, Philadelphia, PA, United States

Wenhui Hu and Jun Yu
Metabolic Disease Research, Inflammation, Translational & Clinical Lung Research, Thrombosis Research, Lewis Katz School of Medicine at Temple University, Philadelphia, PA, United States

Domenico Praticò
Alzheimer's Center, Lewis Katz School of Medicine at Temple University, Philadelphia, PA, United States

Jianxin Sun
Department of Medicine, Center for Translational Medicine, Thomas Jefferson University, Philadelphia, PA, United States

Ruiyan Zhang
Department of Cardiology, Ruijin Hospital, Shanghai Jiao Tong University School of Medicine, Shanghai, China
Institute of Cardiovascular Diseases, Shanghai Jiao Tong University School of Medicine, Shanghai, China

Zeyi Cheng, Yingqiang Guo and Hong Qian
Department of Cardiovascular Surgery, West China Hospital, Sichuan University, Chengdu, China

Tingting Fang
Department of Cardiology, West China Hospital, Sichuan University, Chengdu, China

Jinglei Huang
School of Medicine, Lanzhou University, Lanzhou, China

Mahboob Alam
Division of Cardiovascular Medicine, Department of Medicine, Baylor College of Medicine, Houston, TX, United States

Cun Hua, Xin-Ming Liu and Le-Feng Wang
Heart Center and Beijing Key Laboratory of Hypertension, Beijing Chaoyang Hospital, Capital Medical University, Beijing, China

Li-Rong Liang
Department of Clinical Epidemiology and Tobacco Dependence Treatment Research, Beijing Institute of Respiratory Medicine, Beijing, China

Jiu-Chang Zhong
Heart Center and Beijing Key Laboratory of Hypertension, Beijing Chaoyang Hospital, Capital Medical University, Beijing, China
Department of Clinical Epidemiology and Tobacco Dependence Treatment Research, Beijing Institute of Respiratory Medicine, Beijing, China
Beijing Institute of Respiratory Medicine, Capital Medical University, Beijing, China

Kai-bin Lin, Kan-kai Chen, Shuai Li, Ming-qi Cai, Min-jie Yuan, Yan-peng Wang, Xue Zhang, Meng Wei, Jing-bo Li and Dong Huang
Heart Center, Shanghai Jiaotong University Affiliated Sixth People's Hospital, School of Medicine, Shanghai Jiaotong University, Shanghai, China

Mei-Ling Yan
Department of Cardiology, Huadong Hospital, Fudan University, Shanghai, China

Xin-Xin Ma and Dong-Yan Zheng
Department of Ultrasound in Medicine, Shanghai Jiao Tong University Affiliated Sixth People's Hospital, Shanghai Institute of Ultrasound in Medicine, School of Medicine, Shanghai Jiaotong University, Shanghai, China

Qi-han Wu
NHC Key Lab of Reproduction Regulation (Shanghai Institute of Planned Parenthood Research), Fudan University, Shanghai, China

Keman Xu, Ying Shao, Fatma Saaoud, Charles Drummer IV, Yifan Lu and Yu Sun
Centers of Cardiovascular Research, Inflammation and Lung Research, Philadelphia, PA, United States
Centers for Cardiovascular Research, Lewis Katz School of Medicine at Temple University, Philadelphia, PA, United States

Aria Gillespie
Neural Sciences, Temple University Lewis Katz School of Medicine, Philadelphia, PA, United States

Hang Xi
Departments of Cardiovascular Sciences, Metabolic Disease Research, Thrombosis Research, Philadelphia, PA, United States

Lu Liu and Hong Wang
Departments of Cardiovascular Sciences, Metabolic Disease Research, Thrombosis Research, Philadelphia, PA, United States
Metabolic Disease Research, Inflammation, Translational & Clinical Lung Research, Thrombosis Research, Lewis Katz School of Medicine at Temple University, Philadelphia, PA, United States

Çagla Tükel
Center for Microbiology & Immunology, Temple University Lewis Katz School of Medicine, Philadelphia, PA, United States

Domenico Pratico
Alzheimer's Center, Temple University Lewis Katz School of Medicine, Philadelphia, PA, United States

Xuebin Qin
National Primate Research Center, Tulane University, Covington, LA, United States

Eric T. Choi
Surgery (Division of Vascular and Endovascular Surgery), Temple University Lewis Katz School of Medicine, Philadelphia, PA, United States

Hong-jin Chen, Xiao-xi Pan, Li-li-qiang Ding and Ping-jin Gao
Department of Cardiovascular Medicine, State Key Laboratory of Medical Genomics, Shanghai Key Laboratory of Hypertension, Department of Hypertension, Shanghai Institute of Hypertension, Ruijin Hospital, Shanghai Jiao Tong University School of Medicine, Shanghai, China

Cheng-chao Ruan
Shanghai Key Laboratory of Bioactive Small Molecules, Department of Physiology and Pathophysiology, School of Basic Medical Sciences, Fudan University, Shanghai, China

Ming Wei, Xia Wang, Yanting Song, Dan Qi, Shiyu Jiao, Guomin Xie, Ye Liu, Baoqi Yu and Aijuan Qu
Department of Physiology and Pathophysiology, School of Basic Medical Sciences, Capital Medical University, Beijing China
Key Laboratory of Remodeling-Related Cardiovascular Diseases, Ministry of Education, Beijing, China

Di Zhu and Yuji Wang
School of Pharmaceutical Sciences, Capital Medical University, Beijing, China

Jie Du
Department of Physiology and Pathophysiology, School of Basic Medical Sciences, Capital Medical University, Beijing China
Beijing Institute of Heart, Lung and Blood Vessel Diseases, Beijing, China
Beijing Anzhen Hospital, Capital Medical University, Beijing, China

Rajasekharreddy Pala and Kiumars Shamloo
Department of Biomedical and Pharmaceutical Sciences, Chapman University, Irvine, CA, United States

Farideh Amirrad and Surya M. Nauli
Department of Biomedical and Pharmaceutical Sciences, Chapman University, Irvine, CA, United States
Department of Medicine, University of California, Irvine, Orange, CA, United States

Brian S. Muntean
Department of Pharmacology and Toxicology, Medical College of Georgia, Augusta University, Augusta, GA, United States

Katharina Schimmel, Kenzo Ichimura and Edda Spiekerkoetter
Division Pulmonary, Allergy and Critical Care Medicine, Department of Medicine, Stanford University School of Medicine, Stanford, CA, United States
Vera Moulton Wall Center for Pulmonary Vascular Disease, Stanford University, Stanford, CA, United States
Stanford Cardiovascular Institute, Stanford University, Stanford, CA, United States

Sushma Reddy
Stanford Cardiovascular Institute, Stanford University, Stanford, CA, United States
Pediatric Cardiology, Stanford University, Stanford, CA, United States

Francois Haddad
Vera Moulton Wall Center for Pulmonary Vascular Disease, Stanford University, Stanford, CA, United States
Stanford Cardiovascular Institute, Stanford University, Stanford, CA, United States
Cardiovascular Medicine, Stanford University, Stanford, CA, United States

Index

www.ingramcontent.com/pod-product-compliance
Lightning Source LLC
LaVergne TN
LVHW060538210926
848485LV00005B/1223